New

Dimensions

in Women's Health Fifth Edition

Linda Lewis Alexander, PhD, FAAN

Vice President, Women's Health and Global Advocacy
QIAGEN, Inc.

Judith H. LaRosa, PhD, RN, FAAN

Vice Dean and Professor
Graduate Program in Public Health
SUNY Downstate Medical Center

Helaine Bader, MPH

Director, Women's Health and Global Advocacy
QIAGEN, Inc.

Susan Garfield, SM, MSc

Vice President
Bridgehead International

William James Alexander, MA

Editorial Associate, Ipas

JONES AND BARTLETT PUBLISHERS

Sudbury, Massachusetts

BOSTON   TORONTO   LONDON   SINGAPORE

World Headquarters
Jones and Bartlett Publishers
40 Tall Pine Drive
Sudbury, MA 01776
978-443-5000
info@jbpub.com
www.jbpub.com

Jones and Bartlett Publishers Canada
6339 Ormindale Way
Mississauga, Ontario L5V 1J2
Canada

Jones and Bartlett Publishers International
Barb House, Barb Mews
London W6 7PA
United Kingdom

Jones and Bartlett's books and products are available through most bookstores and online booksellers. To contact Jones and Bartlett Publishers directly, call 800-832-0034, fax 978-443-8000, or visit our website, www.jbpub.com.

Substantial discounts on bulk quantities of Jones and Bartlett's publications are available to corporations, professional associations, and other qualified organizations. For details and specific discount information, contact the special sales department at Jones and Bartlett via the above contact information or send an email to specialsales@jbpub.com.

Production Credits
Chief Executive Officer: Clayton Jones
Chief Operating Officer: Don W. Jones, Jr.
President, Higher Education and Professional Publishing: Robert W. Holland, Jr.
V.P., Sales: William J. Kane
V.P., Design and Production: Anne Spencer
V.P., Manufacturing and Inventory Control: Therese Connell
Publisher, Higher Education: Cathleen Sether
Acquisitions Editor: Shoshanna Goldberg
Senior Associate Editor: Amy L. Bloom
Editorial Assistant: Kyle Hoover
Production Manager: Julie Champagne Bolduc
Production Assistant: Jessica Steele Newfell
Associate Marketing Manager: Jody Sullivan
Composition: Publishers' Design and Production Services, Inc.
Cover Design: Kristin E. Parker
Photo Research and Permissions Manager: Kimberly Potvin
Senior Photo Researcher and Photographer: Christine McKeen
Cover Images: (main) © Jose Luis Pelaez/age fotostock; (side images top to bottom) © Photodisc, © Photodisc, © Photodisc, © Elena Ray/ShutterStock, Inc., © Photodisc, © Courtnee Mulroy, ShutterStock, Inc., © Monkey Business Images/ShutterStock, Inc., © Photodisc
Printing and Binding: Courier Kendallville
Cover Printing: Courier Kendallville

Library of Congress Cataloging-in-Publication Data
New dimensions in women's health / Linda Lewis Alexander . . . [et al.]. —5th ed.
    p. ; cm.
Includes bibliographical references and index.
ISBN: 978-0-7637-6592-7 (pbk. alk. paper)
    1. Women—Health and hygiene. 2. Women—Health and hygiene—Social aspects. I. Alexander, Linda Lewis.
[DNLM: 1. Women's Health. WA 309 N5323 2010]
RA778.A438 2010
613'.04244—dc22   2009020228

6048

Printed in the United States of America
13 12 11 10 10 9 8 7 6 5 4 3 2

BRIEF CONTENTS

CONTENTS

Contents

The *Fifth Edition* of *New Dimensions in Women's Health* discusses health issues as they affect all women: women of all racial and ethnic groups, of all ages, of different sexual orientations, and with various degrees of physical ability. The text presents unbiased, accurate information free from any specific political agenda while allowing its readers to appreciate the range of perspectives that influence how women in the United States and around the world think about health and make decisions that affect their well-being. *New Dimensions in Women's Health* discusses prevention, health promotion, research, clinical intervention, and public policy as well as how these factors interact with and affect rates of different diseases, disorders, and conditions that afflict women. This book is for women, recognizing their outstanding contributions as daughters, sisters, mothers, nurses, doctors, scientists, laborers, advocates, and much more.

Organization of the Book

This book is organized into four parts, each of which covers a different dimension of women's health.

Part One, Foundations of Women's Health, takes a population-based focus. It introduces students to the concepts of women's health, public health, health economics, and issues of health across the lifespan. Chapter 1 provides a brief history of the women's health movement and the political climate around women's health. Chapter 2 is dedicated to the economics of health, including the payer system in the United States, various insurance plans, health-care reform, and the impact on the aging population. Chapter 3 introduces the concepts of health promotion and disease prevention and discusses how these efforts benefit women through the different stages of life.

Part Two, Sexual and Reproductive Dimensions of Women's Health, addresses issues regarding sexual health and sexuality, as well as sexual violence, as a public health problem. Chapter 4 defines sexual health and discusses the cultural, economic, and biological factors that influence women's sexual health. Chapter 5 discusses contraceptive methods, abortion, and information for appropriate decision-making around whether and how a woman wishes to reproduce, and Chapter 6 covers pregnancy, childbirth, breastfeeding, and infertility. Chapter 7 is devoted to the clinical, sociological, and epidemiological dimensions and treatment issues of sexually transmitted infections, including HIV/AIDS. In Chapter 8, menopause is explored as a biological and cultural phenomenon, and the benefits, drawbacks, and effects of hormone replacement therapy are discussed.

Part Three, Physical and Lifespan Dimensions of Women's Health, comprises Chapters 9 through 12. Chapter 9 discusses exercise, nutrition, and weight management. Chapter 10 examines how cardiovascular disease and cancer affect women as well as how these diseases progress and can be prevented, treated, and managed. Chapter 11 discusses other chronic diseases important to women's health, including osteoporosis, arthritis, diabetes, autoimmune diseases, and Alzheimer's disease. Chapter 12 offers definitions of mental health and mental illness, explores the reasons why good mental health is essential, and gives information on various mental disorders.

The final section, Part Four, is titled Interpersonal and Social Dimensions of Women's Health. Chapter 13 discusses substance use and abuse of both legal and illegal drugs. Chapter 14 provides different perspectives on violence, abuse, and harassment, and Chapter 15 discusses current trends and issues for women in the workforce.

Chapter Features

Each chapter reviews an important aspect of women's general health and examines how epidemiological, historical, psychosocial, cultural, ethnic, legal, political, and economic influences shape that topic. *New Dimensions in Women's Health* also discusses how age, ethnicity and race, sexual orientation, and other factors influence women's needs. In addition, special features distributed throughout each chapter highlight and summarize important concepts and promote healthy lifestyle choices:

- **It's Your Health** highlights key facts that help readers improve their own health, such as disease symptoms, screening recommendations, and benefits of healthy behaviors.

- **Informed Decision Making** provides students with detailed information for making appropriate decisions regarding their health and well-being.

- **Self-Assessments** provide exercises to help students determine their risk of disease and need for modifying behaviors.

- **Gender Dimensions**, new to this *Fifth Edition*, discuss how specific health issues, ranging from breast cancer to obesity, vary between the genders.

- **Quotes** from real women offer students experiences, opinions, and thoughts from women of all ages, races, and cultures.

- **Profiles of Remarkable Women** highlight individuals who contributed to the health and well-being of all women. These profiles showcase women as champions of health across all ages and life spans.

- **Topics for Discussion** at the end of each chapter encourage students to consider their own opinions on a topic and to explore the philosophical dimensions surrounding issues of women's health.

- A list of **Web sites** at the end of each chapter enables students to further explore topics of interest.

New to This Edition

The *Fifth Edition* of *New Dimensions in Women's Health* has been expanded, updated, and revised. It presents the most current, accurate, and relevant women's health information in an organized, easily understood manner. New features to this edition include:

- Major content updates for Chapters 1, 4, 5, 6, 7, 10, and 12

- New, straightforward explanations of key concepts such as women's health, mental health, feminism, and health education

- Expanded discussions of women's health from a public health perspective, which cover how disease, environmental factors, and other issues affect populations of women, not just individuals

- New material discussing how the 2008 presidential election, the war in Iraq, and Hurricane Katrina have affected women's health

- New and expanded information on testing and prevention for sexually transmitted infections, including vaccination for HPV

- New quotes from women of all ages and backgrounds discussing their feelings and experiences dealing with anorexia, hormone replacement therapy, birth control, and other issues

The most current guidelines, surveillance, and statistics are included in every chapter. Highlights include:

- The 2008 Physical Activity Guidelines for Americans

- Revised WHO and CDC estimates for the global and national incidence and prevalence of HIV and other sexually transmitted infections

- Updated Youth Risk Behavior Survey data on teenage women's suicide rates, eating habits, drug use, and other factors

- The latest statistics on obesity rates among U.S. women as well as the economic costs that result from obesity

Ancillary Material

New Dimensions in Women's Health, Fifth Edition includes learning tools for students and teaching tools for instructors. ***http://womenshealth.jbpub.com*** offers flashcards, chapter outlines, crossword puzzles, an interactive glossary, practice quizzes, self-assessments, and Web exercises designed to help students learn to evaluate health information found on the Web.

For instructors teaching this course, an instructor's manual, PowerPoint slides, and a TestBank are available online.

Acknowledgments

This edition of *New Dimensions in Women's Health* builds on the success of all previous editions. The authors remain indebted to family and friends for their support, guidance, patience, and sacrifices as we dissected and reconstructed the entire text again. A deep and heartfelt appreciation must be extended to the new member of the author team, William Alexander. In this edition, Will is a formal addition to the author team, and he served as the official taskmaster, researcher, writer, and coordinator for the entire revision. Without his dedication, this new edition simply would not be possible. Will's persistence in data mining, editing, and distilling complex information into our established format is highly valued. More important, he brought a sensitivity and perspective to the gender health issues that we wanted to emphasize in this new presentation of the ever-changing landscape of women's health. Jessica Alexander also provided constant editorial review as well as researching and writing assistance for this new edition, and we are indebted to her support. As ever, we remain grateful to our readers, the professors and students who provide reviews and insights for our continual improvement. Thanks to Kate De-Mayo and Melodie Hunter for their support in the final stages of the revision process. Lastly, we'd like to acknowledge and remember the following remarkable women: Elizabeth Bennett, EdD, RN (1926–1998), Gail Addlestone, MD (1969–2007), and Lucille Dorey Lewis (1915–1993).

Reviewers

We also thank the reviewers of this edition for their valuable suggestions:

Joanne Chopak-Foss, Georgia Southern University

Mary A. Glascoff, MSN, EdD, East Carolina University

Marilyn Grechus, PhD, University of Central Missouri

Joan M. Hall, MS, APRN, CNS, BC, San Diego State University

Robin T. Kelley, PhD, The Washington Center for Internships and Academic Seminars

Laura Kelly, PhD, APRN, BC, Monmouth University

Sylvette A. LaTouche-Howard, MA, NCC, University of Maryland–College Park

Julie A. Lombardi, PED, Millersville University

Leigh Schanfein, BS, Purdue University

Constance T. Skinner, BA, Purdue University

ABOUT THE AUTHORS

Linda Lewis Alexander, PhD, FAAN

Linda Lewis Alexander has an extensive career in public health and women's health. She is currently Vice President, Women's Health and Global Advocacy for QIAGEN Corporation. In this role, Dr. Alexander oversees corporate women's health program efforts in the public sector and advocacy support initiatives in global cervical cancer prevention. Her previous professional experiences included serving as Vice President, Women's Health at Digene Corporation and President and CEO of the American Social Health Association (ASHA). At ASHA she provided national leadership and worked in close partnership with industry and federal leaders to promote national awareness for all sexually transmitted diseases.

Dr. Alexander also is a retired lieutenant colonel with the U.S. Army Nurse Corps. Her military career included assignments in community health nursing in the United States and Europe, and she was a nurse epidemiologist at the Walter Reed Army Institute of Research. As a health educator, she has held academic positions at the University of Maryland–College Park and the Uniformed Services University of Health Sciences. In her position as Vice President for Women's Health and Science with United Information Systems, she provided leadership with the Department of Defense congressionally appropriated research programs in breast cancer, osteoporosis, and ovarian cancer.

Dr. Alexander is nationally known for her leadership in women's health advocacy and has published extensively on women's health issues. Her many honors include appointments to national advisory panels on infectious diseases and women's health; she also is a fellow in the American Academy of Nursing. Dr. Alexander holds a baccalaureate degree in nursing, master's degrees in education/counseling and community health, and a doctoral degree in health education.

Judith H. LaRosa, PhD, RN, FAAN

Dr. Judith LaRosa's career has spanned education, research, and clinical practice. Her present position is vice dean and professor, SUNY Downstate Graduate Program in Public Health, where her current research focuses on cultural perceptions of health and disease.

Prior to this, she served as professor and chair, Department of Community Health Sciences, Tulane University School of Public Health and Tropical Medicine, and Director, Tulane Xavier National Center of Excellence in Women's Health. From 1991 to 1994, she was the first deputy director of the Office of Research on Women's Health, National Institutes of Health (NIH). She is a co-author of the legislatively mandated 1994 NIH Guidelines on the Inclusion of Women and Minorities as Subjects in Clinical Research. From 1978 to 1991, Dr. LaRosa served at the National Heart, Lung, and Blood Institute (NHLBI) as the first coordinator of the NHLBI workplace initiative in cardiovascular disease risk factor reduction. In 1990, she was appointed as the designer and first coordinator of the National Heart Attack Alert Program, a national education program to reduce time to treatment at the first signs of a heart attack.

Dr. LaRosa has served on the Institute of Medicine's Committee on Understanding the Biology of Sex and Gender as well as the Committee on Assessing the Medical Risks of Human Oocyte Donation for Stem Cell Research; the National Institute for Nursing Research's Advisory Council; the Armed Forces Epidemiological Board; and the National Science Foundation/Institute of Medicine Committee on Defense Women's Health Research. She was a member of the U.S. Army Research and Materiel Command/United Information Systems, Inc., core directorate to design and implement the Department of Defense (DoD) breast cancer and defense women's health grant review process. Dr. LaRosa has served as a scientific reviewer for the NIH, CDC, and DoD. She is on the editorial board of the *Journal of Community Health*.

Dr. LaRosa received her bachelor of science degree in nursing and her master of nursing education degree from the University of Pittsburgh and her PhD in health education from the University of Maryland.

Helaine Bader, MPH

Helaine Bader has focused her work in the fields of health communications and women's health. In her present position as Director, Women's Health and Global Advocacy at QIAGEN, Inc., Ms. Bader works to ensure access to cervical cancer screening through developing and implementing advocacy and educational initiatives, with the ultimate goal of eliminating cervical cancer.

Previous to this position, Ms. Bader was with GlaxoSmithKline, where she worked in cardiovascular and women's health communications and was responsible for media relations and community outreach within research and development. Ms. Bader has more than 10 years of experience in women's health research, health communications, and health education, including a breast cancer research fellowship with the National Cancer Institute. She has worked on multimedia and Web-based health campaigns in both the public and private sectors and has developed, implemented, and evaluated health education projects for various issues affecting women and children.

Ms. Bader received her baccalaureate degree in English with a minor in premedical sciences from the University of Pennsylvania and her master's degree in public health from University of Pittsburgh.

Susan Garfield, SM, MSc

Susan Garfield is a market access, reimbursement, and economics strategist, with expertise in demand creation and advocacy. For more than 12 years, her professional career has focused on women's health, innovations in health care, the economics of practice change, and the role of reimbursement and policy to the adoption of new technologies.

Ms. Garfield is currently vice president at Bridgehead International, where she runs the Boston office of the market access consulting practice. At Bridgehead, Ms. Garfield works to help companies navigate the complexities of bringing innovative health-care technologies to market. Prior to joining Bridgehead, Ms. Garfield was the Director of Global Reimbursement Policy and Economic Strategy at QIAGEN, Inc. (formerly Digene Corporation). In this role, she planned and executed a reimbursement strategy that resulted in near universal coverage for the company's leading cancer diagnostic product. In addition, she directed global economic and pricing analyses for the company's clinical diagnostic portfolio. Before QIAGEN, Ms. Garfield was a director at Boston Healthcare Consulting. During her tenure

there, Ms. Garfield worked with biotechnology, medical device, pharmaceutical, and diagnostic firms on market access strategy and execution. In this role she translated primary research with more than 2,000 clinicians, payers, government decision makers, and patients into actionable programs for clients.

Ms. Garfield received her baccalaureate degree in English and women's studies from the University of Pennsylvania, a master's of science in population and development from the London School of Economics, and a master's degree in health policy and management from Harvard University, School of Public Health. Ms. Garfield is currently pursuing her doctorate of public health at Boston University.

William James Alexander, MA

Will Alexander joins the author team for this edition, researching and writing most of the new information and supervising and coordinating the addition of the rest. Mr. Alexander's career and education have centered around health communication and public health, particularly women's health. In his current position as editorial associate at Ipas, an international nonprofit organization dealing with women's reproductive health, he writes, edits, and publishes materials designed to improve women's sexual and reproductive rights and to reduce maternal morbidity and mortality around the world.

Before working at Ipas, Mr. Alexander worked for MEASURE Evaluation, a global organization that helps USAID-funded countries to improve their systems to confront disease, population issues, and poverty. He also has worked for the North Carolina Department of Health and Human Services, the Embassy of Kazakhstan, and the American Social Health Association. Additionally, he has done freelance reporting and writing for several newspapers and magazines.

Mr. Alexander received his baccalaureate degree in English from St. Mary's College of Maryland and his master's degree in medical journalism from the University of North Carolina at Chapel Hill.

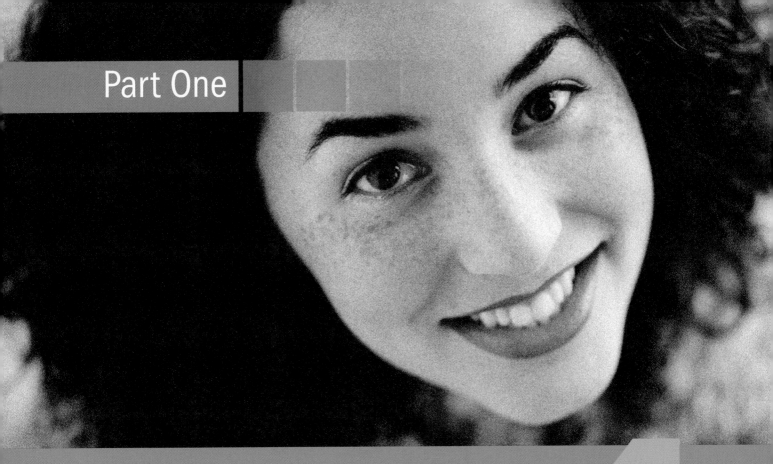

Foundations of Women's Health

1

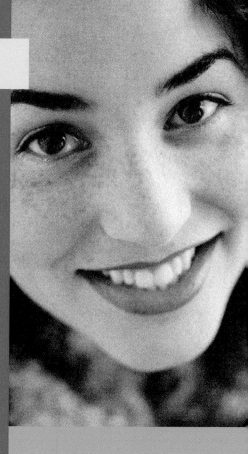

Chapter One

Introduction to Women's Health

Chapter Objectives

On completion of this chapter, the student should be able to discuss:

1. Major ways of thinking about and defining women's health.

2. Government's role in protecting and promoting the health of the public.

3. The responsibilities of the National Institutes of Health and the Office of Research on Women's Health.

4. The federal government's role in funding and conducting research on women's health.

5. The importance of investing in biomedical research and the inclusion of women and minorities in research studies.

6. The concept of gender-based research and basic health differences between women and men.

7. Reproductive rights, the global gag rule, and the effects that restricting abortion has on global health.

8. How lack of access to health care, lack of health insurance, cultural insensitivity, and other obstacles affect the health of women.

9. The need to train health professionals about women's health and cultural sensitivity.

10. Global efforts to support women's health and gender equity.

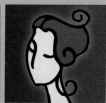

womenshealth.jbpub.com

Women's Health Online is a great source for supplementary women's health information for both students and instructors. Visit http://womenshealth.jbpub.com to find a variety of useful tools for learning, thinking, and teaching.

Introduction

Women's health is a fascinatingly complex area of study. Thousands, even millions, of factors affect the ways women develop, get sick, get well, interact with others, reproduce, age, and receive health care. Some experts in women's health attempt to provide a deep but narrow level of detail by focusing on a few of these factors. This book, however, attempts to explore, or at least introduce, the significant facets of women's health from many different angles. The following paragraphs describe different areas of concern and ways of thinking about women's health and well-being included in the following 15 chapters.

Women's health includes the study of the whole body. Women's health is based on the study of biological characteristics unique to women, the most obvious being the reproductive organs, but also differences in body structure, hormones, and brain chemistry. Yet women's health is also concerned with factors that affect both genders, including the common cold, heart disease, depression, and the benefits of regular physical exercise. Women's health includes the study of disease, but it also examines factors that add to a woman's physical and mental well-being.

Women's health can study populations or an individual woman. Women's health benefits from examining patterns of health and disease in populations; for example, whether women who are exposed to secondhand cigarette smoke have a greater risk for developing lung cancer than women who are not. But women's health also includes the study of how diseases affect individuals, such as ways a woman can reduce her personal risk of getting cancer; what the signs, effects, and treatments of cancer are for an individual woman who has it; and how that woman's unique body acts and reacts to disease.

The entire spectrum of research and social sciences can provide insight into women's health. A full understanding of women's sexual and reproductive health requires biological, cultural, historical, and political perspectives. The physical components of the reproductive system influence a woman's sexual response, but so do cultural mores and traditions that dictate when and how women are supposed to enjoy and think about their sexuality. Women's health includes reproductive health, defined as the well-being of a person's reproductive system, including their ability to decide if and when to have children.[1] Studying reproductive health requires examining the laws, practices, and cultural beliefs that influence when and where women learn about childbirth, family planning, and birth control, and their legal options for ending a pregnancy. Because women's un-equal treatment affects their well-being and lives in many ways, **feminism**, the idea that women should have the same political, economic, and social rights and opportunities as men, is also an important part of women's health. Not all women become mothers, but because all mothers are women, women's health also includes studying pregnancy, fetal development, and mother–infant interactions.

Finally, a variety of sociocultural influences also influence women's health. Women's place in society affects if and how often rape, sexual harassment, and other forms of sexual violence occur. Sociocultural factors also influence where and when women can enter the workforce, as well as what sort of workplace they encounter. Women's health includes women's ability to get and benefit from health care. The study of access to health care has increased dramatically over the past 20 years. Access to health care not only includes whether women can physically get to a doctor or health care provider, but also whether they trust that provider, whether they have insurance or some other way to pay for health care, and whether they know if and when something is wrong. The issue of access to health care and health-care decision making is especially important for women's health, because women are more likely than men to make decisions regarding health care for their relatives and families.

Historical Dimensions: The Women's Health Movement

The following section provides a brief history of the women's health movement and advances in women's health in the United States.

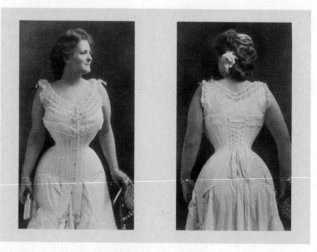

■ During the Popular Health Movement, women were encouraged to eliminate the corset. Corsets were worn as an undergarment or outergarment to support and shape the waistline, hips, and breasts.

1830s and 1840s: The Health Movement

Many historians believe the women's health movement began in the 1830s and 1840s, when small groups of women began advocating to take an active role in preventing disease and staying healthy, rather than completely relying on formally trained physicians for treatment.[2] This first wave of advocacy focused on eating a proper diet, the elimination of the **corset**, and periodic sexual abstinence in marriage to control family size. For the first time, a few middle-class women who became interested in their own health sought entry into the medical profession.[2] Elizabeth Blackwell, for example, entered medical school in 1847 and prompted the opening of several medical schools for women. In 1848, the first women's rights convention was held in Seneca Falls, New York; the convention marked the official beginning of the women's rights movement.

1861–1865: The Civil War

The Civil War prompted many women to volunteer as doctors and nurses to the armies; some women even disguised themselves as men to tend to wounded soldiers on the battlefield. Dorothea Dix and Clara Barton led a national effort to organize a nursing corps to care for the war's wounded and sick.

Women's participation in the war led to the opening of the first training schools for nurses in 1873. By 1890, 35 such schools existed. Although this trend represented advancement for women, the relationship between male doctors and female nurses mirrored the domestic sexual division of labor, with males as the authority figures and females as the subordinates.

Mid- to Late 1800s: The Women's Medical Movement

After the Civil War, educational and employment opportunities, though still severely limited, increased for women. The women's medical movement emerged from the increase in the number of women attending medical schools, their struggles to achieve equal status within the profession, and the popularity of challenging historical notions regarding women's fragility.

1890s–1920s: The Progressive Era

The women's medical movement gave way to the Progressive Era, which advanced the roles of women and women's rights as well as women's health. In 1920, the 19th Amendment to the U.S. Constitution, which guaranteed women the right to vote, was ratified. A few years later, the National Women's Party, formed in 1917, proposed the Equal Rights Amendment (see **It's Your Health**).

During this time, the birth control movement led to the legalization and medical acceptance of contraception. The maternal and child health movement also was working to promote healthy motherhood through prenatal care and child health services. The first birth control clinic in the United States was established in 1916. Soon after, the Shepard Towner Act of 1921 greatly increased the availability of prenatal and child health care.[1]

My grandmother was a physician at a time when all of her peers were men. I have always admired her but now that I am an adult woman, I have a better understanding of the challenges she must have faced at my age in her time.

24-year-old woman

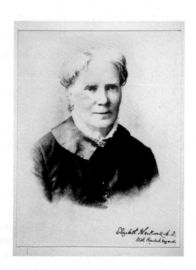

■ Elizabeth Blackwell was responsible for the opening of several medical schools for women in the mid-1800s.

It's Your Health

Equal Rights Amendment

The Equal Rights Amendment was written in 1921 by **suffragist** Alice Paul. It has been introduced in Congress every session since 1923.

Section 1. Equality of Rights under the law shall not be denied or abridged by the United States or any state on account of sex.

Section 2. The Congress shall have the power to enforce, by appropriate legislation, the provisions of this article.

Section 3. This amendment shall take effect two years after the date of ratification.

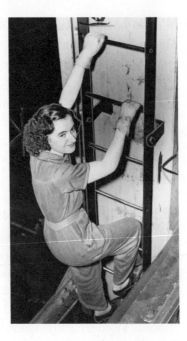

■ The number of women employed in the United States increased by 50% during World War II, but many of these women were forced to leave their jobs when the war ended.

1930s–1950s: World War II and Postwar Years

The United States dramatically increased its production during World War II while millions of male workers were leaving to join the military. Women made a vital contribution to this effort. Twelve million women were working when the United States entered the war; by the time the war ended, 18 million women were employed.[3] Women began receiving more pay and worked in a greater variety of positions, though they were rarely, if ever, employed in skilled labor or managerial positions. When the war ended, women were pressured to leave their jobs and return to being homemakers.

Although many women were using birth control by the 1950s, popular culture still reinforced the idea that sexuality was simply a means for married couples to produce children. The Kinsey reports on human sexuality, issued in 1953, started to dispel this idea by revealing that, for many men and women, marriage was not a prerequisite for sex.

1960s–1970s: The Grassroots Movement

During the 1960s and 1970s, grassroots organizations challenged medical authority in the delivery of health care to women. These groups believed that the overwhelmingly male medical community excluded women from making decisions about their own health care, and they addressed issues such as unnecessary hysterectomies and cesarean sections, postpartum depression, abortion, and childbirth reform from a feminist perspective. The self-help manual *Our Bodies, Ourselves* epitomized this effort. This health book and guide to women's bodies, originally published in 1970,

Before I came to college, I thought that you had to be pretty radical and a little "anti-man" to be a feminist. Now I understand that feminists simply want women to have the same chances to make a name for themselves, have their voices heard, and live a good life as men do. I guess I've always been a feminist, but I just didn't know it.

19-year-old student

was written and self-published by 12 feminist activists. Today the book has been expanded greatly, is in its twelfth edition, and has sold millions of copies worldwide.

Legal reforms during this time gave greater rights to women. The Food and Drug Administration (FDA) approved the birth control pill in 1960. In 1964, Congress passed the Civil Rights Act, including Title VII, which protected women against employment discrimination. In 1972, Congress passed the Equal Rights Amendment, though this amendment fell short of the 38 states needed to ratify it and add it to the Constitution. Also in 1972, legislation known as Title IX forced schools to provide equal funding for men and women in athletic programs.

For decades, the women's health movement had been composed mostly of middle-class white women. During the 1960s and 1970s, this movement began to be more inclusive. Organizations such as the National Black Women's Health Project (now called the Black Women's Health Imperative), the National Latina Women's Health Organization, the National Asian Women's Health Organization, and the Native American Women's Health Education and Resource Center developed to focus on issues and diseases that disproportionately affect women of color.

1980s: Changing Public Policy

In the 1980s, the U.S. Public Health Service's Task Force on Women's Health Issues formed to assess the status of women's health. The Task Force issued recommendations to increase gender equity in **biomedical research** and establish guidelines for the inclusion of women in federally sponsored studies. In 1990, the National Institutes of Health (NIH) strengthened its guidelines and established the Office of Research on Women's Health (ORWH).[4] The ORWH focuses on ensuring women's participation in

I have an inherited condition that affects most of the women in my family. I don't know what we would have done without the support of an advocacy organization that is focused on our condition.

21-year-old woman

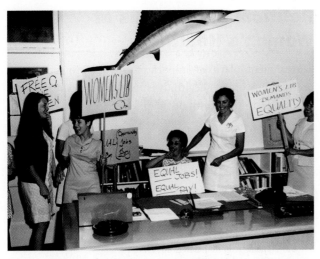

■ During the 1960s and 1970s, women challenged the authorities on many issues regarding gender equality.

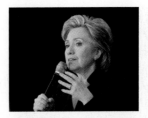
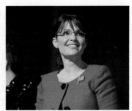
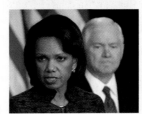
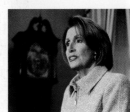

■ The past five years have seen the first major female candidate for president of the United States (Hillary Clinton), the first female vice presidential candidate for the Republican party (Sarah Palin), the first African-American woman as secretary of state (Condoleeza Rice), and the first female speaker of the House of Representatives (Nancy Pelosi).

It's Your Health

Feminism

Feminism is the idea that women should have the same political, economic, and social rights and opportunities as men. Feminism has achieved great advances for women over the past 100 years. Feminism has evolved to help different generations of women, and it will continue to evolve as women face new challenges and opportunities.

The first wave of feminism began in the late nineteenth and early twentieth centuries, when suffragists and abolitionists worked to secure basic rights for women, such as the rights to vote, own property, and inherit property.

The second wave of feminism occurred in the 1960s and 1970s. It fought against specific injustices, such as the lack of reproductive freedom, the lack of equal pay for equal work, and women's inability to receive equal access to jobs and education. The second wave of feminism attempted to highlight ways that society legally and professionally subjugated women, and thus turned women's personal struggles into political action.

The third wave of feminism began in the late 1980s and early 1990s. This new movement addressed domestic violence, access to safe and legal abortions, and sexual harassment, as well as ensuring equal status of women in educational, work, athletic, and social environments. The first two waves of feminism had largely come from a white, middle-class perspective. In this third movement, activists attempted to broaden the scope of feminism to include perspectives of women of color and different social classes. The third feminist wave also looked at all aspects of society, art, and science through a feminist lens. This perspective provided great insights into where inequality persists and how women often contribute to supporting the status quo instead of actively fighting for change. The third wave has also focused on practi-

cal ways to help women achieve equality, such as by promoting flexible work scheduling, demanding the availability of child care, and making time off available for maternity leave and caring for sick family members.

Today, many young women are living out the dreams of the women who started the feminist movement. Women pursue careers and family, demand equality in their relationships, and support feminist political agendas. Although the current generation of women may appreciate advances that feminism has made possible, they do not always feel the same personal connection with the feminist movement that women from earlier generations felt (and feel).

Women in the United States enjoy more power and opportunities than they ever have before. Women's wages have risen, and women now constitute a majority of college and university students. The past five years have seen the first African American woman as secretary of state (Condoleeza Rice), the first female speaker of the House of Representatives (Nancy Pelosi), the first major female candidate for president of the United States (Hillary Clinton), and the first female vice presidential candidate for the Republican party (Sarah Palin). However, women continue to face discrimination at home, in public, and at the workplace because of their gender.

Today, feminism is exploring many aspects of women's lives. Modern feminism acknowledges that gender differences exist even while working to eliminate gender-based favoritism and bias. Feminism acknowledges that women may not all want to focus on their careers, or even have careers (though they continue to be grateful for the opportunity). Feminists come from both genders, and different political and cultural backgrounds, ages, ethnicities, and sexual orientations; in short, they are as diverse a group as women themselves.

clinical trials, strengthening research on diseases affecting women, and promoting the career advancement of women in science. The Women's Health Equity Act also was passed, allocating money to fund health research on particular areas of concern to women, including contraception, infertility, breast cancer, ovarian cancer, HIV/AIDS, and osteoporosis.

1990s: Women's Health at the Forefront

The 1990s brought together government, health-care institutions, academia, and advocacy organizations to analyze and promote women's health and well-being. New women's health offices in federal agencies and in regional public health service offices opened throughout the country. Existing centers broadened their scope beyond reproductive issues to take a more comprehensive look at health and disease among women.

In the 1993 NIH Revitalization Act, Congress required that women and minorities be included as subjects in all human subject research funded by NIH.[3] This decision was a bold and innovative step. The inclusion of women in research has led to the expansion of the scientific knowledge base necessary for developing sex-specific diagnostic techniques, preventive measures, and effective treatments for diseases and conditions affecting women throughout their life span.

The Family and Medical Leave Act, also introduced in 1993, gives employees unpaid medical leave for themselves or for the care of a family member or a newborn or adopted infant. In 1994, the Violence Against Women Act mandated a unified judicial response to sexual crimes committed against women.

The Twenty-First Century

The new millennium has brought many contributions to improving the health of the public—for example, the identification of the **human genome**, the findings from the Women's Health Initiative, improvements in HIV/AIDS medications, public health programs targeting behavior-related health problems, and the inclusion of children in **clinical trials**. Nevertheless, women still face many difficulties in the health-care arena. There has been a rollback of many of the advances made in the 1990s, including curtailment of funding for reproductive health initiatives both domestically and internationally and politicizing of the women's health agenda. Millions of Americans lack health insurance or are underinsured; women are living longer but not necessarily with better quality of life; and women across the United States and the world continue to be victims of individual and societal violence and discrimination.

Political Dimensions of Women's Health

Government plays an important role in protecting and promoting women's health. It is involved in six main areas in relation to the health of the public:[5]

1. Policy making
2. Financing
3. Protecting the health of the public
4. Collecting and disseminating information about health and health-care delivery systems
5. Capacity building for population health
6. Managing of health services

The government exercises control over many of the areas affecting women's health, both directly and indirectly. The federal government ensures that the food supply is safe, provides federal highway funding for states that adopt a legal drinking age, and regulates businesses that provide medications to the public.

During the 1990s, the government established many organizations and agencies devoted to women's health. The Department of Health and Human Services' Office on Women's Health (DHHS-OWH) serves as the coordinating agency for all women's health initiatives throughout the agencies and offices of the U.S. DHHS, including the National Institutes of Health (NIH), Food and Drug Administration (FDA), Centers for Disease Control and Prevention (CDC), and other agencies and departments. OWH finds and addresses inequities in research, health-care services, and education that have placed the health of women at risk.[4]

The Office of Research on Women's Health (ORWH) within NIH is the government's focal point for women's biomedical research.

- ORWH advises the NIH director and staff on matters relating to research on women's health.
- It strengthens and enhances research related to diseases, disorders, and conditions that affect women.
- It ensures that research conducted and supported by NIH adequately addresses issues regarding women's health.
- It ensures that women are appropriately represented in biomedical and behavioral research studies supported by NIH.
- It develops opportunities for and supports recruitment, retention, reentry, and advancement of women in biomedical careers.
- It supports research on women's health issues.

The ORWH has been critical in national and international efforts to make women's health research part of the scientific and educational infrastructure. The ORWH works with scientists, practitioners, legislators, and lay advocates to identify research priorities and set a comprehensive research agenda. The ORWH also encourages research that examines the biological differences between the sexes —that is, gender-based biology—to more fully understand each and thereby enhance knowledge and practice.

The Healthy Women 2000 initiative joined DHHS with other federal agencies, nonprofit organizations, and members of various medical industries to educate women and provide them with the knowledge needed to live long and healthy lives. By identifying diseases that affect women the most, scientists can set future directions and goals for research.

DHHS also has implemented several programs to provide for family planning, prevent sexually transmitted infections, and reduce unintended pregnancies. The Title X program provides funding to millions of people for reproductive health and family planning services. Funding has also increased for research and programs aimed at improving the health of older women, demonstrated in part by the development of a resource center launched by the Administration on Aging to educate older women about issues such as income security, housing, and caregiving. The Administration on Aging has also increased support for community nutrition services to combat nutrition-related illnesses of the elderly.[4]

Investment in Biomedical Research

The federal government plays a critical role in funding biomedical research. NIH is the main federal agency responsible for distributing money to private and public institutions and organizations for conducting medical and health research. Along with the CDC and other agencies, it advances basic research to discover new and better methods of treatment and prevention of numerous health conditions. Funding also comes from the private sector, philanthropic organizations, universities, and voluntary health agencies.

Pharmaceutical companies and private corporations also invest millions of dollars each year to research and develop new drugs, vaccines, and technologies. Investment in biomedical research and new technologies has led to increased **life expectancy**, improved health throughout the life span, and, in many cases, decreased cost of illness.

However, newer medicines, technologies, and equipment are not the only way to improve health. About half the deaths in the United States are directly or indirectly caused by people's behavior choices. Research can also find better ways to educate people about basic health measures, such as preventing disease; eating a healthful, balanced diet; exercising; and avoiding tobacco and other drugs, offering the potential to improve the health of millions of Americans. Promoting healthful behaviors and preventing disease are usually cheaper, more effective methods than intervening after a disease or harmful event occurs. Unfortunately, these types of programs typically receive little funding compared to pharmaceutical drugs or technologies promising the next "miracle cure" (or, for shareholders, the next revenue source).

Research on women's health has seen unprecedented growth over the past 35 years, especially with the push to include women in clinical trials. By demanding that women are included in health research, women as well as men become the studied models for the conditions that affect them and the drugs used to treat these conditions. This trend has led to the integration of women-specific data into clinical practice and the formulation of new questions in regard to women and specific diseases.

Another approach to improving women's health relies on gender-based research—studies that examine the similarities and differences between men and women to learn more about the causes of disease and responses to medication. Gender-based studies identify and examine the biological and physiological differences between men and women. Males and females can manifest different symptoms of a disease, experience the course of a disease differently, or respond in distinct ways to pharmaceuticals. Identifying and studying gender-based differences offers a remarkable potential for understanding disease epidemiology and health outcomes in both men and women. The **Gender Dimensions** box discusses several areas of

The reasons for excluding women from clinical investigations are less obvious than one might expect. In spite of a significant body of opinion to the contrary, the reasons have very little to do with male chauvinism or the gender of the investigating scientist—until the 1990s, female scientists were every bit as likely as men to exclude females from clinical protocols. Even at the most sophisticated academic medical centers, senior investigators taught young scientists that data obtained from male subjects could be extrapolated to women without modification. They assumed that women were essentially small men—identical in all respects except for their reproductive physiology. It is astonishing that in a scientific system that prides itself on its critical sense and accepts no hypothesis as true until it has been rigorously tested, we have tolerated such a leap of faith for so long.[7]

Marianne Legato

Gender Dimensions: Health Differences Between Men and Women

HEALTH DIFFERENCES BETWEEN MEN AND WOMEN

Differences between men and women are not just limited to the reproductive organs. Women and men react differently to certain medications, have distinct reactions and vulnerabilities to disease, and may show disease in different ways.

The following 10 examples show some of the ways that diseases affect men and women differently.

Heart Disease. Heart disease kills 500,000 U.S. women each year—more than 50,000 more women than men. Heart disease also strikes women, on average, 10 years later than men. Compared to men, women are also more likely to have a second heart attack within a year of the first one.

Depression. Depression is two to three times more likely to affect women than men, in part because women's brains make less of the neurotransmitter serotonin, which regulates emotions.

Drug Reactions. Many common drugs, like antihistamines and antibiotics, cause different reactions and side effects in women than in men.

Autoimmune Diseases. Three out of four people suffering from autoimmune diseases, such as multiple sclerosis, rheumatoid arthritis, and lupus, are women.

Osteoporosis. Women have a higher rate of bone loss than men. Four out of five people suffering from osteoporosis are women.

Smoking. Smoking has a more negative effect on cardiovascular health in women than in men. Women have stronger withdrawal symptoms of smoking and are less likely to be able to successfully quit smoking.

Sexually Transmitted Infections. If exposed to a sexually transmitted infection, women are twice as likely as men to become infected.

Anesthesia. Women, on average, wake up from anesthesia after 7 minutes, whereas men, on average, wake up after 11 minutes.

Alcohol. Women produce less of the gastric enzyme that breaks down ethanol (alcohol) in the stomach. Therefore, even after allowing for size differences, women will have a higher blood alcohol content after drinking.

Pain. Some pain medications, such as kappa-opiates, are far more effective in relieving pain in women than in men.

Source: Society for Women's Health Research. http://www.womenshealthresearch.org.

women's health research that have benefited from increased funding and attention. These topics are discussed in greater detail in later chapters of this book.

Fat and body water content, steroidal sex hormone levels, and **genetic phenotype** all affect drug metabolism through pharmacokinetics (concentration of the drug) and pharmacodynamics (ability to metabolize the drug).[8] Medical literature has documented significant differences in the ways that men and women process aspirin, acetaminophen (Tylenol), lidocaine, and other commonly prescribed medications.[9] Differences such as age, hormonal status, race and ethnicity, and socioeconomic status can also affect how women metabolize drugs. The extent to which these differences prevail among the range of drugs used to prevent and treat disease is still not fully known or understood.

Recent FDA guidelines urge drug investigators to account for gender differences in drug metabolism throughout the development process and to include women of childbearing age in both Phase I and Phase II clinical trials (**Table 1.1**). The FDA once excluded women of childbearing potential from clinical trials, but has revised its guidelines to call for gender-specific analyses of safety and effectiveness in new drugs. The FDA also changed its policy of excluding women of childbearing potential from

early drug studies. These measures have helped the FDA acquire better information on drug effects in women.[10]

Gender-based research has posed challenges as well as opportunities for pharmaceutical manufacturers. If research shows that a drug is effecive for only one gender, the potential market for that drug could be limited and diminish the company's profits. However, targeting drugs for women or other specific populations can also allow researchers and pharmaceutical companies to create much more effective products.

Even with advances toward inclusion of women and minority groups in research studies, one major barrier to

Table 1.1   Phases of a Clinical Trial

- **Phase I:** new drug tested in a small group of healthy volunteers (20–80) to evaluate its safety, determine a safe dosage range, and identify side effects.
- **Phase II:** study drug is given to a larger group of people (100–300) to further evaluate its safety and effectiveness.
- **Phase III:** study drug is given to large groups in clinics and hospitals (1,000–3,000) to confirm its effectiveness, monitor side effects, and compare it with other treatments.
- **Phase IV:** study done after drug is marketed to continue collecting information regarding the drug's effects in various populations.

women's participation in biomedical research still exists. Many women are unable to take part in clinical trials because of a lack of insurance coverage. Some states have passed legislation requiring health plans to pay for routine medical care that a person may receive as a participant in a clinical trial. In 2000, **Medicare** began covering **beneficiaries'** patient care costs in clinical trials. Clinical trials still are considered experimental by some insurance companies, however, and therefore are not covered under all standard health policies.[11]

Including women in clinical studies may pose challenges, but leaving them out courts disaster through ignorance. Using women, particularly women of childbearing age, presents challenges to the investigation as the researchers must consider the effect of hormonal cycling on the hypothesis being tested. Furthermore, the potential for pregnancy and possible **teratogenic** effects in the fetus must be considered. These factors weigh heavily in designing and conducting any study.

Reproductive Rights

The history and politics surrounding women's decision to control when and if to have children are long and complex. (See Chapter 5 for more information.) For nearly a century, abortion was illegal in the United States. On January 22, 1973, the landmark Supreme Court decision *Roe v. Wade* legalized abortion; however, this decision has not prevented states from imposing restrictions that limit where and when women may receive abortions.

Roe v. Wade has also not prevented the federal government from imposing abortion restrictions in countries that receive U.S funding. In 1984, President Reagan imposed the Mexico City policy, or "global gag rule." This rule has

been particularly contentious, having been eliminated by President Bill Clinton in 1993, reimposed by President George W. Bush in 2001, and removed once more by President Barack Obama in 2009. This policy withheld U.S. assistance from foreign family planning agencies if they provided the following services, even if U.S. funds were not used for these services:

- Performing abortion in cases of pregnancy that are not life-threatening to the woman or the result of rape or incest
- Providing counseling and referral for abortions
- Lobbying to legalize abortion or increase its availability in the country in which the nongovermental organization (NGO) is operating[12]

The global gag rule's restrictions have had serious effects on women's health in many developing countries. Under this

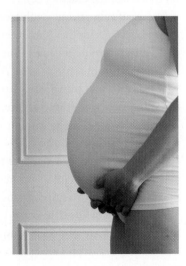

■ The potential for pregnancy and possible teratogenic effects in the fetus must be considered in clinical trials.

It's Your Health

Research Studies

Epidemiologists (scientists who study trends of disease and health in populations) can conduct research studies in many different ways. Each type of study has its own advantages and disadvantages. The following information discusses two of the more common types of studies.

1. **Descriptive studies** attempt to *describe* or *examine* a disease in a population or populations, as well as how that disease or phenomenon is related to variables in those populations, such as race, age, or sex. Descriptive studies can find correlations between the disease and variables, but cannot say one causes the other. So a cross-sectional survey might find that people who work in factories (variable) are more likely than other people to develop cancer (disease), but it could not say that working in a factory causes disease (or vice versa)—there could be some other factor involved. Descriptive studies include population studies, case-report studies, and cross-sectional studies.

2. **Analytic studies** compare people who are exposed to a certain variable to people who are not exposed to a certain variable to see if that variable influences their chances of developing a disease. Unlike descriptive studies, analytic studies *can* find a cause-and-effect ratio, though they are generally more difficult to perform. Studies that have followed otherwise equal groups of smokers and nonsmokers over time and found that smokers were more likely to develop lung cancer were responsible for linking the variable of smoking to the disease of lung cancer. Analytic studies include case-control studies, cohort studies, intervention studies, and clinical trials.

rule, developing countries faced a dilemma: if they agreed to the rule and accept U.S. family planning assistance, they risked seeing death and injuries from unsafe abortions increase because women who cannot obtain safe and legal abortions may visit unqualified practitioners in secret to end their pregnancies. But if these countries rejected U.S. assistance, they lost funding for all areas of family planning, including reducing unplanned pregnancy, preventing HIV, and reducing maternal and infant deaths. This increase in unplanned pregnancies and reduction in the number of safe medical services for pregnant women may have encouraged more women in these countries to seek abortions.

Access to Health-Care Providers, Services, and Health Information

Advances in public health and medicine have created major improvements in the prevention, diagnosis, and treatment of disease. Many people are living longer and healthier lives as a result. Over the years, women have learned to seek out medical information on their own, thereby becoming informed consumers of medicine. As new findings lead to improved methods of prevention, public health officials and health-care practitioners focus on encouraging health-care consumers to practice health promotion and disease prevention.

Unfortunately, health-care promotion and disease prevention are not simple. Many women encounter barriers to adequate health care, such as the following:

- Low socioeconomic status
- Lack of health insurance
- Lack of access to health-care facilities
- Inability to understand medical personnel because of language barriers or illiteracy
- Unfair treatment by medical personnel because of race, ethnicity, or sexual orientation
- Inability to pay for the costs of medications needed for treatment
- Declined coverage for health-care costs that are deemed unnecessary or experimental
- Fear of doctors and avoidance of seeking health care altogether

Lack of adequate access to health-care services and information is a serious issue in the United States, with a lack of health insurance being one of the most formidable barriers. In 2007, 15.3% of Americans (45.7 million) did not have insurance.[13] Millions more were underinsured,

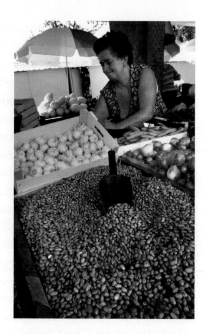

■ Millions of Americans work but do not have access to health care.

meaning their health insurance had limitations that prevented them from receiving necessary services. Health insurance for underinsured Americans may not cover serious illnesses or extended hospital stays, or may require holders to pay large co-payments or deductibles for health services. Under these conditions, when costs for health care are great, insurance or underinsurance can either prevent people from affording health care or force them to devote most of their resources to pay for care. Often, as unemployment rates rise, the number of people covered by insurance steadily declines. **Premiums** for private health insurance are extremely expensive and, therefore, many people opt to take a chance and remain uninsured when an employer does not sponsor them. (For more information on this issue, see Chapter 2.)

A lack of cultural and gender sensitivity, as well as knowledge about specific health concerns of women, also seriously affects women's health. The health needs of women are different from those of men. Additionally, health needs vary from woman to woman, depending on many factors, including her age, ethnicity/race, and sexual orientation. Several steps are being taken to make health-care providers aware of these specific needs. The ORWH has developed coursework for medical students to make them more sensitive toward and aware of women's health issues. Dental, nursing, and pharmacy programs, as well as **osteopathic** and **allopathic schools**, also are developing similar coursework. Health-care providers who receive this training are better equipped to provide care to the diverse population of women in the United States.

Global Perspective on Women's Health

Around the world, women continue to be less likely than men to have access to adequate health care, to have opportunities for economic advancement, and to have political representation. Women who live in the developing world face these challenges and are also much more likely than women in industrialized countries to die or be injured from a variety of illnesses, injuries, and diseases. Global threats to women's health include poverty, underweight and malnutrition, HIV/AIDS, violence, and **maternal morbidity and mortality**. Women are burdened not only by disease, but also by violations of their human rights that directly affect their health. These problems include domestic violence, **female genital mutilation**, **honor killings**, **trafficking**, and barriers to reproductive health services. The social, political, and economic determinants of health greatly affect women and children throughout the world. Access to clean water, nutritious food, and medical care, as well as protection from violence and poor working conditions, are basic rights that should be afforded to all for the improvement of health on a global scale. Social inequalities, such as lack of education, money, and decision-making freedom, pose a greater threat to women than to men. Women consequently have a disproportionately higher burden of disease, poverty, and maternal morbidity and mortality. Women also have the double burden of work and family drawing on them.

The United Nations has worked for the past 30 years to advance the status of women and achieve equity in the treatment, opportunities, and status of both genders. In 1979, the U.N. adopted the Convention on the Elimination of All forms of Discrimination (CEDAW), also referred to as the international bill of rights for women. CEDAW legally binds 165 U.N. member states to take steps to promote women's equity and to report on the steps they have taken. Still, when CEDAW was adopted, the U.N. recognized that even if a country legally recognized women's rights, women in that country were not always able to exercise those rights. Many factors contributed to this discrepancy, including men not working to improve women's place in society, a lack of women in decision-making positions, insufficient childcare support for women, sexist attitudes by people in power, and a lack of educational opportunities for women.[14]

In 1995, the U.N. held a world conference on women in Beijing and identified 12 critical obstacles to women's advancement (**Table 1.2**). Five years later, at the New York

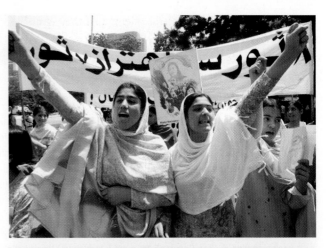

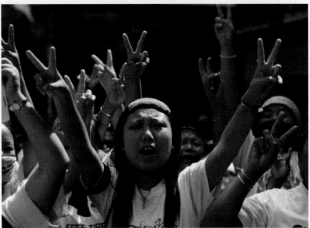

■ Around the world, women are working to improve their lives and make their voices heard.

Table 1.2	U.N. Conference in Beijing: Twelve Critical Areas of Concern for Women's Health

- Women and poverty
- Education and training of women
- Women and health
- Violence against women
- Women and armed conflict
- Women and the economy
- Women in power and decision making
- Institutional mechanisms for the advancement of women
- Human rights of women
- Women and the media
- Women and the environment
- The girl child

Source: United Nations WomenWatch. (2000). The 4 global women's conferences, 1975–1995: Historical perspective. United Nations Department of Public Information: DPI/2035/M.

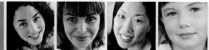

Profiles of Remarkable Women

Susan F. Wood, PhD (1959–)

Dr. Susan F. Wood has dedicated her career to advancing women's health, both by using scientific evidence to make better decisions about health policy and by taking a principled stand against political interference in the scientific process.

Wood studied biology and psychology and graduated with a Bachelor's of Science from Southwestern at Memphis in 1980; she earned a PhD in Biology at Boston University in 1989, and received research fellowship training in neuroscience from Johns Hopkins School of Medicine in 1990. Wood has studied the biochemistry of smells, researched how medications affect women during pregnancy, and advocated for women participating in clinical trial research.

Wood joined the FDA in 2000. She later became the assistant commissioner for women's health, the top agency official for women's health issues. In 2005, Wood resigned from the FDA to protest the agency's continued delays on ruling about the emergency birth control pill known as Plan B. (See Chapter 5 for more information.) Wood believed that decisions to delay the contraceptive were politically motivated.

The FDA's independent, scientific expert advisory committees had recommended that Plan B be approved in 2003, but leadership in the FDA, appointed by President George W. Bush, refused to approve the contraceptive. Before Wood resigned, the FDA regulatory staff, an advisory committee, and the head of the FDA drug center had all found Plan B to be safe and effective, and had recommended that the drug be approved for over-the-counter use. Lester M. Crawford, the head of the FDA during this time, overruled these recommendations and said the decision would be "indefinitely delayed." Wood and many other scientists believed that Crawford's decision amounted to political interference from the Bush administration over a scientific decision.

"I can no longer serve as staff when scientific and clinical evidence, fully evaluated and recommended for approval by the professional staff here, has been overruled," she wrote in an e-mail explaining her decision.[1]

Wood's decision brought immediate national attention to the FDA approval process. In August 2006, less than a year later, the FDA made Plan B available without a prescription to women 18 years of age or older. Wood is currently a research professor in George Washington University's School of Public Health.

[1]FDA Quits over Delay on Plan B, *Washington Post*, September 1, 2005.

conference "Women 2000: Gender Equality, Development and Peace for the 21st Century," the U.N. evaluated the achievements of different governments and new action plans. The U.N.'s Millennium Development Goals specifically look at how the U.N. and other groups can measure countries' progress toward promoting gender equity and empowering women. The U.N. measures progress using factors such as the ratio of boys to girls in elementary, middle, and high schools; the ratio of literate women to literate men; the percentage of women with waged employment; the proportion of seats in parliament held by women; and the percentage of births attended by a skilled health professional.

Many countries have recorded gains in women's life spans, quality of health, and political opportunities; however, women still face discrimination, violence, and marginalization around the world, and women account for the majority of the world's poor.[15] The United Nations' work has created a set of common objectives with the final goal of equity and fair treatment for everyone. Women and men around the world will need to work together to make this goal a reality.

■■■■
Informed Decision Making: Take Action

There are many ways to advocate for women's health. Women's health organizations encourage donating, getting involved by sending letters to legislators and helping to organize events, and educating oneself on women's health issues. Visiting the Internet can be a good first step in learning about organizations and deciding where to focus personal interest and commitment. The Web Sites section of this chapter lists several organizations that offer ways to become involved in promoting women's health.

■■■■
Summary

Women's health is now recognized as a national priority, and tremendous progress has been achieved in expanding the scope and depth of women's health research. Continued success in the women's health movement depends on several factors: political commitment; sufficient funds; ed-

Profiles of Remarkable Women

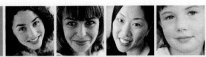

Gloria Steinem (1934–)

Gloria Steinem, well-known feminist leader, activist, and journalist, is the daughter of a newspaperwoman and the granddaughter of the noted suffragette, Pauline Steinem. Steinem studied in India for 2 years, an experience that made her aware of the extent of human suffering in the world. Steinem returned from India strongly motivated to fight social injustice and decided to begin her career as a journalist.

In 1960, Steinem moved to New York and began working as a freelance writer for popular magazines. One of her first major assignments in investigative journalism was a two-part series for *Show* magazine on the working conditions of Playboy bunnies. Steinem worked as a Playboy bunny for three weeks to prepare for the article. The articles she wrote exposed the poor working conditions and meager wages of the Playboy bunnies and the discrimination and sexual harassment that occurred at New York's Playboy Club.

In 1968, Steinem joined the staff of *New York* magazine as a contributing editor and political columnist. During these years Steinem moved into politics, covering everything from the assassination of Martin Luther King, Jr., to demonstrations of United Farm Workers led by Cesar Chavez. She also worked for various Democratic candidates. Steinem's shift to the women's liberation movement and feminism began when she started attending abortion hearings. She found herself deeply moved by the stories, realizing that society oppressed women in many ways.

By the late 1960s, Steinem had positioned herself as a leader of the women's liberation movement through her research, writing, and activism. In 1971, she joined Bella Abzug, Shirley Chisholm, and Betty Friedan to form the National Women's Political Caucus, encouraging women's participation in the 1972 election.

Steinem became friendly with Dorothy Pitman Hughes, an African American childcare pioneer. Steinem and Hughes spoke together publicly throughout the United States to promote women's rights, civil rights, and children's rights, and in 1971 they formed the Women's Action Alliance to develop women's educational programs. Although the alliance folded in 1997, its offshoot WISE (Women Initiating Self-Empowerment) continues.

In 1972, Steinem gained funding for the first mass-circulation feminist magazine, *Ms.* The preview issue sold out, and within five years *Ms.* had a circulation of 500,000. As editor of the magazine, Steinem became an influential spokesperson for women's rights issues, while continuing her active political life. In 1975, she helped plan the women's agenda for the Democratic National Convention, and she continued to exert pressure on liberal politicians on behalf of women's concerns. In 1977, Steinem participated in the National Conference of Women in Houston, Texas. The conference—the first of its kind—drew attention to feminist issues and women's rights leaders.

As a writer and an activist, Gloria Steinem continues to be a leader in the women's rights movement. Steinem's books include *Outrageous Acts and Everyday Rebellions* (1983), *Marilyn: Norma Jean* (1986), *Revolution from Within: A Book of Self-Esteem* (1992), *Moving Beyond Words* (1994), and *Doing Sixty and Seventy* (2006).

---

ucated and interested scientific and lay communities; advocacy by professionals, patients, and the public; and involvement of women, men, and communities in working for equality and recognizing gender differences. These factors have been catalysts driving the explosion in women's health research and are responsible for advances being made both in developed countries and throughout the world. Findings from biological, behavioral, and social sciences all provide insights and important data that can improve women's health and well-being.

■■■■

Topics for Discussion

1. What are some of the different ways of envisioning women's health? What do you think are the most important aspects of women's health?

2. How has the definition of feminism changed over the past 100 years? What elements have remained the same? Do you consider yourself a feminist?

3. What are some of the major differences in how men and women react to medications?

4. Why is it important for women to be included in clinical trials? What is gender-based research, and what areas of health could benefit from further gender-based research?

5. Discuss the ways the government is involved in the following areas in relation to health:

   - Policy making
   - Financing
   - Protecting the health of the public
   - Conducting research
   - Influencing how and where people receive health care

■■■■
Web Sites

Black Women's Health Imperative:
http://www.blackwomenshealth.org

Centers for Disease Control and Prevention:
http://www.cdc.gov/health/womensmenu.htm

The Children's Bureau:
http://www.acf.hhs.gov/programs/cb/

Equal Rights Amendment:
http://www.equalrightsamendment.org

Feminist Women's Health Center: http://www.fwhc.org

Global Health Council: http://www.globalhealth.org

National Organization for Women (NOW):
http://www.now.org

National Women's Health Information Center:
http://www.4woman.gov

Office of Research on Women's Health:
http://orwh.od.nih.gov/owh

Office on Women's Health:
http://www.4woman.gov

Planned Parenthood Federation of America:
http://www.plannedparenthood.org

Society for Women's Health Research:
http://www.womenshealthresearch.org

U.S. Food and Drug Administration (FDA):
http://www.fda.gov

Women's Issues in Congress:
http://www.womenspolicy.org

■■■■
References

1. World Health Organization. (2008). *Reproductive Health*. Available at: http://www.who.int/topics/reproductive_health/en/.
2. U.S. Department of Health and Human Services, Public Health Service, National Institutes of Health. (1999). *Agenda for Research on Women's Health for the 21st Century: A Report of the Task Force on the NIH Women's Health Research Agenda for the 21st Century* (Vol. 1, Executive Summary). Bethesda, MD: Author. NIH Pub. No. 99-4385.
3. Sorensen, Aja. (2004). *Rosie the Riveter: Women Working During World War II*. National Parks Service. Available at: http://www.nps.gov/pwro/collection/website/rosie.htm.
4. Office of Research on Women's Health. (2008). *About the ORWH*. Available at: http://orwh.od.nih.gov/about.html.
5. Hamburg, Margaret A. (2001). National perspective: United States. *Women's Health Issues* 11(4): 282–292.
6. Steen, J. (2007). *The primacy of public health*. American Public Health Association: Community Health Planning and Policy Development. Available at: http://www.apha.org/membergroups/newsletters/sectionnewsletters/comm/spring07/primacyph.htm.
7. Legato, M. J. (1998). Belling the cat: clinical investigation in vulnerable populations (a good idea, but who's going to volunteer?). *Journal of Gender-Specific Medicine* 1(1): 18–22.
8. Owens, N. J., & Hume, A. L. (1994). Pharmacotherapy in women: do clinically important gender-related issues exist? *Rhode Island Medicine* 77: 412–416.
9. Merkatz, R. B., Temple, R., Sobel, S., et al. (1993). Women in clinical trials of new drugs: a change in the FDA. *New England Journal of Medicine* 329: 292–296.
10. U.S. Food and Drug Administration. (2008). *About the Office of Women's Health*. Available at: http://www.fda.gov/womens/programs.html.
11. Howe, J., & Bass, M. (1999). Including women in clinical trials: the need for insurance coverage. *Journal of Gender-Specific Medicine* 2(4): 237–239.
12. Center for Reproductive Rights. (2003). *The Bush Global Gag Rule: Endangering Women's Health, Free Speech and Democracy*. Available at: http://www.reproductiverights.org/pub_fac_ggrbush.html.
13. U.S. Census Bureau (2008). *Health Insurance Coverage: 2007*. Available at: http://www.census.gov/hhes/www/hlthins/hlthin07/hlth07asc.html.
14. Pardes, H. (1998). Changing medical education for the 21st century. *Proceedings of the National Conference on Cultural Competence and Women's Health Curriculum in Medical Education*. Washington, DC: U.S. Department of Health and Human Services, II-4.
15. United Nations Women Watch. (2000). *The 4 Global Women's Conferences, 1975–1995: Historical Perspective*. United Nations Department of Public Information. Available at: http://www.un.org/womenwatch/daw/followup/session/presskit/hist.htm.

Chapter Two

The Economics of Women's Health

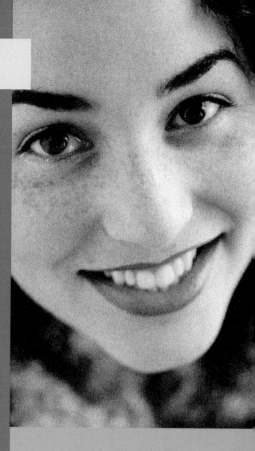

Chapter Objectives

On completion of this chapter, the student should be able to discuss:

1. The third-party payer system.

2. The fee-for-service model versus managed care.

3. Factors to consider when choosing an insurance plan.

4. Types of public health insurance, including Medicare and Medicaid.

5. The significant risks associated with being uninsured.

6. Ways that women as health-care consumers affect demand within the health-care system.

7. Health-care reform and the arguments for and against a universal health system.

8. The financial burden of aging and how it disproportionately affects women.

9. Long-term care and its associated costs.

 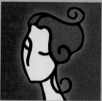

womenshealth.jbpub.com

Women's Health Online is a great source for supplementary women's health information for both students and instructors. Visit

http://womenshealth.jbpub.com

to find a variety of useful tools for learning, thinking, and teaching.

Introduction

In the United States, the economics of health care—how it is financed, what the individual's responsibility for payment is, which services should be paid for, and which social factors influence the availability of care—are the key issues behind most health-care-related decision making and policy. Participants in the health-care system, including physicians, patients, hospitals, health insurers, health education firms, and pharmaceutical, medical device, and diagnostic companies, all work to shape the direction of health care. Although most individuals believe that all people have a right to health care, significant debate has arisen regarding the best pathway to achieving that goal.

Increasingly, health care is becoming a consumer- or patient-oriented industry. As in other markets, goods and services are being developed to court consumers and drive demand for specific services. At the center of the health-care paradigm, the patient is becoming a vital health-care decision maker and is increasingly being targeted by information on diseases and available treatments. Patients are showing a growing willingness to shop around for different providers, an increasing demand for wide access to services, and a growing eagerness to pursue litigation in cases of perceived substandard care.

Understanding the effects of women's growing economic power on women's health and the persistent limitations that marginalized women face in accessing quality women's health care is critical. A discussion of the way in which the health-care system is funded identifies how the system functions and leads to an examination of the factors that create inequities in women's health care. Other important issues include the economics of aging and the effects of an aging population on women's health, public policy that influences the economics of health care, and the roles that women as caregivers have in the delivery of health care.

Paying for Health Care

Health care functions within the parameters of a market setting, offering goods and services that carry costs to health-care consumers and patients. Unlike in other markets, like real estate or retail, all individuals are health-care consumers at one stage or another of their lives. People do not have control over the degree to which they need to interact with the health-care system in the same way that they do when deciding whether to purchase a TV. If a woman has heart disease and needs to go to a cardiologist,

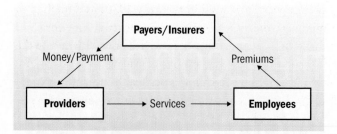

Figure 2.1

The third-party payer system.

she has very little choice except to purchase the services needed or go without care. In addition, a patient must trust her physician to tell her which goods and services she needs instead of making that decision on her own. The necessity of health care, and an individual's inability to have full information to make purchasing choices, make health care a unique market from an economic perspective.

In the United States, the health-care system is based on a **third-party payer system** in which most individuals do not pay directly for the delivery of care (**Figure 2.1**). Instead, many have health insurance, which, in return for a monthly or yearly payment called a premium, provides coverage for health-related goods and services. Before third-party payers became a mainstay of the U.S. system, patients would pay out-of-pocket for health care, either to their doctor or to hospitals. Medical care was purchased and delivered much like most other commodities. Private health in-

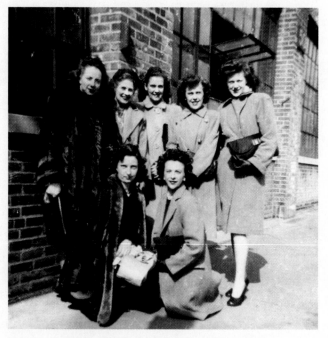

■ Before World War II, few Americans had health insurance.

surance was introduced in the early 1930s as a method to minimize the risk associated with hospital care costs. At that time, if an individual became sick or was injured on the job, the financial repercussions of paying for medical care could be significant. In response, health insurance was developed and based on an **indemnity** or **fee-for-service** system. Through this system, hospitals were reimbursed by health insurers based on a list of charges for services rendered. As the third-party payer system matured, it grew to include fee-for-service payments to physicians and other outpatient providers of health care (**Table 2.1**).

Today, most people (71%) are covered by private health insurance either provided by their employer or purchased individually. Much of private health insurance is now structured within a managed care plan. **Managed care** was introduced as a method to control costs by changing how the delivery of care is coordinated and how health care is reimbursed. In contrast to a fee-for-service model, managed care requires patients to go to specific providers, have access to care only when certain criteria are met, and, in some cases, the payer pays physicians a lump sum for all care delivered as opposed to a fee for each service rendered.

Table 2.1	Paying for Health Care Time Line

1900s	▪ American Medical Association (AMA) becomes a powerful national force.
	▪ In 1901, AMA reorganizes as the national organization of state and local associations. Membership increases from about 8,000 physicians in 1900 to 70,000 in 1910—half the physicians in the country. This period is the beginning of "organized medicine."
	▪ Doctors are no longer expected to provide free services to all hospital patients.
	▪ The United States lags behind European countries in finding value in insuring against the costs of sickness.
	▪ Railroads are the leading industry to develop extensive employee medical programs.
1910s	▪ U.S. hospitals are now modern scientific institutions, valuing antiseptics and cleanliness, and using medications for the relief of pain.
	▪ American Association for Labor Legislation (AALL) organizes first national conference on "social insurance."
	▪ Progressive reformers argue for health insurance and seem to be gaining support.
	▪ Opposition from physicians and other interest groups, plus the entry of the United States into the war in 1917, undermine the reform effort.
1920s	▪ Consistent with the general mood of political complacency, there is no strong effort to change health insurance.
	▪ Reformers now emphasize the cost of medical care instead of wages lost to sickness. The relatively higher cost of medical care is a new and dramatic development, especially for the middle class.
	▪ The cultural influence of the medical profession grows—physicians' incomes are higher and prestige is established.
	▪ General Motors signs a contract with Metropolitan Life to insure 180,000 workers.
	▪ Penicillin is discovered. It will be 20 years before this antibiotic is used to combat infection and disease.
1930s	▪ The Depression changes priorities, with greater emphasis being placed on unemployment insurance and "old age" benefits.
	▪ The Social Security Act is passed, omitting health insurance.
	▪ There is a push for health insurance within the Roosevelt Administration, but politics begins to be influenced by internal government conflicts over priorities.
	▪ Against the advice of insurance professionals, Blue Cross begins offering private coverage for hospital care in dozens of states.
1940s	▪ Prepaid group health care begins; it is seen as radical.
	▪ During World War II, wage and price controls are placed on U.S. employers. To compete for workers, companies begin to offer health benefits, giving rise to the employer-based system in place today.
	▪ President Roosevelt asks Congress for an "economic bill of rights," including the right to adequate medical care.
	▪ President Truman offers a national health program plan, proposing a single system that would include all of U.S. society.
	▪ Truman's plan is denounced by the American Medical Association (AMA), and is called a Communist plot by a House subcommittee.
1950s	▪ At the start of the decade, national health-care expenditures are 4.5% of the gross national product.
	▪ Attention turns to the Korean War and away from health reform; the United States will have a system of private insurance for those who can afford it and welfare services for the poor.
	▪ Federal responsibility for the sick poor is firmly established.
	▪ Many legislative proposals are made for different approaches to hospital insurance, but none succeeds.
	▪ Many more medications are available now to treat a range of diseases, including infections, glaucoma, and arthritis, and new vaccines become available that prevent dreaded childhood diseases, including polio. The first successful organ transplant is performed.

(continues)

(continued)

1960s	■ In the 1950s, the price of hospital care doubled. In the early 1960s, those outside the workplace, and especially the elderly, have difficulty affording insurance.
	■ More than 700 insurance companies sell health insurance.
	■ Concern about a "doctor shortage" and the need for more "health manpower" leads to federal measures to expand education in the health professions.
	■ Major medical insurance endorses high-cost medicine.
	■ President Lyndon Johnson signs Medicare and Medicaid into law.
	■ "Compulsory health insurance" advocates are no longer optimistic.
	■ The number of doctors reporting themselves to be full-time specialists grows from 55% in 1960 to 69% by 1969.
1970s	■ President Richard Nixon renames prepaid group health-care plans as health maintenance organizations (HMOs), with legislation that provides federal endorsement, certification, and assistance to them.
	■ Health-care costs are escalating rapidly, partly due to unexpectedly high Medicare expenditures, rapid inflation in the economy, expansion of hospital expenses and profits, and changes in medical care, including greater use of technology, medications, and conservative approaches to treatment. U.S. medicine is now seen as in crisis.
	■ President Nixon's plan for national health insurance is rejected by liberals and labor unions, but his "War on Cancer" centralizes research at NIH.
	■ The number of women entering the medical profession rises dramatically. In 1970, 9% of medical students are women; by the end of the decade, the proportion exceeds 25%.
1980s	■ Corporations begin to integrate the hospital system (previously a decentralized structure), enter many other health-care-related businesses, and consolidate control. Overall, there is a shift toward privatization and corporatization of health care.
	■ Under President Reagan, Medicare shifts to payment by diagnosis (DRG) instead of by treatment. Private plans quickly follow suit.
	■ Growing complaints are voiced by insurance companies that the traditional fee-for-service method of payment to doctors is being exploited.
	■ "Capitation" payments to doctors become more common.
1990s	■ Health-care costs rise at double the rate of inflation.
	■ Expansion of managed care helps to moderate increases in health-care costs.
	■ Federal health-care reform legislation fails again to pass in the U.S. Congress.
	■ By the end of the decade 44 million Americans, 16% of the nation, have no health insurance at all.
	■ The Human Genome Project to identify all of the more than 100,000 genes in human DNA gets under way.
	■ By June 1990, 139,765 people in the United States have HIV/AIDS, with a 60% mortality rate.
2000s	■ Health-care costs are on the rise again.
	■ Medicare is viewed by some as unsustainable under the present structure and must be "rescued."
	■ Changing demographics of the workplace lead many to believe the employer-based system of insurance cannot last.
	■ The Human Genome Project was completed a full two years ahead of schedule, in 2003.
	■ Direct-to-consumer advertising for pharmaceuticals and medical devices is on the rise.
	■ Medicare expands to include a prescription drug benefit as of January 2006.
	■ Employers continue to cut down on health insurance benefits in an attempt to address persistent increases in costs.
	■ Medical savings accounts become common.
	■ President George W. Bush unsuccessfully tries to privatize Social Security.
	■ Congress passes a major expansion to State Children's Health Insurance Program (SCHIP), which will provide insurance for an additional 4 million low-income children, in 2009.

Source: Adapted from *Healthcare Crisis: Who's at Risk?* Healthcare Timeline, PBS. Produced by Issues TV, 2000. Reprinted with permission.

Managed care has been perceived both as a driver of positive change by keeping costs down and providing broad access to services and as a villain by placing limits on care. It is blamed for decreased access to care, shorter physician office visits, higher co-payments, and more restrictions on which doctors patients can see. Managed care is not a static concept; in fact, the types of products that are offered are continually evolving to meet the changing needs and demands of patients, employers, and providers.

The limitations on access that lead patients and physicians to vilify managed care ended up slowing the rate at which health-related expenditures grew in the United States in the 1990s (see **Figure 2.2**). This goal was accomplished by managed care organizations asking for more

Employment-based health benefit programs have existed in the United States for more than 100 years. In the 1870s, for example, railroad, mining, and other industries began to provide the services of company doctors to workers. In 1910, Montgomery Ward entered into one of the earliest group insurance contracts. Prior to World War II, few Americans had health insurance, and most policies covered only hospital room, board, and ancillary services. During World War II, the number of persons with employment-based health insurance coverage started to increase for several reasons. When wages were frozen by the National War Labor Board and a shortage of workers occurred, employers sought ways to get around the wage controls in order to attract scarce workers, and offering health insurance was one option. Health insurance was an attractive means to recruit and retain workers during a labor shortage for two reasons: unions supported employment-based health insurance, and workers' health benefits were not subject to income tax or Social Security payroll taxes, as were cash wages. Under the current tax code, health insurance premiums paid by employers are deductible for employers as a business expense, and are excluded, without limit, from workers' taxable income.[1]

It's Your Health

Drive-Through Deliveries

In the 1990s, HMOs and other managed care plans shortened average maternity stays for normal births. Such programs were dubbed "drive-through deliveries." Because women were being discharged from hospitals only 24 to 48 hours after giving birth, many lawmakers, alarmed that the practice would endanger newborns, adopted laws to require insurance coverage for at least 48 hours of care after delivery.

In a study conducted at Harvard Medical School, researchers found that newborns needed the same number of later emergency room visits and hospital readmissions, regardless of whether they had longer initial stays or shorter ones. In essence, the shorter stays were not adding risk to the newborns, even though the "common sense" of many women and legislators suggested that it would. The study looked at 20,366 normal deliveries in the 1990s. During the period studied, newborn visits to emergency rooms kept steady at an average of about 1% every three months. Hospital readmissions hovered around 1.5%. The same pattern held for a more vulnerable group of young, lower-income mothers with less education.

In an article on this subject published by the Associated Press (December 18, 2002), Larry Akey, a spokesman for the Health Insurance Association of America, said that short-stay programs were designed "not entirely as cost-saving measures, but an opportunity for the mother to get home" faster. The debate continues among women's advocacy groups, health insurers, and hospitals.

stringent proof of medical necessity before services are paid for—for example, by requiring physicians to get prior authorizations from the payer before certain care is rendered. Another method for controlling costs has been to allow members to get care only from a specific network of physicians who have contracted with the payers to offer low-cost care, or to make patients pay higher co-payments if they see doctors who are not members of the network. By controlling the supply of health-care resources, however, managed care organizations have been able to provide patients

with access to a wider range of services at a relatively reasonable cost, such as pharmaceuticals and rehabilitation services, than fee-for-service models are now able to offer. More recently, health care as a share of the gross domestic product (GDP) has begun to rise fairly rapidly.

Managed care plans differ based on the level to which they control what services are provided to patients. Types of managed care plans include preferred provider organizations (PPOs), health maintenance organizations (HMOs), and point-of-service (POS) plans. **Table 2.2** describes the various types of managed care plans. Almost all health insurers today offer some form of managed care products or include elements of managed care products such as physician networks or tiered co-payments into their existing product lines.

In paying for health care, insurers decide which types of services they will cover (see **Figure 2.3**). Hospital care, outpatient care, physician office visits, diagnostic tests, preventive services, prescription drugs, mental health services, durable medical equipment like wheelchairs, and home health care are all elements of health care that most people would consider important; however, all of these are separate services that may or may not be covered under a given

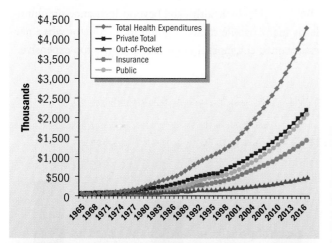

Figure 2.2

National health expenditures: 1965–2017 (projected).

Source: Centers for Medicare & Medicare Services, Office of the Actuary. National Health Expenditures data. Released January 2008.

Table 2.2	Managed Care Plans

Health Maintenance Organization (HMO): An HMO is a managed care plan that offers a full range of services for a fixed prepaid fee, rather than charging patients for each service provided. Patients normally pay only a small co-payment for care. With some plans and for some services, patients also have to satisfy a deductible. Usually, patients don't have to file claims.

HMO plans typically fall into one of two categories:

- **Staff Model:** A staff model HMO has salaried physicians who provide services only to plan members. They offer care at a hospital, clinic, or health center in the community.

- **Independent Practice Association (IPA):** An IPA maintains contracts with a number of physicians and/or physician group practices. These physicians see patients in their own offices.

Point-of-Service (POS) Plan: POS plans function much like IPAs. Patients select a primary care physician who coordinates all care within the participating provider network, including specialist referrals.

Preferred Provider Organization (PPO): A PPO plan functions much like a POS plan, but it eliminates the primary care physician. As with the POS plan, patients can use a health-care provider outside of the preferred provider network for an additional cost. Patients can usually see any participating provider—whether a primary care physician or a specialist—without a referral, at no additional cost.

High Deductible Health Plan (HDHP) with a Health Savings Account (HSA) or a Health Reimbursement Arrangement (HRA): An HDAR/HSA or HRA provides traditional medical coverage and a tax-free way to build savings for future medical expenses. It gives patients flexibility and discretion over how health-care benefits are used. The HDHP features higher annual deductibles than other plans (usually $1,000 to $2,000) and usually has some upper limit on out-of-pocket liability. HDHPs make consumers share the financial burden of health-care utilization. Most plans' coverage doesn't kick in until a large deductible is met, though many plans will pay for routine preventive care before the deductible is met.

■ A co-pay is the amount of money that a patient is responsible for paying to receive health-care services; co-pays are either a fixed amount of money or a percentage of the overall charge for a given service.

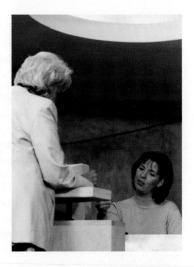

insurance plan. As patient demand evolves, many alternative therapies and preventive care services, such as massage, acupuncture, and chiropractic care, are beginning to be covered by health insurance.

Choosing an Insurance Plan

When people choose between different insurance options, their choices are often influenced by which services are covered or what percentage of the total cost the insurer will pay. If a woman thinks that she is unlikely to use many services, as a 26-year-old woman without any existing medical conditions might, she may opt for a less expensive insurance program like an HMO that has more restricted coverage. Regardless of the insurance program selected, an individual is at significant financial risk if her insurance does not cover or only partially covers the services that she uses. The inability to pay for health care, beyond insurance premiums, leads many people to avoid going to the doctor when necessary or to cut short therapy if it becomes too expensive.

Figure 2.3

Health insurance coverage of nonelderly Americans by source of coverage, 2006.

Source: Employee Benefit Research Institute estimates from the March Current Population Survey, 2007 Supplement.

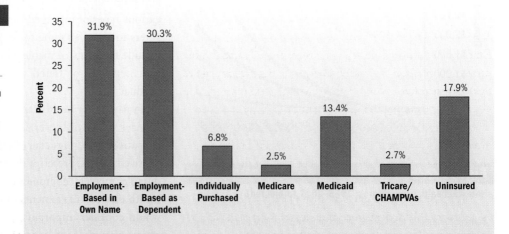

As a method to manage rising costs, patients are increasingly being required to pay out-of-pocket for a portion of their health care. A **co-payment** (or **co-pay**) is the amount of money a patient is responsible for paying to receive health-care services. Co-pays can be either a fixed amount of money, like a $10 or $20 co-pay for a routine office visit, or a percentage of the overall charge for a given service (referred to as a co-insurance), like the popular 80% covered/20% patient responsibility payment schemes.

With prescription drugs, many payers have introduced a tiered co-pay system, in which different levels of payment are required for different types of medications. Most tiered co-pays try to reward patients for purchasing lower-cost generic drugs, as opposed to more expensive brand-name drugs. **Generic drugs** are the chemical equivalents of brand-name drugs, but are far less expensive. Within a tiered co-pay system, for example, a patient may pay $5 for a generic antibiotic, $15 for a preferred brand-name drug, and $25 for the premium-cost brand-name drug. Women often are forced to make significant co-pays for birth control pills, with many prescriptions falling into the highest co-pay tier. As a result, a woman may have to pay $20 to $40 per month to control her fertility. Health insurers have lists of drugs for which they provide reimbursement called **formularies**, which describe to patients and doctors which drugs are covered, into which tier each drug falls, and how much each drug will cost the patient.

Out-of-pocket costs to women continue to be a significant barrier to appropriate care and compliance with taking medication. A report by the Kaiser Family Foundation found that one in five (21%) nonelderly women did not fill a prescription because of the cost, compared with 13% of men.[1] This issue was also a problem for 40% of uninsured women, 27% of women with Medicaid, and 15% of privately insured women.

Types of Health Insurance

Employer-sponsored health insurance, as well as health insurance purchased by individuals, is considered **private health insurance**. Most private health insurance in the United States is purchased and subsidized by employers. When an individual has a full-time job, health insurance is often a central benefit. Employer-sponsored health insurance can often be extended to cover the family of the insured individual.

Public health insurance is insurance provided by the government. The federal government is the largest health insurer in the United States through its Medicare, Medicaid,

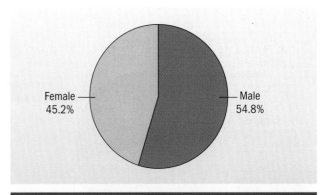

Figure 2.4

Uninsured nonelderly adult population by gender, 2006.

Source: Employee Benefit Research Institute estimates from the March Current Population Survey, 2007 Supplement.

Veterans Administration, Department of Defense, and Bureau of Indian Affairs insurance programs (see **Figure 2.4**). Medicare is the result of a bill enacted by Congress in 1965 to provide health insurance at a reasonable cost to Americans aged 65 and older. Medicare is provided in several parts:

- Part A is provided to all enrollees and covers inpatient hospitalization.
- Part B is optional and covers outpatient services.
- Part D is optional and covers a portion of prescription drug costs.

Since 1965, the program has grown to cover disabled individuals and patients with end-stage renal disease. Most recently, it has grown to include a portion of prescription drug coverage. Medicare's prescription drug coverage is expected to have a significant impact on who pays for prescription drugs in the United States (see **Figure 2.5**).

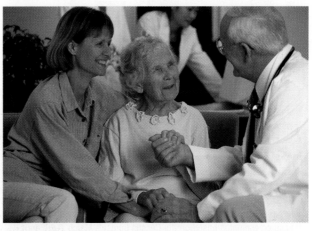

■ Due to the aging population and the fact that women live longer than men, an increasing majority of Medicare beneficiaries are women.

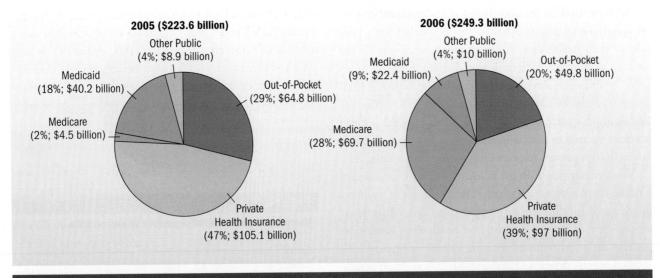

Figure 2.5

Projected prescription drug spending, by payer, 2005 and 2006.

Source: Centers for Medicare & Medicaid Services, Office of the Actuary, National Health Statistics Group.

Today, Medicare is the largest single insurer in the United States, covering more than 42 million people, 56% of whom are women. Due to the aging of the population and the fact that women live longer than men, an increasing majority of Medicare beneficiaries who are the oldest of the old are women (**Figure 2.6**).

Medicaid is a program jointly administered by federal and state governments that provides health insurance for low-income Americans. Whereas Medicare is a federally

controlled health system, Medicaid is largely run at the state level. In some states, such as California and Tennessee, Medicaid has a state-specific name (MediCal, TennCare). The vast majority of Medicaid recipients are low-income women and their children; the children are covered through State Children's Health Insurance Programs (SCHIPs). Medicaid and the benefits it provides are fundamental to the provision of health care to economically disadvantaged women and children in the United States. In 2009, legislation passed by Congress, and signed by President Barack Obama, expanded SCHIP to provide coverage to an additional four million low-income children. Funded by an increased federal cigarette tax, the new SCHIP will insure a total of 11 million low-income children.

Currently, Medicaid covers nearly 52 million people. Individuals qualify based on income status, level of disability or need for long-term care, or by being a dependent of a Medicaid recipient. Medicaid is accepted as a payment method by all hospitals and most physicians, although some private physicians refuse Medicaid patients due to the lower reimbursement rates the system provides as compared to private insurance. All states cover the following basic services for Medicaid recipients:

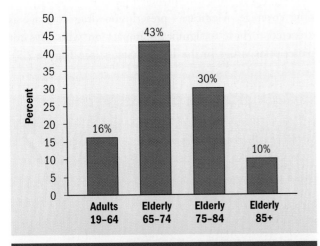

Figure 2.6

Medicare population by age.

Source: Urban Institute and Kaiser Commission on Medicaid and the Uninsured estimates based on the Census Bureau's March 2007 and 2008 Current Population Survey (CPS: Annual Social and Economic Supplements).

- Inpatient and outpatient medical care
- Laboratory and X-ray services
- Chronic care facilities for persons older than 21 years
- Home health care for those eligible for nursing facility services

- Services provided by a physician or nurse practitioner
- Necessary transportation

States may provide optional services to eligible patients, including prescription drugs, case management, dental care, prosthetic devices, medical transportation, intermediate care facilities, optometry, and tuberculosis-related services. Federal law requires the delivery of services that are "medically necessary," but states exercise substantial independence in determining the amount and duration of services covered by establishing criteria for medical necessity and utilization control.

In addition to Medicare and Medicaid, the federal government provides health insurance to veterans through the Veterans Administration (VA), active-service military personnel through the Department of Defense (DOD), government workers through the government's own health insurance program, and Native Americans through the Indian Health Services. These programs are all separately adminis-

tered and have differing organizational structures. For example, the VA is not only a payer for health care, but also a network of providers. Veterans covered within this system are eligible for care at VA hospitals and clinics. This approach is similar to how the DOD provides health insurance and health-care services to active-duty military personnel.

Uninsured Americans

In addition to those people with private insurance and those with public insurance, 45.7 million Americans were uninsured for all of 2007[2]—more than the populations of Texas, Florida, and Connecticut combined (**Figure 2.7**). A larger number of people are uninsured for a portion of the year. In one recent report, that figure almost doubles the number of people uninsured for the whole year. That means that close to one in three Americans were uninsured for all or part of the period studied. Of those, two-thirds were uninsured for six months or longer. [3]

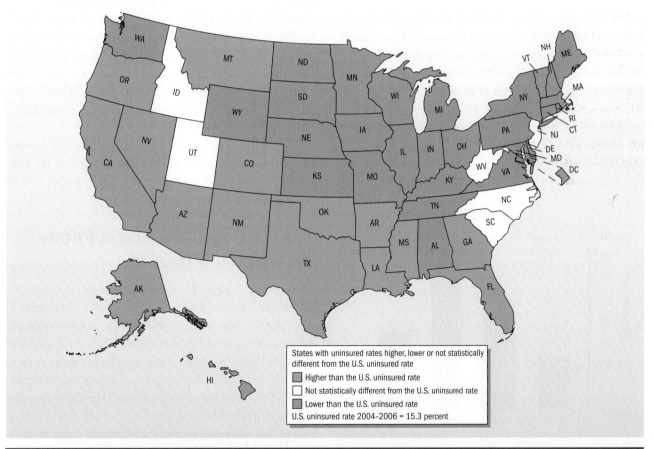

States with uninsured rates higher, lower or not statistically different from the U.S. uninsured rate

☐ Higher than the U.S. uninsured rate
☐ Not statistically different from the U.S. uninsured rate
☐ Lower than the U.S. uninsured rate
U.S. uninsured rate 2004-2006 = 15.3 percent

Figure 2.7

Uninsured rates by state, using three-year average: 2004[1]–2006.

Source: U.S. Census Bureau, Current Population Survey, 2005 to 2007 Annual Social Economic Supplements.

[1] The 2004 and 2005 data have been revised since originally published. See www.census.gov/hhes/www/hlthins/usernote/schedule.html.

The uninsured are men, women, and children, though today, men are more likely to be uninsured than women. Uninsured individuals are more likely to have poorer health, have significantly less access to care, and die prematurely than their counterparts with insurance. Nearly one in five families has at least one uninsured member. Most uninsured individuals are younger than age 30. In fact, 11.7% of children are uninsured.

People without health insurance are at significant financial risk if they get sick or have an accident that requires emergency medical care. Because the uninsured must pay out-of-pocket for medical services, such as doctors' office visits or prescription drugs, they often avoid preventive care or proper follow-up care due to cost concerns. In addition, the uninsured end up paying more for medical care because they are not eligible for the discounted pricing structures that health insurance companies negotiate with hospitals and doctors. As a result, the cost of care often strains family finances, jeopardizing families' physical, emotional, and economic health.[4] Long-term implications from being uninsured may include worsening of health status due to lack of appropriate care and not being accurately monitored by a physician, leading to suboptimal care.

Minorities, including African Americans and Hispanic Americans, have higher rates of uninsurance than white or Asian Americans (see **Figure 2.8**). Although lower-income people have the highest rates of being uninsured, the profile of who lacks health insurance is changing. Only 7.1% of people in the $75,000-plus income bracket are uninsured, compared to 35.7% of people with family income

below $10,000. Unemployment has increased significantly due to a weakening U.S. economy and rising health-care costs for employers; as a result, many individuals who were formerly covered by their employers have suddenly lost their health insurance. A decline in coverage through employer-based health plans, rising out-of-pocket costs associated with these plans, and skyrocketing costs for insurance premiums are seen as major drivers of this trend.

Lack of health insurance affects access to health services and contributes to poorer health, higher hospitalization rates, and more advanced disease states by the time health services are finally received. Although more than 1 in 10 children still lack health coverage, the expansion of Medicaid and the State Children's Health Insurance Program is helping. Nearly 20% of uninsured Americans—8.7 million individuals—are children. The likelihood that a child is uninsured fell from 13.9% in 1998 to 10.5% in 2004 (**Figure 2.9**). It has since increased to 11.7% in 2006. Federal health insurance coverage of children through the 2009 expansion of SCIP may eventually reduce this number, but these changes will likely take years for their full effects to be felt. Although children are more likely to be insured than nonelderly adults, health insurance is particularly important for children. Uninsured children are more likely than insured children to lack a usual source of health care, to go without needed care, and to experience worse health outcomes.[1]

Overall, the scope of the uninsured problem is vast and requires significant attention by the U.S. public if the goals related to equity in delivery of and access to health care are to be achieved.

Preventive Care and a Focus on Women's Health

Managed care plans have been successful at using evidence-based medicine and economic analysis to determine the value of new medical technologies, procedures, and drugs to the plan and its members. A positive outcome of this trend has been widespread support for many preventive services, such as mammograms, cervical cancer screening, and smoking cessation programs. The old saying that "an ounce of prevention is worth a pound of cure" has been proven true in most studies. (See Chapter 3 for more on primary, secondary, and tertiary prevention.) Payers have been shown that investing in preventive services and education leads both to members with fewer major medical problems, such as heart disease, and to the ability to diagnose diseases, such as breast cancer, at an earlier stage. Through their positive effects on health-care outcomes,

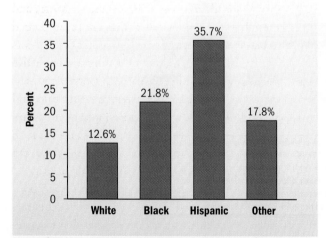

Figure 2.8

Percentage uninsured among the nonelderly population by race and ethnic origin, 2005.

Source: Employee Benefit Research Institute estimates from the March Current Population Survey, 2007 Supplement.

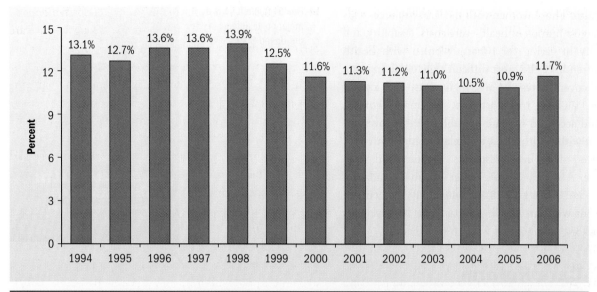

Figure 2.9

Percentage of children under age 18 without health insurance, 1994–2006.

Source: Employee Benefit Research Institute estimates from the March Current Population Survey, March 1995–2007 Supplement.

Note: 1994–2003 data are adjusted for Census correction announced in March 2007.

many preventive and educational services have shown their ability to decrease overall health-care costs.

Preventive services and health education are the cornerstones of women's health. As awareness and support of these and other women-specific health issues increase, many payers have established whole departments dedicated to women's health. These departments help to ensure that patients and physicians are educated about best practices and newly available treatments specifically for women; they also analyze the benefits of new technologies. Women's health departments within payer organizations have enjoyed success in prioritizing women's health issues—for example, by supporting prenatal check-ups and strict monitoring regimens for pregnant women, promoting women's cardiac health, and ensuring universal coverage of gynecological exams.

Women as Health-Care Consumers

Women have been recognized as the primary decision makers relating to health care and as a growing economic force to be courted. In one large survey, women were reported to make 90% of health-related decisions for their families.[5] As a group, women have seen their economic power and ability to affect the overall demand within the health-care system increase significantly. They have in-

creased their participation in the workforce, in government, and in decision-making positions over the last 40 years. In the United States, women earn more than $1 trillion annually, and according to a study by the Commonwealth Institute, more than 68% of women say they manage the bills in their household, compared to 55% of men. Women's growing economic power has made them increasingly important in the eyes of pharmaceutical, medical device, and diagnostics manufacturers. More and more, research and development dollars are being poured into discovering both necessary and voluntary treatments for women. In addition, women are taking a more active role in their own health care, by learning more about their health status, by taking part in preventive health care, and by articulating their needs to providers, payers, manufacturers, and legislatures. Together, these factors work to raise awareness of women's health issues and force the health-care industry to make women's health a priority.

Although women's overall economic position has been improving, many women still find themselves in economically disadvantaged circumstances. Whether due to being unemployed or underemployed, not having adequate childcare support, lacking education, being in poor health, lacking access to resources, or just not having adequate support, they do not have the decision-making freedom that other women with greater access to resources enjoy. Today, lower-income women are disproportionately affected by poor health. Those women with the least resources thus carry the largest burden of health-care costs, disability, and responsibility in caring for others. Women with health problems often have the most difficult time obtaining care because of coverage restrictions, high costs, and logistical barriers, such as transportation. For many women, coverage and access to care are unstable. Health coverage, involvement with health plans, and relationships with doctors are often short lived, resulting in spotty and fragmented care. A survey by the Kaiser Family Foundation found that one quarter (24%) of nonelderly women delayed or went without care in the past year because they could not afford it, compared with 16% of men.[6]

■ Health-care reform is a major political topic in the United States.

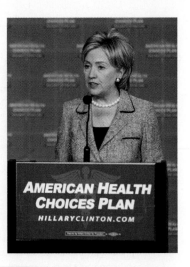

Health-Care Reform

In many countries, such as Canada and the United Kingdom, the government provides health insurance to all citizens through a system of **universal health insurance**. Universal health-care systems are aimed at allowing all citizens access to a minimum level of care that is deemed acceptable. Individuals are then allowed to purchase supplementary insurance to pay for items not covered under the national health systems. Proponents of these types of systems argue that health care is a right, not a privilege, and should therefore be available to all citizens. Their opponents counter that universal health care is an overly costly approach and prefer that the private sector manage and fund health care through a free-market approach. In the early 1990s, President Bill Clinton led a major drive for establishing universal health insurance in the United States. Although those efforts ultimately failed, health-care reform has remained a major political topic. (See **It's Your Health** for more information.) President Barack Obama has promised to make health-care reform one of the top priorities of his administration.

In the future, health care is likely to be significantly affected by the research and development of new technologies. Major advances in women's health issues are likely to arise from research into genetic engineering, stem cell research, microscopic surgical techniques, and molecular diagnostics. How the system will pay for these advancements and make them accessible to the majority of people remains a challenge.

To ensure the ongoing improvement of our health-care system in general, and in women's health issues in particular, health-care reform must take into account the disparities in care and outcomes related to the socioeconomic positions of patients. The U.S. public must identify their

It's Your Health

Universal Health Care

The lack of health-care coverage is detrimental to individuals, their families, and the community at large. Due to the high costs of health care, uninsured individuals and their families have difficulties getting quality health care when they are sick. They tend to delay treatments until their illnesses become serious, and they are less likely to seek routine preventive health services that can avert or detect major illnesses early on. As a result, they tend to die sooner than people with health insurance.

The lack of health insurance aggravates the financial burden placed on the community as a whole. Because the uninsured tend to delay necessary treatment, they are often sicker and therefore more expensive to treat when they finally seek care. Also, they frequently turn to the nearest hospital emergency room, which is an expensive and inefficient way to get care. Furthermore, the primary providers of care to the uninsured—such as public hospitals, teaching hospitals, academic health centers, and nonprofit community hospitals—incur heavy losses from high rates of uncompensated care. In turn, these providers are forced to cut back on their services to all patients or even close their facilities.

The American Public Health Association has advocated the following:

- Universal coverage for everyone in the United States, to include comprehensive benefits, affordable prices, and quality services

- Organization and administration of health care through publicly accountable mechanisms to assure maximum responsiveness to public needs, with a major role for federal, state, and local government health agencies

- Attention in the organization, staffing, delivery, and payment of care to the needs of all populations, including those confronting geographic, physical, cultural, language, and other nonfinancial barriers to service.

Source: American Public Health Association; www.apha.org. Related APHA Policy: Support for a New Campaign for Universal Health Care. 20007, 9502.

Gender Dimensions

HEALTH DIFFERENCES BETWEEN MEN AND WOMEN

The population of the United States is getting older as disease prevention, health promotion, and innovative treatments prevent or delay disease and prolong life. In 2006, the average life expectancy for all Americans was 78.1 years of age: 76 years for white men and 70 years for black men, and 81 years for white women and 76.9 years for black women.[7] On average, women now live six years longer than men. In 2000, there were only 70 men per 100 women over age 65; there were only 41 men per 100 women age 85 or older (see **Figure 2.10**). Note, however, that these figures are an aggregate of all U.S. women. When examined by race and ethnicity, life expectancy varies among both women and men.

As a result, most of the burden of aging rests on women, and increasingly women are aging into their oldest years without the support or help of spouses.[8] The aging trends have enormous economic ramifications. As women age, they become more likely to suffer from chronic disease such as heart disease, cancer, and arthritis. These illnesses create significant morbidity as well as costs to affected individuals.[9] Currently, Medicare provides health insurance for all Americans over the age of 65, ensuring that all older Americans have at least some access to health care. Because Medicare covers only 80% of costs, however, a significant financial burden is often imposed on older patients when seeking care.[10]

The economic realities faced by elderly women also affect women's health. As women age, they are likely to need increased access to

prescription drugs, perhaps specialty medical assistance, durable medical equipment (such as walkers and orthopedic beds), and other expensive goods and services.

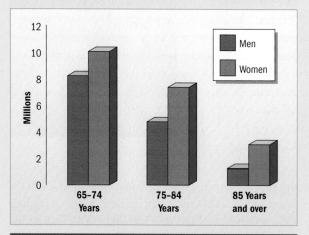

Figure 2.10

Population 65 years and over by age and gender, 2000.

Source: U.S. Census Bureau, U.S. Census 2000 Summary File.

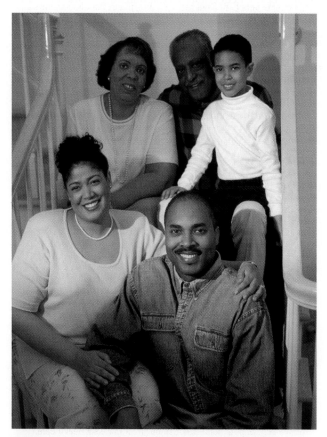

■ Many women are "sandwiched" with requirements for elder care and child care.

priorities as they relate to health care, whether that entails equity, access to new technology, or improved outcomes. Reform should attempt to manage rising costs while recognizing and addressing the diverse needs of women within the system.

Taking Care of the Population: Long-Term Care and Women as Caregivers

Once an individual or her family becomes unable to take care of an elderly or disabled person any longer, long-term care or assisted living communities are available. In direct correlation to the percentage of women and men in the oldest age categories, the vast majority of residents in these facilities are women.

Long-term care provides ongoing care for people who need lengthy or even lifelong assistance with daily living due to an illness, injury, or severe cognitive impairment (such as Alzheimer's disease). It can be provided either in a nursing home, in an assisted living facility, or at the patient's home. According to the Federal Long-Term Care Insurance Program, sponsored by the U.S. Office of Personnel Management, the average annual cost for home care substantially exceeds $20,000. The national average

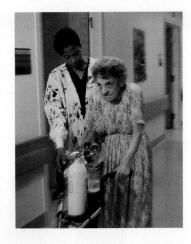

■ Most older women in nursing homes spend down their life savings to pay for services until Medicaid begins to cover the remaining costs of care.

annual cost for care in a nursing home exceeds $75,190 for a private and $52,000 for a semi-private room, according to a recent survey by MetLife's LifePlans. This was an increase of 6% from the year before. Costs are expected to continue to increase dramatically, with a semi-private room costing $190,600 by 2030.[11] Two insurance options are available to cover these expenses:

■ Private long-term care insurance programs are very expensive and are predominantly purchased by wealthier Americans.

■ Medicaid covers Americans in long-term care facilities once they have spent out all other resources. Most older women in nursing homes spend down their life savings to pay for services until Medicaid begins to cover the remaining costs of care.

As the U.S. population ages and life spans increase, informal caregiving by family members has become a vital component of the health-care delivery system in general and elder care in particular. One national study estimates the value of unpaid caregiving at approximately $350 billion per year. That is twice as much as is spent on home care and nursing home services.[12] Women continue to provide the majority of this informal caregiving today, even though most working-age women now participate in the labor force. As a result of shouldering the stress and burden for caregiving, women caregivers tend to suffer more adverse health events than non-caregivers.[9] According to the Commonwealth Fund, one-fourth (25%) of women caring for a sick or disabled family member rate their own health as fair or poor, compared with one-sixth (17%) of other women. More than half (54%) of women caregivers have one or more chronic health conditions, compared with two-fifths (41%) of other women. In addition, half

(51%) of all caregivers exhibit high depressive symptoms and sleeplessness, while 38% of other women do so.

■■■■

Informed Decision Making

Choosing health insurance is often a baffling undertaking, with many options meaning little to the individual other than being associated with different monthly premiums. Most people receive their health insurance through their employers, so they usually have a small menu of plans from which to pick.

When choosing a health insurance plan, it is important to consider the following:

■ *Deductibles.* Often different plans have a certain amount that the individual must pay out-of-pocket before the benefit kicks in. For example, if a woman has a $500 deductible on her insurance plan, she must pay for the first $500 worth of health-care services she receives before the insurance plan will begin to pick up the cost. Usually, the less expensive the plan, the higher the deductible. Deductibles are common in all types of insurance programs.

■ *Benefits.* Look closely at the list of covered services. For example, does the insurance plan cover prescription drugs? Does it cover open access to relevant specialists or provide medical equipment needed for specific health problems?

■ *Network.* Consider the implications of a restrictive network to the costs of care and access to care. Does the insurance plan restrict access to a specific network of physicians? Is the preferred doctor a member of that network? If not, what are the costs for going to a doctor that is out of the network? Are the major local hospitals part of the health plan's network?

■ *Co-insurance.* Many plans today require patients to pay a set percentage of charges, often 10–20%. While this can keep premiums affordable, patient costs can be very high if hospitalization or long-term care is required. Consumers should inquire whether their insurance plan has a maximum amount that a patient is required to pay if a hospitalization or other high-cost event occurs.

■ *Emergency Services.* Often health insurance programs have very restrictive criteria for use of emergency ser-

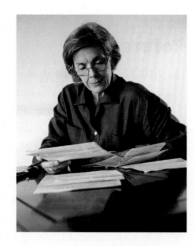

■ Choice of health insurance plans is often a baffling undertaking; there are many important factors to consider other than simply the monthly premium.

vices. What is the process for receiving emergency services? Is prior authorization needed before going to the emergency room?

■ *Co-payments.* Co-payments are fixed amounts of money a patient is required to pay to receive health-related goods or services. Co-pays usually have to be paid out-of-pocket, either at the doctor's office, at the pharmacy, or at the hospital.

■ *Benefit Cap.* Is there a maximum amount of money for which the insurer is liable, after which the patient has to pay for services? This is usually only a concern for very ill people, or people who have very serious accidents.

By considering these factors when choosing health insurance, a woman is more likely to get a package that is right for her and her family.

■■■■

Summary

The delivery of and access to health care in the United States is significantly affected by the way it is funded. The U.S. system includes both public and private health insurance that helps individuals to afford high-quality health care. The way health insurance is structured affects the amount that individuals have to pay out-of-pocket for health-care goods, such as prescription drugs, and services, such as physician office visits. There are still significant inequity issues within the health-care system, as demonstrated by the fact that more than 47 million Americans do

Profiles of Remarkable Women

Katherine Swartz (1950–)

Katherine Swartz is a Professor of Health Policy and Economics at the Harvard School of Public Health. She is a demonstrated leader in health policy research, with a focus on the issue of the uninsured. She has been involved in research concerning health insurance issues since she graduated from college and went to work at what was then the U.S. Department of Health, Education, and Welfare (now the Department of Health and Human Services). For the last 20 years, Prof. Swartz's research interests have focused on the population without health insurance and efforts to increase access to health-care coverage. Her research contributed to policy makers' understanding that people without health insurance are not all alike—many different types of people lack insurance. Prof. Swartz also was the first researcher to show that people differ in terms of the length of time they may go without health insurance. In fact, many spells without health insurance last less than six months but a significant percentage of uninsured spells last more than two years. The dynamic nature of health insurance coverage means that over the course of a year, many more people are at risk for the financial costs of medical care than the number estimated to be uninsured when a survey is conducted.

　　Prof. Swartz's interest in how health insurance might be made more affordable and more accessible to the uninsured has led her to analyze the markets for health insurance, particularly for individuals who may not be covered through work in a group insurance plan. This research has focused on insurance companies' fear of being left with the sickest and therefore most expensive people in these markets. Findings from her research have emphasized the need for government policy to reduce such fears so as to allow the nongroup insurance markets to expand health insurance coverage. One such policy that Prof. Swartz has proposed is that government act as the reinsurer and take responsibility for the extremely high-cost people each year in the nongroup markets. Her most recent book, *Reinsuring Health: Why More Middle-Class People Are Uninsured and What Government Can Do,* was published in 2006.

not have health insurance. Among the elderly population, issues of access to and payment for health-care goods and services continue to be a major problem. Although most are covered by Medicare and Medicaid, the elderly, who are predominantly women, face a unique set of economic challenges in managing their health.

■■■■
Topics for Discussion

1. How can a person's health insurance status affect his or her health status?

2. Should everyone have access to health insurance, even if she can't afford it?

3. Is access to health care a right or a privilege?

4. What are some common health-related items that often are not covered by health insurance?

5. What role do employers have in the delivery of health care?

6. What are potential implications of Medicare becoming more like a managed care program and less of a fee-for-service program?

7. How can health insurance status be affected by women's different stages of life?

8. What are some central issues related to the elderly population's health-care needs?

■■■■
Web Sites

Academy Health: http://www.academyhealth.org

America's Health Insurance Plans: http://www.ahip.org

Center for Medicare and Medicaid Services: http://www.cms.hhs.gov

Kaiser Family Foundation: http://www.kaisernetwork.org

National Center for Quality Assurance: http://www.ncqa.org

■■■■
References

1. *EBRI Databook on Employee Benefits* (4th ed.). (1997) updated June 2008. Washington, DC: Employee Benefits Research Institute; and Fronstin, P. (2007) *The Future of Employment-Based Health Benefits: Have Employers Reached a Tipping Point?* Washington, DC: National Academies Press.

2. U.S. Census Bureau. (2007). *Current Population Reports, P60-233, Income, Poverty, and Health Insurance Coverage in the United States: 2006.* Washington, DC: U.S. Government Printing Office.

3. Families USA. (2007). *Wrong Direction: One Out of Three Americans Are Uninsured.* Publication 07-108.

4. Collins, S., Kriss, J., Davis, K., Doty, M., & Holmgren, A. (2006). *Squeezed: Why Rising Exposure to Health Care Costs Threatens the Health and Financial Well-Being of American Families, Prepared by the Commonwealth Fund.* Washington, DC: The Commonwealth Fund.

5. Shaller, D. (2005). *Consumers in Health Care: The Burden of Choice, Prepared for the California HealthCare Foundation.* Sacramento, CA: California Hospital Association.

6. Fronstin, P., & Collins, S. (2008). *Findings from the 2007 EBRI/Commonwealth Fund Consumerism in Health Survey.*

7. Heron, M., Hoyert, D., Xu, J., Scott, C., & Tejada-Vera, B. (2008). Deaths: preliminary data for 2006. *National Vital Statistics Reports* 56(16): 2008–2010.

8. National Alliance for Caregiving, & AARP. (2004). *Caregiving in the U.S.* Washington, DC: National Allliance for Caregiving.

9. Johnson, R. W., & Wiener, J. M. (2006). *A Profile of Older Americans and Their Caregivers* (Occasional Paper Number 8). Washington, DC: The Urban Institute.

10. Banthin, J., Cunningham, P., & Bernard, D. (2008). Financial burden of health care, 2001–2004. *Health Affairs* 27(1): 188–195.

11. MetLife Mature Market Institute. (2006). *The MetLife Market Survey of Nursing Home & Home Care Costs, September 2006.*

12. Gibson, M., & Houser, A. (2007). *Valuing the Invaluable: A New Look at the Economic Value of Family Caregiving.* Washington, DC: AARP Public Policy Institute.

Chapter Three

Health Promotion and Disease Prevention

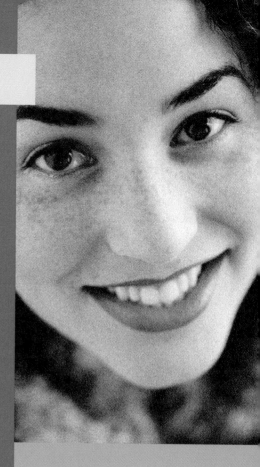

Chapter Objectives

On completion of this chapter, the student should be able to discuss:

1. Concepts of health promotion and disease prevention.

2. Definitions of epidemiology, incidence, prevalence, morbidity, and mortality.

3. Primary, secondary, and tertiary levels of prevention.

4. Diversity of women based on factors such as race, ethnicity, age, and sexual orientation.

5. Diversity as a barrier to health-care access.

6. Global health issues and the variations in the burden of disease in less economically developed versus more economically developed countries.

7. Differences in life expectancy according to gender and race.

8. Health-care concerns and preventive measures for adolescents.

9. Health-care concerns and preventive measures for young adults.

10. Health-care concerns and preventive measures for women in midlife.

11. Health-care concerns and preventive measures for senior women.

12. Taking responsibility for one's own health.

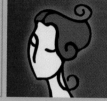

womenshealth.jbpub.com

Women's Health Online is a great source for supplementary women's health information for both students and instructors. Visit

http://womenshealth.jbpub.com

to find a variety of useful tools for learning, thinking, and teaching.

Introduction

Just as major biological and social differences exist between men and women, differences also exist between numerous overlapping subgroups of women. These subgroups can be described in many ways: racial, ethnic, social, economic, physical, and psychological. When examining women's issues and health-related needs, one should consider these factors:

- The cyclic variability of women of reproductive age

- The changes in women throughout their life span as adolescents, pregnant women, premenopausal women, postmenopausal women, and older women

- The different needs of women of varying racial, ethnic, cultural, socioeconomic, and demographic backgrounds

Recognizing the diversity of the female population is important for understanding factors influencing causes, diagnoses, progression, and treatment of disease. These differences create a need for tailored approaches to the delivery of health education and health-care services. Some women, including women with disabilities or chronic diseases, women in prison, and lesbians, are systematically mistreated or have their needs ignored. This marginalization often prevents their different perspectives from being considered. Some groups of women, such as elderly women, black women, and Hispanic women, have organized to find a collective voice to influence health-related decision making and to draw attention to health needs important for these women.

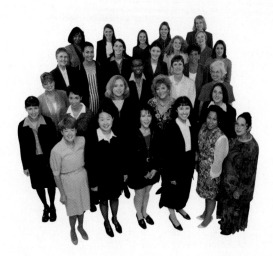

■ Women are not a homogenous population.

Political Dimensions

There are many players in the health system, including government agencies, international agencies, national health education associations, hospitals, and volunteer groups. The federal health infrastructure starts with the Secretary of Health. The Assistant Secretary for Health, who is the principal advisor to the Secretary on public health and scientific issues, is supported by the Surgeon General. The Surgeon General's responsibilities include protecting and advancing the nation's health through educating the public, advocating for effective disease prevention and health promotion programs and activities, and providing a highly recognized symbol of national commitment to protecting and improving the public's health. Reports, workshops, conferences, and calls to action from the Surgeon General on issues including the adverse health consequences of smoking, nutrition and health, mental health, violence, overweight and obesity, suicide, and sexual health, have heightened awareness of important public health issues and generated major public health initiatives. One of these initiatives, Healthy People 2010, grew out of the 1979 Surgeon General's report, *Healthy People—The Surgeon General's Report on Health Promotion and Disease Prevention.* Healthy People 2010 is a set of national disease prevention and health promotion objectives for the United States to achieve over the first decade of the new century. Healthy People 2020, which will build these initiatives for the next 10 years, will be released in 2009–2010.

The Department of Health and Human Services (HHS) is the U.S. government's principal health agency and includes more than 300 programs. HHS works with state, local, and tribal governments, and provides funding for some services offered at the local level. Eleven HHS operation divisions—eight agencies in the U.S. Public Health Service and three human service agencies (**Figure 3.1**)—administer the HHS's programs.

The eight agencies of the U.S. Public Health Service have different mandates:

- *National Institutes of Health (NIH).* NIH is the world's premier medical research organization, supporting some 35,000 research projects nationwide in diseases such as cancer, Alzheimer's disease, diabetes, arthritis, cardiovascular disease, and AIDS.

- *Food and Drug Administration (FDA).* FDA assures the safety of foods and cosmetics, and the safety and efficacy of pharmaceuticals, biological products, and medical devices.

■ Healthy People 2010 is a set of national disease prevention and health promotion objectives for the United States to achieve in the first decade of the century. Healthy People 2020, its successor, will be released in 2009-2010.

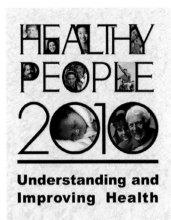

Understanding and Improving Health

■ *Centers for Disease Control and Prevention (CDC).* Working with states and other partners, CDC provides a system of health surveillance to monitor and prevent disease outbreaks, implement disease prevention strategies, and maintain national health statistics.

■ *Agency for Toxic Substances and Disease Registry (ATSDR).* ATSDR helps prevent exposure to hazardous substances from waste sites on the U.S. Environmental Protection Agency's National Priorities List, and it develops toxicological profiles of chemicals found at these sites.

■ *Indian Health Service (IHS).* The IHS provides health services to nearly 1.5 million American Indians and Alaska Natives of 557 federally recognized tribes in 35 states.

■ *Health Resources and Services Administration (HRSA).* HRSA provides access to essential health services for people who are poor, who are uninsured, or who live in rural and urban neighborhoods where health care is scarce. Working with state and community organizations, HRSA also supports programs that ensure healthy mothers and children, increase the number and diversity of health-care professionals in underserved communities, and provide supportive services for people fighting human immunodeficiency virus (HIV) infection and acquired immune deficiency syndrome (AIDS) through the Ryan White Care Act.

■ *Substance Abuse and Mental Health Services Administration (SAMHSA).* SAMHSA works to improve the quality and availability of substance abuse prevention, addiction treatment, and mental health services. This agency provides federal block grants to the states to support and maintain substance abuse and mental health services.

■ *Agency for Healthcare Research and Quality (AHRQ).* AHRQ supports research designed to improve the quality of health care, reduce its cost, improve patient safety, address medical errors, and broaden access to essential services. It provides evidence-based informa-

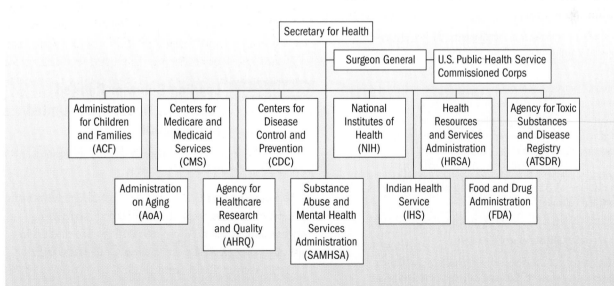

Figure 3.1

The U.S. Department of Health and Human Services (DHHS).

tion on health-care outcomes; quality; and cost, use, and access.

The Assistant Secretary for Health oversees these eight health agency divisions of HHS as well as the Commissioned Corps, a uniformed service of more than 6,000 health professionals who serve at HHS and other federal agencies. The Surgeon General is head of the Commissioned Corps.

The HHS also includes three human service agencies:

■ *Centers for Medicare and Medicaid Services (CMS).* CMS administers the Medicare and Medicaid programs, which provide health care to approximately one in every four Americans. Medicare provides health insurance for more than 42 million elderly and disabled Americans. Medicaid, a joint federal–state program, provides health coverage for nearly 52 million low-income individuals, as well as nursing home coverage for low-income elderly people. The State Children's Health Insurance Program (SCHIP), expanded in 2009, will cover 11 million children.

■ *Administration for Children and Families (ACF).* ACF is responsible for some 60 programs that promote the economic and social well-being of families, children, individuals, and communities. This agency administers

the state–federal welfare program, the national child support enforcement system, and the Head Start program.

■ *Administration on Aging (AoA).* AoA supports a nationwide aging network, providing services to the elderly, such as home meal delivery and transportation services, that enable them to remain independent.

Economic Dimensions

People's behavioral choices cause half of the deaths in the United States.[1] Public health policies, health-promotion efforts, and prevention campaigns can help people make healthier decisions and reduce the burden of illness, enhance quality of life, and increase the lifespan. Additionally, public health efforts that focus on changing behavior are usually much less expensive than later medical intervention.

Unfortunately, these types of programs are critically underfunded. In 2005, total medical expenditures came out to more than $7,000 per person, yet only $60 per person was spent on public health efforts.[1] **Table 3.1** lists the major behavior-related causes of death in the United States.

One major health problem in the United States is the growing number of people who are overweight or obese. One recent estimate of the direct medical costs of treating obesity and overweight in the United States, after adjusting for inflation for 2009 dollars, was $123 billion per year (**Figure 3.2**).[2] The indirect costs are also great: obesity may cost U.S. employers $45 billion a year in lost productivity

---

It's Your Health

Cost Benefits of Prevention Programs

Some examples from the National Center for Chronic Disease Prevention and Health Promotion show the cost benefits of prevention programs:

■ One quality-adjusted year of life is saved for the cost of a smoking cessation program ($1,109 to $4,542).

■ For each $1 spent on a school HIV, other sexually transmitted infection (STI), and pregnancy prevention program, roughly $2.65 is saved on medical and social costs.

■ For every $1 spent on preconception care programs for women with diabetes, $1.86 can be saved by preventing birth defects among their offspring.

■ A mammogram every two years for women ages 50-69 years costs only about $9,000 per year of life saved.

■ For the cost of 100 Papanicolaou (Pap) tests for low-income elderly women, about $5,907 and 3.7 years of life are saved.

Source: United States Department of Health and Human Services, Centers for Disease Control and Prevention, National Center for Chronic Disease Prevention and Health Promotion. Available at http://www.cdc.gov/nccdphp/index.htm.

Table 3.1   **Leading Behavior-Related Causes of Death in the United States, 2000**

Cause	Number of Deaths	Percentage of Total Deaths
Tobacco	435,000	18.1
Poor diet and inactivity	365,000	15.2
Alcohol consumption	85,000	3.5
Motor vehicle accidents	43,000	1.8
Firearm (gun) accidents	29,000	1.2
Sexual behavior	20,000	0.8
Illegal drug use	17,000	0.7

Source: Steen, J. (2007). *The primacy of public health.*

and health expenditures.[3] By changing individual behaviors, such as modifying diet and increasing exercise, individuals can improve their own health and greatly reduce health-care costs down the road. But education efforts and policies that promote healthy behaviors are also important to help people make better decisions. Improving education about the importance of regular exercise and a healthy diet, or helping to fund local farmer's markets so that people can purchase fresh fruits and vegetables, for example, are two ways to encourage healthful decision making.

Total costs associated with diseases are often significantly less for people who take part in preventive care measures, because disease is often detected at earlier stages. For example, according to the American Cancer Society, the five-year survival rate for cervical cancer detected at the earliest invasive stage is 92%. The costs and associated morbidity of treating women with early cellular changes, or minor cervical cancers, is significantly lower than that associated with treating women for invasive disease. Total costs should be considered in terms of both true financial costs and human costs counted in pain, suffering, and anxiety.

Some health insurers have grown to understand the economic value of health promotion and preventive care, and they recognize their importance by increasingly covering these services. These insurers now offer some benefit for joining a health club, or provide some payment or reimbursement for alternative therapy services such as massage or chiropractic adjustments.

Important Terms

Epidemiology is the study of patterns of disease in the population. Although many people think of health and disease as issues relating to individuals, epidemiologists examine the health of communities, specific populations, and entire countries. It is concerned with the frequency and types of diseases in groups of people and the factors that influence the distribution of disease. The following list defines some of the terms used to describe the epidemiology of a given disease within a population:

- **Incidence:** new cases of a condition that occur during a specified period of time.
- **Prevalence:** the total number of people affected by a given condition at a point in time or during a period of time.
- **Mortality rate:** the incidence of death in a given population during a particular time period. It is calculated by dividing the number of deaths in a population by the total population.
- **Morbidity rate:** the incidence of illness in a given population during a particular time period. Morbidity rate is calculated in a similar manner to mortality rate.

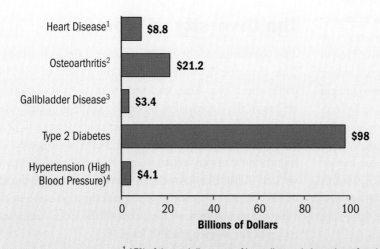

1 17% of the total direct cost of heart disease, independent of stroke.
2 Direct cost: $5.3 billion; indirect cost: $15.9 billion.
3 Direct cost: $3.2 billion; indirect cost: $187 million.
4 Direct cost: $4.1 billion—17% of the total cost of hypertension.

Figure 3.2

Cost burden of obesity-related conditions to society and the health industry.

Source: The Endocrine Society and The Hormone Foundation. (2004). *The Endocrine Society Weighs In: A Handbook of Obesity in America* 43. Available at http://www.obesityinamerica.org. Reprinted with permission.

It's Your Health

Important Epidemiological Terms

Measures of Morbidity (illness)

$$\text{Incidence} = \frac{\text{number of new cases of a disease during a given period of time}}{\text{total population at risk}}$$

$$\text{Prevalence} = \frac{\text{number of existing cases of a disease at a given point in time}}{\text{total population at risk}}$$

Measures of Mortality (death)

$$\text{Mortality rate} = \frac{\text{number of deaths in a population in a given period of time}}{\text{total population}}$$

Analyzing incidence and prevalence rates allows epidemiologists to examine trends in how diseases or conditions progress. A condition with a high prevalence and a low incidence (a common condition with few new cases), for example, might eventually stabilize or drop within a population, whereas a condition with a low prevalence but a high incidence (a rare condition with many new cases) may indicate a major public health concern for the future. Morbidity and mortality rates can be calculated across the entire population or within a specific subpopulation, such as age, gender, or race, to show relevant variations across those groups.

Health education and health promotion are two important public health concepts. Health education can be defined as efforts to improve people's knowledge and awareness about health. Health education can focus on teaching individuals, communities, or entire populations. Health education can cover any health-related topic, including prenatal care, improving physical fitness, or recognizing signs of stroke. Health promotion focuses on actually getting people to change their behavior. Health promotion includes health education as well as policies designed to improve the public health. (New York City's recent ban of trans fats in foods in restaurants is one such policy.) Health promotion deals primarily with lifestyle and chronic disease factors, such as smoking, drinking, use of primary care facilities, and sexual activity.

Many diseases and conditions are a result of lifestyle factors, such as poor nutrition or smoking, and are therefore preventable. Health promotion efforts attempt to allow individuals and populations to make informed decisions regarding lifestyle behaviors and disease prevention

practices. Prevention is practiced at three different levels—primary, secondary, and tertiary.

- **Primary prevention** is prevention of disease or injury by reducing exposure to a risk factor that may lead to the disease or injury. Primary preventive measures include healthy nutrition, regular physical activity, cessation of smoking, and safe sexual practices.

- **Secondary prevention** refers to early detection and prompt treatment of disease. Screening tools such as mammography and cervical cancer screening are considered examples of secondary prevention because they may detect disease before it spreads, thereby preventing further complications or disease progression. The use of medications and lifestyle behaviors to control chronic diseases that cannot be prevented, such as diabetes or asthma, are also examples of secondary prevention.

- **Tertiary prevention**, which takes place once a disease has advanced, involves alleviating pain, providing comfort, halting progression of an illness, and limiting disability that may result from disease. It consists of rehabilitation in situations where a person can work on restoring certain functions, such as those lost after suffering a stroke.

Primary prevention is largely the responsibility of the health-care consumer. Secondary prevention requires both the guidance of the health-care provider and the compliance of the consumer. Tertiary prevention remains a goal of both health-care providers and caregivers.

The Diversity of Women

The population of the United States continues to change. This changing diversity is seen in the growth of the Hispanic and Asian American sectors of the population, as well as in the increased numbers of people of mixed racial backgrounds. By 2030, 1 in 5 American women will be of Hispanic heritage, and 1 in 14 will be Asian (**Figure 3.3**). Significant diversity exists among women based on age as well. By 2030, 1 in 4 American women will be over the age of 65.[4] Because a majority of the elderly population in the United States is female, the needs of the elderly represent a significant women's health issue.

Women's increased educational attainment adds to the diversity of the population. Educated women tend to be more educated health-care consumers. Differing education levels create heterogeneity among women, as women with little or no education and women with advanced education

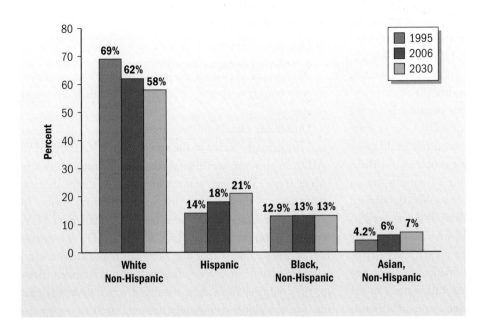

Figure 3.3

Projected U.S. population by race and Hispanic origin, 1995–2030.

Source: U.S. Census Bureau. (2004). U.S. interim projections by age, sex, race, and Hispanic origin. Available at http://www.census.gov/ipc/www/usinterimproj/.

may have differing health and health education needs. The increased number of women in the workforce also presents new opportunities in women's health, providing another venue for disseminating health education information to women. Women work in a variety of settings, creating differences in their health-care needs. For example, women working at home, in factories, in offices, in agriculture, and in retail will encounter different work-related health issues.

Another area of diversity relates to the ways and stages of life in which women become mothers. Many women are delaying marriage and family to focus on careers, and thus are having children at a later age. This trend creates new issues surrounding childbirth, fertility, and parenting that target women in their thirties, forties, and fifties as opposed to solely focusing on women in their twenties. Other women are having children at younger ages, becoming teenage mothers. Many of these women are either working to raise children alone or having their parents take a leadership role in childrearing responsibilities by raising their grandchildren. Some women choose not to have children, instead pursuing careers and other opportunities.

Diversity also is reflected in women of different sexual orientation. Health concerns specific to lesbian women are often overlooked, leaving many women without proper guidance and medical attention. Lesbians share many health concerns and risks with heterosexual women, but misconceptions about the health needs of lesbians by health-care providers and lesbians themselves often create barriers to receiving adequate care. Both lesbians and health-care providers often believe that women who have sex with women do not need cervical cancer screening, routine gynecological care, or information about sexually transmitted infections (STIs), including HIV/AIDS. Other barriers to health care may include homophobia among providers and lack of health insurance coverage, because many lesbians are unable to share their partner's benefits or are eligible for less complete benefit coverage than a heterosexual spouse would be.[5]

Incarcerated women face special health-related challenges. Many have unmet medical needs that relate to drug addictions, mental health, and reproductive health.[5] Women in prison complain of "lack of regular gynecological and

■ By 2030, one in five American women will be of Hispanic heritage.

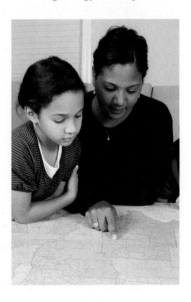

breast exams and argue that their medical concerns are often dismissed or overlooked."[5] Many women in prison are survivors of physical and sexual abuse, putting them at increased risk for high-risk pregnancies, HIV/AIDS, hepatitis C, and cervical cancer. Pregnant incarcerated women also face special challenges to their health.[6]

Women with disabilities have, until recently, been the focus of less research and clinical attention than is warranted. Physical barriers, such as inaccessible facilities or examination equipment, present major problems for these women in obtaining adequate health care. Communication barriers may pose a problem if a patient has visual, hearing, or verbal disabilities. Women with disabilities, as well as uninformed health-care professionals, may have the misconception that they are less likely to acquire diseases or infections. Many times, health-care providers focus on the woman's disability and associated issues, rather than on basic routine health-care needs.[6] Whether a woman's disability is a mobility, vision, hearing, speech, or cognitive challenge, greater levels of research, support, and compassion are needed to adequately address her health concerns.

Differences in race, ethnicity, socioeconomic status, geographic location, sexual orientation, country of origin, and employment status contribute to the diversity of women's needs. As the medical community has begun to embrace the diversity of women, significant emphasis has been placed on health promotion and disease prevention efforts targeted toward specific populations of women.

Global Health Issues for Women

In developing countries, the health needs of women are extensive and often differ from the needs of U.S. women. According to *The World Health Report 2004*, a report from the World Health Organization (WHO), 10 factors globally account for more than 40% of the disease burden worldwide[7] (**Table 3.2**). Major behavioral and environmental risk factors that contribute to death and disease worldwide include the following:

- Underweight
- Unsafe sex
- High blood pressure
- Tobacco consumption
- Alcohol consumption
- Unsafe water, sanitation, and hygiene
- Iron deficiency

- Indoor smoke from solid fuels
- High cholesterol
- Obesity

All ages are at risk for **underweight**, but this condition is most common among children younger than five years of age.

Unsafe sex closely follows underweight as a risk factor and is the major factor in the spread of HIV/AIDS. HIV/AIDS is now the world's fourth leading cause of death. More than 15 million women are living with the disease; two-thirds of these women live in sub-Saharan Africa. In 2007, 2.7 million people were newly infected with HIV, and 2 million people died from AIDS.[8] AIDS is a devastating disease that is affecting both adults and children and wreaking havoc on already fragile health systems in many of the countries most dramatically affected. Over the past decade, the global community has organized an unprecedented campaign to fight the spread of HIV and to treat people who are affected. This effort has made enormous progress, but much works needs to be done.

Antiretroviral therapy (ART), though not a cure, can greatly increase the quality of life and life expectancy for people living with HIV. Yet, for years, these treatments were prohibitively expensive for the vast majority of people living in the developing world. Recent efforts have mobilized billions of dollars to provide treatment and to prevent transmission of HIV; however, deciding how to most effectively spend these funds remains an important concern. Private companies are working with both **nongovernment organizations (NGOs)** and governments to address the issue. The World Bank defines NGOs as "private organizations that pursue activities to relieve suffering, promote the interests of the poor, protect the environment, provide basic social services, or undertake community development." In wider usage, the label NGO can be applied to any nonprofit organization that is independent from government, including a large charity, community-based self-help group, research institute, church, professional association, or lobbying group.

Risk factors caused by exposure to tobacco and influenced by unhealthy eating, such as high blood pressure, high cholesterol, and obesity, affect people throughout the world. The conditions they produce were once considered diseases of excess, but now they affect people in low-resource settings as well as their counterparts in wealthy communities. Diseases caused or influenced by the local environment, such as cholera and tuberculosis, are often caused by people not having access to clean water or regu-

Table 3.2 Leading Causes of Disease Burden for Males and Females Age 15 Years or Older

Males	% DALYs	Females	% DALYs
1 HIV/AIDS	7.4	1 Unipolar depressive disorders	8.4
2 Ischemic heart disease	6.8	2 HIV/AIDS	7.2
3 Cerebrovascular disease	5.0	3 Ischemic heart disease	5.3
4 Unipolar depressive disorders	4.8	4 Cerebrovascular disease	5.2
5 Road traffic injuries	4.3	5 Cataracts	3.1
6 Tuberculosis	4.2	6 Hearing loss, adult onset	2.8
7 Alcohol use disorders	3.4	7 Chronic obstructive pulmonary disease	2.7
8 Violence	3.3	8 Tuberculosis	2.6
9 Chronic obstructive pulmonary disease	3.1	9 Osteoarthritis	2.0
10 Hearing loss, adult onset	2.7	10 Diabetes mellitus	1.9

Note: DALYs are disability-adjusted life years, a measure used to calculate the total amount of healthy life lost to a given cause.

Source: *The World Health Report 2004.*

lar trash removal, and lack of regulations providing bacteria-free meat and food sources. People in developed countries often take for granted the infrastructures that make these systems available and reliable in their countries. In contrast, many developing countries have no system in place for sanitation and often use the same polluted water sources for bathing, drinking, and washing clothes. Parasitic infections from contaminated water and food sources are major causes of morbidity and mortality in countries throughout the world. Increasing access to preventive care, vaccinations, safe drinking water, and proper sanitation has been a primary focus of global health initiatives. Additionally, the developing world faces a chronic shortage of trained health-care providers, particularly physicians. The World Health Organization and various NGOs have played leadership roles in trying to effect change in countries that do not have adequate resources.

In almost every country in the world, women are the primary caregivers for children and elderly family members. Although family composition varies from culture to culture, women consistently shoulder the burden of reproduction and feeding, clothing, and caring for children and elderly across the world. The health risks associated with motherhood in developing countries are astronomically higher than those experienced by women in more developed countries. Iron deficiency, one of the most prevalent nutrient deficiencies in the world, most severely affects young children and their mothers because of the high iron demands of infant growth and pregnancy. Sources of iron, such as meat, fish, and beans, are not always regularly available to families living in developing countries. Indoor smoke from solid fu-

els also directly affects women in developing countries because they are inside cooking for their families and working in the home far more often than men. In developing countries, about 700 million people—mainly women and children in poor rural areas—inhale harmful smoke from burning wood and other fuels. They are increasingly at risk from acute respiratory infections, especially pneumonia.[10] According to the World Health Organization:

> In some communities, inequality of girl children and women is the transcending risk factor that explains the prevalence not only of maternal mortality and morbidity, but also of higher vulnerability of girls to childhood mortality. Risk factors like malnutrition of girl children resulting in anemia, and early marriage resulting in premature pregnancy, can be traced to the fact that women do not enjoy the status and significance in their communities that men enjoy. . . . Barriers to improving women's health are often rooted in social, economic, cultural, legal and related conditions that transcend health considerations. Social factors, such as lack of literacy and of educational or employment opportunities, deny young women alternatives to early marriage and early childbearing, and economic and other means of access to contraception. Women's vulnerability to sexual and other abuses, in and out of marriage, increases risks of unsafe pregnancy and motherhood.[9]

By creating guidelines for prevention and developing health promotion programs, practitioners, policy makers, and health-care activists are encouraging women both in the United States and abroad to become empowered and knowledgeable health-care consumers.

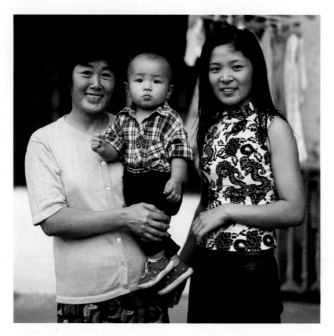

■ Health risks and concerns change as a woman develops from a child to an adolescent, from a young adult to an older adult.

Table 3.3	Primary Preventive Measures Throughout the Life Span

Avoid tobacco and other drugs.

Reduce alcohol intake.

Consume a healthy diet.

Participate in regular physical activity.

Learn appropriate and effective weight-management techniques.

Practice safe behaviors, such as using seat belts, wearing motorcycle and bicycle helmets, not driving under the influence of alcohol, and not riding with someone under the influence of alcohol.

Learn nonviolent measures to achieve conflict resolution.

If engaging in sexual activity, use condoms to reduce the risk of STIs, HIV/AIDS, and pregnancy.

Maintain an overall sense of well-being through stress reduction techniques, relaxation methods, socializing with friends and family, and seeking counseling if needed.

Strive to balance work, school, family, friends, and time for oneself.

Stages of Life

Health risks and concerns change as a woman ages, but some factors remain constant at any age. Good nutrition, regular physical activity, and adequate sleep are essential for health at all stages of life. Healthy living also encompasses avoidance of harmful substances, such as tobacco, drugs, and excessive alcohol. Mental health is equally as important as physical health. Maximizing mental health requires recognizing signs and symptoms of mental health threats, such as depression, drug or alcohol abuse, and physical or mental abuse. In addition, healthy sexuality and responsible sexual behavior are important for a woman's overall health. Healthy sexuality is expressed throughout life by exploring one's sexuality in adolescence, establishing long-term intimate relations in adulthood, and maintaining sexual pleasure in the senior years.

Health risks and concerns change as a woman develops from a child to an adolescent, and then from a young adult to an older adult. Aspects of health promotion must be accompanied by methods of disease prevention. The risk of disease often varies throughout life, and, therefore, the methods of prevention differ depending on one's age as well as multiple other factors. **Table 3.3** highlights the major primary preventive measures that should be taken throughout one's life span. Nevertheless, the need for one practice remains constant for all women: Women should

learn, understand, and listen to their bodies and empower themselves by becoming informed health-care consumers.

Adolescence

The transition from childhood to adolescence is a time of major change. Adolescence begins with the onset of puberty and continues until the approximate age of 17, when adult physical development is generally realized. During adolescence, a girl becomes a woman and begins to form her identity and sense of independence. As girls set off on this journey, they face a host of issues that threaten their physical and mental well-being. It is important for parents to provide guidance and support during this time and to help their children make appropriate decisions. Adolescents should be encouraged to learn on their own and begin to understand how to take responsibility for oneself and one's actions.

Puberty encompasses changes in nearly every aspect of development, from physical to intellectual maturation. During this period in life, girls begin to differ in appearance from boys. Secondary sexual characteristics appear, such as widening hips, breast development, height and weight gain, and bodily hair growth. Perspiration and body odor increase, and vaginal discharge creates a new awareness of sexuality for girls. Menstruation, the onset of a woman's reproductive capability, also begins. As these changes occur, adolescents begin to separate from their

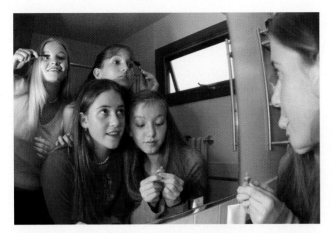

■ Adolescence is a time when friends become an important influence in a girl's life.

parents and assume greater independence. Teens may display rebelliousness, with friends often influencing decision making. Peer pressure may also affect self-esteem and self-perception. Adolescent girls often focus on and define themselves through their relationships with both friends and romantic interests. Their concerns often revolve around popularity, attractiveness, and body weight. They face many challenges as they adjust to their sexual maturation and their increased independence.[10]

Specific Health Concerns for Adolescents

In the United States, the top four causes of death for females ages 15 to 19 are accidents (unintentional injuries), cancer, assault, and suicide (see **Table 3.4**). Mortality rates for boys in the same age group are more than twice as high as for girls.[11] Behaviors such as not using seat belts, not wearing motorcycle helmets and bicycle helmets, riding with a driver who has been drinking alcohol, and driving after drinking alcohol are responsible for many of the injuries that result in death. Homicide is the third leading cause of death for adolescents ages 15 to 19 years and the sixth leading cause of death for adolescents ages 10 to 14 years.[11] Current statistics show that guns kill 10 to 12 children (ages 0–19) in the United States every day on average. Two or three of these children take their own lives, and the other deaths are homicides or unintentional injuries. In contrast, in the developing world, major health issues for young people typically involve infections, diarrheal diseases, and other communicable diseases like tuberculosis.

Although many adolescents display moody behavior and signs of rebelliousness (normal behaviors during the teenage years), this should not be confused with depression, a significant concern during adolescence. As girls reach adolescence, there is a noted increase in the rate of depression and the rate of suicide attempts. At any given time, between 10% and 15% of children and adolescents have some symptoms of depression. After age 15, depression is two times as common in girls and women as in boys and men.[12] Suicide is the second leading cause of death for adolescents ages 15–19 years and the third leading cause of death for younger adolescents.[11] According to the 2007 Youth Risk Behavior Survey (YRBS), 15% of students had seriously considered attempting suicide and 7% of students had attempted suicide. Of the students surveyed, girls were more likely than boys to have considered attempting suicide (15% versus 10%) and more likely to actually attempt suicide (9% versus 5%).[13]

Trying new behaviors is a key aspect of the period of adolescence and is essential for healthy development; however, risky behaviors may lead to negative health consequences. Sexual experimentation is one example of a behavior that has potentially life-altering consequences. Almost half of high school students (48%) have had sex at least once, and more than one-third (35%) are currently sexually active. Sexual relations often occur before adolescents have experience and skills in self-protection and in setting and expressing the kinds of behaviors they feel comfortable with, before they have acquired adequate information about sexually transmitted infections (STIs), and before they have access to health services and supplies

Table 3.4   Leading Causes of Death for U.S. Females, 2004

Ages 10–14

Cause	Percentage of Total Deaths
1. Accidents	35.2
2. Malignant neoplasms (cancer)	14.1
3. Suicide	6.2
4. Congenital and chromosomal abnormalities	5.3
5. Heart disease	4.6
6. Assault	4.3
7. Chronic respiratory disease	1.8
8. Cerebrovascular disease (stroke)	1.3
8. Influenza and pneumonia	1.3
10. Benign and in situ neoplasms	1.1

Ages 15–19

Cause	Percentage of Total Deaths
1. Accidents	51.7
2. Suicide	8.8
3. Assault	7.5
4. Malignant neoplasms (cancer)	7.3
5. Heart disease	3.1
6. Congenital and chromosomal abnormalities	2.8
7. Pregnancy and childbirth	0.9
8. Chronic respiratory diseases	0.7
8. Cerebrovascular disease (stroke)	0.7
10. Influenza and pneumonia	0.6

Ages 20–24

Cause	Percentage of Total Deaths
1. Accidents	40.5
2. Assault	8.4
3. Malignant neoplasms (cancer)	8.0
4. Suicide	7.6
5. Heart disease	4.6
6. Pregnancy and childbirth	2.7
7. Congenital and chromosomal abnormalities	1.9
8. HIV/AIDS	1.4
9. Cerebrovascular disease (stroke)	1.4
10. Diabetes	1.2

Source: Heron, M. (2007). *Deaths: Leading causes for 2004*. Hyattsville, MD: National Center for Health Statistics.

(such as condoms). This problem is often amplified in developing countries, where girls typically have even less access to health care and information. Each year, approximately 1 million teenagers become pregnant, though teen pregnancy rates dropped for much of the 1990s and into the 2000s.[14] According to the National Center for Health Statistics, increased condom use, the adoption of the effective injectable and implantable contraceptives, and the leveling off of teen sexual activity are some of the factors believed to be driving this downturn in teen pregnancies.

Despite these positive trends, only 38.5% of students who were currently sexually active reported that they had used a condom during their last act of sexual intercourse,[13] putting themselves at risk for various STIs, including HIV infection. Approximately 3 million cases of STIs occur an-

nually among teenagers.[15] HIV infection is the eighth leading cause of death among persons ages 20 to 24 years in the United States, but its incidence varies greatly among races. Chlamydia infection during adolescence is more likely to result in pelvic inflammatory disease and, potentially, lead to infertility.

Globally, more than half of all new HIV infections affect members of the 15–24 age group. According to UNAIDS, "7,000 girls and women become infected with HIV every day. In South Africa, Zambia, and Zimbabwe, young women (ages 15–24) are 5 to 6 times more likely to be infected than young men of the same age."[16] In one study in Zambia, more than 12% of the 15- and 16-year-olds seen at antenatal clinics were already infected with HIV. Girls appear to be especially vulnerable to infection.

It's Your Health

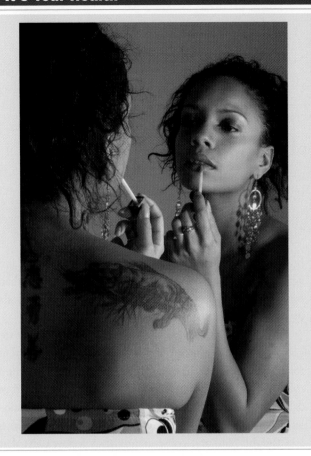

Tattoos

The following advice has been prepared by professional tattooists working with local, state, and national health authorities.

1. Always insist that *you see* your tattooist remove a new needle and tube set-up from a sealed envelope immediately prior to your tattoo.

2. Be certain that *you see* your tattooist pour a new ink supply into a new disposable container.

3. Make sure your artist puts on a new pair of disposable gloves before setting up tubes, needles, and ink supplies.

4. Satisfy yourself that the shop furnishings and tattooist are clean and orderly in appearance—much like a *medical facility*.

5. Feel free to question the tattooist about any of his or her sterile procedures and isolation techniques. Take time to observe the tattooist at work and do not hesitate to inquire about his or her *experience and qualifications* in the tattoo field.

6. If the tattooist is a qualified professional, he or she will have no problem complying with standards above and beyond these simple guidelines.

7. If the artist or studio does not appear up to these standards or if the person becomes evasive when questioned, seek out a different professional tattooist.

Source: Alliance of Professional Tattooists, www.safe-tattoos.com. Reprinted with permission.

Adolescents may also engage in substance use, another risky behavior.[20] Alcohol and drug use are detrimental activities on their own (see Chapter 13), but they also lead to other situations that may compromise one's health. According to the latest YRBS, 45% of high school students had drunk alcohol within the past month, and 26% had drunk five or more drinks in a row in the past month. Almost a quarter (23%) of sexually active students had had at least one drink the last time they had intercourse. One in ten (11%) students had driven a car or other vehicle while drinking, while 3 in 10 (29%) had been in a car while the driver had been drinking.[13] Alcohol and drug use can also both increase the likelihood that a person will choose casual sex and reduce the chance that a person will use prophylactics. Another harmful behavior that can cause illness later in life is smoking. Most adults who smoke regularly began the habit as adolescents and consequently are at greatest risk of diseases attributed to smoking. The 2007 YRBS found that 50% of students in grades 9–12 reported having tried cigarettes and 20% were engaging in current cigarette use.[13]

Recently there has been a dramatic increase in overweight and obesity among adolescents (**Figure 3.4**). Obese children are at risk for type 2 diabetes, low self-esteem, and many other adverse health outcomes. In 2007, 13% of high school students were obese, and 16% were overweight. Nearly half (45%) of high school students were attempting to lose weight. Although male students are more likely than female students to be overweight, female students are twice as likely to attempt to lose weight. Female students are also more likely than male students to try to lose weight using dangerous, unhealthy methods (going more than a day without food, vomiting or taking laxatives, or taking diet pills, powders, or liquids).[13]

Tattoos and piercings have also become popular with adolescents. These activities hold inherent risks of infection and have been associated with serious complications. Increasingly, people are choosing to have body parts such

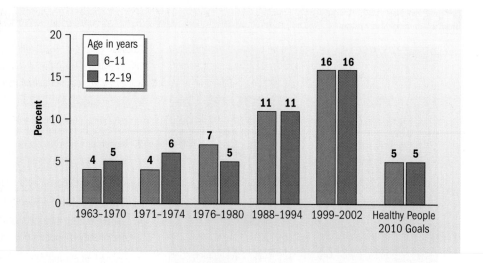

Figure 3.4

Prevalence of overweight among children and adolescents ages 6–19 years.

Source: CDC/NCHS, NHES, and NHANES.

as the lips, eyebrows, septums, or genitalia pierced, in addition to the more standard ear piercing. These piercings increase risks of infections, scarring, and nerve damage. Individuals can minimize the risks associated with these behaviors by choosing experienced professionals who uphold high safety and cleanliness standards. For more information, individuals can contact organizations like the Association of Professional Piercers and the Alliance of Professional Tattooists, which have created tattoo, piercing, and jewelry guidelines. In many cases, primary care physicians have ear-piercing kits and can perform the service in the safety of a clinical setting. To further ensure safety, anyone getting either a piercing or a tattoo should be fully sober.

Preventive Behaviors

Behavioral decisions are by far the greatest influence on adolescent health. Harmful behaviors include smoking, alcohol and drug use, unhealthy dietary behaviors, inadequate physical activity, and risky sexual behaviors. Many of them contribute to today's major killers, such as heart disease, cancer, and injuries.

Two especially important aspects of health promotion for adolescents are regular physical activity and good nutrition. There are numerous benefits of regular physical activity, as discussed in Chapter 9. Just over one-third (35%) of U.S. high school students met the recommended levels of physical activity (were active for a total of 60 minutes or more for at least five days in the past week). An equal percentage of high school students watched three or more hours of television a day. Nationwide, 25% of high school students did not exercise for one hour or more in any given day in the past week.[13] Female students were significantly less likely than male students to be physically active. In 2007, just 21% of

high school students had eaten five servings of fruits and vegetables per day during the previous week. More than one-third (34%) of students had had at least one can of soda or pop per day during the same period.[13]

Although all of the essential nutrients are important for good health, the mineral calcium is especially important for adolescent girls. Girls need to consume enough calcium to develop good bone health and protect themselves from osteoporosis in their later years. Unfortunately, many adolescent girls become concerned about their widening hips and weight gain, and consequently they follow diets that lack sufficient nutrients. The average calcium intake of adolescent girls is about 800 mg per day, considerably less than the Recommended Dietary Allowance for adolescents of 1,200 mg per day.[17] Even more devastating are the numbers of teenage girls who develop eating disorders as a result of poor body image, unhealthy eating habits, and dangerous purging behaviors (discussed further in Chapters 9 and 12).

Heavy sun exposure during early life has been strongly correlated with an increased lifetime incidence of both **melanoma** and **nonmelanoma** skin cancers. Tanned skin remains fashionable, however, and most teenagers continue to regularly visit beaches or tanning salons. A major study of more than 10,000 young people found that sunscreen use was low (about 35%), but was likely to be higher among girls than boys. At least one sunburn during the previous summer was reported in 83% of survey respondents, and 36% of respondents reported three or more sunburns. About one-tenth of teenagers indicated use of tanning beds. This use was mostly among girls and increased in prevalence as the girls approached age 18.[18]

Generally, adolescence is a period of good health; however, millions of teens suffer from the special health con-

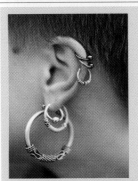

Safe Piercing

Here are 10 things to look for that will help you choose a safe piercer or piercing studio.

1. **Cleanliness:** A good studio should have a separate counter, waiting room, piercing room, bathroom, and an enclosed sterilizing room. All of these, as well as studio staff, should be neat and clean.

2. **An autoclave and spore tests:** Studios should have an autoclave (a steam sterilizer) and a spore test to check whether the autoclave is working correctly. Chemical soaks or "dry heat" systems do not provide adequate sterilization.

3. **Single-use needles:** Needles should be opened while you are present, as well as individually packaged, sterile, and single use. Needles should go into an approved sharps container.

4. **Good piercing room practices:** Ideally, watch the piercer prepare for the piercing. Beforehand, the piercer should wash his or her hands and then wear latex gloves, changing gloves if he or she touches anything nonsterile.

5. **No ear-piercing guns:** In many cases, ear-piercing guns can't be adequately sterilized.

6. **Knowledgeable staff:** Ask the staff questions. Do they seem knowledgeable and friendly? How long has the piercer been doing his or her job? Does he or she seem well informed?

7. **An after-care sheet:** Studios should have a sheet that explains how to best take care of your new piercing. Make sure this sheet is up to industry standards.

8. **Listen to your instincts (and friends):** Have your friends had experience with a given studio or piercer? What did they think, and how does their piercing look? Do you feel comfortable with the studio/piercer? If not, go somewhere else.

9. **A license:** States and cities have different requirements for a studio or piercer, usually requiring regular inspections. Call your local health department to find the standards in your area.

10. **APP recognition:** Studios or piercers that have joined the Association of Professional Piercers have agreed to standards of cleanliness and jewelry quality set forth by the organization. APP members should have a membership certificate displayed on premises; make sure this certificate is up to date.

cerns for adolescents mentioned above. The cognitive development occurring during adolescence assists many teenagers in considering the future and understanding the consequences of their present behaviors on their future health. Therefore, it is an excellent time for health-care providers to guide parents in encouraging health promotion in their children and to offer adolescents a sense of self-empowerment by encouraging them to make healthy and sensible choices (**Table 3.5**).

Young Adulthood

As adolescents become adults, they generally become independent of their parents and gain rights that were not afforded to them as children. Yet, the age of adulthood is often confusing considering that one can vote and can enlist in the military service at the age of 18, yet cannot legally drink alcohol until age 21. Postsecondary school and the high financial burdens associated with advanced education keep many people dependent on their parents well into their twenties. Nevertheless, as a woman ages, her increased independence and inevitable increase in age bring new health challenges and risks.

For some women, the first stage of young adulthood occurs in college. College can be an extension of adolescence in the sense that many women continue to experiment with new behaviors and explore their sense of self. Other women begin to turn their focus toward choosing a career path. Some find that the freedom of being away from home allows them to engage in behaviors that were not

Table 3.5 **Secondary Preventive Measures for Adolescents**

Pap test three years after onset of sexual activity or by age 21.

Annual STI screening for sexually active adolescents.

HIV screening for high-risk adolescents with their consent.

Annual preventive services visit to screen for depression, risk of suicide, abuse (emotional, physical, and sexual), eating disorders, learning or school problems, and drug use.

Physical exam recommended at least once between ages 11 and 14, once between 15 and 17, and once between 18 and 21.

Annual screening for high blood pressure, cholesterol (if risk factors are present), and tuberculin test (PPD) if risk factors are present.

Annual screening for anemia if any of the following risk factors are present: heavy menstruation, chronic weight loss, nutritional deficit, or excessive athletic activity.

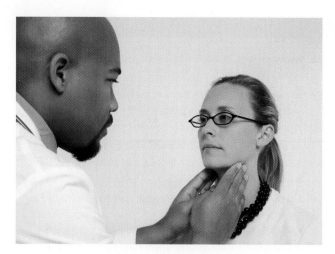

■ Many young women avoid routine health examinations.

permitted in high school. Young women experience many of the same health threats that affected them as adolescents, including drug and alcohol use, smoking, violence (such as date rape), risky sexual behaviors, poor nutrition, and lack of exercise. For those women who graduate from high school and then directly enter the workforce or begin parenting, as well as for women after graduation from college, different health challenges await.

Specific Health Concerns for Young Adults

For women between the ages of 15 and 24, accidents, assault, and suicide are the top three causes of death, followed by heart disease and cancer. As women reach their mid-twenties, however, deaths from heart disease, cancer, and other chronic diseases increase.

Chronic diseases (as opposed to **acute diseases**) are diseases or conditions that are not short-lived. They include heart disease and cancer, as well as diabetes, HIV/AIDS, and **autoimmune diseases**. Although chronic diseases are generally thought of as afflictions of the elderly, they are significant causes of death for all age groups; additionally, healthful behavior choices and prevention strategies begun early in life can often prevent these diseases from developing later in life, or reduce the harm that these diseases cause.

Causes of death for young adult women vary dramatically by race and ethnicity. These variations are especially pronounced during the young adult years. HIV-related diseases are the leading cause of death for black women ages 25–34, but only the seventh-leading cause for Hispanic women, and the tenth-leading cause for white and Asian American women in that same age group (see **Table 3.6**).[11] White women ages 25–34, meanwhile, are more likely to die from suicide or accidents than other women in

this age group. Black women are more likely than any other racial or ethnic group to die during these years, followed respectively by white, Hispanic, and Asian women.[11] Cultural, economic, social, and individual factors all contribute to these differences.

In developing countries, young adult women are at high risk from reproductive health–related disease and infectious disease. The top causes of death for young adult women in developing countries in this age group are six infectious diseases:

- Pneumonia
- Tuberculosis
- Diarrheal diseases
- Malaria
- Measles
- HIV/AIDS

Young adulthood can be rewarding as well as stressful. During this time, many women seek or develop long-term intimate relationships. They may be starting a family and having children. Women may be defining their career path, advancing within their career, or still searching for the right career. Many women face obstacles along the way, such as lack of adequate child care and the juggling of family and work responsibilities. Women with disabilities may encounter new challenges as they enter the workforce, including discrimination from employers and employees, lack of accessibility throughout the workplace, and adjustment to new tasks. Some women find it difficult to cope as their friends transition into different stages of life while they feel as if they are standing still. Managing stress and maintaining emotional well-being are important for achieving a healthy perspective.

■ Women with disabilities may face condescending attitudes or discrimination when visiting health-care providers.

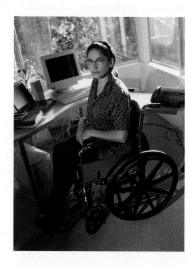

Table 3.6 Leading Causes of Death for U.S. Females, 2004

Ages 25–34		Ages 35–44	
Cause	Percentage of Total Deaths	Cause	Percentage of Total Deaths
1. Accidents	25.3	1. Malignant neoplasms (cancer)	26.2
2. Malignant neoplasms (cancer)	15.1	2. Accidents	15.1
3. Heart disease	8.2	3. Heart disease	12.4
4. Suicide	7.5	4. Suicide	5
5. Assault	5.8	5. HIV/AIDS	4.3
6. HIV/AIDS	4.4	6. Cerebrovascular disease (stroke)	3.5
7. Pregnancy and childbirth	2.3	7. Liver disease and cirrhosis	2.8
7. Cerebrovascular disease (stroke)	2.3	8. Diabetes	2.4
9. Diabetes	2.1	8. Assault	2.4
10. Congenital and chromosomal abnormalities	1.5	10. Chronic respiratory disease	1.4

Source: Heron, M. (2007). *Deaths: Leading causes for 2004.* Hyattsville, MD: National Center for Health Statistics.

Although women and men report similar levels of stress, causes of stress and coping mechanisms often differ between women and men. A study of 1,600 Americans found that women are more apt to attribute stress to family and health issues than are men. Most women surveyed (52%) were personally concerned about the effect of stress on their health and 30% (versus 24% of men) said that they found it "very challenging" to manage the stress and tension they confront. Men were more likely than women to report watching more television (42% versus 36%) and drinking alcohol (29% versus 18%) as a way of dealing with the stress in their lives. Women report either increased eating of "comfort foods" or decreased contact with the stressor as common strategies of coping.[19]

Alcohol and drug abuse affect the lives of many young women, including women who have children. An estimated 6 million children younger than 18 years of age have a parent who has used illicit drugs in the past month. Marijuana is the drug parents are most likely to use. Heavy drinking, defined as consumption of five or more drinks at one time on at least three occasions in the past 30 days, was reported by 5.2 million parents (3% of mothers and 14% of fathers).[20]

Young women deal with of health-related issues associated with dating and sexual relationships, including sexual violence, STIs, and pregnancy. Consider these statistics:

- Almost 18% of the women in the United States have been the victim of rape or attempted rape that occurred at some point during their lives.

- In college, one in four female students is a rape survivor; experts estimate about 60% of the victims in reported rapes know their assailant.

- Of the estimated 333 million new cases of STIs that occur in the world every year, at least 111 million occur in young people under 25 years of age.

- According to Planned Parenthood International, nearly 4 in 10 pregnancies are unplanned.

- The WHO estimates that between 8 and 30 million unplanned pregnancies result from inconsistent or incorrect use of contraceptive methods, or from method-related failure.

Women who desire to have children may face fertility problems or other complications regarding pregnancy or childbearing. Infertility can lead to physical and emotional stress, financial burdens, and the anxiety and discomfort that often accompany fertility tests and treatment (see Chapter 6). Women with disabilities may face attitudinal barriers from health-care poviders as well as friends and family members who feel they should not have children. Lesbians who want to have children may run into opposition while they explore options for sperm donors or adoption agencies.

Preventive Behaviors

Because many chronic diseases can be prevented or controlled by behavioral changes, it is important for a young woman to continue following a healthful diet, participate

■ Physical activity is important for both physical and mental well-being.

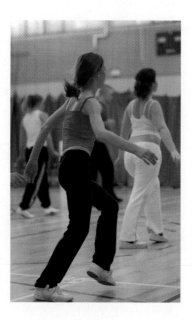

in regular physical activity, avoid smoking and drug abuse, and moderate her intake of alcohol. Secondary preventive measures, such as screenings for cancer, Pap and human papillomavirus (HPV) tests, and blood pressure screenings, are essential during this time as well (see **It's Your Health**).

As in all stages of life, positive mental well-being is essential for a young woman's overall health. Finding ways to cope with stress and addressing any mental health issues will help to establish a more balanced sense of well-being. Physical activity, healthy relationships with an intimate partner as well as close friends, and participation in enjoyable activities are all effective ways of reducing stress.

Young adulthood is often a time when women are meeting and dating new people as they try to establish long-term intimate relationships. As such, they must face the challenge of not putting themselves in risky situations,

It's Your Health

Preventive Services Throughout a Woman's Life

Mammograms. Have a mammogram every one to two years starting at age 40.

Cervical cancer screening. Have a Pap test every one to three years if you have been sexually active or are older than 21. If you are 30 or older, you can have a Pap test and HPV test together.

Cholesterol checks. Have your cholesterol checked regularly starting at age 45. If you smoke, have diabetes, or heart disease runs in your family, start having your cholesterol checked at age 20.

Obesity. Have your body mass index (BMI), a measure of body fat based on height and weight, calculated to screen for obesity. A BMI calculator table is included in Chapter 9.

Blood pressure. Have your blood pressure checked at least every two years.

Colorectal cancer tests. Have a test for colorectal cancer starting at age 50. Your doctor can help you decide which test is right for you. If you have a family member who has had colon cancer, you should begin screening earlier and should consult your doctor.

Diabetes tests. Have a test to screen for diabetes if you have high blood pressure or high cholesterol.

Depression. If you've felt "down," sad, or hopeless, and have felt little interest or pleasure in doing things for two weeks straight, talk to your doctor about whether he or she can screen you for depression.

Osteoporosis tests. Have a bone density test at age 65 to screen for osteoporosis (thinning of the bones). If you are between the ages of 60 and 64 and weigh 154 pounds or less, talk to your doctor about whether you should be tested.

Sexually transmitted Infections. Have a test for chlamydia, HIV, and other STIs if you are 25 or younger and sexually active. If you are

older, talk to your doctor to see whether you should be tested. Also, talk to your doctor to see whether you should be tested for other sexually transmitted diseases.

Immunizations. Stay up-to-date with your immunizations:

■ Have a flu shot every year if available.

■ Have a tetanus-diphtheria shot every 10 years.

■ Talk to your doctor about whether you need hepatitis B shots.

Don't smoke. If you do smoke, talk to your doctor about quitting. You can take medicine and get counseling to help you quit. Make a plan and set a quit date. Tell your family, friends, and co-workers you are quitting. Ask for their support. If you are pregnant and smoke, quitting now will help both you and your baby.

Eat a healthy diet. Eat a variety of foods, including fruits, vegetables, animal or vegetable protein (such as meat, fish, chicken, eggs, beans, lentils, tofu, or tempeh), and grains (such as rice). Limit the amount of saturated fat you eat.

Be physically active. Walk, dance, ride a bike, rake leaves, or do any other physical activity you enjoy. Start small and work up to a total of 20-30 minutes most days of the week.

Stay at a healthy weight. Balance the number of calories you eat with the number you burn off by your activities. Remember to watch portion sizes. Talk to your doctor if you have questions about what or how much to eat.

Drink alcohol only in moderation. If you drink alcohol, one drink a day is safe for women, unless you are pregnant. If you are pregnant, you should avoid alcohol completely. Because researchers don't know how much alcohol will harm a fetus, it's best not to drink any alcohol while you are pregnant.

Source: *Preventive Services.* AHRQ Publication No. APPIP03-0008. Updated February 2007.

while simultaneously living as independent and open individuals. It is not healthy for women to consider themselves victims or targets for violence at all times, but education about how to avoid compromising situations and how to fight off an attack if it should occur can help women to maintain their independence and peace of mind while dating.

During this period of life, some women have multiple sexual partners or may be sexually involved with someone who has multiple partners. These women are at high risk for contracting STIs if they do not protect themselves by using latex condoms or other barrier contraception methods. Most sexually transmitted infections, such as chlamydia and gonorrhea, can cause irritating and often painful symptoms immediately and cause infertility and other health problems (see Chapter 7).

Many women in their twenties and thirties experience pregnancy for the first time. Roughly half of all pregnancies are unplanned, causing anxiety and difficult choices for many women. Whether a woman is in a relationship or dealing with a pregnancy on her own, an unplanned pregnancy can be an enormously stressful experience. Seeking advice and counseling from friends, family, health-care poviders, and knowledgeable reproductive health agencies can assist women with their decision-making process.

For a woman who is planning to become pregnant, proper nutrition and consumption of essential vitamins and minerals like folic acid are important measures to prevent birth defects. For a woman who is sexually active and does not want to become pregnant, effective birth control and risk reduction for STIs become very important preventive health behaviors. Other lifestyle choices become significant preventive health choices as well, such as wearing sunblock, reducing unnecessary stress, and making sure that routine medical appointments are made. In the case of

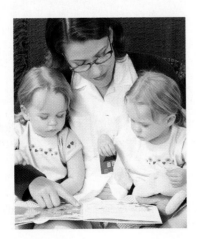

■ Many women no longer choose to begin their families in their twenties.

skin cancers, routine visits to the dermatologist or primary care physician for full body checks are important for all women, but vital for women with fair skin or a family history of skin cancer.

Midlife

As women move into their forties, many have completed their families and either remain at home or continue working outside of the home. Some have established productive careers, whereas others struggle to find and maintain a job with decent wages, advancement opportunities, and a satisfactory work environment. Women in this stage of life are often busy raising children, possibly caring for elderly parents, and working to keep their relationships healthy. As they reach their fifties and sixties, many must deal with the mortality of their parents as well as their own aging. Some may be fearful of getting older, whereas others are looking forward to retirement. Some grandparents, often women in their fifties and sixties, are raising their grandchildren. The parents of these children, for various reasons, have left the responsibility of childrearing with the grandparent, creating a different dimension of aging for these women.

Thanks to increasing physical fitness and greater access to effective medical treatment, many women discover midlife to be an ideal time to focus on themselves. They realize some of the benefits of the healthier lifestyles they have adopted over the past 20 years and consequently find their retirement years to be filled with physical activity, travel, healthy sexuality, and relaxation.

Specific Health Concerns for Women During Midlife

Between the ages of 45 and 64, the top five causes of death for women are chronic diseases. Cancer, heart disease, cerebrovascular disease (stroke), chronic obstructive pulmonary disease, and diabetes all benefit from behavioral changes (**Table 3.7**). In developing countries, the leading causes of death for women in this age group are a mix of infectious diseases, diseases of the reproductive system, and chronic diseases. Chronic diseases such as cancer and heart disease are increasingly dominant causes of death for women in this age group in developing countries as well.

Menopause, the cessation of the menstrual cycle, is a significant transition for women during their midlife years (see Chapter 8). For some women, menopause is a welcome change, eliminating their menstrual cycle and the need for contraception. Other women experience bothersome

Table 3.7   Leading Causes of Death for U.S. Females, 2004

Ages 45–54

Cause	Percentage of Total Deaths
1. Malignant neoplasms (cancer)	36.2
2. Heart disease	15.8
3. Accidents	7.4
4. Cerebrovascular disease (stroke)	4.2
5. Diabetes	3.3
6. Liver disease and cirrhosis	3.2
7. Suicide	2.7
8. Chronic respiratory disease	2.6
9. HIV/AIDS	1.6
9. Septicemia	1.6

Ages 55–64

Cause	Percentage of Total Deaths
1. Malignant neoplasms (cancer)	41.5
2. Heart disease	18.6
3. Chronic respiratory disease	5.4
4. Diabetes	4.3
5. Cerebrovascular disease (stroke)	4.2
6. Accidents	2.9
7. Liver disease and cirrhosis	1.9
8. Kidney disease	1.7
8. Septicemia	1.7
10. Influenza and pneumonia	1.2

Ages 65 and older

Cause	Percentage of Total Deaths
1. Heart disease	30.3
2. Malignant neoplasm (cancer)	19.3
3. Cerebrovascular disease (stroke)	8.5
4. Chronic respiratory disease	5.7
5. Alzheimer's disease	4.8
6. Influenza	3.1
7. Diabetes	3.1
8. Kidney disease	1.9
9. Accidents	1.8
10. Septicemia	1.5

Source: Heron, M. (2007). *Deaths: Leading causes for 2004.* Hyattsville, MD: National Center for Health Statistics.

symptoms or more serious health concerns associated with menopause and have difficulty finding an effective therapy. Women entering menopause today are encountering more confusion than in the past due to recent controversy surrounding hormone replacement therapy (HRT). The controversy has limited the medical options for dealing with the distressing side effects of menopause. Women in perimenopause, the period just before menopause, may find themselves experiencing discomfort during sex or lack of libido.

As women live longer and many postpone marriage, some are finding themselves sandwiched between the demands of their children and their parents. Due to difficult economic times, more children are living at home to attend college, and an increasing number of adult children are returning home after a divorce or loss of job. These

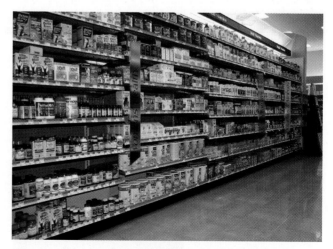

■ Significant controversy and confusion remain over the use of hormone replacement therapy and dietary supplements for perimenopause and menopause.

"boomerang" children change the dynamics of life for many women in their middle years who assumed their children would grow up, leave home, and live as independent, self-supporting adults. Instead, many women must deal with a child at home again precisely at the time when their caregiver roles increase for their own parents.

Preventive Behaviors

Healthful eating, regular physical activity, and avoidance of smoking are primary preventive measures that should be continued through all stages of life. As a woman ages, secondary preventive measures, such as mammograms and colonoscopies, become extremely important to ensure early detection of disease and, consequently, timely treatment. **Table 3.8** lists secondary preventive behaviors for women in this stage of life.

As in other stages of life, maintaining mental wellness is of significant importance in midlife. Women who are caregivers for children, elderly relatives, or both often find themselves suffering from severe stress, depression, and anxiety. Many of these women may see the effects spill over from their home life into their work life. Finding support groups, seeking professional help, and establishing time to

Table 3.8	**Secondary Preventive Measures for Women During Midlife**

Annual screening for high blood pressure.

Periodic height and weight measurement to monitor for overweight and obesity.

Clinical breast examinations yearly.

Periodic screening for high cholesterol levels, at least once every five years.

Behavioral assessment to detect depression and other problems.

Annual fecal occult blood test plus sigmoidoscopy every five years or colonoscopy every 10 years or barium enema every 5-10 years; a digital rectal examination should also be performed at the time of screening—for adults age 40 years or older with a family history of colorectal cancer and all adults age 50 years or older.

Annual mammography for women at high risk beginning at age 35 and for all women after age 50. Some authorities recommend screening mammograms every one to two years for women 40 to 49 years of age.

Annual Pap test or HPV test; after three or more consecutive normal exams, the Pap test may be performed less frequently in low-risk women at the discretion of the patient and clinician.

Counseling about the benefits and risks of postmenopausal hormone replacement therapy.

Bone density measurements for women at risk of osteoporosis.

take care of oneself are effective means for improving the mental health of many women.

Discussing options with a health-care provider can help improve sexual functioning and desire, if necessary. Many women may still require contraception for preventing pregnancy or STIs if they are not in a mutually monogamous relationship.

The Senior Years

Over the past century, the average life expectancy in the United States has increased by about 30 years.[1] Public health initiatives are responsible for about 25 of those years; all the medical advances over the past century have only increased the average life expectancy by about four years.[1] Increasing life expectancies have led to a "graying" of the U.S. population. Today, nearly one out of seven people in the United States is 65 or older, and the fastest growing section of the population is people over age 85. Because of their longer life expectancies, women constitute a majority of both these populations.

In 1900, the average life expectancy at birth for women was 48.3 years. By 1970, it had increased to 68.3 years, and by 2004 it had increased to 76.3 years. (The life expectancy for men in 2004 was 69.5 years.)[21] The U.S. National Center for Health Statistics projects that the average life expectancy for women born in 2015 will be 79.9 years.[21]

Life expectancy also has increased for women at age 65 and 85. On average, women who live to age 65 can expect to live to age 84.5; those who live to 85 can anticipate living to age 92.[4] The increase in life expectancy at these ages is partly due to decreased mortality rates, specifically from heart disease and stroke. Despite decreases in mortality rates, heart disease remains the number one killer of women in the United States for women age 65 or older.

Life expectancy also varies by race (**Figure 3.5**). In 2004, life expectancy at birth was four and a half years

It's Your Health

Contributors to Improved Life Expectancy for Women

Identification, treatment, eradication, and control of some infectious and parasitic diseases

Better prenatal and antenatal care

More efficient, effective methods for assisting childbirth

Greater awareness, identification, and control of threats to health and ways to promote and maximize health

Improved protection from environmental and workplace toxins and hazards

Figure 3.5

Life expectancy for black women and white women, 1900–2002.

Source: National Center for Health Statistics. (2004). *Health, United States 2004 with Chartbook on Trends in the Health of Americans.* Hyattsville, MD.

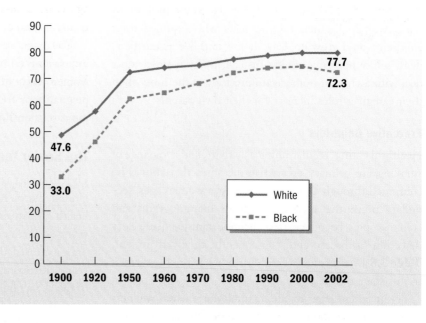

longer on average for white women than for black women. These differences shrink as women age, however. By age 65, white women live an average of 1.6 years longer than black women, and by age 85, life expectancy for black women is nearly equal that for white women. By 2030, one in four American women will be older than 65. The population over the age of 85 is projected to more than double from nearly 4 million in 1995 to more than 8 million in 2030. In 2050, an estimated 18 million people over the age of 85 will live in the United States, accounting for 4.6% of the U.S. population. The aging of the population presents a unique challenge to both society and individual health-care providers, along with opportunities to allow this growing population to live healthier, more satisfying lives.

Health Concerns During the Senior Years

Women 65 or older face a spectrum of health issues. Many women remain healthy into their eighties and beyond. Other women struggle with continual health issues as they age. From the age of 65 on, chronic diseases are the leading cause of death for women in the United States.[3] For women ages 65–74, the five leading causes of death are cancer, heart disease, chronic lower respiratory diseases, stroke, and diabetes. For women ages 75–84, heart disease moves up to number one as the leading cause of death. For women age 85 or older, heart disease remains the number one killer, but Alzheimer's disease and influenza and pneumonia move into the top five causes of death, surpassing chronic lower respiratory diseases and diabetes. Chronic obstructive lung disease, largely caused by tobacco use or exposure, is a leading cause of death and disability worldwide.

Diseases such as osteoporosis and arthritis may also make it harder for women to maintain their independence. Fall-related fractures are a major concern for anyone, but they can be extremely detrimental to a woman whose bone health is suffering (see Chapter 11). Arthritis can make it difficult for a woman to perform daily activities, such as opening jars, lifting objects, bending to pick up an item that has fallen, or lifting herself from the toilet seat. A woman also may begin having problems with vision or hearing, creating new challenges in performing everyday tasks and maintaining independent living.

■ Living a healthy life from childhood on may lead to fulfilling and enjoyable senior years.

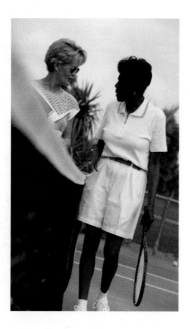

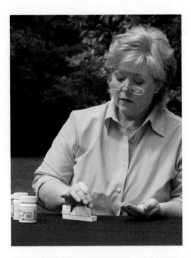

■ A major health concern related to aging is the side effects of taking multiple drugs.

Women over the age of 65 often take multiple medications on a regular basis. The combination of these drugs may produce serious side effects. The risk of side effects is especially high for women who have multiple conditions or who take a medication that requires other medications to treat side effects it causes. Health-care providers are not always aware of harmful drug interactions. Harmful effects of drug interaction may include, but are not limited to, abnormal heart rate and/or rhythm, depression, dizziness and imbalance, constipation, blood pressure increase, and confusion.

Health-care providers and other caregivers can also harm elderly people by treating them with a lack of respect. This lack of respect is not necessarily deliberate. It can include a nurse withholding medical information from an elderly woman on the assumption that a woman "won't understand" the information, or a physician who calls her elderly patients names like "dear" or "sweetie" in an effort to be friendly. Recent research has found that these kinds of habits reduce elderly patients' self-esteem and perceptions of themselves; these reduced perceptions in turn actually lower patients' life expectancies.[22]

The loss of a spouse and close friends may affect a woman's well-being as she ages. The number of women who are widowed doubles after the age of 65. Learning to cope with grief and loss is essential for physical and mental well-being. Maintaining independence and fostering social relationships may help women deal with feelings of grief, sadness, and loneliness.

Diagnosable depression, however, is not the same as sadness, grief, or the emotional effects of loss. Depression is a significant health concern for aging women and may result from medication interactions, chronic disease, pain, or loneliness; it should not be viewed as a normal part of

aging. An estimated 6% of Americans age 65 or older suffer from diagnosable depression in any given year.

Today, women most frequently bear the responsibility of caring for their parents or loved ones when they need help. Women account for more than 80% of the family caregivers for chronically ill elders, and 73% of these women caregivers are 65 or older.[23] The value of services caregivers provide is estimated to be more than $350 billion per year. Some women may experience cognitive decline and depression as a result of being the primary caregiver for a partner, relative, or friend. Health-care providers also need to be aware of the possibility of abuse by a relative or caregiver and help provide protection when a woman is unable to or afraid to protect herself (see Chapter 14).

As women age, their skin becomes thinner, loses some of its elastic quality, suffers injury more easily, and heals more slowly. Women who have spent a lot of time in the sun during their lives often experience the development of skin cancers at this stage of their lives. Most skin cancers can be removed safely and easily with a simple procedure. If left untreated, however, they can pose a very serious health risk. Proper attention to skin care throughout life can prevent serious consequences as women age.

Sexuality also remains an issue for older women. Although many health-care poviders do not view their patients as sexual beings at this age, many women continue to desire sexual relations and may need advice for maintaining healthy sexuality as they age. A study conducted by the American Association of Retired People (AARP) reported that 44% of women 75 years of age or older believe that "a satisfying sexual relationship" is important to their quality of life.[25] This issue is discussed in more depth in Chapter 4.

Preventive Behaviors

The early senior years can be a time of relaxation and fulfillment for women who are fortunate enough to have achieved financial stability, who have maintained their physical and mental health, and who are surrounded by

■ Flu immunizations significantly reduce the chance of an older woman getting influenza or pneumonia.

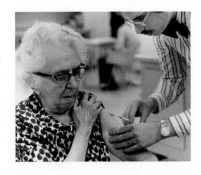

Gender Dimensions

On average, a woman born in the United States can expect to live almost seven years longer than a man born under the same conditions. Two major contributors to this discrepancy are women's lower rates of death for accidents and suicide. In 2004, accidents caused 6.1% of total deaths for males, but only 3.3% of deaths for females.[11] More than 2% of men, but only 0.6% of women, died of suicide in the same year.[11] Suicide and accidents dramatically reduce life expectancy because they typically happen while men are relatively young. A man who dies at age 25 from a work-related accident reduces the average life expectancy for males far more than a woman who dies from a heart attack at age 70.

Compared to men, women are significantly more likely than men to die of stroke (7.5% of deaths versus 5% of deaths) and Alzheimer's disease (3.9% versus 1.6%), in large part because women are likely to reach the ages at which these diseases typically strike.[11]

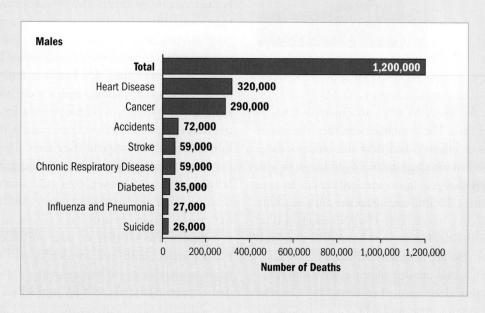

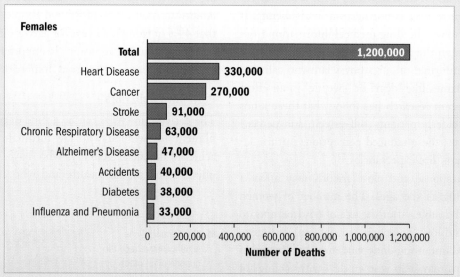

Leading causes of death for U.S. males and females, 2004.

Source: Heron, M. (2007). *Deaths: Leading causes for 2004*. Hyattsville, MD: National Center for Health Statistics.

loving family and friends. Other women may be less fortunate and experience considerable concerns regarding their future. Planning for one's future and maintaining one's health from childhood on may help women to have an easier time in their later years.

As throughout life, good nutrition, exercise, and avoidance of harmful substances continue to provide protection from harmful diseases in old age. Regular health-care screening and preventive checkups are essential, as is continual monitoring for drug interactions and signs or symptoms that may signal a health concern. Additionally, women living in their senior years may wish to consider lifestyle changes, such as making safety arrangements to reduce the danger of falling, thus reducing their risks of accidents while maintaining their independence. Getting a flu vaccination and paying close attention to colds and minor illnesses can help keep a woman safe from pneumonia and influenza (**Table 3.9**). Women should also take special care of their skin as they age, using proper moisturizers and barriers to protect against skin breakdown. In addition, women should get bone density screenings to make sure they are not at risk for developing osteoporosis.

Informed Decision Making

To take personal responsibility for their own health and wellness, all women should educate themselves about their health status. Integrating primary prevention methods into one's daily life can improve both present and future health (see Self-Assessment 3.1). By understanding their own secondary prevention needs, such as the appropriate screening methods for women at certain ages, women can better inform their health-care poviders about their health status and demand the health-care services that they require and deserve.

The Internet has evolved into a valuable resource for health information. Yet the quality of health information on Web sites is extremely variable and difficult to assess. Evaluating the information can be a significant challenge, even for an experienced Web user. Being able to identify the validity of the material in a given Web site is crucial, as it could potentially affect health outcomes for millions of people. Most content on the Web is posted without any

Table 3.9   Secondary Preventive Measures for Seniors

Annual screening for high blood pressure.

Cholesterol screening every three to five years or as recommended by the health-care provider.

Periodic height and weight measurement to monitor for overweight and obesity.

Clinical breast examinations yearly or as recommended by one's health-care provider.

Initial assessment of cognitive function and monitoring of changes as part of a routine preventive visit.

Behavioral assessment to detect depression and other problems.

Annual fecal occult blood test plus sigmoidoscopy every 5 years or colonoscopy every 10 years or barium enema every 5 to 10 years; a digital rectal examination should also be performed at the time of screening.

Routine mammography screening as recommended by the health-care provider.

Periodic evaluation for hearing loss and visual acuity.

Thyroid-stimulating hormone test every three to five years.

Bone mineral density test as recommended by the health-care provider; counseling on fall prevention.

Annual influenza and pneumococcal pneumonia vaccines.

Self-Assessment 3.1

Rate Your Preventive Practices

Answer the following questions:

1. Do you eat a healthful diet consisting of the appropriate servings of fruits and vegetables, grains, protein, vitamins, and minerals?

2. Do you participate in moderate-intensity physical activity at least four days a week?

3. Do you get enough sleep so that you do not feel tired throughout the day?

4. Do you avoid using tobacco products and drugs?

5. If you consume alcohol, do you do so in moderation?

6. If you are sexually active, do you use condoms or other barrier contraceptives to protect against STIs?

7. Do you employ methods to reduce stress, find time to socialize with friends and relax, and maintain an overall sense of mental wellness?

8. Do you practice safe behaviors, such as using seat belts, wearing motorcycle and bicycle helmets, not driving under the influence of alcohol, and not riding with someone under the influence of alcohol?

9. Do you use nonviolent methods of conflict resolution?

10. Do you receive routine preventive care from a health-care provider?

The more questions to which you answered "yes," the better off you are! If you answered "no" to any questions, try to change that behavior to achieve a better state of overall health.

form of approval or review for accuracy and reliability, or it is posted by a company having a financial stake in the information being communicated (for example, pharmaceutical firms or physicians offering specific surgical procedures). A number of organizations are working to credential health-related Web sites, by providing "stamps of approval" so consumers can have independent validation that the content is valid; however, this practice is not widespread across cyberspace. In the absence of these content authentication measures, health-care consumers must often rely on their own common sense and judgment. Following some basic guidelines will help women evaluate the quality of information they find online. In addition, women should understand that open communication with their physicians is their right. Better communication between physicians and patients can improve both the quality of the care women receive and their health promotion knowledge base.

■■■■
Summary

Primary prevention is the first step toward health promotion and disease prevention for women at all stages of their lives. Many women have already taken the first steps by reclaiming their bodies and taking responsibility for their own health; however, many women remain unable or unwilling to make these changes.

Women can take important preventive health actions throughout their lives. Some tests and behaviors are specifically indicated starting at a given age. Becoming familiar with the appropriate health promotion and prevention activities across a woman's life span is especially valuable. Women can empower themselves by recognizing the central role that proper access to health care for them and their families plays in creating stability in their lives. Around the world, inequities in access to proper health care, specifically preventive services, medical treatments, surgical interventions, family planning, or proper maternal and child health threaten and reduce women's quality of life. These services are essential to women who seek to lead active, healthy, and happy lives at all stages of life.

In addition, around the world, women tend to be the main health observers and resource attainers in the family. Women who are better educated about their and their family's needs can improve the well-being of their family and community.

Communities, health-care poviders, workplaces, and educators need to effectively reach underserved women

Profiles of Remarkable Women

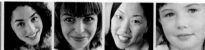

Margaret Chan (1947–)

Margaret Chan is the Director-General of the World Health Organization (WHO), the United Nations organization that directs global health efforts.

Chan, born in the People's Republic of China, obtained her medical degree from the University of Western Ontario in Canada. She started working in public health in 1978, when she joined the Hong Kong Department of Health.

Chan became Director of Health of Hong Kong in 1994. There, Chan introduced initiatives to improve recording of and response to disease outbreaks, train public health professionals, and improve relationships between Hong Kong's public health department and local and international groups. She effectively managed outbreaks of avian influenza (bird flu) and of severe acute respiratory syndrome (SARS).

Chan's position leading public health efforts in Hong Kong required difficult decisions on a daily basis. To avoid a possible outbreak of influenza among humans, Chan ordered the slaughter of 1.5 million chickens in Hong Kong.[26] Chan had no way of knowing at the time how many chickens were infected, or if the outbreak would occur. The decision to destroy Hong Kong's poultry population also brought considerable economic consequences. But the consequences of a new influenza outbreak, both for Hong Kong and the world, would have been catastrophic. Today, many public health experts believe that Chan's actions may have prevented a global disease outbreak.

In a 2007 interview, Chan said, "In public health, especially when you're dealing with new and emerging infections, science is always lagging behind time and in the absence of solid evidence. But based on the best available information and evidence, one has to make difficult and often times unpopular decisions. Of course the recommendation . . . was a very difficult decision we took, but all in all, that was the right decision."[27]

Chan joined WHO in 2003 and was nominated as Director-General in November 2006. Her term runs through June 2012.

with health-care services and education. Women must also work to educate one another about the important health-related information that they learn throughout their lives, so as to expand the rich network of communication from which women around the world benefit. By improving access to health care for all women and providing appropriate guidelines for care to both health-care poviders and consumers, women will be better equipped for remaining healthy throughout their life span.

■■■■
Topics for Discussion

1. How can parents, health-care poviders, and health educators encourage adolescents to follow healthy behaviors? How can they convince adolescents that their present behaviors will have a significant impact on their future health?

2. What are some ways in which you can improve your health? Are there preventive practices from which your parents can benefit that they are not practicing?

3. How do the health needs of women in developing countries differ from those of women in the United States? How are they similar?

4. What are some preventive measures for lesbians? for physically challenged women?

5. Some health behaviors are detrimental to well-being. Should policies such as restricting smoking or mandating bicycle helmets be mandatory or voluntary?

■■■■
Web Sites

Administration on Aging: http://www.aoa.gov

Administration for Children and Families: http://www.acf.hhs.gov

Agency for Healthcare Research and Quality: http://www.ahrq.gov

Centers for Disease Control and Prevention: http://www.cdc.gov

Centers for Medicare and Medicaid Services: http://www.cms.hhs.gov

Food and Drug Administration: http://www.fda.gov

Health Resources and Services Administration: http://www.hrsa.gov

Healthy People 2010: http://www.healthypeople.gov

Indian Health Service: http://www.ihs.gov

National Institutes of Health: http://www.nih.gov

Office of the Surgeon General: http://www.surgeongeneral.gov

Substance Abuse and Mental Health Services Administration: http://www.samhsa.gov

U.S. Department of Health and Human Services: http://www.hhs.gov

U.S. Public Health Service Commissioned Corps: http://www.usphs.gov

■■■■
References

1. Steen, J. (2007). *The Primacy of Public Health*. American Public Health Association: Community Health Planning and Policy Development. Available at: http://www.apha.org/membergroups/newsletters/section newsletters/comm/spring07/primacyph.htm.

2. Finkelstein, E., Fiebelkorn, I., & Wang, G. (2003). National medical spending attributable to overweight and obesity: How much, and who's paying? *Health Affairs*. Available at: http://content.healthaffairs.org/cgi/content/full/hlthaff.w3.219v1/DC1. (*Adjusted for inflation by authors for 2009.*)

3. Barrington, L., & Rosen, B. (2008). Weights and Measures: What Employers Should Know about Obesity. New York: The Conference Board.

4. National Center for Health Statistics. (2004). *Health, United States 2004 with Chartbook on Trends in the Health of Americans*. Hyattsville, MD: Department of Human Services.

5. Solarz, A. L. (Ed.). (1999). *Lesbian Health: Current Assessment and Directions for the Future. Committee on Lesbian Health Research Priorities. Institute of Medicine*. Washington, DC: National Academy Press.

6. Weiner, S. (1999). *A Provider's Guide for the Care of Women with Physical Disabilities and Chronic Medical Conditions*. Raleigh, NC: Office on Disability and Health.

7. World Health Organization. (2004). *The World Health Report 2004*. Geneva.

8. Joint U.N. Programme on HIV/AIDS. (2008). *2008 Report on the Global HIV/AIDS Epidemic*. New York: UNAIDS.

9. World Health Organization. (2001). *Advancing Safe Motherhood Through Human Rights*. Geneva.

10. Benderly, B. L., for the Institute of Medicine. (1997). *In Her Own Right: The Institute of Medicine's Guide to Women's Health Issues*. Washington, DC: National Academy Press.

11. Heron, M. (2007). Deaths: leading causes for 2004. *National Vital Statistics Reports* 56(5), Hyattsville, MD: National Center for Health Statistics.

12. Substance Abuse and Mental Health Services Administration Center for Mental Health Services, in partnership with the National Institute of Mental Health, National Institutes of Health. (1999). *Mental Health: A Report of the Surgeon General*. U.S. Department of Health and Human Services.

13. Centers for Disease Control and Prevention. (2008). *2007 Youth Risk Behavior Survey*. Atlanta: Eaton, D., et al.

14. Ventura, S., Abma, J., Mosher, W., & Henshaw, S. (2006). *Recent Trends in Teenage Pregnancy in the United States, 1990–2002. Health E-stats*. Hyattsville, MD: National Center for Health Statistics.

15. Centers for Disease Control and Prevention. (2000). *Tracking the Hidden Epidemic: Trends in STDs in the United States 2000*. Atlanta: CDC.

16. UNAIDS Global Coalition on Women and AIDS. (2005). *2005 Progress Report*. Available at: http://data.unaids.org/Publications/IRC-pub07/JC1210-GCWA-ProgressReport-2005_en.pdf.

17. Centers for Disease Control and Prevention. (2000). *Promoting Lifelong Healthy Eating: CDC's Guidelines for School Health Programs*. Division of Adolescent and School Health. Atlanta: CDC.

18. Geller, A. C., Colditz, G., Oliveria, S., et al. (2002). Use of sunscreen, sunburning rates, and tanning bed use among more than 10,000 U.S. children and adolescents. *Pediatrics* 109(6): 1009–1014.

19. The Tension Tracker 2002. Based on 1,805 interviews among a representative sample of Americans 18 years or older. Harris Interactive conducted interviews from April 29, 2002, to May 8, 2002.

20. Centers for Disease Control and Prevention. (2005). *Summary Health Statistics for U.S. Adults: National Health Interview, 2004 Survey*. Atlanta: CDC.

21. *Expectation of life at birth, 1960–2004, and projections, 2010 and 2015. National Center for Health Statistics*. (August 21, 2007). *National Vital Statistics Reports*, 55(19): 246–254.

22. Leland, John. (October 6, 2008). In "Sweetie" and "Dear," a hurt for the elderly. *New York Times*. Available at: http://www.nytimes.com/2008/10/07/us/07aging.html.

23. Hooyman, N. R., & Kiyak, H. A. (1996). *Social Gerontology* (4th ed.). Boston: Allyn and Bacon.

24. Gross, Jane. (October 14, 2008). Who cares for the caregivers? *New York Times*. Available at: http://newoldage.blogs.nytimes.com/2008/10/14/who-cares-for-the-caregivers/.

25. AARP/Modern Maturity. (1999). AARP/Modern Maturity Sexuality Survey. Atlanta: NFO Research.

26. Associated Press (November 8, 2006). Margaret Chan rose to prominence in Hong Kong's battle with bird flu. *International Herald-Tribune*. Available at: http://www.iht.com/articles/ap/2006/11/08/news/UN_GEN_UN_WHO_Chan_Profile.php.

27. CNN. (April 16, 2007). Interview with Dr. Margaret Chan. Available at: http://www.cnn.com/2007/WORLD/asiapcf/04/13/talkasia.chan.script/index.html.

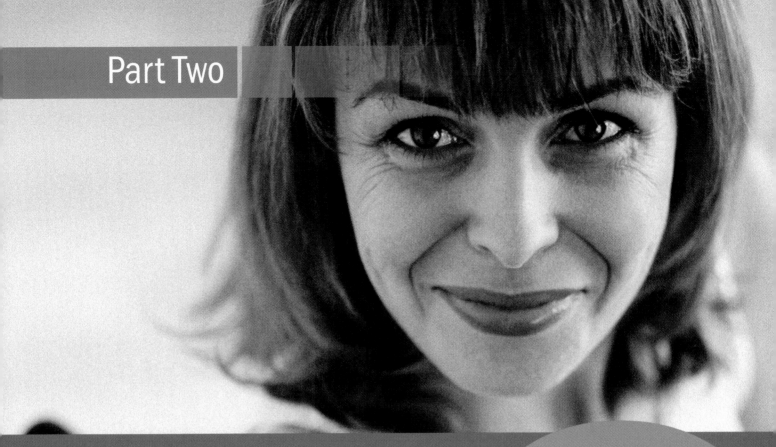

Part Two

Sexual and Reproductive Dimensions of Women's Health

Chapter Four

Sexual Health

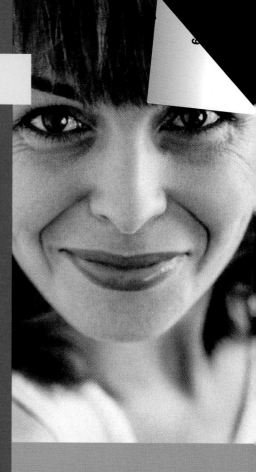

Chapter Objectives

On completion of this chapter, the student should be able to discuss:

1. The ways that cultural values, stereotypes, and socialization define or influence sexual behavior.

2. The economic, legal, and political dimensions of sexual health.

3. The significance of research on sexual behavior and major contributors to this body of research.

4. The difference between sex and gender and the concepts of gender identity and gender role.

5. Homosexual, heterosexual, and bisexual orientation and issues surrounding homophobia.

6. The location and function of the major external and internal female genital structures.

7. The three phases of the menstrual cycle.

8. The four basic phases of the female sexual response cycle.

9. Several examples of sexual expression.

10. The importance of the gynecological examination and the procedures involved.

11. The major areas of sexual dysfunction in women.

12. The ways in which sexuality is expressed throughout a person's life span.

13. Sexual violence as a public health problem.

14. The significance of communication in intimate relationships and with a woman's health-care provider.

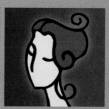

womenshealth.jbpub.com

Women's Health Online is a great source for supplementary women's health information for both students and instructors. Visit

http://womenshealth.jbpub.com

to find a variety of useful tools for learning, thinking, and teaching.

Introduction

Sexual health refers to the physical, psychological, social, cultural, and emotional facets of sexual human interactions. The World Health Organization defines sexual health as

> . . . a state of physical, emotional, mental and social well-being related to sexuality; it is not merely the absence of disease, dysfunction or infirmity. Sexual health requires a positive and respectful approach to sexuality and sexual relationships, as well as the possibility of having pleasurable and safe sexual experiences, free of coercion, discrimination, and violence. For sexual health to be attained and maintained, the sexual rights of all persons must be respected, protected, and fulfilled.[1]

Both scientific and psychological perspectives are needed to understand sexual health. Sexual health entails the need for responsible sexual behavior to avoid sexually transmitted infections (STIs), unintended pregnancy, and sexual abuse, coercion, or violence. Positive sexuality requires thoughtful and respectful discussion of issues that may be difficult or awkward for some people to vocalize. Learning about the physical and emotional aspects of sexuality and respecting the variations in forms of sexual behavior can improve sexual health and responsible sexual behavior.

Perspectives on Sexual Health and Sexuality

When different cultures are examined, it becomes readily apparent that society, as well as physiology, influences how men and women interact sexually. Vast differences in sexual norms exist across cultures. The question arises as to what causes people to assume specific sexual roles and preferences. The hypothesis that sexual behavior is simply a reproductive function is not substantiated across generations or across cultures.

Cultural and Religious Dimensions

Cultural values often define sexual behavior. Tremendous cultural diversity throughout the world creates a spectrum of sexuality issues, including normative sex roles, accepted types of sexual activity, preferences for sexual arousal, and the sanctions and prohibitions on sexual behavior. One consistent theme exists, however—that of "marriage" in some form or another. Within all cultures, marriage provides sanctioned sexual privileges and obligations. Social scientists have recognized that every society shapes, structures, or constrains the development and expression of sexuality in all of its members.

Some cultures have strong values that warn against premarital sex; people, especially women, participating in sexual activity before marriage bring shame to a family and may be ostracized from a community. Other cultures insist on extreme modesty and sexual restraint for females, but have a greater acceptance for male sexual behavior. Many cultures ignore the sexuality and sexual needs of people with disabilities, while stigmatizing people involved in same-sex relationships. Other cultural influences extend into contraception decision making. In some cultures, it is acceptable for a woman to decide what form of birth control to use, as well as to purchase condoms and ask her partner to use them. In other cultures, men take charge of this decision and consider it disrespectful for a woman to mention the use of contraception to her partner. The tremendous cultural diversity in the United States results in a spectrum of perspectives, values, and messages to women about sexual practices.

Economic Dimensions

Historically, marriage represented the exchange of property between two families—usually in the form of a daughter. The daughter was either purchased from the maternal family through the exchange of goods or, in some cultures, the father of the girl would offer a dowry to the groom's family to compensate for the financial burden of taking the girl into their house or clan.

Throughout history, and even today in some parts of the world, the value of a bride often depends on her virginity. A girl who has lost her virginity before marriage, either

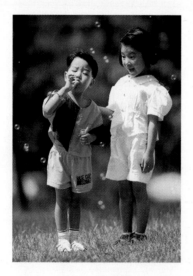

■ Society expects little boys to grow up to be men and do what men do, and little girls to grow up to be women and do what women do.

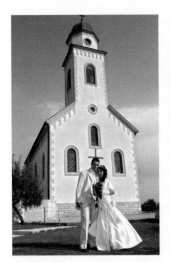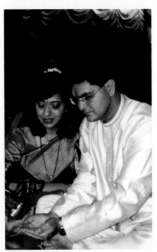

■ Marriage is a central social underpinning of most societies.

either cultural or individual factors, the less able she is to control a given sexual encounter. Significant power imbalances, like those seen between rich and poor, educated and noneducated, and young and old, have been strongly associated with sexual violence and abuse. For example, within the commercial sex industry in Bangkok, Thailand, the highest incidence of sexual violence is documented between Western adult males and native girl sex workers under the age of 12. Social and economic factors that give men power over women can undermine women's abilities to say "no" to unwanted sexual advances or aggression. Initiatives that educate women about how to achieve more parity in the power distribution of their relationships have helped reduce sexual violence and empower women in contraceptive decision making.

willingly or unwillingly, can lose significant value to both her family and the groom's family she is entering. In the United States and other Western countries, it has become extremely common for young women to have sex before marriage. Rates for U.S. teens ever having sexual intercourse have decreased over the past 15 years, but during this same period, the percentage of teenagers who are sexually active has remained relatively constant (**Figure 4.1**).

Sexuality can be viewed within a frame of power and economic dynamics. The less power a woman has, based on

One direct relationship between sexuality and economics occurs between a commercial sex worker, or prostitute, and a sex consumer. In this relationship, sexual acts are delineated and certain price points are attached to them. Some intellectuals have argued that prostitution creates the ultimate power inversion, whereby women take control of sexuality and reap the financial rewards of performing sexual acts. The reality for most sex workers is quite different. The vast majority of sex workers are working under some level of indentured servitude for a male pimp who takes a portion of their earnings in exchange for protection

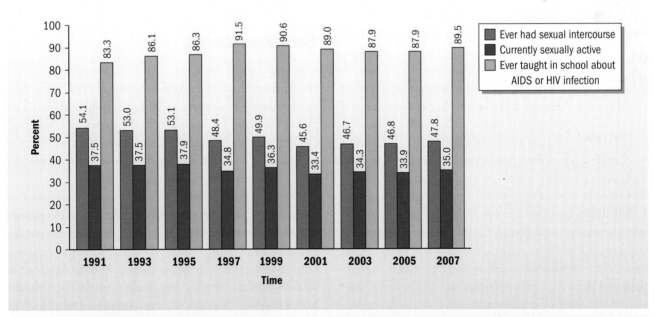

Figure 4.1

Trends in sexual behaviors among U.S. youth, 1991–2007.

Source: Centers for Disease Control and Prevention. (2008). Trends in the Prevalence of Sexual Behaviors, National YRBS: 1991–2007.

and limiting competition. Pimps are individuals who act as brokers and supposed protectors for sex workers. They often require their sex workers to perform sexual acts on them for free, and they use physical abuse and threats to maintain power in the relationship.

Legal Dimensions

Laws criminalizing sexual intimacy once existed in all 50 states. These laws were enacted to impose norms on the lives of the nation's citizens and, sometimes, to prevent sexual activity not intended for procreation. Cohabitation, or unmarried sexual partners sharing a living space, and fornication, defined as sexual intercourse between unmarried partners, were also illegal in most states. Although these laws exist in a handful of states, they are rarely enforced today. Cohabitation is common today. By age 30, about half of U.S. women have cohabitated outside marriage.[2]

A sodomy law is a law that defines certain sexual acts as sex crimes. In 2003, the Supreme Court struck down state laws that ban sodomy, calling them an unconstitutional violation of privacy. The precise sexual acts meant by the term *sodomy* were spelled out in the law, but courts typically interpreted the term to include any sexual act that does not lead to procreation, such as oral sex, anal sex, and bestiality; in practice such laws were rarely enforced against heterosexual couples.

Same-sex partners face discrimination when it comes to legalizing their partnership. Same-sex marriages are currently legal in only a few countries around the world. In the United States, six states currently recognize gay marriages, but the federal government does not. In 2008, voter initiatives specifically banning same-sex marriages passed in California, Arizona, and Florida. Some countries and U.S. states recognize civil unions, which offer some, but not all, of the rights of a civil marriage.

A civil-union license makes the couple eligible for the same state-provided benefits, protections, and responsibilities that are granted to spouses in a marriage. A couple in a civil union becomes subject to laws regarding annulment; separation and divorce; child custody and support; and property division and maintenance. However, a civil union does not provide access to federal benefits of marriage, nor does it guarantee recognition of the union outside of the state or country that has granted the union. Likewise, many states ban recognition of marriages of same-sex couples should they be permitted in another state or country.

Political Dimensions

Controversy about school-based sex education programs has been intense for over a decade. Starting with President Bill Clinton, and continuing with President George W. Bush, the federal government has endorsed abstinence-only until marriage (AOUM) as the primary approach to sex education. Federally funded AOUM programs must promote abstinence from sexual activity and limit discussion of condoms and contraception. The AOUM programs exist despite evidence that comprehensive sexuality education effectively promotes sexual health and that parents support these programs in public schools.[3] The federal government has provided states with more than $1.5 billion for AOUM programs over the past decade. However, no research has shown that they are effective at preventing teen pregnancies or sexually transmitted infections (STIs), and many of the programs contain misleading and medically inaccurate information.[4,5]

Proponents of AOUM programs have argued that comprehensive sex education might lead to an increase in teens having sex; however, research shows that these types of programs either delay or have no effect on initiation of sexual activity. Studies have shown that teaching about contraception was not associated with increased risk of adolescent sexual activity or STIs. Adolescents who received comprehensive sex education had a lower risk of pregnancy than adolescents who received abstinence-only or no sex education.[6]

Sex Research

Despite its importance, there has been less systematic, scientific research on the sexual behavior of Americans than on most other health and social topics of importance. The AIDS epidemic has improved the accuracy and increased the availability of information on sexual behavior, but the collection of scientific information on sexual matters continues to face much political opposition.

Researchers attempting to understand sexual behavior face many of the same problems that handicap all research into human social behavior. Human subjects cannot be placed in a laboratory setting where variables that influence outcome measures can be controlled. Human behavior is infinitely more complex, and studies, particularly on human behavior, are prone to many types of contamination and bias. Sex is considered a private arena and as such is even more limited than other areas of behavioral research. Clearly, many problematic issues arise with any attempt to

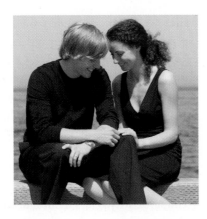

■ An array of intimate behaviors may be included in a personal definition of virginity.

understand the prevalence and nature of contemporary sexual behavior.

Even with these limitations, there are still ways to study sexual behavior, including case studies, direct observation, experimental laboratory research, and surveys. There are many ways to measure or analyze sexual activity. Sexual research can be addressed directly, as in determining the actual prevalence of certain sexual behaviors such as oral sex or types of sexual activity such as the prevalence of homosexual activity. Indirect assessments, such as adolescent pregnancy rates or sexually transmitted disease rates, provide insight into the consequences of sexual behavior.

Definitions create another technical difficulty in research. "Premarital sex" has been traditionally defined as penile-vaginal intercourse that takes place before a couple is married. This definition is misleading because it excludes many of noncoital heterosexual and homosexual activities. Heavy petting can include extensive types of sexual contact, often resulting in orgasm. "Virginity," therefore, may not reflect a lack of sexual activity. The term "premarital" has inherent connotations that may be inappropriate to some individuals, especially to couples in same-sex relationships or relationships in cultures that offer commitments equal to marriage. Not all couples who engage in sexual activity have marital intentions with that partner. Any review of sex studies must consider the inherent limitations of such research.

Well-Known Studies

Several important studies on sexual behavior have provided valuable information and insight into sexual practices, behaviors, and attitudes.

■ In 1948 and 1953, Kinsey conducted the most comprehensive taxonomic surveys of human sexual behavior to date.[7,8] The 1948 study researched sexual behavior in the human male, and the 1953 study researched sexual behavior in the human female. Both studies at-

tempted to present objective data on sexual behavior. The researchers interviewed thousands of people of various socioeconomic status, educational levels, marital status, and sex education experiences. The results showed how factors such as age, religious adherence, and gender influenced the incidence, frequency, and patterns of sexual behavior.

■ Masters and Johnson are perhaps the best-known sex researchers. In 1966, through direct observation techniques, they observed and recorded more than 10,000 completed sexual response cycles.[9] Before their work, no significant empirical data had been gathered about male and female sexual arousal. Masters and Johnson were considered pioneers in sexual research for determining the four phases of the sexual-reponse cycle: excitement, plateau, orgasm, and resolution.

■ The *Redbook* Survey (1977) was a questionnaire sent to more than 100,000 women that examined sexual behavior and attitudes of U.S. women.[10] This survey documented women's sexual fulfillment in respect to their marital status, age at sexual initiation, and sexual fidelity.

■ In 1976, the Hite Report, a questionnaire survey on female sexuality, also provided extensive narrative answers to several important questions about the sexual practices of American women.[11]

■ Blumstein and Schwartz (1983) elicited excellent information about a variety of sexual and nonsexual components of relationships from a large national sample.[12]

In a 2004 poll, the vast majority of respondents said they were monogamous and that they were happy about it. The random telephone survey queried a national sample of adults about sexual activities, fantasies, and attitudes.[13] Of the respondents:

■ 57% said they have had sex outdoors or in a public place

■ 42% call themselves sexually adventurous

■ 29% said they have had sex on a first date

■ 15% of men said they have paid for sex

■ 50% of women said they have faked an orgasm

Although each study has been criticized for over-representing or under-representing certain population segments, these studies provide valuable information and insight into sexual behavior and attitudes. They demonstrate, however, that in evaluating any study of sexual behavior, it

Call to Action to Promote Sexual Health and Responsible Sexual Behavior

Individual responsibility includes the following duties:

- Understanding and awareness of one's sexuality and sexual development
- Respect for oneself and one's partner
- Avoidance of physical and emotional harm to oneself or one's partner
- Ensuring that pregnancy occurs only when welcomed
- Recognition and tolerance of the diversity of sexual values within any community

Community responsibility includes assurance that its members have the following characteristics:

- Access to developmentally and culturally appropriate sexuality education as well as sexual and reproductive health care and counseling
- The latitude to make appropriate sexual and reproductive choices
- Respect for diversity
- Freedom from stigmatization and violence on the basis of gender, race, ethnicity, religion, or sexual orientation

Source: *The Surgeon General's Call to Action to Promote Sexual Health and Responsible Sexual Behavior.* (2001). U.S. Department of Health and Human Services.

is important to consider the quality of the study method and the sampling techniques employed.

In 2001 the Surgeon General's Call to Action to Promote Sexual Health and Responsible Sexual Behavior expanded the research base, helping to provide a foundation for promoting sexual health and responsible sexual behavior.[14] The Call to Action was the first time that the promotion of responsible sexual behavior and the improvement of sexual health were addressed as significant public health challenges (see **It's Your Health**).

Sex and Gender

Gender refers to the economic, social, and cultural attributes and opportunities associated with being male or female, whereas the term **sex** refers to an individual's biological status as male or female. Issues surrounding sex and gender differences in health have been evolving for the past several decades.

In 2001, the Institute of Medicine published, *Exploring the Biological Considerations of Human Health: Does Sex*

Matter?[15] The report underscored the importance of understanding sex and gender differences in health and disease across the life span and the myriad factors that influence such differences, from genetics to hormones to the environment. Yet, as expected, the study posed as many questions as it answered. The publication highlighted the need for additional research into both sex-based biology and gender-based medicine.

Gender Identity

Gender identity refers to an individual's personal, subjective sense of being male or female. Biological sex clearly influences gender indentity, which is determined by a complex set of variables; however, a person's gender identity is not necessarily consistent with his or her biological sex.

The genetic material in a fertilized egg is organized within structures known as chromosomes. Chromosomes give rise to the process of sexual differentiation, whereby an individual develops distinct physical male or female characteristics. The physical femaleness or maleness is not just a result of this chromosome mix, however, but rather the result of processes that occur at various levels of sexual differentiation. In early prenatal development, male and female external genitalia are undifferentiated and will remain so unless a specific gene on the Y chromosome involved in sex determination is present and is activated. This gene is necessary for the development of the testes, so it is involved in initiating the male sexing process. Through a series of complex interactions involving gonadal sex hormones, both the internal and the external sex structures differentiate into male or female genitalia. Because the external genitals, gonads, and some of the internal structures of males and females originate from the same embryonic tissues, it is not surprising that they have homologous, or corresponding, parts (**Figure 4.2**).

Scientists have found important structural and functional differences in the brains of males and females. The process of sex differentiation of human brains occurs largely, if not exclusively, during prenatal development. Sex differences in the brain and different sex hormones contribute to differences in processes such as thinking, remembering, language use, and ability to perceive spatial relationships. Other gender differences such as sensory perception and emotional responses may also affect sexual behavior. Clearly, these differences also can be significantly influenced by environmental factors and psychosocial factors. It is premature to suggest which factors play the most important role in determining these female–male differ-

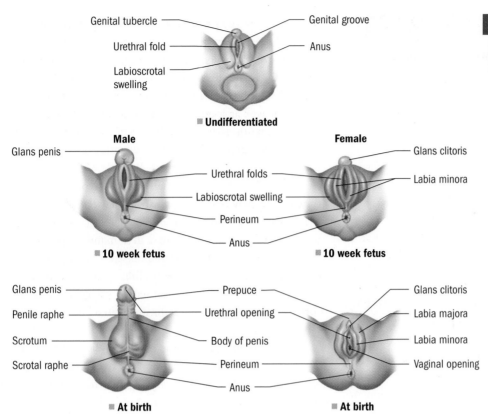

Figure 4.2

External genital differentiation: male and female.

ences. Some individuals experience considerable confusion and stress in their efforts to establish their gender identity.

Gender Roles

Gender role refers to the public expression of one's gender identity, as well as cultural expectations of male and female behaviors. Gender-role expectations are culturally defined and vary from society to society; they can also change as a culture develops.

Social-learning theory suggests that the identification with either feminine or masculine roles or a combination (androgyny) results primarily from the social and cultural models and influences to which the individual is exposed from birth. Parents typically dress boys and girls differently. Children grow up with toys specifically designed for their gender and receive reinforcement for gender-expected behaviors. At some point, most children develop a firm sense of being a girl or a boy, as well as a strong desire to adopt behaviors that are considered by society appropriate for their sex. Socialization refers to the process whereby society conveys behavioral expectations to the individual. Parents, peer groups, schools, textbooks, and the media frequently help develop and reinforce traditional gender-role assumptions and behaviors. Gender-role con-

ditioning affects all facets of an individual's life, perhaps most importantly in influencing sexuality.

Gender-role expectations and their resulting stereotypes have clearly influenced the ability of women to succeed in traditional male arenas such as sports and professional careers. Stereotyping also influences the sexual health and behavior of women, who naturally find conflict with assumptions and expectations that they be passive, submissive, dependent, emotional, and subordinate. Stereotypical expectations of men and women clearly influence gender-role expectations. These expectations actually hinder both men and women in maximizing their individual capabilities and in establishing fulfilling relationships. Despite the constraints associated with rigid, stereotypical gender roles, many men and women behave in a manner that is remarkably consistent with the norms that these roles establish (see **It's Your Health**).

I used to feel confused about what was feminine or what was masculine. I finally decided that it didn't matter. What mattered is what I wanted to do. I really enjoy nontraditional activities. That really does not make me less of a woman.

18-year-old student

Androgyny refers to having characteristics of both sexes. This term is often used to describe flexibility in gender roles. Androgynous individuals have integrated aspects of traditional masculinity and femininity into their lifestyles. Androgyny offers the option of expressing whatever behavior seems appropriate in a given situation instead of limiting responses to those traditionally considered gender appropriate. Androgynous individuals of both sexes are more likely to engage in behavior typically ascribed to the other sex than are gender-typed individuals.

Transgender

Transgender is an umbrella term that refers to anyone whose behaviors, thoughts, or traits differ from those traditionally ascribed to the person's sex. It is used to describe several groups of people who use other terms to self-identify, including transsexuals and cross-dressers. Like other people, transgender people can be straight, gay, lesbian, or bisexual. A transsexual is a person whose gender identity is opposite to her or his biological sex. A *transsexual* should not be confused with a transvestite, an individual who obtains sexual excitement from putting on clothes of the opposite sex. The American Psychiatric Association classifies transsexualism as a gender identity disorder (GID), a mental disorder characterized by strong and persistent cross-gender identification; however, significant controversy exists regarding the classification of transsexuality as a mental disorder.

Gender dysphoria is the overall psychological term used to describe negative or conflicting feelings about one's sex or gender roles. Almost all transgendered people suffer from some degree of gender dysphoria. **Transitioning** is the process in which transsexuals work to change their appearance and societal identity so as to match their gender identity. To acknowledge their transition, transsexuals self-identify as male to female (MTF) or female to male (FTM). Changes are often medical, via surgery and hormones, as well as legal, through name and sex changes on legal documents and forms of identification.

No clear understanding of the nature and causes of transsexualism has yet emerged. Possible explanations include both biological and social-learning hypotheses. Data support the view that transsexualism may reflect a form of brain hermaphroditism, meaning that structures in the brain are sexually differentiated in a manner opposite to the transsexual's genetic and genital sex.[16] As described by one transgender group, these findings propose "a medical model of transsexuality as an 'obscured' congenital intersex condition in which the genitalia are spared but the brain is not."[17]

Intersexuality refers to the sexual physiology of an individual. A person who is born intersexed is born with sex chromosomes, external genitalia, or internal reproductive organs that are not considered "standard" as male or female. This condition can be manifested as a girl without ovaries, a boy without testes, or a child with genitalia that may appear as neither a vagina nor a penis.

Health care is a major challenge for transgender and intersex individuals. The research describing their health-care needs is in its infancy, and much remains to be done to design effective medical and mental health programs and interventions.[18] For intersex individuals, recent activism has drawn attention to harmful childhood surgeries performed to "assign" a sex to an infant.

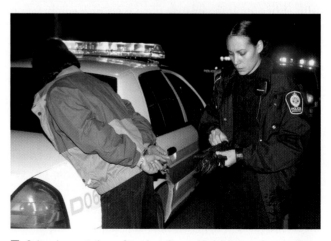

■ Cultural expectations of gender roles and behaviors evolve over time.

Sexual Orientation

Sexual orientation refers to a person's erotic, romantic, and affectional attraction to people of the same sex, to the opposite sex, or to both sexes. **Homosexual** orientation is attraction to same-sex partners, and **heterosexual** orientation is attraction to other-sex partners. A **bisexual** person is attracted to both sexes.

Although these concepts imply a clear distinction between the terms, the actual delineation is not always so precise. Kinsey described a seven-point continuum that ranged from exclusive contact with and attraction to the other sex to varying degrees of heterosexual and homosexual orientation.[7,8] Although Kinsey's methodology and conclusions have been criticized, the continuum of orientation provides a model for understanding differences in sexual orientation in society. The presumption that most people are heterosexual and the idea that heterosexuality and homosexuality represent sharply distinct behaviors are inconsistent with the complex, often unpredictable arena of human behavior.

A homosexual is defined as a person whose primary erotic, psychological, emotional, and social interest is in a member of the same sex. *Gay* is another word often used to describe homosexual men or women as well as social and political concerns related to homosexual orientation.

Homosexual women are often referred to as *lesbians.* There is no profile that fits all lesbian women. Lesbians are of varied socioeconomic status and ethnicity. They may be single, married, divorced, teenagers, middle-aged, or seniors. Many self-identified lesbians exhibit a variety of sexual practices, including heterosexual and bisexual activity. Many misconceptions exist about lesbian sexual expression

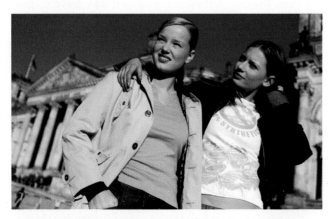

■ There is no profile of a lesbian woman. Lesbians may be teenagers, middle-aged, or seniors and of varied socioeconomic status and ethnicity.

I am a lesbian. I am still "in the closet." I would like to be more open about my identity, but I am afraid. I hear jokes and comments about homosexuals that really hurt me. I am continually confronted with misunderstandings and fear about homosexuality. If I could erase anything in this world, it would be homophobia.

27-year-old woman

and lifestyles. The extent to which a lesbian decides to be secretive or open about her sexual orientation has a significant effect on her lifestyle. There are various degrees of being "in the closet" and several steps in the process of "coming out." These steps are usually incremental and include self-acknowledgment, self-acceptance, and disclosure. These steps are particularly difficult because of homophobia.

Homophobia, an irrational fear or hatred of homosexuality, leads to many problems, including discrimination in medical care.[19] Misconceptions about health needs also present with health-care providers and patients. For example, many health-care providers, as well as women who identify themselves as lesbians, believe that lesbians are not at risk for sexually transmitted infections, gynecological infections, or cancers, and therefore do not require contraception education, regular cervical cancer screening, or pelvic exams. Some health-care providers do not address the issue of sexual orientation and assume that any sexually active woman of reproductive age should practice methods of birth control to prevent pregnancy. After encountering physicians who either ignore the facts or respond negatively, many lesbians hesitate to disclose their sexual orientation or even to visit a health-care practitioner regularly. Better awareness and training among health-care providers would allow lesbians to receive better preventive services, health care, and health education.[20]

Biological Basis of Sexual Health

Female Sexual Anatomy and Physiology

External Structures

Unfortunately, many women not only harbor misconceptions about their bodies, but also are unfamiliar with their own genitalia. Gaining knowledge and understanding of how her body functions and performs is an important aspect of a woman's sexual health and well-being. One way

Gender Dimensions

Role Conflict

Researchers continue to study role-conflict issues and challenges for women. Over the past 30 years, many women have assumed traditional male roles in the workplace, often becoming the primary breadwinners for their families; others have proven their abilities to succeed in historic male bastions such as athletics. The migration of women into these traditional male environments has been largely studied from the perspectives, needs, issues, and challenges of working women. Researchers are appreciating now that women's intrusion into these domains has created significant disruption and confusion for many men.

Men with deeply entrenched expectations of gender roles for themselves are most affected. Traditional career men have more conservative gender role attitudes for themselves and for women. They are more likely than other men to believe in traditional masculine ideol-

ogy. As a result, they are more likely to experience gender role conflict with their female colleagues, friends, and sometimes their partners. Adherence to traditional gender roles and the societal pressure to conform can lead to high levels of internal conflict and conflict with others.

A "traditional male ideology" typically includes three core beliefs. First, a man's work is the measure of his masculinity. Second, male power, control, and competition are the way to success and respect. Third, intimacy should be avoided. The more that men embrace these concepts, the greater their potential for gender-role conflict, and resultant stress and negative feelings, when females enter the workplace or assume positions of power.

Further research into the understanding of gender role attitudes and beliefs will be essential to successfully integrate men and women into the work environment.

to begin understanding female sexual anatomy is to examine the vaginal area with a mirror.

All women have the same genital structures, but there are individual variances in terms of color, shapes, and textures (**Figure 4.3**). The **vulva** encompasses all the female external genital structures, including the pubic hair, folds of skin, and urinary and vaginal openings. The **mons veneris,** or "mound of Venus," is the area covering the pubic bone. It consists of pads of fatty tissue between the bone and the skin. Numerous nerve endings in this area are responsible for the pleasure sensations from touch and pressure. At puberty, the mons becomes covered with pubic hair that varies in color, texture, and thickness.

The **labia majora** consist of the outer lips that extend downward from the mons and extend toward each side of the vulva. The color of the labia majora is usually darker than the color of the thighs. The nerve endings and underlying fatty tissue are similar to those in the mons. The **labia minora,** or inner lips, are located within the outer lips and often protrude between them.

The **clitoris** consists of an external shaft and glans and parts known as internal crura; its function is sexual arousal. The shaft and glans of the clitoris are located just below the mons area, where the inner lips converge. They are covered by the clitoral hood, or prepuce. Initially, it may be easier for a woman to locate her clitoris by touch rather than by sight or location because of its sensitive nerve endings and small size. The external part of the clitoris, although tiny, has about the same number of nerve endings as the head of the penis.

The vestibule is the area of the vulva inside the labia minora. It is rich in blood vessels and nerve endings. Its tissues are also sensitive to touch. Both the urinary and the vaginal openings are located within the vestibule.

The urinary opening is also called the urethral opening. Urine collected in the bladder passes out through the body via this opening. The **urethra** is the short tube connecting the bladder to the urinary opening, located between the clitoris and the vaginal opening.

The vaginal opening, known as the introitus, is located between the urinary opening and the anus. The **hymen,** a thin piece of tissue, partially covers the introitus. It is typically present at birth and usually remains intact until first penetration, although the vaginal opening is partially open and flexible enough to insert tampons before the hymen has been broken. Although the hymen may serve to protect the vaginal tissues early in life, it has no other known function. Nevertheless, many cultures have traditionally placed great significance on its presence or absence. A common misconception is that a woman's virginity can be proved or disproved by the pain or bleeding that may occur with initial coitus. Although discomfort and spotting sometimes occur with first coitus, the hymen can be partial, flexible, or thin enough for there to be no discomfort or bleeding. This very sensitive tissue also may stretch or break while performing activities such as bike riding, horseback riding, and gymnastics.

The **perineum** refers to the area of smooth skin between the vaginal opening and the anus. This tissue is rich with nerve endings and very sensitive to touch.

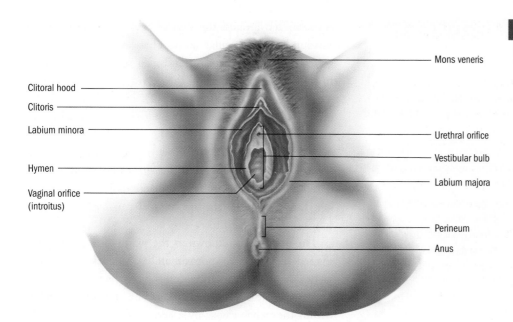

Figure 4.3

External female sexual anatomy.

Mons veneris

Clitoral hood

Clitoris

Labium minora

Urethral orifice

Vestibular bulb

Hymen

Labium majora

Vaginal orifice
(introitus)

Perineum

Anus

Internal Structures

Several structures lie along the vaginal opening. The vestibule refers to the area of the vulva inside the labia minora. The vaginal walls are lined with a vast network of bulbs and vessels that engorge with blood during sexual arousal. The vestibular bulbs alongside the vagina also fill with blood during sexual excitement, causing the vagina to increase in length and the vulvar area to become swollen. These bulbs are similar in structure and function to the tissue in the penis that engorges with blood during male sexual arousal and causes penile erection.

The **Bartholin's glands** are located on each side of the vaginal opening. They secrete a liquid that lubricates the tissues at the vaginal opening. The glands are usually not noticeable. Occasionally, the duct from the gland becomes blocked and enlargement results. Medical intervention may be indicated if the condition does not subside within a few days.

In addition to the glands, a complex musculature underlies the genital area. The pelvic floor muscles have a multidirectional design (**Figure 4.4**) that permits the vaginal opening to expand during childbirth and to contract after delivery. These muscles can lose muscle tone during childbirth or over time. A series of exercises known as **Kegel exercises** can help restore the muscular tone, reduce involuntary urinary incontinence, and enhance sexual sensations (see **It's Your Health**).

Internal female sexual anatomy consists of the vagina, cervix, uterus, fallopian tubes, and ovaries (**Figure 4.5**). The **vagina** opens between the labia minora and extends

upward into the body, angling toward the lower back. The vagina is approximately 3 to 5 inches in length when not aroused. The folded walls of the vagina are known as rugae and form a flat tube. These walls are warm, soft, and moist, and they normally produce secretions that help maintain the chemical balance of the vagina.

The vagina consists of three layers of tissue—mucous, muscle, and fibrous tissue—all of which are richly endowed with blood vessels. The mucosa is a layer of moist membrane inside the vagina. During sexual arousal, lubricating fluid exudes through the mucosa. The muscular tissue is

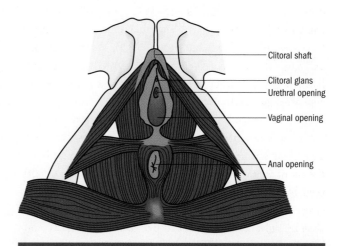

Clitoral shaft

Clitoral glans
Urethral opening

Vaginal opening

Anal opening

Figure 4.4

Pelvic floor muscles.

It's Your Health

Kegel Exercises

To identify the pelvic floor muscles:

1. Try stopping a flow of urine in midstream while urinating. The muscles that are tightened in this effort are the muscles of the pelvic floor.

2. Tighten the ring of muscles around the rectum, as if trying to stop a bowel movement. The muscles that are tightened in this effort are also muscles of the pelvic floor.

3. While lying down, place a hand over the abdomen. Tighten all of the muscles of the abdomen and pelvis. Notice that the hand will move. These are *not* muscles of the pelvic floor, and they should be relaxed during Kegel exercises. During the first few practice sessions, it is helpful to check with a hand to make sure that the abdominal muscles are relaxed.

To practice Kegel exercises:

1. Take deep breaths—do not forget to breathe.

2. Tighten the anal muscle, pulling inward and outward.

3. Tighten the vaginal muscle, pulling inward and outward.

4. Hold these muscles tight, counting slowly to 10, and then relax.

Do Kegel exercises in sets of 5 to 10 at a time, several times a day. Build up to being able to hold the contraction for 20 seconds at a time.

concentrated around the vaginal opening. Fibrous tissue surrounds the muscular layer. This layer aids in vaginal contraction and expansion and also serves as connective tissue to other structures in the pelvic cavity.

The **cervix**, located at the back of the vagina, is the mouth of the uterus and actually looks like a small, pink, glazed doughnut. Glands line the cervical canal and produce a constant downward flow of mucus to protect the uterine cavity from bacterial invasion. The cervix is composed of fibrous tissue that is capable of dramatic stretching. During childbirth, the cervical canal is 50 or more times its normal width.

The **uterus**, also known as the womb, is a thick, pear-shaped organ. It is approximately 3 inches long and 2 inches wide in a woman who has never had a child. After a pregnancy, it is somewhat larger. The uterus is suspended within the pelvic cavity by a series of six ligaments. The alignment of these ligaments permits some movement of the uterus within the cavity.

The uterine wall consists of three layers: the endometrium, the myometrium, and the perimetrium. The endometrium is the lining of the uterus, which, in preparation for fertilization, thickens in response to hormone changes during the monthly menstrual cycle. In addition, the endometrium is a source of hormone production. The

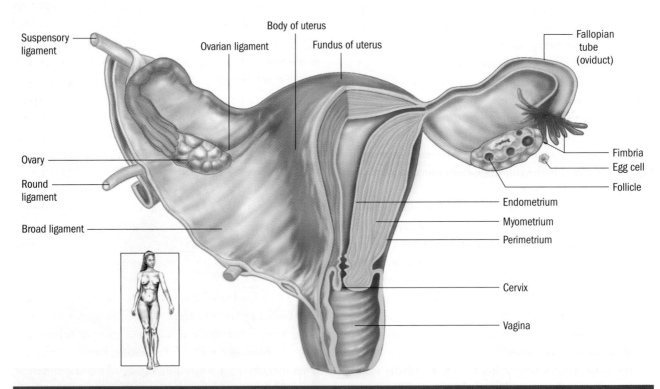

Figure 4.5

Internal female sexual anatomy.

myometrium, the middle layer, consists of the longitudinal and circular muscle fibers of the uterus. The muscle fibers are interwoven and enable the uterus to expand during pregnancy and contract during labor and childbirth. The myometrium is covered by a thin membrane known as the perimetrium. The perimetrium functions as the external surface of the uterus.

The **fallopian tubes**, which are thin, pale, pink filaments, connect the uterus with the ovaries. The outside end of each tube is like a funnel, with fingerlike projections called fimbriae that draw the egg from the ovary into the tube. The **ovaries** are located at the end of the fallopian tubes and are about the size of a small walnut in premenopausal women. The ovaries are endocrine glands that produce two classes of sex hormones: estrogens and progesterones. The estrogens influence the development of female physical sex characteristics and help regulate the menstrual cycle. The progesterones help regulate the menstrual cycle and stimulate development of the uterine lining in preparation for pregnancy. During puberty, these hormones play a critical role in the maturation of the reproductive organs and the development of secondary sex characteristics, such as pubic hair and breasts.

The Menstrual Cycle

Women usually begin to menstruate in their early teens. During the **menstrual cycle**, the body prepares the uterine lining for implantation of a fertilized egg. If **conception** does not occur, the lining sloughs off and is discharged as menstrual flow. This menstrual discharge consists of blood, mucus, and endometrial membranes that sometimes present as small clots. The amount of menstrual flow varies, but is usually 6 to 8 ounces in volume per cycle (about half a can of soda). The cycle is often 28 days in length but can vary from 21 to 40 days.

The menstrual cycle is regulated by a complex series of interactions between the hypothalamus and the pituitary gland in the brain, the adrenal glands on top of the kidneys, the ovaries, and the uterus. The hypothalamus produces and secretes hormones and releasing factors that act directly on the pituitary gland. One such releasing factor, gonadotropin-releasing hormone (GnRH), is responsible for reproductive hormone control. GnRH varies in amount and frequency during each menstrual cycle. In addition, this hormone plays a role in the timing of puberty. Alterations in the GnRH pulse release may be the mechanism by which stressors such as athletic training or dieting influence menstrual cycles.

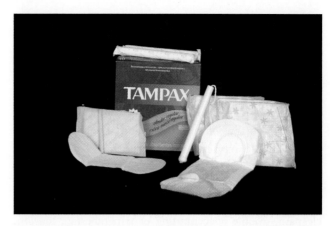

A wide variety of products are available for use during menustration, including many different styles, sizes, and absorbencies of sanitary napkins or pads, tampons, and menstrual cups.

The menstrual cycle is a self-regulating and dynamic process in which the level of a particular hormone impedes or increases the production of the same and other hormones.

Problems with Menstruation

For most women, menstruation creates no medical problems, but some women experience certain physical and emotional difficulties. **Dysmenorrhea**, meaning "painful menstrual flow," is a term for what most women call "cramps." It may be caused by the normal production of prostaglandins that produce strong contractions of the uterus (primary dysmenorrhea) or by problems in the uterus, fallopian tubes, or ovaries (secondary dysmenorrhea). Women with primary dysmenorrhea experience pain in the lower abdomen and back, whereas those with secondary dysmenorrhea often feel pain during urination and bowel movements. Relief from primary dysmenorrhea may be found through regular aerobic exercise, stress reduction techniques, adequate sleep, and decreased fat, caffeine, and sodium in the diet. Some women with primary or secondary dysmenorrhea may need anti-inflammatory medications or oral contraceptives to relieve the pain. Secondary dysmenorrhea is treated based on the underlying condition.

Premenstrual syndrome (PMS) is a group of symptoms linked to the menstrual cycle. PMS symptoms occur in the week or two weeks before the menstrual period, and they usually dissipate after menstruation starts. PMS can affect menstruating women of any age. It is also different for each woman. Most women of reproductive age have some physical discomfort, but about 5–8% of women suffer from severe premenstrual syndrome, where symptoms interfere with daily activities.[21] Although the root causes of PMS are not known, PMS is clearly linked to changing hormones during the menstrual cycle. Stress and emotional problems do not seem to cause PMS, but they may make it worse.

Diagnosis of PMS is usually based on a woman's specific symptoms, when they occur, and how much they affect her life. Symptoms include acne, breast swelling and tenderness, feeling tired, having trouble sleeping, upset stomach, bloating, constipation or diarrhea, headache or backache, appetite changes or food cravings, joint or muscle pain, trouble concentrating or remembering, tension, irritability, mood swings, crying spells, anxiety, and depression. Tracking the severity of these premenstrual problems daily on a calendar can assist clinicians with diagnosing PMS.[22]

PMS is more likely to present in women who are between their late 20s and early 40s, have at least one child, and have a family history of depression or a history of either postpartum depression or a mood disorder. Research also suggests that cigarette smoking, especially in adolescence and young adulthood, may increase the risk of moderate to severe PMS.[23]

A single universal treatment is not yet available for PMS. Experts recommend basic health measures such as a nutritious diet, getting adequate sleep, daily exercise, a daily multivitamin that includes 400 micrograms of folic acid, a calcium supplement with vitamin D, and cessation of cigarette smoking to reduce PMS symptoms. (All of these measures are also excellent steps for improving general health.) Over-the-counter pain relievers such as ibuprofen, aspirin, or naproxen may ease cramps, headaches, backaches, and breast tenderness. In more severe cases of PMS, prescription medicines can ease symptoms. One approach has been to use drugs such as birth control pills to stop ovulation from occurring. Women on the pill report fewer PMS symptoms, such as cramps and headaches, as well as lighter periods. Further research is needed to ascertain the efficacy of this approach.[24]

Premenstrual dysphoric disorder (PMDD) is a severe form of PMS. The condition can be disabling with emotional symptoms such as intense sadness, despair, tension, anxiety, mood swings, irritability, anger, and physical symptoms consistent with PMS. There is evidence that a brain chemical called serotonin plays a role in PMDD. Studies have found continuous dosing regimens of selective serotonin reuptake inhibitors (SSRIs) to be effective in treating these symptoms.[25] Studies also suggest that cognitive behavioral therapy in the forms of individual counsel-

ing, group counseling, and stress management may also help relieve symptoms.[26]

Amenorrhea is the lack of menstrual flow. Primary amenorrhea occurs in women who have not yet begun menstruation and may result from hormone-related problems or extremely low body fat. Secondary amenorrhea is the lack of blood flow for three or more consecutive months, except during pregnancy, breastfeeding, and perimenopause; it may result from conditions such as anorexia nervosa, ovarian cysts or tumors, substance abuse, stress, or use of oral contraceptives. Health-care providers will want to work with a woman to first establish the cause of her amenorrhea and then consider options for treatment.

Physical Health and the Gynecological Examination

A gynecological examination usually begins with a medical history and a general physical examination, including a breast examination, and is followed by a pelvic examination. The pelvic exam provides the woman and her clinician with essential basic information about her gynecological health. It should be timed to avoid the menstrual period. It is also advisable to avoid douching at least 24 hours before an examination; some clinicians recommend avoiding vaginal intercourse for at least 48 hours before the examination as well. These precautions ensure a more accurate visualization of the cervix and greater likelihood of diagnosing an infection if it is present.

For the pelvic exam, the woman lies on her back with her bottom at the very end of the examining table and her legs supported in foot stirrups. The pelvic examination consists of three phases:

- The first phase is the external examination, in which the clinician inspects the vulva and perineum visually for any evidence of infection or injury.
- The second phase involves the use of a speculum, a device that holds the vaginal walls apart to permit visual inspection of the cervix. The speculum is inserted with the blade closed. Once inside the vagina, the blades are opened and locked into place at the correct width.

■ The speculum permits visual examination of the vagina and cervix during a gynecological visit.

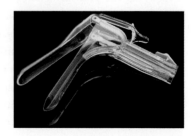

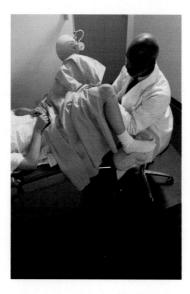

■ The pelvic examination is an important part of a woman's health visit.

With the speculum open, the clinician inspects the vaginal walls and cervix for any redness, irritation, unusual discharge, or lesions. Specimens for laboratory tests are collected while the speculum is in place. After the specimens are collected, the speculum is removed.

■ The third phase of the examination is the bimanual examination, which involves the insertion of two gloved fingers of one hand into the vagina while the other hand presses downward on the abdomen. The purpose of this activity is to locate and feel the size, consistency, and shape of the uterus and ovaries and to check for any abdominal masses or tender areas.

A rectal examination also may be performed to evaluate the muscular wall separating the rectum and vagina, the position of the uterus, and any possible masses or tenderness in the area.

A pelvic examination takes only a few minutes, and it provides a starting point to ascertain any gynecological or sexual health concerns. Pelvic examinations should be arranged at regular intervals throughout a woman's adult life (see **It's Your Health**).

Sexual Arousal and Sexual Response

Sexual arousal and response are highly individualized physical, emotional, and mental processes. The female sexual response is not a geographically isolated phenomenon of the vaginal area. Instead, the brain, senses, and hormones all play an integrated role in the response cycle.

The brain plays an important role in sexual arousal by mediating thoughts, emotions, and fantasies that provide the psychological "stage" for the sexual experience. Hearing, touch, smell, sight, and taste provide stimuli that can significantly influence the level of sexual arousal. In addition to performing their primary role of regulating the menstrual cycle, hormones also play a role in sexual arousal. The function of certain hormones in the sexual response cycle—specifically, estrogens and androgens—has been studied extensively for many years. Estrogens promote cell growth and replication in the vaginal cells, increase blood flow in the vagina and urethra, and maintain vaginal lubrication in postmenopausal women. Androgens affect the brain by influencing sexual behavior and libido. Data are conflicting, however, regarding the role of androgens for improving libido and well-being in postmenopausal women.[27] Additional studies are needed to determine the specific roles of estrogen and androgen and the effects of estrogen–androgen therapy on a woman's health.

The sexual response cycle has been described in several ways, most notably by Masters and Johnson.[9] This cycle represents only a composite of many possible physiological reactions; from person to person there can be tremendous variability and differences in sexual response. Masters and Johnson reported three variations among women in the sexual response cycle, as shown in **Figure 4.6**. Pattern #1 demonstrates that some women are able to have one or

Figure 4.6

Female sexual response cycle.

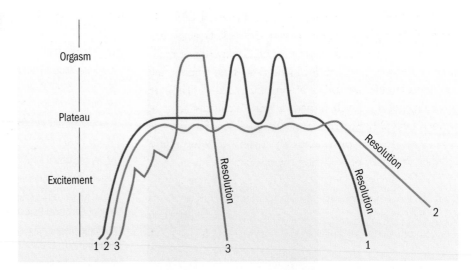

more orgasms without dropping below the plateau level of sexual arousal. Pattern #2, a variation of this response, includes an extended plateau with no orgasm. Pattern #3, which most closely resembles the typical male cycle, describes a rapid rise to orgasm with no definitive plateau and a quick resolution.

Each pattern distinguishes four phases: excitement, plateau, orgasm, and resolution. In the excitement phase of the female sexual response cycle, the clitoris swells with blood engorgement. This change ranges from very slight to quite noticeable. The clitoral glans is highly sensitive. Some women find that the entire sexual response cycle can be set into motion and maintained to orgasm by light stimulation of the glans alone. The glans is so sensitive that women usually stimulate the area with the hood covering the clitoris to avoid direct stimulation. In addition to clitoral swelling, the labia majora flatten and separate during the excitement phase. The labia minora increase in size, and lubrication begins.

Lubrication is a unique feature of the vagina and an important aspect of sexual arousal. It is often the first physiological sign of sexual arousal in women. Vaginal lubrication serves two primary functions. First, it enhances the possibility of conception by helping to alkalinize the normally acidic vaginal chemical balance. Sperm are able to move faster and survive longer in an alkaline environment. Second, vaginal lubrication helps to increase sexual pleasure.

Also during the excitement phase, the uterus elevates and becomes engorged with blood, and the breasts enlarge. Superficial veins in breast tissues may become more visible during this time.

During the plateau phase of the female sexual response cycle, the clitoris withdraws under its hood and shortens in length. The labia majora remain unchanged from the ex-

citement phase, while the labia minora intensify in color. An orgasmic platform develops from further vasocongestion of the outer third of the vagina. Lubrication from the vagina slows, and the uterus is fully elevated in position. Breast tissue remains swollen.

As effective stimulation occurs, many women move from the plateau phase to the orgasmic phase of the sexual response cycle. In contrast to men, who almost always experience orgasm after reaching the plateau level, women may obtain plateau levels without the orgasmic release. Many women cannot reach orgasm by penis insertion alone, and therefore prefer other forms of stimulation in addition to coital stimulation. The "G" spot, or Grafenberg spot, has been identified as a sensitive area that can lead to orgasm when stimulated. Orgasm is the shortest phase of the sexual response cycle, although female orgasms often last slightly longer than male orgasms. Orgasmic experiences vary widely in intensity, frequency, and duration among both men and women. The female physiological responses in the orgasmic phase include an elevated blood pressure, heart rate, and breathing pattern. Orgasmic platform contractions are rhythmical, beginning at high intensity and then becoming weaker and slower. The uterus usually contracts at orgasm. These physiological responses are consistent whether they originate from direct clitoral stimulation or from coital stimulation, although women report wide differences in subjective feelings and preferences.[10,12]

The resolution phase is the final phase of the sexual response cycle. During this phase, the sexual systems return to the nonexcited state. If no additional stimulation occurs, the resolution begins immediately after orgasm. Skin coloration quickly subsides, and vital signs return to normal levels. The clitoris, labia majora, and labia minora return to their unaroused sizes and positions.

A significant male–female response difference occurs in the resolution period. After orgasm, the male typically enters a refractory period—a time when no amount of additional stimulation will result in orgasm. This time period has considerable variability among men and depends on physiological and psychological factors. In contrast to men, women generally experience no comparable refractory period. Thus they are physiologically capable of returning to another orgasmic peak during the resolution phase.

The female sexual response cycle described here is simply a framework for understanding the physiological events of sexual response. Sexual response cycles of individual women can vary considerably from these models.

Forms of Sexual Expression

Society has traditionally placed restrictions on the "appropriate" forms of sexual expression. Missionary (vaginal intercourse with the male on top of the female) heterosexual sex is only one of many sexual expression options. Women may elect different forms of sexual expression under different circumstances or at different times in their lives.

Masturbation refers to erotic self-stimulation, usually to the point of orgasm. Historical records indicate that both genders have engaged in masturbation since ancient times. Masturbation practices begin early in life with infants exploring their genitals and receiving pleasure from touching them. Often self-stimulation continues throughout life, whether or not the individual is a partner in an intimate relationship. Studies vary greatly regarding masturbation statistics, although all studies show that this practice is more common in males than females.

Even though masturbation is widespread, many women feel ashamed or embarrassed about the practice. Folklore has falsely labeled masturbation as sinful, evil, and even physically or mentally harmful. Such ideas are entirely false, and many therapists and sex experts believe that masturbation can be helpful as a sexual outlet and as a means to become comfortable with one's own body.

Petting is defined as erotic stimulation of a person by a sexual partner, without actual sexual intercourse. It can include kisses, genital caresses, and oral-genital contact. Petting may culminate in orgasm. During adolescence, petting is often a way to experience intense sexual excitement without actually engaging in intercourse. Petting is carried over into adult sexual experiences as foreplay or for sexual variety.

Oral-genital stimulation, also known as oral sex, takes two basic forms. **Cunnilingus** is the act of sucking or licking the vulva, particularly the clitoris. **Fellatio** is the act of

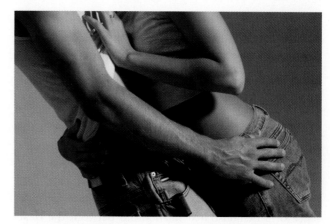

■ During adolescence, petting is a way to experience intense sexual excitement.

sucking or licking the penis and scrotum. A common sexual practice among both heterosexual and homosexual couples, oral sex is often believed to be a "safe" sexual activity. Sexually transmitted infections such as genital herpes, human papillomavirus, gonorrhea, and HIV all can be transmitted through oral-genital sex.[28]

Anal intercourse is another form of sexual expression. Because the anal opening is richly endowed with nerves, this area can be very sensitive and sexually arousing. A couple needs to be careful, however, in performing anal intercourse for many reasons. The anal sphincter tends to be tight and when stimulated can tighten even more, resulting in pain on penetration. In addition, the anal region has no natural lubrication of its own, which increases the possibility of both pain and injury. Usually anal intercourse can be accomplished without discomfort if precautions are taken. A water-based lubricant (not petroleum-based products, which weaken condoms) should be used. Care should be taken to avoid contamination of the vaginal area once anal penetration has occurred. It must be emphasized that anal intercourse is not without risks. This kind of sexual activity has been associated with the transmission of sexually transmitted infections, including HIV. Anyone engaging in anal intercourse should use a latex condom and never use a petroleum-based lubricant. In addition, after anal penetration, the genitals should be washed thoroughly before resuming vaginal or oral sex.

Sexual Dysfunction

Sexual dysfunction is defined as the inability of an individual to function adequately in terms of sexual arousal, orgasm, or in coital situations. A recent national survey found about 40% of U.S. women report sexual problems, but only about 12% are distressed about it.[29] Older women experienced both the highest prevalence of sexual dysfunction and a reduced level of associated distress. The most distress occurred at mid-life; younger women had the lowest prevalence of problems and associated distress.[29]

The medical and scientific community once classified women's sexual problems under the general label of "frigidity." These problems were severely misunderstood and thought to be symptomatic of a neurosis or some other psychological disorder that required long-term psychiatric therapy. This traditional approach persisted despite the absence of a demonstrated relationship between the treatment and the alleviation of the sexual problem. More recently, however, the pharmaceutical industry has become more interested in understanding and treating female sexual problems with the hopes of uncovering a new market as lucrative as that for male-targeted medications such as Viagra.

Today, four major areas of sexual dysfunction are defined for women: sexual desire disorders, sexual arousal disorders, orgasmic disorders, and sexual pain disorders. Treatments for each of these conditions require an understanding of the complex relationships between physiological and psychological considerations. Any form of sexual dysfunction or discomfort with intercourse or sexual stimulation should be evaluated to rule out any underlying pathology (see **Self-Assessment 4.1**). In addition, the evaluation should include efforts such as counseling or therapy, if needed, to seek resolution of the condition.

Sex Therapy

Professional help may be indicated in cases where individualized efforts, couple efforts, or both do not produce the desired effects. Sex therapy has evolved as a legitimate method for understanding sexual problems and increasing sexual satisfaction. In many cases, communication about sexual issues and finding ways to solve problems are critical but often difficult steps toward achieving a satisfying

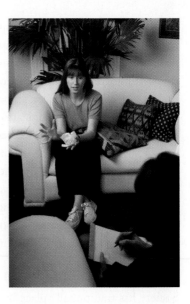

■ A trained counselor or clinician can often provide valuable assistance for a woman who is experiencing sexual dysfunction.

sex life. Sex therapy often can make such communication easier. Strategies with a therapist may range from expanding self-knowledge to sharing more effectively with a partner.

Therapy can also benefit individuals or couples by providing them with information. By providing specific accurate and reassuring information, a therapist is often able to address thoughts and feelings that may be interfering with the person's ability to enjoy or respond to sexual activity. A therapist is also able to provide specific activities or homework "assignments" that enable the client to reduce anxiety, enhance communication, and learn new sexually enhancing behavioral techniques. Intensive therapy may be indicated in some situations in which personal emotional difficulties or significant relationship problems interfere with sexual expression.

I used to fake orgasms. I am not sure why, but somehow I felt it was necessary. My current partner figured it out, and we have spent a lot of time talking about this. I am seeing a therapist. With a few sessions, I was able to climax with masturbation, and I know that I am much more comfortable with my sexuality. I know that "faking it" was not fair to me or my partner.

35-year-old woman

Self-Assessment 4.1

Self-Evaluation for Sexual Dysfunction

1. Do you experience pain or discomfort during intercourse?
2. Do you lack interest in or desire for sex?
3. Do you feel anxious when you begin to engage in sexual activity?
4. Do you lack pleasure when sexually stimulated?
5. Do you have difficulty achieving orgasm?

Answering yes to one or more of these questions may signify a sexual problem. Communication with one's partner may help resolve some of the issues. If not, women should seek medical attention to rule out any underlying causes and consider therapy to address ways to enhance sexual satisfaction.

Sexuality Through the Life Span

In many Western societies, childhood has traditionally been seen as a time of unexpressed sexuality and behavior, and adolescence has been viewed as a time to restrain immature sexual drives. The opinion that adolescent sexual behavior should be curtailed or restricted receives considerable support from multiple sectors of U.S. society. However, current evidence suggests that sexuality and sexual capacity are not "awakenings" that suddenly appear at a definitive time in development, but rather that both male and female infants are born with the capacity for sexual pleasure and response.

Childhood

Individuals experience considerable variation in sexual development during childhood and adolescence. The pleasures of genital stimulation are generally discovered in the first few years of life. Besides self-stimulation, prepubescent children often engage in play that may be viewed as sexual in nature. The activities may range from exhibition and inspection to simulating intercourse by rubbing genital regions together. Both natural childhood curiosity and curiosity about what is forbidden probably play a role in these behaviors. As children get older, they become more keenly aware of and interested in body changes, particularly those involving the genitals and secondary sex characteristics.

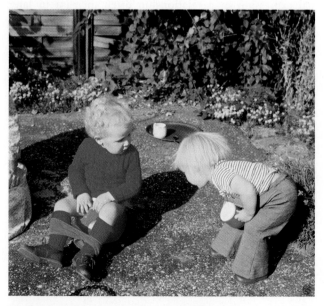

■ Children are innately interested in their bodies.

Adolescence

Adolescence, the period from about 12 to 19 years of age, is the most dramatic stage for physiological changes and social-role development. The first few years of adolescence are known as puberty, and this is a time of dramatic physiological change. Over the past 20 years, the average age of puberty appears to have decreased, with some girls seeing physical changes as young as the age of seven.[30] The onset of puberty generally occurs two years earlier in girls than in boys. Secondary sex characteristics appear at this time in response to higher levels of hormones. In females, estrogen levels result in pubic hair growth and breast budding. African American females seem to experience puberty earlier than white adolescents. Obesity appears to influence earlier onset, although researchers caution other genetic or environmental factors also appear to be important.[31]

Hormone stimulation during adolescence causes addtional internal changes. Vaginal walls gradually become thicker, and the uterus becomes larger and more muscular. The vaginal pH changes from alkaline to acidic as vaginal and cervical secretions increase in response to the changing hormone status. Eventually, menstruation begins. The first menstrual period is known as menarche. Initial menstrual cycles may be irregular and occur without ovulation. Most girls menstruate at about the age of 12 or 13, but there is considerable variation in this timing.[30,31]

The difficulties of adjusting to new physical characteristics pale in comparison to the psychological adjustments of adolescence. This period is characterized by evolving responsibilities and assimilation of societal expectations. In Western cultures, these expectations include inherent double standards for women. Sexual overtones are blasted through the media in everything from ads for jeans to magazine photos, to television shows, yet the message also prevails for young women to maintain their virginity. In contrast, the expectations for young men are more tolerant of experimentation and overt sexual behavior.

Young to Middle Adulthood

Both personal and cultural factors influence sexual behavior in adults. Several factors have contributed to a dramatic increase in single, sexually active adults over the past 50 years:

- The trend toward marriage at a later age
- An increase in the number of women who never marry
- More women placing career goals before marriage
- An increase in the number of cohabiting couples
- A rise in divorce rates

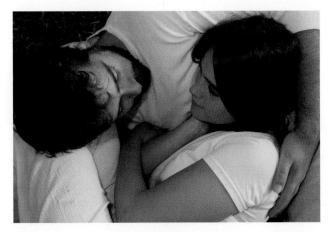

■ Communication contributes greatly to the satisfaction of an intimate relationship.

- A greater emphasis on advanced education
- An increase in the number of women who no longer must depend on marriage to ensure their economic stability

Sexual behavior is not always confined to marital arrangements. Instead, contemporary developments and changes in sexual mores and behavior of young adults are often discussed in the context of nonmarital, marital, or extramarital activities. An *extramarital relationship* describes the sexual interaction experienced by a married person with someone other than his or her spouse. Data evaluating these arrangements are incomplete and biased at best.

■ Many women are placing career goals before marriage.

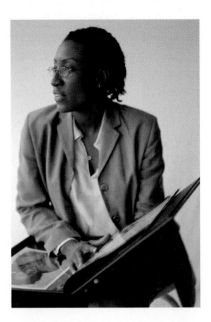

In the absence of data, it is difficult to draw conclusions about these arrangements.

Older Adulthood

The term **climacteric** refers to the physiological changes that occur during the transition period from female fertility to infertility. At about age 40, the ovaries begin to slow the production of estrogen and androgens. **Menopause**, one of the climacteric events, refers to the cessation of menstruation and generally occurs at about 45 to 55 years of age (see Chapter 8). The hormonal changes of menopause affect the sexual response of most women. In general, all phases of the response cycle continue at a decreased intensity. The depletion of hormones associated with menopause can result in several vaginal changes, including dryness, thinning of the walls, and delayed or absent lubrication during sexual excitement. For many women, hormone replacement therapy may help; however, it is not a solution for every woman (see Chapter 8). For some women, prescription estrogen creams applied directly to the vagina may help prevent dryness and thinning. Water-soluble lubricants and vaginal moisturizers can help solve problems related to dryness. Kegel exercises can help make sex more pleasurable by toning the pelvic floor muscles that support the bladder and uterus, which tend to relax as estrogen declines.

Although the general focus on sexual response in later years tends to highlight a decline in frequency and intensity of sexual activity, in fact the opportunities for sexual expression in a relationship often increase in later years, as pressures from work, children, and fulfilling life's goals may be reduced and more time becomes available for sharing with a partner. Couples may increasingly emphasize quality rather than quantity of sexual expression, and intimacy may find new and deeper dimensions in later years.

The perception that old age and sex are incompatible is totally erroneous. All too often, women dismiss sexual problems as a consequence of aging. In truth, most people can enjoy an active sex life no matter how old they are. This misconception about aging may have evolved for a number of reasons. The United States is still influenced by the philosophy that equates sexuality with procreation. For older people who are neither capable of nor interested in the reproductive facets of life, this viewpoint offers little sensitivity or insight into their personal needs. Society also sends the message via the media that love, sex, and ro-

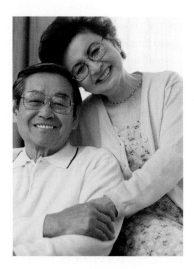

■ Sexuality is an important dimension of aging.

mance are only for the young and "sexy." The implicit message is that this scenario excludes older individuals.

A recent comprehensive national survey of seniors found that most people from the ages of 57 to 85 think of sexuality as an important part of their lives. The study also found that many older adults are sexually active and that sexual activity was closely related to overall health.[32] Societal expectations can complicate sexual communication with older adults. Elders who are single may meet with disapproval from their family and friends when dating or engaging in sexual relations. People in long-term care facilities may feel deprived of their right to privately engage in sexual behavior. Studies have found that sexual expression in older adults can provide relaxation, reassurance, and companionship and can also reduce depression and social isolation.[33]

Sexual Violence as a Public Health Problem

Sexual violence against women violates a woman's fundamental human rights and freedoms. Sexual violence can occur against young girls, women during midlife, and elderly women. The perpetrator is often someone the woman knows and can be a family member or friend, a respected member of the community, a colleague at work, or someone in a health facility or educational institution. Sexual violence can also occur in the highly organized and lucrative form of forced prostitution or trafficking.

Sexual Assault and Rape

Sexual assault and rape are crimes of aggression. **Sexual assault** often refers to forced sexual contact. **Rape** is usu-ally defined as an event occurring without consent, involving the use of force or the threat of force to sexually penetrate the victim's vagina, mouth, or rectum. Rape may occur among strangers or intimates; it can also happen in a marriage, during a legal separation, or after a divorce. In addition, rape can occur between people of the same sex. Women are disproportionately affected by such sexual violence. One out of every six U.S. women and 1 in 33 men will be sexually assaulted in their lifetimes. College women are four times more likely to be sexually assaulted. These numbers translate into someone in the United States being sexually assaulted every two minutes.[34]

Rape and sexual assault crimes occur throughout the world. In the United States, many women who are raped or assaulted blame themselves for the attacks. In some cultures, especially in countries where women have a low place in society, families blame the girl or woman who is raped. Every year, as many as 5,000 women and girls are murdered by members of their own families in honor killings, for the "dishonor" that the rape has brought to the family.[35] Chapter 14 provides more information on sexual violence, abuse, and harassment.

Female Genital Mutilation

Female genital mutilation (FGM) is also known as female circumcision and female genital cutting. The practice includes all procedures that involve partial or total removal of the external female genitalia, or other injury to the female genital organs for nonmedical reasons. The practice is usually performed on women by traditional circumcisers, who often play other central roles in communities, such as attending childbirths. Increasingly, however, FGM is performed by medically trained personnel. FGM is nearly always carried out on minors without their consent or under coercive pressures.[36]

These practices, which destroy or cripple a woman's ability to feel sexual pleasure, are usually performed for cultural or religious reasons. Girls or infants suffer short-term and long-term consequences, including infections and other conditions from lasting psychological harm to death. Globally, between 100 million and 130 million women have suffered FGM as young girls, and every year, an estimated 2 million girls are at risk in Africa, South and East Asia, and in parts of Europe, North America, and Australia. FGM is now illegal in the United States, but more than 100,000 women have undergone FGM or are currently at risk.[37]

Forced Sterilization

Forced sterilization, performed throughout the world for population control and eugenics (the Darwinian notion of producing a "perfect" race of humans), is a violent crime against the reproductive rights of both women and men. People targeted for surgeries may be poor and/or illiterate; they may suffer from alcoholism, chronic disease, or mental and physical challenges. In countries with high rates of poverty, forced sterilization is used to control population growth. Women are often bribed with payments of food, clothing, or money. Women also may be unknowingly sterilized during childbirth or other medical procedures. Forced sterilizations have occurred all over the world, including Nazi-run Germany, Sweden, Japan, Peru, and the United States.

■■■■
Informed Decision Making

Sexual well-being encompasses far more than sexual arousal and response. It includes effective decision making across the spectrum of issues affecting sexual health. A gynecological checkup is a good place to start for guidance in reproductive and sexual health matters, as well as preventive health screening. A woman can maximize the benefits of a gynecological examination by selecting a clinician who is sensitive to her needs. Often that means changing clinicians until the "right" one is found. Even so, it is better to "shop" while feeling well than to wait until a pressing medical problem requires immediate attention.

Understanding personal feelings, thoughts, and symptoms and articulating concerns and questions are essential for effective personal communication and preventive health. Communication is a critical component of promoting sexual health and responsible sexual behavior. Being able to talk about needs, feelings, concerns, and fears is an essential component of a healthy relationship. Sexual communication can contribute greatly to the satisfaction of an intimate relationship. Unfortunately, American language lacks a comfortable sexual vocabulary. Available language seems to be either "clinical" or "medical" in nature, which may be perceived as too cold and unfeeling, or "street language," which may be perceived as too crass or juvenile. Beyond the handicaps imposed by socialization and language limitations, difficulties in sexual communication may be rooted in fears of too much self-exposure. Any sexual communication involves a degree of risk and vulnerability to judgment, criticism, or rejection. The willingness to take risks may be related to the amount of trust that exists within a relationship.

Responsible sexual behavior is essential for promoting positive sexual health. Children look to their parents as a first resource; a healthy, loving, committed relationship can serve as a blueprint for children. Although communication between parents and children can be helpful, many parents find it difficult to discuss sexual health issues. Some parents are unsure of their own knowledge about sexual health and therefore they may not benefit the child by sharing their own experiences and information.

As girls grow up, they begin picking up information from television, movies, books, magazines, and friends. Although this is a natural behavior, parents should maintain an open dialogue with their children to ensure that they continue to learn facts and not myths. Although television and radio often suggest sexual behavior, the media typically depict sexual behavior in short-lived romances without the use of contraception. According to the Institute of Medicine's publication *No Time to Lose*, "The Code of Silence has resulted in missed opportunities to use the mass media to encourage healthy sexual behavior."[38] It is important to realize that sexual relationships should include negotiation and communication skills, safe sex practices, and healthy and positive relationships.

Health-care providers also can be a good source of information for adolescent girls and women. It is critical for women to articulate the reason for their doctors' visits and to address specific questions or concerns. Clinicians will not necessarily ask a standard set of questions or ascertain by examination the nature of a sexual concern or automatically detect an underlying fear or anxiety. Insisting that all questions be answered and persisting when answers are not clear are equally important avenues for maximizing the effectiveness of the visit. Women are often eager to please their health-care providers and will nod as if understanding when in actuality they do not. This behavior results in more confusion and an increased likelihood of problems. Many women find it helpful to write down their questions and concerns and deal with them one by one with the clinician in the office before clothes are removed and the examination begins. Unfortunately, many health-care providers do not address important topics regarding sexual health and appear uncomfortable when questions are asked of them. Health-care providers need to find ways to broach the subject in a respectful, culturally sensitive manner.

Profiles of Remarkable Women

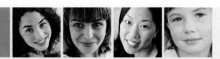

Eve Ensler (1953–)

Eve Ensler is a playwright and an activist whose work grows out of her own personal experiences with violence. Ensler's Obie-Award-winning play, *The Vagina Monologues*, is based on her interviews with more than 200 women about their intimate anatomy. The piece celebrates women's sexuality and strength and exposes the violations that women endure throughout the world. Glenn Close, Calista Flockhart, Rosie Perez, and other actresses have performed in *The Vagina Monologues*. The play has been translated into more than 45 languages and has been performed in theaters all over the world, including sold-out runs both at Off-Broadway's Westside Theater and on London's West End (2002 Olivier Award nomination, Best Entertainment).

V-Day originated out of Ensler's conversations with women who approached her after early performances of *The Vagina Monologues* to tell her of their own experiences of violence. Ensler began to use performances of the play to raise funds for organizations working to stop violence.

Today, V-Day is a global movement that helps antiviolence organizations continue and expand their core work on the ground, while drawing public attention to the larger fight to stop worldwide violence (including rape, battery, incest, female genital mutilation, and sexual slavery) against women and girls. In 2001, V-Day was a sellout at Madison Square Garden, a first for a women's event at a major sports arena. In 2008, more than 3,700 V-Day benefit events—produced by local volunteer activists and performed in theaters, community centers, houses of worship, and college campuses—took place around the world, educating millions of people about the reality of violence against women and girls and raising funds for local groups within their communities. V-Day has raised more than $50 million over nine years.

Another of Ensler's plays, *Necessary Targets*, is set in a Bosnian refugee camp and based on a collection of stories from victimized female refugees. The play opened Off-Broadway at the Variety Arts Theater in February 2002, after a hit run at Hartford Stage. Other plays include *Conviction, Lemonade, The Depot, Floating Rhoda and the Glue Man*, and *Extraordinary Measures*.

Ensler is an executive producer of *What I Want My Words to Do to You*, a documentary about the writing group she has led since 1998 at the Bedford Hills Correctional Facility for Women. The film premiered at the 2003 Sundance Film Festival, where it received the Freedom of Expression award; it also premiered nationally on PBS's *P.O.V.* in December 2003.

■■■■
Summary

Sexuality pervades every aspect of a person's life. It is a continually evolving issue throughout the life span, from the beginnings of sexual urges in girlhood to maintaining a fulfilling sexual life into old age. Understanding the biological, psychological, power, and sociological dimensions of sexual health enhances total wellness. Women must understand the unique facets of their own sexuality, from their physiology to their desires. Both positive and negative sexual experiences can affect a woman's overall well-being. Communication and awareness of sexuality are key factors to resolving these experiences in a healthy way. Incorporating open communication and awareness of sexuality into personal relationships, informed decision making, and preventive health care can enhance a woman's sexual health throughout her life span.

■■■■
Topics for Discussion

1. How do the sexual norms of a society restrict individuals? How do they benefit society?

2. Should sex education be taught in the nation's public schools, and, if so, what kind of education should be provided? Which topics do you think are appropriate for school-based sex education courses?

3. Explain the terms *gender* and *sex* in your own words. Can a person be of female sex but have a male gender identity?

4. A paradox is that women appear to have a greater capacity for orgasm and can experience orgasm from a wider range of stimulation, yet seem to have more difficulty experiencing orgasm than men. Is this true? If so, which factors may contribute to this paradox?

5. How is homophobia displayed in modern society?

6. In addition to Masters and Johnson's sexual response cycle, a number of other researchers have proposed non-linear models of sexual response patterns. Identify two of these models.

7. What are ways to maintain healthy relationships while being aware of risks of sexually transmitted disease, pregnancy, and rape?

■■■■
Web Sites

American Civil Liberties Union (ACLU):
http://www.aclu.org

American College of Obstetricians and Gynecologists (ACOG): http://www.acog.org

American Society for Reproductive Medicine:
http://www.asrm.org

Association of Reproductive Health Professionals (ARHP): http://www.arhp.org

Centre for Development and Population Activities (CEDPA): http://www.cedpa.org

Engender Health: http://www.engenderhealth.org

Gay and Lesbian Alliance Against Defamation (GLAAD):
http://www.glaad.org

Go Ask Alice:
http://www.goaskalice.columbia.edu/Cat7.html

Guttmacher Institute: http://www.guttmacher.org

Human Rights Campaign (HRC): http://www.hrc.org

Intersex Society of North America (ISNA):
http://www.isna.org

Kinsey Institute: http://www.kinseyinstitute.org

National Gay and Lesbian Task Force:
http://www.thetaskforce.org

Parents, Families and Friends of Lesbians and Gays (PFLAG): http://community.pflag.org

Sexuality Information and Education Council of the United States (SIECUS): http://www.siecus.org

World Health Organization (WHO):
http://www.who.int/reproductive-health/gender/sexualhealth.html

■■■■
References

1. World Health Organization. (2006). *Defining Sexual Health*. Report of a technical consultation on sexual health 28–31 January 2002, Geneva. Available at: http://www.who.int/reproductive-health/publications/sexual health/index.html.

2. Centers for Disease Control and Prevention. (2002). *Cohabitation, Marriage, Divorce, and Remarriage in the United States*. Series Report 23, Number 22. Available at: http://www.cdc.gov/nchs/pressroom/02news/div_mar_cohab.htm.

3. Eisenberg, M. E., Bernat, D. H., Bearinger, L. H., & Resnick, M. D. (2008). Support for comprehensive sexuality education: perspectives from parents of school-age youth. *Journal of Adolescent Health* 42(4): 352–359.

4. Duffy, K., Lynch, D., & Santinelli, J. (2008). Government support for abstinence-only-until-marriage education. *Clinical Pharmacology and Therapeutics* 10(15). Available at: http://www.nature.com/clpt/journal/vaop/ncurrent/full/clpt2008188a.html.

5. Ott, M. A., & Santelli, J. S. (2007). Abstinence and abstinence-only education. *Current Opinions in Obstetrics and Gynecology* 19(5): 446–452.

6. Kohler, P. K., Manhart, L. E., & Lafferty, W. E. (2008). Abstinence-only and comprehensive sex education and the initiation of sexual activity and teen pregnancy. *Journal of Adolescent Health* 42(4): 344–351.

7. Kinsey, A., Pomeroy, W., & Martin, C. (1948). *Sexual Behavior in the Human Male*. Philadelphia: W. B. Saunders.

8. Kinsey, A., Pomeroy, W., Martin, C., & Gebhard, P. (1953). *Sexual Behavior in the Human Female*. Philadelphia: W. B. Saunders.

9. Masters, W., & Johnson, V. (1966). *Human Sexual Response*. Boston: Little, Brown.

10. Tavris, C., & Sadd, S. (1977). *The Redbook Report on Female Sexuality*. New York: Delacorte Press.

11. Hite, S. (1976). *The Hite Report: A Nationwide Study of Female Sexuality*. New York: Dell Books.

12. Blumstein, P., & Schwartz, P. (1983). *American Couples: Money, Work and Sex*. New York: William Morrow.

13. ABC News. (2004). *Primetime Live Poll: The American Sex Survey.* Available at: http://abcnews.go.com/images/Politics/959a1AmericanSexSurvey.pdf.

14. U.S. Department of Health and Human Services. (2001). *The Surgeon General's Call to Action to Promote Sexual Health and Responsible Sexual Behavior.* Hyattsville, MD: Department of Health and Human Services.

15. Wizemann, T. M., & Pardue, M. L. (Eds.). (2001). *Exploring the Biological Contributions to Human Health: Does Sex Matter?* Washington, DC: National Academies Press.

16. Johnson, C. V., Mimiaga, M. J., & Bradford, J. (2008). Health care issues among lesbian, gay, bisexual, transgender and intersex (LGBTI) populations in the United States: introduction. *Journal of Homosexuality* 54(3): 213–224.

17. Kruijver, F. P., Zhou, J. N., Pool, C. W., Hofman, M. A., Gooren, L. J., & Swaab, D. F. (2000). Male-to-female transsexuals have female neuron numbers in a limbic nucleus. *Journal of Clinical Endocrinology and Metabolism* 85(5): 2034–2041.

18. Gooren, L. (2001). Gender identity and sexual behavior. In: DeGroot, L. J., and Jameson, J. (Eds.). *Endocrinology*, Philadelphia: W. B. Saunders, p. 2039.

19. Jackson, N. C., Johnson, M. J., & Roberts, R. (2008). The potential impact of discrimination fears of older gays, lesbians, bisexuals, and transgender individuals living in small- to moderate-sized cities on long-term health care. *Journal of Homosexuality* 54(3): 325–339.

20. Marrazzo, J. M. (2004). Barriers to infectious disease care among lesbians. International Conference on Women and Infectious Diseases. *Emerging Infectious Diseases* 10(11): 1974–1978.

21. Yonkers, K. A., O'Brien, P. M., & Eriksson, E. (2008). Premenstrual syndrome. *Lancet* 371(9619): 1200–1210.

22. Borenstein, J. E., Dean, B. B., Yonkers, K. A., & Endicott, J. (2007). Using the daily record of severity of symptoms as a screening instrument for premenstrual syndrome. *Obstetrics and Gynecology* 109: 1068–1075.

23. Bertone-Johnson, E. R., Hankinson, S. E., Johnson, S. R., & Manson, J. E. (2008). Cigarette smoking and the development of premenstrual syndrome. *American Journal of Epidemiology* 168(8): 938–945.

24. Lopez, L. M., Kaptein, A. & Helmerhorst, F. M. (2008). Oral contraceptives containing drospirenone for premenstrual syndrome. *Cochrane Database System Review.* Jan 23(1): CD006586.

25. Shah, N. R., Jones, J. B., Aperi, J., Shemtov, R., Karne, A., & Borenstein, J. (2008). Selective serotonin reuptake inhibitors for premenstrual and premenstrual dysphoric disorder. *Obstetrics and Gynecology* 111: 1175–1182.

26. Busse, J. W., Montori, V. M., Krasnik, C., Patelis-Siotis, I., & Guyatt, G. H. (2008). Psychological intervention for premenstrual syndrome: a meta-analysis of randomized controlled trials. *Psychotherapy and Psychosomatics* 78(1): 6–15.

27. Garefalakis, M., & Hickey, M. (2008). Role of androgens, progestins and tibolone in the treatment of menopausal symptoms: a review of the clinical evidence. *Clinical Interventions of Aging* 3(1): 1–8.

28. American College of Obstetricians and Gynecologists. (2008). Addressing health risks of noncoital sexual activity. *Obstetrics and Gynecology* 112: 735–737.

29. Shifren, J. L., Monz, B. U., Russo, P. A., Segreti, A., & Johannes, C. B. (2008). Sexual problems and distress in United States women. *Obstetrics and Gynecology* 112: 970–978.

30. Hillard, P. J. (2002). Menstruation in young girls: a clinical perspective. *Obstetrics and Gynecology* 99, 655–662.

31. Kaplowitz, P. B., Slora, E. J., Wasserman, R. C., Pedlow, S. E., & Herman-Giddens, M. E. (2001). Earlier onset of puberty in girls: relation to increased body mass index and race. *Pediatrics* 108(2): 347–353.

32. Lindau, S. T., Schumm, L. P., Laumann, E. O., Levinson, W., O'Muircheartaigh, C. A., & Waite, L. J. (2007). A study of sexuality and health among older adults in the United States. *New England Journal of Medicine* 357(8): 762–874.

33. Laumann, E. O., Anirudda, D., & Waite, L. J. (2008). Sexual dysfunction among older adults: prevalence and risk factors from a nationally representative U.S. probability sample of men and women 57–85 years of age. *Journal of Sexual Medicine* 5(10): 2300–2311.

34. Rape, Abuse, and Incest National Network (RAINN). (2008) *Statistics.* Available at: http://www.rainn.org/statistics.

35. United Nations Population Fund. (2000). *The State of World Population 2000 Report. Lives Together, Worlds Apart: Men and Women in a Time of Change.* Available at: http://www.unfpa.org/swp/2000/english/index.html.

36. World Health Organization. (2008). *Female genital mutilation.* Factsheet #241. Available at: http://www.who.int/mediacentre/factsheets/fs241/en/print.html.

37. United States Congress. Report on Female Genital Mutilation as required by Conference Report (H. Rept. 106-997) to Public Law 106-429 (Foreign Op-erations, Export Financing, and Related Programs Appropriations Act, 2001). Prevalence of the practice of Female Genital Mutilation (FGM); laws prohibiting FGM and their enforcement; recommendations on how to best eliminate FGM. Available at: http://www.state.gov/documents/organization/9424.pdf.

38. Institute of Medicine (IOM). (2001). *No Time to Lose: Getting More from HIV Prevention.* Washington, DC: National Academies of Science.

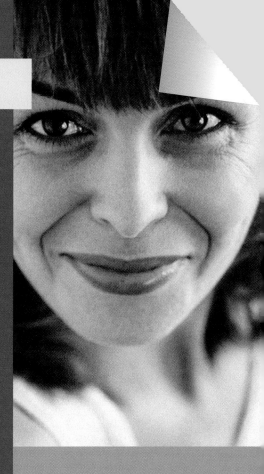

Chapter Five

Reproductive Health

Chapter Objectives

On completion of this chapter, the student should be able to discuss:

1. The four primary mechanisms by which birth control can be accomplished.

2. Contraceptive efforts from a historical perspective.

3. Ways in which sociocultural considerations influence contraceptive decision making.

4. The prevalence of contraceptive use among American women today.

5. Economic issues associated with contraception.

6. The concept of fertility awareness.

7. The mechanisms, risks, benefits, side effects, and contraindications of hormonal, barrier, permanent, and other methods of contraception.

8. The options available for an unplanned pregnancy.

9. The difference between induced and spontaneous abortion.

10. Abortion from a historical perspective.

11. The pro-life, pro-choice, and middle ground positions on abortion.

12. Abortion from an epidemiological perspective.

13. The major types of abortion procedures.

14. Reasons why the assessment of risks, benefits, and contraindications is an integral component of contraceptive decision making.

15. The strategies in effective contraceptive decision making.

16. The importance of careful decision making regarding abortion.

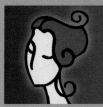

womenshealth.jbpub.com

Women's Health Online is a great source for supplementary women's health information for both students and instructors. Visit

http://womenshealth.jbpub.com

to find a variety of useful tools for learning, thinking, and teaching.

Introduction

A woman's ability to control her reproductive functioning is a necessary part of her health, career preparation, and family growth management. Approximately 70% of reproductive-age women in the United States use some form of birth control. The two most popular forms of birth control are female sterilization and the birth control pill (**Figures 5.1** and **5.2**). Many methods of **contraception** are available today, and no one method is perfect. Ultimately, contraception is a shared responsibility. The best method is one that a woman and her partner feel comfortable using and one that they will use correctly and consistently. The risk for sexually transmitted infections, including HIV, should also play an essential part in a couple's decision.

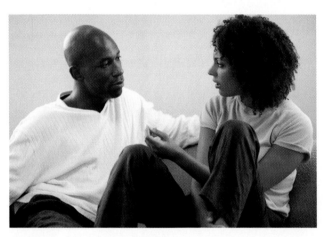

■ Choosing the right contraception is a decision that couples should make together.

Perspectives on Contraception

Although the terms "birth control" and "contraception" are often used interchangeably, each conveys a slightly different perspective on **fertility** control. *Contraception* is a specific term for any procedure used to prevent fertilization of an ovum. *Birth control* is an umbrella term that refers to procedures that prevent the birth of a baby, so it would include all available contraceptive measures as well as sterilization, the **intrauterine device** (IUD), and abortion procedures. Contraceptive methods do not necessarily provide protection from sexually transmitted diseases.

There are four primary mechanisms by which birth control can be accomplished:

1. Preventing sperm from entering the female reproductive system. Strategies that use this mechanism include abstinence, withdrawal, the condom, and male sterilization.

2. Preventing sperm from fertilizing an ovum once it has entered the female reproductive system. Strategies that use this mechanism include the diaphragm, cervical cap, contraceptive sponge, and spermicides.

3. Preventing ovulation and/or preventing the ovum from reaching the sperm. Strategies that use this mechanism include oral contraceptives, hormone implants, hormone injectables, hormone patch, vaginal ring, and female sterilization.

4. Preventing progression of a fertilized egg. Strategies that use this mechanism include the IUD, some forms of oral contraceptives, emergency birth control, and abortion.

Figure 5.1

Percentage of U.S. women ages 15 to 44 using certain contraceptive methods, 2002, by age group.

Source: Mosher, W.D., Martinez, G.M., Chandra, A., Abma, J.C., and Wilson, S.J. (2004). Use of contraception and use of family planning services in the United States, 1982–2002. *Advance Data from Vital Health Statistics*, no. 350. Hyattsville, MD: National Center for Health Statistics.

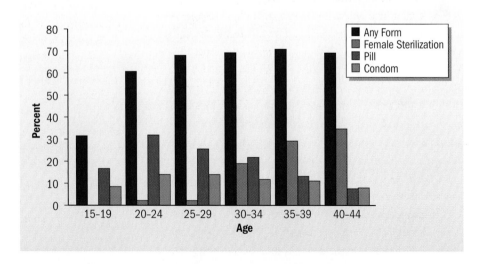

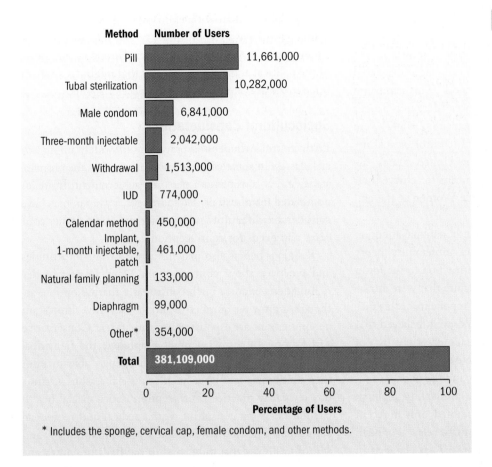

Figure 5.2

Contraceptive method choice among U.S. women using contraception, 2002.

Source: The Alan Guttmacher Institute. (2005). Contraceptive Use: Retrieved online January 16, 2006, from http://www.guttmacher.org/pubs/fb_contr_use.html.

Method | Number of Users

Pill — 11,661,000
Tubal sterilization — 10,282,000
Male condom — 6,841,000
Three-month injectable — 2,042,000
Withdrawal — 1,513,000
IUD — 774,000
Calendar method — 450,000
Implant, 1-month injectable, patch — 461,000
Natural family planning — 133,000
Diaphragm — 99,000
Other* — 354,000
Total — 381,109,000

Percentage of Users

* Includes the sponge, cervical cap, female condom, and other methods.

The decision to have sex or intercourse is a major decision for every person. The risks of unprotected sex include pregnancy and infections. Some couples may elect to practice **oral sex**, outercourse, or other forms of sexual intimacy before engaging in sex. Oral sex, or oral–genital contact, does not result in pregnancy but can result in the transmission of sexually transmitted infections, or STIs (see Chapter 7 for more information). Outercourse is the sharing of sexual intimacy with behaviors such as kissing, petting, and mutual masturbation. The advantages of outercourse include no risk of pregnancy without penile–vaginal penetration and the behaviors permit emotional bonding and closeness. These activities can result in STI transmission if fluids are exchanged or if genital skin comes in contact with another person's genitals, mouth, or anus. Couples who practice outercourse require strong and motivated discipline. Ejaculation on, next to, or inside the vaginal opening has real risk for pregnancy and requires contraception if pregnancy is not desired.

Contraceptive decision making is not easy. Couples are often faced with a choice between highly effective contraceptive methods that have a number of side effects and other methods that have few side effects but may detract from sexual enjoyment and may have a higher failure rate.

Historical Overview

Throughout history, women have attempted to control their fertility status by using many different methods. Records indicate that ancient Egyptian and Greek women made primitive diaphragms by inserting paste-like mixtures into their vaginas. Women from many ages and cultures have consumed various teas and septic solutions with the hopes that they would prevent unwanted pregnancy. Early attempts at spermicidal agents included mixtures of acid, juice, honey, alcohol, opium, and vinegar.

Until the introduction of the birth control pill in 1960, diaphragms and condoms were the primary forms of contraception. Early condoms were probably made from linen

I am dependent on our local family planning clinic for birth control. We can't afford a private doctor.

26-year-old mother of three

sheaths. The cervical cap was introduced in the early 1800s, and the diaphragm was introduced later in the same century. In the mid-nineteenth century, feminists in the United States began a birth control campaign associated with the slogan "Voluntary Motherhood." This campaign advocated birth control by abstinence. Margaret Sanger (1879–1966) and Mary Coffin Dennett (1872–1947) were early promoters of contraceptive birth control (sexual intercourse without pregnancy) in the United States, although the two advocated different means to achieve their goals (see the **Profiles of Remarkable Women** at the end of this chapter).

Birth control remained at the center of national attention for many years. "Race suicide" was an antifeminist theory developed between 1905 and 1910 in reaction to the lower birth rates and changes in family structure that were attributed to the birth control movement. Proponents of this theory, including President Theodore Roosevelt, believed that upper-class, educated women were failing society by not having large families and that they were allowing the upper classes to be overtaken by immigrants and the poor.

Although women today take the availability of birth control devices and information for granted, only in recent years has it been legal to use them. Fifty years ago, birth control pills were illegal in some states. That changed in 1965 with the Supreme Court's landmark decision, *Griswold v. Connecticut,* which struck down a statute that made the use of birth control illegal and criminalized spreading information about its use. Justice William Orville Douglas found the strength for the decision in the fact that the case involved "the intimate relationship of husband and wife" and contraceptives were a logical extension of the marital relationship. In 1972, the Court invalidated a Massachusetts law that had made it a felony to give contraceptives to anyone other than a married person.

Recent legal victories in the contraceptive movement have mandated increased women's access to contraception through their health insurers. Federal employees won mandated coverage for contraception via an act of Congress in 1998. More recently, women's advocacy groups have pressured insurers and employers to include oral contraception in covered prescription drug benefits. More than three-quarters of women age 18–44 rely on private insurance to defray their medical expenses.[1] Until recently, many insurers did not offer reimbursement for oral contraception, leaving many women to pay for their "pill" out of pocket.

Federal restrictions on contraceptive development have resulted in the United States lagging behind many countries in this arena, leaving U.S. couples with fewer contraceptive options than couples in other developed nations. U.S. women have a responsibility to stay informed as contraceptive technology continues to evolve and to stay aware of the political and economic forces that might facilitate or impede the availability of these devices or agents.

Sociocultural Considerations

Birth control attitudes and practices vary widely among social classes. In some cultures, motherhood has the ultimate status and is considered a personal achievement. In male-dominated relationships and marriages, a woman may have considerable difficulty in expressing and asserting her concerns and needs for contraception.

Religious beliefs also may influence a woman's attitudes and practices about contraception. Many Protestant denominations endorse birth control as a marital option, although a growing number of ultraconservative Protestant denominations are espousing limiting its use. Conservative and Reform Judaism teachings emphasize the individual choice of the married couple, with couples able to limit their family size for either health or social reasons. Orthodox Jews may practice contraception under special health circumstances by consulting with medical and rabbinical authorities. The Roman Catholic Church traditionally and still officially accepts only rhythm methods of contraception. According to its teachings, the primary purpose of sexual intercourse is procreation, and any interference with procreation is considered to be a violation of natural law. Studies show that significant numbers of Catholics do use contraceptives, but this practice in violation of church teachings creates emotional difficulties for some Catholic women. White women raised as fundamental Protestants are more likely to report any sterilization operation than their black or Hispanic counterparts.[2] The Muslim faith also forbids contraception, because reproduction is seen as both a sacred duty and a gift. Although Muslims, on average, have the highest birth rates in the world, many Muslim couples use contraception, and some Islamic scholars approve of its use.

Use of family planning services has increased in recent years from 33% in 1995 to 42% in 2002. The National Survey of Family Growth, conducted by the U.S. federal

I am really concerned about birth control. My family expects me to be a virgin when I marry. But we aren't ready to get married yet and I am not a virgin. I am afraid that my family will not understand this problem.

20-year-old Hispanic American woman

government, revealed that in 2002, 42% of women 15 to 44 years of age had at least one family planning service in the past year.[3] However, white non-Hispanic women were more likely to receive family planning from private doctors or HMOs and less likely to receive their family planning from clinics, which deliver services to people with lower incomes and often have fewer resources.[3] The underlying reasons for these differences are complex, but may in part be because black and Hispanic women are less likely than white women to have health insurance or sufficient monetary means to pay private practitioners. The geographical distribution of clinics and private practitioners' offices may also help explain disparities in contraceptive use.

The same study compared specific contraceptive behaviors among these three groups of women. It found that white non-Hispanic women were more likely to use some form of contraception than black or Hispanic women (64.5% versus 57.4% and 59.0%, respectively). The most commonly used contraceptive method also differed among racial and ethnic groups. White women were most likely to rely on birth control pills, whereas black and Hispanic women were most likely to rely on female sterilization. However, male sterilization was much more common among white couples than it was among black or Hispanic couples (**Figure 5.3**). In a study to evaluate availability

trends and use of publicly funded family planning clinics in the United States, researchers found that contraceptive services grew from 1994 to 2001. More than 6.7 million women received services, an 8% rise in clinics and a 2% rise in clients since 1994. However, the authors noted considerable variability in the states' ability to provide needed services, especially for low-income women.[4]

Economic Perspective

Contraceptives have costs for both individuals and societies. At the personal level, the cost of different contraceptive methods is an important consideration for couples considering adopting a new method. The costs of using different contraceptive methods vary significantly, both for the initial purchase and for how often (if at all) the method needs to be repurchased. Birth control pills and diaphragms, for example, both have required office visit costs, but pills may cost about $35 per month, whereas a diaphragm may have

We are happily married, and someday we wish to have children, but right now our goals are to establish our careers. It would be really difficult for me to establish myself professionally if I become pregnant during the next three years.

26-year-old attorney

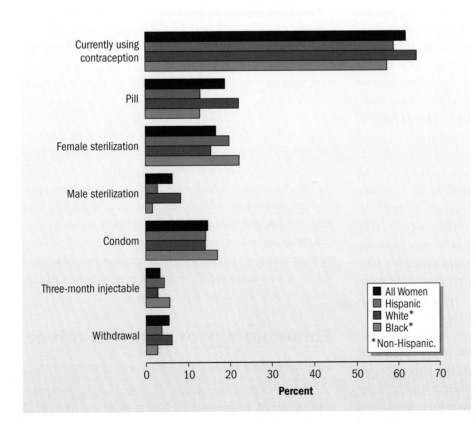

Figure 5.3

Percentage of U.S. women, ages 15 to 44 years, using certain methods of contraception, distributed by ethnicity/race, 2002.

Source: Mosher, W.D., Martinez, G.M., Chandra, A., Abma, J.C., and Wilson, S.J. (2004). Use of contraception and use of family planning services in the United States, 1982–2002. *Advance Data from Vital and Health Statistics*, no. 350. Hyattsville, MD: National Center for Health Statistics.

a one-time cost of about $100. Additional costs are often associated with some methods. For example, contraceptive jelly or cream must be used with a diaphragm, and insertion and removal fees should be considered with an IUD. Understanding all the cost considerations should be part of any personal decision about contraceptive use.

Contraceptive failures also present cost considerations. Emergency contraception may require a prescription and office costs. The expenses associated with pregnancy or a child are part of the larger personal economic consideration when determining contraceptive costs. STI risk and the costs of STI screening and treatment also contribute to the costs of contraceptive failure. Additionally, there are personal emotional costs to contraceptive failure. If a woman is not prepared to handle an unwanted pregnancy or STI, her behavioral and contraceptive choices should reflect this personal priority.

As **Table 5.1** shows, contraceptive costs vary considerably in private and public settings. Couples may be able to save on contraceptive costs by using a publicly funded facility. Publicly funded family planning clinics currently provide care for more than one-quarter of the more than 20 million women who obtain contraceptive services from a medical provider.[5] Health insurance can sometimes also help defray contraceptive costs. Currently 27 states have laws that require insurers that provide coverage for prescription drugs in general to provide coverage of the full range of FDA-approved contraceptive drugs and devices.[5] Some states still permit employers or insurers to refuse to cover contraceptives on religious or moral grounds. Federal law requires insurance coverage of contraceptives for federal employees and their dependents. A 2002 study found that most insurance plans purchased by employers for their employees cover a full range of prescriptive contraceptives,[6] but half of women in the United States live in states that do not require insurers to provide coverage. About half of all Americans who do have employer-based health insurance obtain coverage from employers that self-insure, and self-insured plans are exempt from state coverage requirements. Additionally, one in six (17%) nonelderly women in the United States are uninsured.[7] Women who are Latina, low-income, single, and young are particularly likely to be uninsured. Insurance coverage remains an important cost determinant for personal contraceptive decision making.

Societal costs are an important economic dimension of contraception. Unintended pregnancy is a major public health and societal health problem in the United States. Roughly half of the 6 million pregnancies that occur in the United States every year are unintended. As a result of these unintended pregnancies, 1.4 million unplanned

Table 5.1 Contraceptive Costs*

Low Cost/Low Reliability	Cost Per Use
Fertility awareness	No cost
Male condom	$.50–$3.00
Female condom	$.50–$3.00
Spermicides	$.50–$3.00

Higher Initial Cost/ Higher Reliability	Cost for Method and Fitting
Diaphragm	$100–$200 plus spermicide per use
Cervical cap	$100–$200 plus spermicide per use

Hormonal Options/ High Reliability	Monthly Cost
Combined pills	$20–35 plus examination costs
Progestin-only pills	$20–35 plus examination costs
Transdermal contraceptive patch	$25–30 plus examination costs
Injectables	$60–$75 (for 3 months) plus examination costs
Vaginal ring	$35–$40 plus examination costs

Long-Term Contraceptives	Cost
Implants	$450–$750 for 5 years
IUDs	$430 for up to 10 years
Intrauterine system (IUS)	$395 for 5 years

Permanent Contraception	Cost
Female sterilization	$1,200
Vasectomy (for males)	$250–$400

*These are approximate costs for public-sector settings. Private settings have significantly higher costs.

Source: Association of Reproductive Health Professionals. (2008). Comparison chart of average costs of contraception, http://www.arhp.org/crc/compare-methods.html.

births and 1.3 million abortions occur each year.[8] Universal access to contraceptives will be key to reducing both these numbers and their associated financial, emotional, and societal costs. From state to state, there have been vastly different levels of progress in service availability, laws and policies, and public funding to support access to contraceptive services. Together the personal and societal costs of contraceptive use, as well as contraceptive misuse and the lack of contraceptive use, play an enormous role in many areas of life in the United States.

Epidemiology of Contraceptives

Contraceptive Use

Most reproductive-age women in the United States use some form of contraception. Ninety-eight percent of all women who have ever had intercourse have used at least one method of birth control.[3] The pill is the leading method of choice; female sterilization is the second-leading method. The National Surveys of Family Growth from 1982, 1995, and 2002 provide useful insights into trends and contraceptive practices among U.S. women. From 1982 to 2002, the percentage of women whose male partner had ever used a condom increased from 52% to 90%. Contraceptive use at the first premarital intercourse increased from 43% in 1982 to 79% in 2002. Contraception use varies among racial and ethnic groups. Non-Hispanic black and Hispanic women are more likely to use female sterilization than non-Hispanic white women. White women are more likely to rely on male sterilization. When male and female sterilization rates are considered together, there are minor differences in the three groups (see **Figure 5.4**).

Contraceptive decision making is a complex task for a woman and her partner. Men and women have somewhat different priorities when choosing a contraceptive method. According to a study conducted by the Kaiser Family Foundation, women consider the following characteristics to be "very important" when choosing a contraceptive method:[9]

- Effectively prevents pregnancy (90%)
- Effectively protects against sexually transmitted diseases (77%)
- Provides no health risk (77%)
- Is easy to use (51%)
- Requires no advance planning (45%)

Together these factors influence which contraceptive method is chosen, how regularly it is used, and ultimately how effective a contraceptive strategy will be for a woman.

Contraceptive Efficacy

Consistency and correct use are the two most important factors that determine contraceptive efficacy—how well a particular method is likely to work. However, even if used consistently and correctly, some methods are more likely to work than others. Contraceptive failure rates provide important information in the selection of a birth control method. Failure rates are determined by following large groups of couples who use specific methods of birth control for a specified time and then counting the number of pregnancies that occur. The larger the number of study participants, the more reliable the study results. A failure rate of 2% means 2 pregnancies per 100 women per year studied.

Two types of failure rates exist:

- The lowest observed failure rate represents a method's absolute top performance, the highest efficacy ever achieved in a reputable clinical trial. This rate is often referred to as the failure rate with perfect use.

- The failure rate for typical users is an average rate based on an analysis of a range of reputable studies. The failure rate for typical users is usually lower than the best observed failure rates (**Table 5.2**).

In 2001, the U.S. government's *Healthy People 2010* initiative set a goal of reducing contraceptive failure during the first year of use from 13% in 1995 to 7% by 2010. Researchers found that in 2002, 12.4% of all episodes of contraceptive use ended with a failure within 12 months after they were started. The study showed no clear improvement in contraception effectiveness between 1995 and 2002.[10]

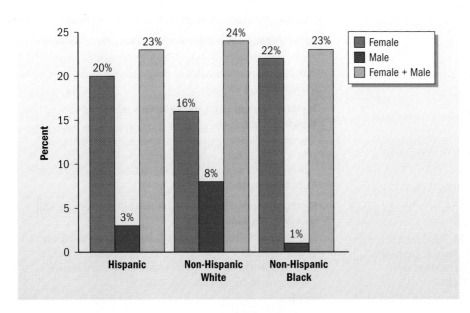

Figure 5.4

Percentage of U.S. women 15–44 years of age and their partners using sterilization for contraception by race and Hispanic origin, United States, 2002.

Source: Adapted from: Mosher, W.D., Martinez, G.M., Chandra, A. Contraception and use of family planning services in the United States, 1982–2002. *Vital Health Statistics*, Hyattsville, MD: National Center for Health Statistics.

Age influences the efficacy of the birth control method, with married older women generally being more successful contraceptors than unmarried younger women. The reasons for this discrepancy are not totally understood. It may be that younger women are less experienced with careful planning, are less likely to follow a routine, may be more fertile, may have intercourse more often, or may experience a combination of these factors. At any rate, young women who wish to avoid pregnancy need to take extra care with contraception.

Several methods of contraception have demonstrated high levels of effectiveness, defined as a failure rate of two or fewer pregnancies per 100 couples per year. These methods include pills (oral contraceptives), Norplant (hormone implants), Depo-Provera and Lunelle (hormone injectables), IUDs, spermicidal condoms (if used correctly), NuvaRing (vaginal hormone ring), Ortho Evra (hormone patch), and sterilization. Methods that have lower rates of effectiveness include diaphragms, cervical caps, sponges, and spermicidal agents, such as foams, creams, gels, suppositories, and vaginal contraceptive film. The effective-

ness of a birth control method depends in large part on how carefully and consistently it is used. A diaphragm does not work when it is left in a drawer, pills may be forgotten, and condoms may break or leak.

Special Population: Adolescents

Teens and young adults often harbor many myths and misconceptions about contraception (see **Table 5.3**). Teenage girls tend to rely on their male partners for contraceptive implementation (withdrawal and use of condoms) during early sexual intercourse experiences and later adopt prescription methods. The average delay between first inter-

---

Table 5.2 | **Contraceptive Efficacy Rates: Percentage of Women Experiencing an Accidental Pregnancy in the First Year of Use**

Method	Perfect Use	Typical Use
Pill (combined)	0.3	8.0
Tubal sterilization	0.5	0.5
Male condom	2.0	15.0
Vasectomy	0.1	0.2
Withdrawal	4.0	27.0
IUD (copper-T)	0.6	0.8
IUD (Mirena)	0.2	0.2
Periodic abstinence	3.0–5.0	25.0
Implant	0.05	0.05
Patch	0.3	8.0
Diaphragm	6.0	16.0
Sponge: parous women	20.0	32.0
Sponge: nulliparous women	9.0	16.0
Female condom	5.0	21.0
Spermicides (alone)	18.0	29.0
No method	85.0	85.0

Source: Trussell, J. (2007). Contraceptive efficacy. In Hatcher, R.A., Trussell, J., Nelson, A.L., Cates, W., Stewart, F.H., Kowal, D. *Contraceptive Technology.* 19th rev. ed. New York: Ardent Media. Modified from http://www.contraceptivetechnology.com/table.html.

Table 5.3 | **Myths and Misconceptions About Contraceptives**

There are perhaps as many myths and misconceptions about contraceptives as there are facts. A few of the more common ones are summarized below:

Myth: Birth control pills make a woman fat.

Some women may gain a few pounds while taking the pill; some women may lose weight.

Myth: A woman needs to take a break from the pill every year.

There is no medical reason to have a break from the pill; it can be taken for many years without a break.

Myth: IUDs make sex uncomfortable for men.

IUDs are rarely felt by the male partner.

Myth: Wearing two condoms will provide twice as much protection.

Using more than one condom actually increases the risk of tearing due to friction.

Myth: Condoms detract from sexual pleasure.

Some condoms are designed to increase sensitivity. Not using a condom increases the risk of sexually transmitted infections.

Myth: Plastic wrap can be a substitute for a condom.

Plastic wrap, balloons, and plastic bags do not work as protection during sexual intercourse. They do not fit and can be easily torn or displaced during sex.

Myth: A woman can't get pregnant while she is breastfeeding.

Breastfeeding will delay ovulation and will reduce the chance of getting pregnant, but it is not a guarantee. Nursing mothers who are sure they do not want to become pregnant should use an additional form of birth control.

Myth: Douching, showering, or urinating after sex will prevent pregnancy.

Douching is not effective, and there is some evidence that it may increase the risk for pregnancy by propelling the semen toward the cervix. Showering or urinating will not stop the sperm that have already entered the uterus through the cervix.

course and the first visit for medical consultation is about one year, and this visit is often motivated by a pregnancy scare. Among single female adolescents using contraceptives, however, the pill and condom are the most popular methods. Teen contraceptive use does appear to be improving. Compared to teenagers in 1995, teenagers in 2002 were more likely to use contraception the first time they had intercourse. Teenagers in 2002 also were more likely to have used condoms or injectable methods of birth control and were less likely to use no method of contraception at all.[3] Unprotected adolescent sexual activity poses a risk not only for unintended pregnancy, but also for sexually transmitted infections (see Chapter 7).

Contraceptive Methods

Fertility Awareness Methods

Methods of fertility awareness include the calendar method, basal body temperature, and cervical mucus or ovulation method. These methods are based on avoidance of sexual intercourse during a woman's fertile time of the month, which includes the days previous to, during, and immediately following ovulation. An understanding of the female menstrual cycle is an essential foundation for using fertility awareness methods. Couples using fertility awareness tend to have more accidental pregnancies than couples using most other contraceptive methods (Table 5.2).

One of the most important changes during the menstrual cycle is the cyclical variations of hormones from the anterior pituitary and the ovaries. The cyclical variations in these hormones cause biological alterations throughout the cycle. These cyclical hormones cause fluctuations in basal temperature patterns and variations in the type of cervical mucus produced. Many women are able to feel these changes during their fertility cycles and use methods of fertility awareness as either contraceptive techniques or methods for contraception.

The calendar method requires determining when ovulation occurs by calculating the length of consecutive menstrual cycles. It is not reliably effective, especially for women who do not have regular menstrual cycles. Measuring the body's daily temperature (basal body temperature)

Well, I am proof that you need to follow directions. I thought that using a diaphragm was enough. I don't like that spermicidal stuff, and I thought a diaphragm alone was good protection. So I am pregnant. I can't believe that this is because I didn't follow directions.
21-year-old pregnant woman

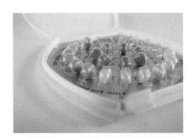
One type of birth control pills.

is another way to determine that ovulation has occurred. When progesterone is released immediately after ovulation, the body's temperature increases a small amount; however, women need to be certain that other factors, such as sexual activity, illness, or infection, are not causing these temperature fluctuations. Women also may determine the most fertile phase of the menstrual cycle by monitoring the change in the quality of the cervical mucus. During the fertile phase, women experience an increase in discharge and change in color and consistency of the mucus.

Fertility awareness methods have the advantage of causing no side effects, and anyone can use them. Also, a couple using fertility awareness with another contraception method has a lower risk of unintended pregancy than a couple using either method alone. These methods help a woman understand her body and her cycles. It also empowers her with practical knowledge. This method may be used with other barrier forms of contraception. Fertility awareness methods have many drawbacks, however, including limited effectiveness, the need to abstain from sexual intercourse during many days of the month, and the lack of protection against sexually transmitted infections. For a woman who absolutely does not wish to become pregnant, fertility awareness methods for contraception have inherent liabilities. Timing of ovulation is not the only critical dimension of fertility awareness. Women can get pregnant a few days before and a few days after ovulation. Sperm can be viable for as long as five days, and eggs are viable for 24 hours. Fertility awareness methods depend on complex calculations, personal discipline, and good luck. Couples who rely on fertility awareness methods should plan on eventual failure of these methods.

Hormonal Methods

Oral Contraceptives

Currently about 19% of women 15 to 44 years of age who use contraception take oral contraceptives, or birth control pills, making them the most commonly used nonsurgical method of birth control (see Figures 5.1 through 5.3). Since its introduction in the United States in the 1960s, the birth control pill has been one of the most extensively studied pharmacological preparations. The pill has changed considerably since its initial launch into the marketplace. Although the specific hormones are the same or similar, the dosages and formulations have undergone tremendous changes.

Oral contraceptives are now available in packets of 21, 28, or 91 pills to be taken once a day, preferably at the same time each day. It is important to take the pills as prescribed. There are many brands, which can have different hormone levels; different women find that they prefer different formulations of pills. Talking with a health-care provider about symptoms and concerns may help a woman find the pill that best suits her individual needs. Pills are usually started on the first or fifth day of a menstrual cycle. Sometimes women need to use a back-up contraceptive for the first few days of starting the pill. Back-up contraception should also be used when a pill user has extended vomiting or diarrhea.

Birth control pills offer many benefits, in addition to contraception, for women. Oral contraceptives are associated with lighter and less painful periods, decreased symptoms of premenstrual syndrome (PMS), and improved skin conditions. They may also provide some protection against benign breast disease, ovarian cysts, pelvic inflammatory disease (PID), ovarian cancer, and endometrial cancer. Long-term use of oral contraceptives also increases a woman's bone density, thereby protecting her against osteoporosis. Many perimenopausal women also receive benefits from oral contraceptives, such as decreased complaints associated with menopause. Although generally safe, birth control pills may be a health risk for some women, primarily smokers or women at risk for high blood presure.

With birth control pills, the woman's own reproductive hormone cycle is generally suppressed, and the synthetic estrogen and progestin of the pill produce an artificial cycle to replace it. Without the natural signals, the egg follicle in the ovary cannot mature, and ovulation cannot occur. Another way the pill prevents pregnancy is by inducing development of thick cervical mucus, in contrast to the profuse, slippery mucus associated with ovulation. The thick cervical mucus impedes sperm movement through the cervical canal and inhibits chemical changes in sperm cells that would permit them to penetrate the outer layer of the egg. The pill also acts as a contraceptive by preventing the uterine lining from thickening as it normally does in the menstrual cycle. Thus, even if ovulation and conception did manage to occur, successful implantation would be quite unlikely.

Overall, birth control pills are highly effective in preventing pregnancy. Effectiveness rates of 99% can be expected when they are taken properly.

Side Effects

Several side effects have been associated with birth control pills. They may include both negative and positive changes:

1. Shorter, lighter, and more regular menstrual periods. The reduced amount of uterine lining results in reduced blood loss.

2. Reduction or elimination of menstrual cramps. Cramping is often associated with ovulation; because ovulation does not occur with use of birth control pills, cramping is reduced or eliminated. Steady progestin exposure with birth control pills tends to reduce or eliminate cramps and menstrual discomfort.

3. Mood changes. Some women may experience diverse reactions to birth control pills, such as irritability, depression, or mood swings. Some women, particularly those with a history of depression or premenstrual syndrome (PMS), may find these mood-related changes intolerable and choose to discontinue the pill.

4. Reduction or elimination of premenstrual symptoms. In many women, PMS tends to be significantly reduced or eliminated with birth control pills.

5. Decreased libido. For some women, birth control pills may increase sex drive by reducing anxiety about pregnancy and alleviating discomfort or distaste at having to "get ready" for sex. From a biochemical perspective, however, some women may experience adverse reactions to birth control pills and experience a decrease in sex drive, depression, irritability, or mood swings.

6. Spotting or bleeding between periods. The estrogen level maintained in the body by the pill is often lower than the natural level produced by the ovaries. This lower level may trigger slight uterine bleeding, which is generally referred to as "breakthrough bleeding." Such bleeding is more likely to occur when a pill is taken late or forgotten.

7. Weight changes. Some birth control pill users gain weight with the pill; others lose weight with its use.

8. Acne improvement. Most women who have acne notice significant improvement when they take birth control pills, and some brands of pills are used to treat acne in some patients. However, birth control pills may cause chloasma, the darkening of skin pigment on the upper lip, under the eyes, and on the forehead. These effects are not common and

disappear when use of the birth control pills is discontinued.

Other effects associated with birth control pills include nausea, tender or larger breasts, headaches, and fluid retention.

Risks and Complications

Risks and complications are a major concern for oral contraceptive users, although many of these fears are unfounded. Safety issues concerning oral contraceptives are mainly based on the use of pills with high levels of hormones (current brands contain less than 50 micrograms of estrogen) and the risks associated with smoking and use of oral contraceptives.

One concern about oral contraceptives has been that they may increase the risk of venous thromboembolism, or the formation of abnormal blood clots. Current evidence indicates that this increased risk is very small, and may not actually exist. In a recent meta-analysis study, only 10 of 16 studies examining oral contraceptives' influence on venous thromboembolism found "good" evidence for an increased risk.[11]

An increased risk of high blood pressure, especially for older women and obese women, also has been associated with use of birth control pills. Other concerns identified by earlier studies of high-dose oral contraceptives include an increased risk of stroke and heart attack. Recent studies show that there is no increased risk for either condition in women without preexisting risk factors, regardless of age. There is, however, an increased risk if the woman smokes or has hypertension. For women with cardiovascular risk factors or for women who smoke, nonhormonal methods of birth control may be the best option.[12]

Concerns have been raised about a possible connection between the pill and cancer in women. Because the pills were introduced five decades ago, sufficient time has elapsed to permit long-term studies on the possible association between the pill and cancer. Because some cancers depend on naturally occurring sex hormones, researchers have wondered if the hormones in oral contraceptives affect cancer risk. To date, hundreds of studies have been conducted. The results have not always been consistent. Researchers have learned that taking oral contraceptives *reduces* a woman's chances of getting endometrial and ovarian cancers, but some studies have shown an *increased* risk for breast and cervical cancers. Other studies have shown no increased risk for breast cancer among pill users.[13,14,15]

Some evidence has shown that long-term use of birth control pills is associated with changes in the surface of the cervix. These changes may make pill users more vulnerable to cervical cancer and sexually transmitted diseases of the cervix, particularly chlamydia. Confounding factors, however, make it very difficult to draw conclusions based on this evidence. Contradictory studies have shown no significant alterations of the cervix that would lead to associated risks. Women who have more than one sexual partner or who are at risk of transmission of sexually transmitted diseases should consider using condoms in combination with birth control pills.

Several drugs can reduce the contraceptive effectiveness of the pill and increase the risk of bleeding between periods. These drugs include barbiturates, some anticonvulsants, antifungal medications, phenytoin (Dilantin), and certain antibiotics such as isoniazid, rifampin, and possibly tetracycline. It is probably wise for any woman using birth control pills to employ a backup form of contraception while taking any of these medications. Oral contraceptives also may prolong the effects of caffeine, theophylline, and benzodiazepines (e.g., Librium, Valium, and Xanax).

Advantages

Birth control pills provide the maximum protection possible with a temporary contraceptive method. They do not require any additional supplies or equipment, and they do not interfere with the spontaneity of lovemaking. Also, they provide freedom from heavy menstrual cramps and excessive menstrual bleeding, and often relieve premenstrual symptoms. Menstrual periods become regular and predictable. Birth control pills provide some benefits as well as pregnancy prevention. For example, women who take birth control pills have a lower prevalence of ovarian and endometrial cancers, and benign breast disease and ovarian cysts are less common in them. Women who take the pill also may be at lower risk for developing PID, iron-deficiency anemia, and osteoporosis.

Contraindications

A contraindication is a medical condition that renders a treatment or procedure that otherwise might be recommended inadvisable or unsafe. Women who are contemplating use of birth control pills should carefully review and evaluate the contraindications before deciding to proceed with them. Absolute contraindications—meaning that the pills absolutely should not be taken—specified by the FDA include the following conditions:

- Known cardiovascular disorder, now or in the past, such as thrombophlebitis, stroke, heart attack, coronary artery disease, or angina pectoris
- Impaired liver function

- Known or suspected cancer of the breast, uterus, cervix, or vagina
- Known or suspected estrogen-dependent neoplasia (abnormal tissue growth)
- Current or suspected pregnancy
- Abnormal vaginal bleeding
- Jaundice during previous pill use or pregnancy
- Malignant melanoma, now or in the past
- Smoking in women older than 35 years of age

Oral contraceptive use when breastfeeding has generated concern for infant safety. Studies are limited and although there is no evidence of harm, the question cannot be definitively answered. The American Academy of Family Physicians noted that the existing low-quality research evidence suggests that combined oral contraceptives may reduce the volume of breast milk but does not affect infant growth.[16]

Types of Birth Control Pills

There are currently more than 50 birth control pill brands available in monophasic (each cycle provides 21 identical hormone-containing pills), biphasic (two-phase), and triphasic (three-phase) formulations. Triphasic pills, the most recently introduced combination pills, contain three different **progestin** doses for different parts of each pill cycle. The primary advantage of triphasic pills is that the overall amount of progestin in a cycle is lower than it is with regular, identical-dose pills.

Traditionally, oral contraceptives have been prescribed in 21-day cycles of active hormone pills followed by a 7-day placebo or pill-free interval that produces predictable withdrawal bleeding in most users. Some women who follow this regimen, however, experience nuisance breakthrough bleeding, spotting, or amenorrhea. New formulations of continuous oral contraceptive therapy provide continuous hormonal dosing without periods of menstrual flow. The most commonly prescribed regimen for extended therapy is 84 days of active pill use followed by a 7-day hormone-free interval. Patient satisfaction studies indicate that many women prefer continuous therapy, as it provides fewer and lighter bleeding days and less bloating and menstrual pain.[17] Most clinicians do not feel that prescribed withdrawal bleeding has benefits or is necessary.[18,19]

Estrogen dose is generally considered to be the most important factor in selecting a pill. Side effects and complications are reduced with lower estrogen doses. Minipills are estrogen-free birth control pills that provide a continuous, low dose of progestin. They are slightly less effective than the phasic pills and often cause irregular menstrual patterns. Minipills do not totally suppress hormone production. Natural estrogen and progesterone production usually remains sufficient to trigger menstrual periods. There is less margin of error with these oral contraceptives, however. The likelihood of pregnancy increases substantially with just one or two missed tablets. Although menstrual periods tend to be less predictable with the minipills, women who use them generally experience fewer premenstrual symptoms, lighter or absent menstrual periods, decreased menstrual cramps, and less pain during ovulation.

Like other oral contraceptives, the minipill requires a prescription and does not protect against STIs, including HIV/AIDS. The minipill must be taken at the same time every day, and it may be less effective when taken with some drugs. Women on the minipill face an increased risk of functional ovarian cysts and ectopic pregnancies. Menstrual bleeding may be irregular.

Hormonal Implants

A hormonal implant is a matchstick-like small rod that releases a small, steady dose of hormones under the skin. Implants work like oral contraceptives, providing progestin that prevents ovulation. Progestin also thickens cervical mucus, preventing sperm from migrating through the cervix to the uterus. The implant is usually inserted under the skin of the upper arm, and it provides contraceptive protection for three years or until it is removed. The insertion procedure usually lasts about five minutes. A local anesthetic is used, and the procedure is usually painless. Hormonal implants are more than 99% effective in preventing pregnancy, but like other hormonal birth control products, they do not provide any protection against STIs. Hormonal implants are not as widely available as other forms of hormonal contraception because of the training that is needed for insertion and removal.

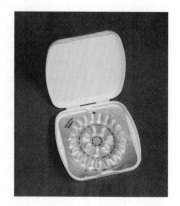

■ The minipill can be an effective form of birth control, but it must be taken every day, preferably at a consistent time.

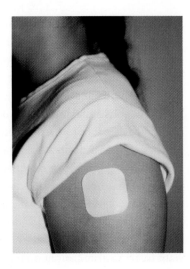

■ The contraceptive patch is worn on the skin for one week and replaced on the same day of the week for three consecutive weeks.

Irregular menstrual bleeding is the most common side effect reported with the implant. This usually occurs in the first few months of use. After one year on the implant, most women report that they have fewer and lighter menstrual periods, and some women stop having periods entirely. Some women will report longer and heavier periods. Another possible side effect is difficulty in removing the implants, but this is minimized with an experienced practitioner. Fertility is not affected after the implant is removed. Benefits, cautions, and contraindications for implants are similar to those for the minipill. Studies have shown that the implant is safely tolerated and does not increase the risk for cardiovascular disease.[20,21]

The hormonal implant is highly convenient. Candidates for a hormonal implant include those women who do not desire children for at least three to five years and who are seeking a highly effective and convenient form of birth control. Women for whom other methods may be contraindicated or for whom contraceptive compliance is an issue may find the implant appealing. Women who are pregnant, or who have unexplained vaginal bleeding, serious liver disease, or a history of breast cancer should not use a hormonal implant. Although the initial cost of the implant can be several hundred dollars, this cost provides pregnancy protection for three years, making it a cost-effective solution in the long run. Many insurers will cover the cost of the hormonal implant.

Hormonal Delivery Methods: Injectables, Patches, and Vaginal Rings

Other hormonal forms of contraception besides the pill and the implant include injectables, patches, and vaginal rings. They are all similar in that they provide steady and predictable doses of contraceptive hormones that prevent ovulation and thicken the cervical mucus.

The most common hormonal injectable, or "shot," is Depo-Provera. This injection of progestin is given intramuscularly, and it lasts three to four months. It has both a theoretical and actual-use effectiveness of almost 100%. It works best with a regular schedule of getting the injection every 12 weeks. In a study comparing the injectable and the pill, the injectable protected against bloating and mood swings but had an increased association with weight gain, bleeding episodes of more than 20 days, and missed periods.[22] Some women experience a delayed return to fertility after discontinuing the injections. Women who cannot take estrogen or women who are breastfeeding are not good candidates for the injectable. The risk of STI transmission presents with the injectable. One study found that women using Depo-Provera were more likely to develop gonorrhea or chlamydia than comparable women using oral contraceptives or other forms of birth control.[23] Women who use injectable contraception and who have multiple sex partners (or exposure to multiple partners through their partner) may wish to use condoms during sex to reduce their risk of infection.

The contraceptive patch is an adhesive patch that delivers hormones to the body. It is worn on the skin for one week and then is replaced on the same day of the week for three consecutive weeks. The fourth week is patch-free, and then the patch-use cycle resumes. The patch is durable and does not break away from the skin during warm weather, bathing, or vigorous exercise. Contraceptive patch users are exposed to higher doses of estrogen than pill users. Side effects to the patch are similar to oral contraceptives, though patch users report increased transient breast tenderness. The patch is less effective in women weighing 198 pounds (90 kilograms) or more.[24]

Vaginal rings are a relatively new hormonal contraceptive. One vaginal ring, the NuvaRing, is inserted in the vagina for three weeks and then removed for a week of menstruation. A new ring is inserted after the menstrual week. The ring releases a gradual and steady dose of

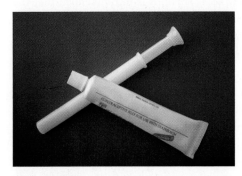

■ Several contraceptive choices are available today.

hormones. Women must learn to correctly insert the ring. Most women do not feel the ring when it is properly inserted. It can occasionally dislodge when a tampon is removed, but the ring can be rinsed and reinserted if this happens. Less than 1 out of 100 users will become pregnant using the ring as directed. Typical use results in 8 out of 100 users becoming pregnant each year with the ring.[25]

Barrier Methods

Barrier methods of contraception were the primary forms of contraception before the pill and IUD. After the introduction of the latter "high-tech" birth control measures, barrier methods were seen as messy, unromantic, and less sophisticated. Barrier methods do offer several advantages over other contraceptives. The condom has reemerged, particularly as a result of the AIDS epidemic, as a major form of protection against HIV infection as well as other sexually transmitted infections, such as herpes and gonorrhea. In addition, the diligent and proper use of condoms has demonstrated pregnancy protection rates fairly comparable to those seen with the pill and IUD. Another major compelling reason for the return to barrier methods is that they have virtually no associated health risks, with the exception of rare allergic responses or localized irritation.

Barrier methods, as the name implies, provide a physical or chemical barrier that prevents sperm from fertilizing eggs. All barrier methods (except plain condoms) are used with **spermicide**, a chemical that breaks down the cell membranes of sperm. Most barrier methods are used inside the vagina to cover the cervix and prevent sperm from entering the uterus. Male condoms are protective sheaths that enclose the penis during intercourse and ejaculation. Female condoms line the inside of the vagina and prevent semen from coming in contact with the vagina.

Barrier methods are very safe for the user, and problems and risks tend to be rare. One rare but important risk from barrier methods is toxic shock syndrome (TSS), which may be associated with the diaphragm, cap, and sponge. Although the TSS risk is small, it is recommended that the diaphragm, sponge, or cervical cap not be used during a menstrual period or when any type of vaginal bleeding occurs. Further recommendations include delaying using these devices four to six weeks after having a baby or until all postpartum bleeding completely stops. TSS risk also can be minimized by not leaving the devices in place in the vagina for longer than the recommended time period.

Vaginal birth control devices are also associated with some other complications. A **diaphragm**, sponge, or **cervical cap** may cause a vaginal bacterial infection if it is left in place for more than 24 hours. A foul-smelling discharge is an indication of such an infection and should be evaluated by a clinician. The diaphragm and cervical cap also may increase the risk of urinary tract infections, indicated by painful and frequent urination.

Although the diaphragm and cervical cap require fitting by a clinician, the other barrier methods may be conveniently purchased in pharmacies. With the exception of abstinence, condoms are the only contraceptive method that can reliably reduce the risk of transmission of sexually transmitted infections, including HIV. Barrier methods are seen as noninvasive contraceptive measures by those women who do not want to have an IUD inside their uterus and who do not want to manipulate their hormonal system. They may also be used as backup contraceptive measures for a woman who has forgotten a pill or who questions an IUD's effectiveness. Some couples have intercourse sporadically or infrequently and find that barrier methods are appealing because they are effective but have to be used only when necessary. Older women and careful users find barrier methods to be more effective than do younger women, women who have frequent intercourse, and those who are not careful users.

Spermicides

Spermicidal agents are available as creams, foams, films, suppositories, or gels. Foams, creams, and jellies are inserted into the vagina via an applicator (**Figure 5.5**). Suppositories are soft capsules that melt into a thick spermicidal liquid agent after being inserted into the vagina. Contraceptive film contains spermicide in a small, thin sheet of glycerine that is placed over the cervix. It melts in response to body temperature, and the spermicide in the film is released into the vagina. Spermicides are available without prescription in drugstores or from online retailers. Spermicides do provide some protection as mechanical barriers, by spreading over the surface of the cervix and blocking access to the cervical opening. More importantly, though, the active ingredient in most spermicides, nonoxynol-9 (N-9) inactivates sperm by breaking down the surface of the sperm cells on contact. To be effective, spermicides must be inserted deep into the vagina.

Spermicidial agents have the advantage of being effective immediately upon use, and they may provide some level of protection against STIs. They do have time limits, and their effectiveness varies. It is important to carefully read and comply with the timing instructions of each type of spermicide. An additional application of spermicide is needed for each round of lovemaking, and the product should be left in place with no douching for at least six

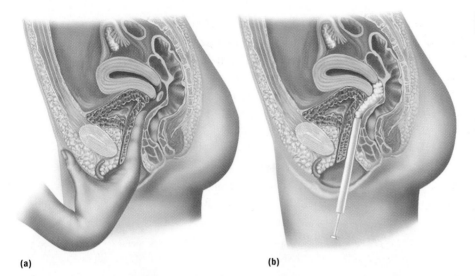

(a)   (b)

Figure 5.5

Spermicidal agents.
Hints: (1) Woman should lie down after insertion; spermicide will leak out and have reduced effectiveness if she is in a vertical position. (2) No douching for 6 hours. (3) Keep extra supplies available—it is not possible to measure residual amounts of foam in containers. (4) Repeat intercourse requires repeat application of spermicide. (5) Wash reusable applicators with soap and water after use. Follow directions carefully for amounts and frequency of use.

hours after each round. Spermicidal agents may be used alone or with diaphragms, cervical caps, or condoms. Contraceptive protection is more effective when the agent is used with a barrier method. Spermicides have been found safe to use for extended periods. Studies have shown that exposure to different formulations and doses of spermicides containing N-9 is unlikely to cause harmful changes to cervical cells.[24]

Diaphragm

A diaphragm is a dome-shaped latex cup rimmed with a firm but flexible band or spring (**Figure 5.6**). It must be first coated with a spermicidal agent before being inserted into the vagina before intercourse. The spermicidal agent is important because it creates a tighter seal around the cervix and kills sperm on contact. The diaphragm is anchored in place by the pubic bone, and it is sized to fit each woman. Because the diaphragm must fit the cervix it is to cover, this contraceptive method requires clinician examination, fitting, and prescription. During the fitting, it is important to evaluate the comfort of the diaphragm as well as to practice its insertion and removal.

Diaphragm effectiveness depends on proper fit and diligent use. A diaphragm that is too small may not stay in place and slip off the cervix; one that is too large may press on the urethra and cause a urinary tract infection. Application of the spermicidal cream or gel and insertion of the diaphragm can occur as long as six hours before intercourse. If intercourse occurs more than once, it is important to use an additional application of spermicide for each event, regardless of how short a time the diaphragm has been in place. The diaphragm should not be removed or dislodged to add the cream or gel for a follow-up round of lovemaking; spermicide can be inserted directly into the vagina.

Like the cervical cap, the diaphragm may be inserted as long as six hours before intercourse and need not interrupt or interfere with lovemaking. It should be left in place for a minimum of six hours after intercourse to allow the spermicide to kill all of the sperm. Douching should not occur during that time. A diaphragm is not recommended during menstruation.

The diaphragm should not remain in place longer than 24 hours. After removal, the diaphragm should be washed with warm water and soap, rinsed, and dried with a towel. Petroleum jelly or oil-based lubricants should not be used with a diaphragm for lubrication because they will weaken the latex. If additional lubrication is desired, a water-soluble lubricant, such as K-Y Jelly or Astroglide, may be used.

■ A diaphragm is a dome-shaped latex cup rimmed with a firm but flexible band or spring.

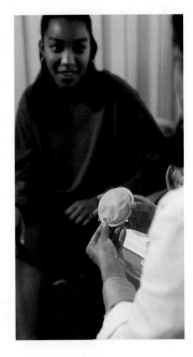

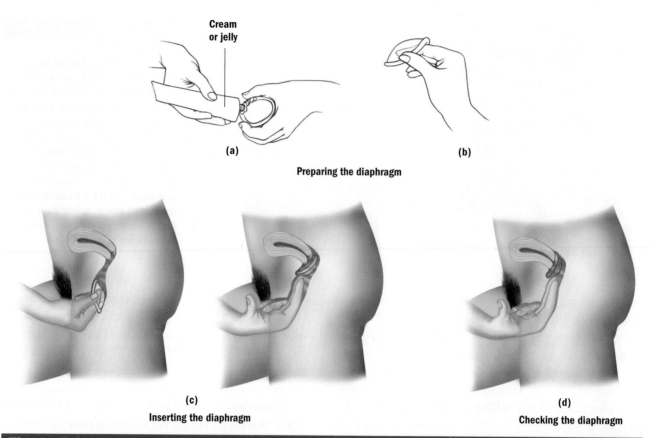

Cream
or jelly

(a)

(b)

Preparing the diaphragm

(c)

Inserting the diaphragm

(d)

Checking the diaphragm

Figure 5.6

Diaphragm. *Hints:* (1) Apply 1 to 2 tsp of spermicide to diaphragm rim and inside dome. (2) Insert the diaphragm by holding it in one hand, squeezing rim together in center. With other hand, spread labia and insert diaphragm. (3) Diaphragm is inserted deep into vagina with the anterior rim tucked into place last. (4) Check for proper placement of the diaphragm. Cervix is felt through dome—feels like tip of the nose. (5) To remove the diaphragm, assume the squatting position and break the suction by placing index finger between diaphragm and pubic bone. Hook finger behind anterior rim, bear down, and remove.

Side effects with the diaphragm are infrequent. An allergic response to the latex of the diaphragm or to the spermicide is possible but rare. Urinary tract infections are another possible side effect of the diaphragm. Some diaphragm users feel bladder pressure, rectal pressure, or cramps when the diaphragm is left in place six hours after intercourse. A smaller diaphragm or a different rim type might help relieve this side effect. Women with poor muscle tone of the vagina, a vaginal or cervical infection, vaginal bleeding, or a history of toxic shock syndrome should not use a diaphragm. After childbirth, weight loss or gain of more than 10 pounds, pelvic surgery, or a miscarriage or an abortion, women should have their diaphragms refitted to ensure proper size.

Cervical Cap

The cervical cap, shown in **Figure 5.7**, looks and works like a small, deep diaphragm. It is made of latex and is used with a spermicidal agent. The cap fits snugly over the

■ The cervical cap looks and works much like a small, deep diaphragm; it is made of latex and is used with a spermicidal agent.

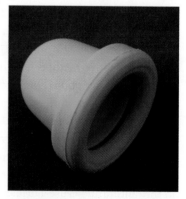

cervix and is held in place by suction. Caps require a clinician's examination, fitting, and prescription. A cervical cap should be replaced each year for best protection. Due to normal anatomical variances, not every woman can be properly fitted with a cervical cap. Because it is smaller than a diaphragm, some women find that insertion and removal of the cap is more frustrating and time consuming than using a diaphragm.

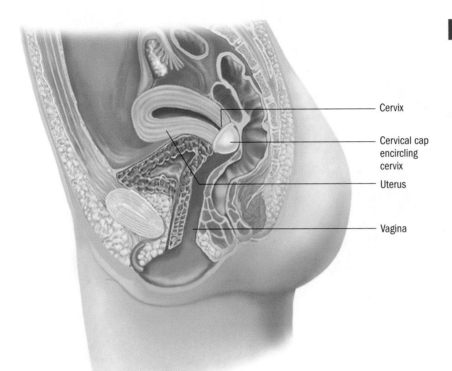

Figure 5.7

Cervical cap. *Hints:* (1) Fill cap approximately two-thirds full of spermicide. (2) Insert the cap by holding it in one hand, squeezing rim together in center. With other hand, spread labia and insert cap. (3) Cap is inserted deep into vagina. Use the index finger to press cap around the cervix until dome covers the cervix. (4) To avoid odor and reduce the risk of complications, remove within recommended time. (5) To remove the cap, break the suction by placing index finger between cap and pubic bone. Grasp dome and pull down and out.

Cervix

Cervical cap encircling cervix

Uterus

Vagina

The cap's effectiveness depends on proper fitting and placement each time it is used. Like the diaphragm, the cap may be inserted hours before lovemaking, but unlike the diaphragm, it can be left in place up to 48 hours. Fresh spermicidal agent should be used with each round of sex. Women should check the seal of the cap before sex and reposition it over the cervix if it has become dislodged. If the cap has moved during sex, additional spermicide should be used. A woman should not douche while the cap is in place, and a cervical cap should not be used during menstruation.

Side effects of the cervical cap are rare, but some women or their partners are allergic to latex. After childbirth, weight loss or weight gain of 10 pounds or more, pelvic surgery, a miscarriage, or an abortion, women should have their cervical caps refitted to ensure proper sizing. The cap is not recommended for women who have a history of toxic shock syndrome or a history of reproductive tract infections. Unlike the diaphragm, women with poor vaginal muscle tone or a history of urinary tract infections can use a cervical cap.

Vaginal Shield

The vaginal shield, also known as Lea's shield, is a new form of barrier contraception now available in the United States. It is a soft silicone cup with a loop used to facilitate removal from the vagina. Like the diaphragm and cap, it is reusable and covers the cervix. However, the shield is not held in place by the cervix; the shield works by volume and is held in place by the vaginal muscles. Because it does not depend on vaginal length or cervical size, one size of the shield fits all women.

Like other vaginal barrier methods, the shield works by completely covering the cervix. It is inserted like a tampon, and the air trapped between the cervix and the shield creates a snug fit in the vagina. Like other vaginal barrier methods, it is recommended that spermicides be used with the shield. Most women have little or no difficulty inserting and removing the shield. Most women do not feel the shield when it is in place but occasionally a male partner can feel the device. The shield should not be used during menstruation. The shield requires a prescription and is not available over-the-counter in drugstores.

Condom

Condoms (Figure 5.8) recently have resurfaced as a popular barrier contraceptive. Women are now responsible for nearly 40% of total condom sales, and condoms are advertised in women's magazines. Condoms are available with lubricants and spermicides and come in a variety of colors and textures. Condoms are portable, disposable, and easy to purchase. They may be discreetly carried and are, therefore, easily available when necessary. Women do not experience any post-intercourse vaginal leaking, and condoms permit the male partner to take an active role in birth control. Latex and polyurethane condoms are also the only

Figure 5.8

Condom use. *Hints:* (1) Avoid prolonged heat or pressure—condoms should not be stored in glove compartments or wallets. (2) Use only once and throw away. (3) If condom should break, use an extra dose of spermicide. (4) Put condom on an erect penis *before* it comes into contact with the vagina, pinching the tip of the condom to prevent air from becoming trapped. (5) Hold onto the rim of the condom as the penis is withdrawn from the vagina. (6) Do not use petroleum-based lubricants with condoms. (7) Latex condoms are more impermeable to the AIDS virus, though some individuals are sensitive or allergic to latex.

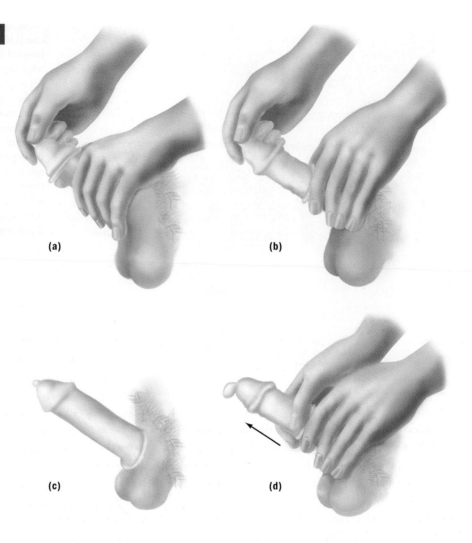

(a)   (b)

(c)   (d)

methods that effectively prevent STIs, including HIV infection. For couples who want to be especially diligent in their birth control efforts, condom use can supplement other forms of contraception.

Condoms should be stored in a cool, dry place, because storage in a heated area (such as a glove compartment) can result in their deterioration. Latex condoms should not be lubricated with an oil-based lubricant (such as Vaseline), which can weaken the latex. If extra lubrication is desired, a water-soluble lubricant (such as K-Y Jelly or Astroglide) or prelubricated condoms can be used. Prelubricated condoms may also help to reduce friction during intercourse and reduce the risk of vaginal or penile irritation.

If a couple selects condoms as their method of birth control, it is essential that a condom be used for every love-making event. Effective use of this contraceptive method requires commitment and discipline. A spermicide-coated condom affords the most effective birth control protection and offers additional protection from STIs. The clear fluid that collects on the end of an erect penis may contain live

sperm, so the condom should be placed on the penis before the penis comes near the vagina. It is important that room be left at the end of the condom to collect the semen. A person should pinch the tip of the condom before putting it on; this will ensure that there is room for the semen and will prevent air bubbles, which increase the risk for breakage, from forming. A condom that is stretched very tightly over the head of the penis is more likely to break or to force the seminal fluid along the shaft of the penis and out the upper end of the condom. The penis should be withdrawn from the vagina before the erection subsides, and the condom should be held during this withdrawal of the penis. As the penis begins to lose its erection, the condom will collapse and the contents of the condom may spill within the vagina. A quick visual inspection to ensure that the contents are inside and that no spill or leakage has occurred is a good idea.

Couples should use condoms both during and after treatment for any reproductive tract infection as a precaution against reinfection. Use of a latex or polyurethane con-

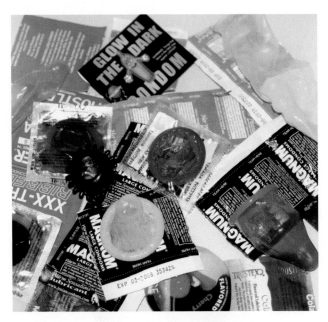

■ Condoms can be latex, polyurethane, or lambskin. Latex and polyurethane condoms offer better protection from sexually transmitted diseases than other types of condoms.

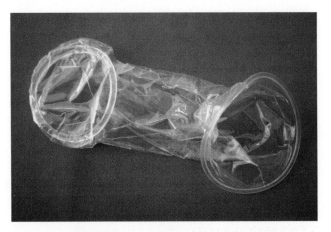

■ The female condom works by lining the entire vagina, thereby preventing the penis and semen from coming in direct physical contact with the vagina.

dom is encouraged for women who are at risk for sexually transmitted diseases—even for those who are using an effective form of birth control, such as the pill. Lambskin and novelty condoms do not protect against diseases. Condoms also should be used on any items that are used during sexual activity that penetrate both partners. Examples would include shared sex toys, such as vibrators and dildos. In such cases, condoms should be changed between insertions if penetrating both vaginal and anal regions. Couples should not use more than one condom at a time, and condoms should never be reused.

Female Condom

The **female condom** is another form of barrier contraception. It is the only female-initiated contraceptive method currently available that can prevent pregnancy and sexually transmitted infections. The female condom, approved by the FDA in 1993, is now available in many countries and is often promoted as a woman-controlled device for HIV protection. In spite of the educational details necessary for individual use, the female condom has enormous potential for improving women's choices for contraception and STI prevention, both in the United States and around the world. Twelve million female condoms are distributed annually, but this represents less than 1% of global male condom distribution.[27] The condom lines the entire vagina, preventing the penis and semen from coming in direct

physical contact with the vagina. It consists of a sheath with a closed ring at one end and an open ring at the other. The female condom covers part of the external genitals, providing extra protection from semen leakage. Although lubricant is contained inside the female condom, additional lubricant is provided, and it should be used.

The female condom gives the woman more control and a sense of freedom with her personal protection. A woman does not need to see a clinician because the female condom is available in some drugstores and through online retailers. It is safe and fairly effective in preventing both pregnancy and sexually transmitted infections. The female condom can make rustling noises during sex, but additional lubricant will help diminish this effect. The size and shape of the condom are unappealing to some women. Proper insertion of the penis into the condom is essential for the condom's effectiveness. Because the female condom is made of polyurethane, not latex, it may be more appealing to individuals who have latex allergies, and because polyurethane transmits heat well, some couples find increased pleasure with the female condom. The female condom is not as widely available as the male condom and it costs more. The female condom can be inserted as long as eight hours before sex. A study comparing the efficacy of the male and female condoms found that although mechanical problems are more common with the female condom, both devices involve a similar risk of semen exposure.[28]

Use of the female condom requires paying attention to details, as well as patience and practice (see **Figure 5.9**). Before insertion, the sides of the female condom should be rubbed together to evenly distribute the lubrication inside the pouch. The female condom should be stored in a cool, dry place and it should be used only once. It should not be

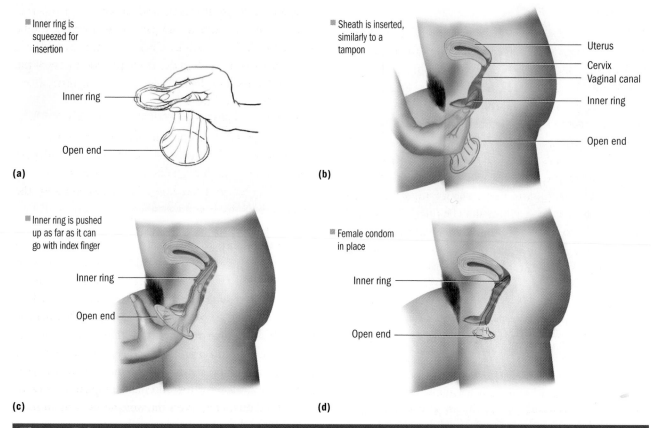

■ Inner ring is
  squeezed for
  insertion

Inner ring ———

Open end ———

(a)

■ Sheath is inserted,
  similarly to a
  tampon

——— Uterus
——— Cervix
——— Vaginal canal
——— Inner ring

——— Open end

(b)

■ Inner ring is pushed
  up as far as it can
  go with index finger

Inner ring ———

Open end ———

(c)

■ Female condom
  in place

Inner ring ———

Open end ———

(d)

Figure 5.9

The female condom.

used with a male condom, diaphragm, cervical cap, or sponge. The only side effect to the female condom is possible allergy to the lubricant.

Contraceptive Sponge

The **contraceptive sponge** is a barrier method that acts as both a cervical barrier and a source of spermicide; it also absorbs ejaculated semen. The sponge is a soft disk-shaped device made from polyurethane foam. One side of the sponge has a dimple that fits up against the cervix, and the other side has a nylon loop that facilitates removal. The sponge is relatively inexpensive, available without a fitting or a prescription, and available in drugstores and online retailers. The sponge is portable, disposable, and can be inserted a few hours before having sex. It does not interrupt lovemaking. The sponge is designed for 24 hours of use, and it should remain in place for 6 hours after the last round of sex. It does not require repeat applications of spermicide for additional sex, and it is less messy than some other forms of spermicidal agents. Because the sponge covers the cervix, it may offer some protection against

STIs, but this protection should not be considered to be reliable. The effectiveness of sponge birth control, like all methods, varies depending on how it is used. The sponge is more effective in women who have never given birth than in women who have. Individual sponges cannot be reused. The sponge can be easy to use, although some women may have difficulty learning to properly insert and remove it.

■ The contraceptive sponge
  acts as both a cervical
  barrier and a source of
  spermicide. It absorbs
  ejaculated semen.

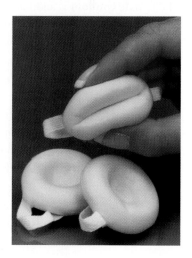

Permanent Methods

Healthy men and women usually have many years of fertility after they have completed their childbearing. Surgical **sterilization** offers permanent birth control for individuals who do not wish to have any more children. Female sterilization is second only to oral contraceptives in overall popularity as a method of birth control (see Figures 5.1 and 5.2). Today, advantages of sterilization include a very high rate of effectiveness and relatively quick, simple procedures that have minimal complications and side effects. An important disadvantage of sterilization as a form of birth control is that although it can sometimes be surgically reversed (a much more complicated procedure than sterilization), it should be considered a lifetime permanent choice to end childbearing. Also, sterilization, for men and women, provides no protection against STIs.

One of the most important decisions for a couple is which partner will undergo permanent sterilization. Women have the option of a having a tubal ligation (tubes "tied"), and men have the option of a vasectomy. The most common choice is for a tubal ligation. This may be due to several factors. Many couples don't realize that a vasectomy poses far less risk to men than the risks associated with tubal ligation for women. Men may also be reluctant to have the procedure. A vasectomy is usually performed in a physician's office and a ligation requires a hospital setting.

Female Sterilization (Tubal Ligation)

Trends among contracepting older reproductive-age U.S. women show a dramatic increase in sterilization rates. Sterilization of women has been made much easier in recent years by the development of new instruments and new techniques that have replaced laparotomy, which involves surgically opening the abdomen and tying off the fallopian tubes. Because a significant number of unwanted subsequent pregnancies occurred with this procedure, newer techniques were developed that destroy or remove part of the fallopian tube.

We have three children and that is our family. The decision for sterilization was not difficult once we realized that we did not wish to become pregnant again. Our sex lives have improved—there is no need to worry about birth control anymore.

35-year-old woman

Laparoscopic sterilization, also known as "band-aid" surgery, is one of these techniques. A laparoscope, a tube equipped with light and magnification lenses (see **Figure 5.10**), is inserted into the abdomen to provide a view of the uterus and tubes. The doctor uses a cauterizing instrument, rings, or clips to seal the fallopian tubes.

Minilaparotomy is the latest technique for tubal ligation. It requires a small abdominal incision and is performed under local or general anesthesia. The fallopian tubes are lifted out through the incision, cut, sealed, and replaced. The entire procedure takes a few minutes; the woman is able to go home after a few hours of recovery and observation.

A new, less invasive form of female sterilization, called Essure, has been available since 2002. It is performed in an ambulatory clinic setting. The procedure requires the insertion of a small plug through a hysteroscope into each of the fallopian tubes. The plugs cause a local inflammatory process that results in tubal occlusion within three months of insertion. A back-up form of birth control is needed for three months; a radiologic confirmation test then is performed to confirm that the tubes are completely blocked. The method offers high sterilization efficacy without incisions, general anesthesia, or a prolonged recovery period for the woman.[29] The procedure has also been found to be more cost-effective than laparoscopic tubal ligation.[30]

Male Sterilization (Vasectomy)

A **vasectomy**, a 30-minute surgical procedure usually performed under local anesthesia in a physician's office, can permanently sterilize a man. In most cases, one or two small incisions are made just through the skin of the scrotum. The vas deferens is lifted through the incision and the two ends are tied or cauterized to seal them. Most men are able to return to work and normal activities the day after surgery but are advised to avoid strenuous activities, such as straining and lifting, for the first week after surgery.

Vasectomy does not provide immediate contraceptive protection. Live sperm may remain in semen temporarily because mature sperm are stored in the vas deferens above the surgical site. As a consequence, men often are advised to use backup contraception for approximately 15 to 20 ejaculations.

Vasectomy offers several advantages. It is extremely effective as a permanent form of birth control and has a very low risk of complications compared to temporary forms of birth control or tubal ligation for women. Vasectomy does not cause any change in hormone levels or in the

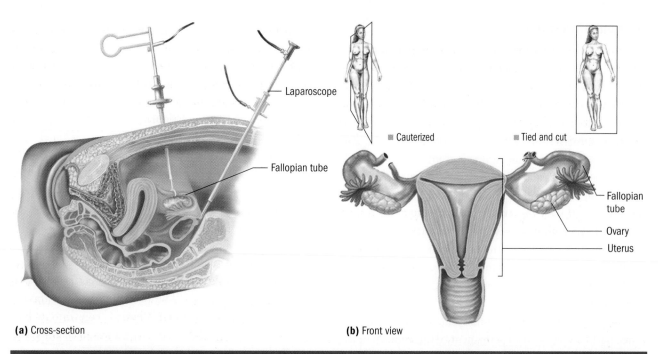

Laparoscope

Fallopian tube

■ Cauterized   ■ Tied and cut

Fallopian tube

Ovary

Uterus

(a) Cross-section   **(b)** Front view

Figure 5.10

Female sterilization. *Hints:*
(1) Resume normal activity slowly after procedure. (2) Most sutures are dissolvable. (3) Take mild analgesic for discomfort. (4) Resume sexual activity when comfortable. (5) Seek medical attention if temperature rises above 100°F, or if acute pain, discharge from incision, or bleeding is experienced.

appearance or volume of semen. It also permits the male partner to take an active role in contraceptive responsibility.

Other Forms of Contraception

Not all contraceptive methods are appropriate for general use. Some methods are valid approaches to birth control, yet are associated with fairly high failure rates. **Abstinence** refers to no penis-in-vagina intercourse and depends on a couple's sustained willpower. Some couples consider oral sex or mutual masturbation, which do not result in pregnancy, a form of abstinence. In theory, abstinence is 100% effective; unfortunately, this method requires considerable sacrifice and has a high rate of failure in practice.

Withdrawal, also known as coitus interruptus, refers to interrupting lovemaking before ejaculation of semen. Al-

He told me that he knew what he was doing. It was the first time that I had sex. He pulled out but I still got pregnant. I was so foolish to think that I would not or could not get pregnant.

16-year-old student

though it may seem logical that conception requires semen and therefore requires ejaculation, withdrawal often fails as a form of birth control when the man is unable to remove his penis in time or because some sperm are released before ejaculation. The failure rate for withdrawal as a form of birth control is fairly high because it is difficult for a man to know exactly when ejaculation will occur. It also is mentally and physically difficult to suddenly stop in the midst of lovemaking. Withdrawal does not protect either partner from sexually transmitted infections.

Lactational Amenorrhea Method (LAM)

Breastfeeding women may use the lactational amenorrhea method, alone or with other forms of contraception, for the first six months postpartum. For LAM to be effective, the woman must be breastfeeding exclusively on demand, be amenorrheic (no vaginal bleeding after eight weeks postpartum), and have an infant younger than six months. The failure rate of this contraceptive method is reported to be less than 2% if these criteria are met.[31] If pregnancy is not desired, another method of contraception must be used as soon as menstruation resumes, breastfeeding is decreased, or the baby reaches six months of age.

Intrauterine Devices

An intrauterine device (IUD) is a small object that a clinician inserts into a woman's uterus. Today, the IUD is the most widely used contraceptive in the world.[32] The IUD, however, is not as popular in the United States as it is in the rest of the world. For example, a recent study in California found that although the IUD is available at no cost from the state family planning program for low-income women, only 1.3% of female patients obtain IUDs annually.[33] Modern forms of the IUD provide very effective and reversible long-term protection from unwanted pregnancy without increasing the risk of reproductive tract infections. Although initial costs for an IUD may be higher than other forms of contraception, their long-term effectiveness is an important consideration, and IUDs yield a very low cost over time.

There is not yet scientific consensus about how IUDs prevent pregnancy, and their different designs present different theories for their effectiveness. The horizontal arms of some designs contain copper that is slowly released into the uterine cavity, preventing sperm from successfully reaching eggs from a woman's ovaries. Other types contain a progestin hormone that is slowly released, causing a thickening of the cervical mucus that prevents sperm migration to the egg. All IUDs are believed to establish a chronic sterile inflammatory reaction in the uterus that interferes with sperm function so that fertilization is less likely to occur. IUDs also interfere with implantation, but the extent to which this contributes to their contraceptive effectiveness is not known.[32]

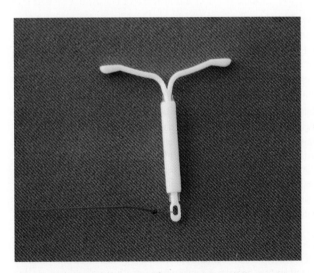

■ An intrauterine device (IUD) is a small object placed in the uterus through the cervix by a clinician.

There are currently two highly effective forms of IUDs available in the United States. One form is the Copper T-IUD, which is effective for at least 10 years. This long-term effectiveness presents a good alternative to a younger woman who might be contemplating sterilization. The other available IUD is the LNG-IUS, which may be left in the uterus for up to seven years. It is more effective than the copper IUD and is sometimes used as a treatment for endometriosis or as an alternative to hysterectomy for menorrhagia, a condition characterized by abnormally heavy and prolonged menstrual periods at regular intervals. Both IUD forms rival surgical sterilization in their effectiveness in preventing pregnancy. Less than 1% of users will experience an accidental pregnancy in the first year. These IUDs prevent ectopic pregnancies, and they provide some protection against endometrial cancer. Menstrual cramping is decreased with the IUDs, and menstrual blood flow is often dramatically reduced. It has been suggested that IUDs may not be offered to young women as often as hormonal contraceptives due to provider educational and training issues.[33]

Emergency Birth Control

Contraceptive methods are not universally effective, and accidents can occur with any method or any couple. A bout of a gastrointestinal illness can reduce the effectiveness of the pill; condoms may break; a cervical cap can become dislodged; and a diaphragm can be removed too early. These unintended consequences can lead to an unplanned pregnancy. Women, their partners, and clinicians have often had a need for measures that can provide immediate additional back-up protection. Emergency contraception (EC) is known by several other names, including emergency birth control (EBC), the morning-after pill, and postcoital contraception. These terms all relate to a therapy or a procedure used to prevent pregnancy after an unprotected or inadequately protected act of sexual intercourse. A recent review by the Cochrane Group found several interventions are available for emergency contraception. Their review concluded that the copper IUD inserted after

I did not know that my regular birth control pills could be used for emergency contraception. I had missed a couple of them because I forgot to take them with me on a weekend trip. My pharmacist was very helpful in explaining my EC options.

20-year-old college student

unprotected intercourse was effective in providing emergency contraception. Of the hormonal methods, the group concluded that 25–50 mg of mifepristone was superior to other hormonal regimens. Other hormonal regimens and dosages were also effective.[34]

EC is not intended for routine use, but as a backup in the event of unprotected sex or a contraceptive failure. Emergency contraception should not be confused with medical abortion. A medical abortion is used to terminate an existing pregnancy. EC is effective only before a pregnancy is established. *EC is not a medical abortion drug.* EC works by inhibiting or delaying ovulation or by preventing the implantation of a fertilized egg in the uterus. EC is ineffective after implantation. Studies indicate that EC confers no increased risk to an established pregnancy or harm to the developing embryo.[35]

In the United States, the availability of hormonal emergency contraception has been a political story as much as a medical story. Conservative groups have organized heavy resistance to the availability and use of the product. In 1999 the Food and Drug Administration (FDA) approved a form of EC for use with a doctor's prescription. In 2003, a combined panel of the FDA's Advisory Committee on Reproductive Health Drugs and the Advisory Committee on Nonprescription Drugs concluded that the EC regimen was safe for nonprescription status. However, EC was not available for over-the-counter (OTC) sales until 2006. The approved form is a prepackaged dose of progestin hormones, the same hormone used in daily oral contraceptives.

Plan B is the only dedicated EC product currently available in the United States. It is a two-dose regimen that should be taken within 120 hours of unprotected sex in order to be effective. Previously available only by prescription, it is now available in most major pharmacies. Plan B is not stocked on the shelves, but is available from the pharmacist. Men or women 18 years old or over may purchase Plan B. Early data indicate that availability of Plan B increased after it was awarded OTC status.[36] Some insurance plans will provide coverage and reimbursement for Plan B; however, most will require a prescription from a clinician. Although Plan B is the only dedicated product specifically marketed for emergency contraception in the United States, specific dosages of 21 brands of oral contraceptives on the market today can also be used for emergency contraception.

Many women still do not understand EC. Survey data show that many women are unaware of EC, misunderstand its use and safety, do not have convenient and prompt access to it, or do not use it when a need arises.[37] Some groups have argued that EC availability would lead to increased sexual behavior risk taking; others have argued that EC would lead to lower unintended pregnancy rates. Long-term studies are not yet available to answer these important concerns. One study compared women seeking EC and women seeking family planning to be quite different. The EC group had higher levels of education, were more likely to have been protected at their last intercourse, and were less likely to have a previous STI.[38]

Gender Dimensions

CONTRACEPTION

Historically, contraceptive options have been largely for women. This may be due in part to the reality that women, not men, get pregnant, or the fact that family planning research and contraceptive services have focused disproportionately on women. The female reproductive system has been extensively studied for centuries. Studies on male contraceptives have been seriously limited. Today, options for the male range from mildly effective (withdrawal) to highly effective (vasectomy). It could be argued that the remarkable effectiveness of modern hormonal contraceptives for women has given women high levels of protection, but that it has absolved men from participating in contraceptive protection and decision making. Men are often silent partners in preventing unwanted pregnancies.

Several factors contribute to the dominant role women play in contraceptive decision making and the availability of services for them. Modern medical care services provide ready access to contraceptive information and options for women. Women are taught and encouraged to see a gynecologist in their teens. There is not a parallel system for

men. Society educates girls and young women early that the penalty of unprotected sex will be an unwanted pregnancy, shame, and economic hardships. The educational message to boys and young men is not the same, although legal issues surrounding paternity and child support in recent years have introduced the penalty concept to an unwanted pregnancy.

Multicultural surveys demonstrate that men are willing to participate in contraception, and their female partners trust them to do so.[41] Male contraceptive research includes hormonal and nonhormonal methods. Today the most significant barriers for expanded use include limited delivery methods and perceived regulatory obstacles. New reversible hormonal advances in oral, implant, and injectable androgen methods are promising options for men.[42] Recent international clinical studies have shown 90–95% efficacy rates for male hormonal methods.[41] Nonhormonal male contraceptives include products that target sperm motility. Although considerable progress has been made in clinical research on male contraception, no new product is currently available or likely to be so in the near future.

Providing EC in advance of need gives women rapid access to the medication in case of unprotected intercourse or contraceptive failure. Studies have examined the availability of an advance supply of EC to see how it would affect contraceptive use. Results are early and also somewhat mixed. One study found that advance provision of EC significantly increased use without reducing use of routine contraception.[39] Another meta-analysis found that advance provision of emergency contraception did not reduce pregnancy rates and did not negatively affect sexual and reproductive health behaviors. The authors acknowledge that many variables need further study to better understand the behavioral and social issues surrounding the failure to use emergency contraception even when it is readily available.[40]

Time is critically important for EC to be effective. To help make accurate and sensitive information readily available to women, information is available on the Internet from the Office of Population Research at Princeton University and from the Association of Reproductive Health Professionals at http://ec.princeton.edu/get-ec-now.html. The site has no connection with any pharmaceutical company or for-profit organization, and the information is peer reviewed by a panel of independent experts.

Handling an Unplanned Pregnancy

Women who experience an unplanned pregnancy must face a difficult decision. They may decide to terminate the pregnancy, to carry the baby to term and keep the child, or to carry the baby to term and have the child adopted. A woman must consider the implications of each decision and feel comfortable with her choice. Having a baby brings major changes to a woman's life, and it may cause many difficulties for a woman who is young and single. Plans for future education, careers, or relationships may have to be sacrificed to raise a child. All of these issues must be considered so that a woman does not resent her child based on a decision she has made. A woman may be concerned about financial and emotional support during the pregnancy, especially if she does not have support from the baby's father or from family and friends. Many family planning clinics, crisis pregnancy centers, and health departments have programs set up to meet the needs of these women.

Unplanned pregnancies are not always unwanted pregnancies. Often, a couple is not planning to have a child at the time that they become pregnant, but they want a child and happily decide to proceed with the pregnancy.

If a woman decides that she would like to carry the baby to term but not raise the child, she should look into adoption. Adoption can be "open," where the birth mother has some role in the child's future, or "closed," where the whole process remains confidential. Both public and private adoption services are available. Public adoption services are usually less costly but may be very competitive and require long waits. Parents often have to be more flexible about the age or race of child they are willing to take. Private adoptions usually involve a financial arrangement negotiated by an agency or lawyer between the adoptive parents and the birth mother. Private adoptions can be faster and allow adoptive parents and birth mothers to have more options in selecting each other. Adoptions also can be domestic or international, though adoption laws vary from country to country. In all adoptions, a host of legal and ethical factors must be considered by all parties involved. Many adoption agencies can help match the child with an adoptive family and may be able to arrange for the adoptive parents to pay for the mother's health-care costs during the pregnancy.

Other women choose to terminate their pregnancies. In these cases, a decision should be made as early as possible to ensure a safe abortion.

Perspectives on Abortion

Abortion may be defined as the spontaneous or induced expulsion of an embryo or fetus before it is viable or can survive on its own. This can occur without human interference. Natural complications of fetal development, perhaps due to genetic, medical, or hormonal problems, can result in the spontaneous termination of the pregnancy. This termination of pregnancy is called a miscarriage or a spontaneous abortion (see Chapter 6). In contrast to a spontaneous abortion, an induced abortion involves a decision to terminate a pregnancy by medical procedures.

Abortions are one of the most common medical procedures undergone by women of reproductive age. Each year, about 1.2 million women in the United States end their pregnancies through abortion. This number represents almost 20% of the 6.4 million annual pregnancies in the

I am an organized and responsible person. I was a victim of contraceptive failure. It was impossible for me to have a child at that time in my life. It would have destroyed everything that I had worked years for. So I had an abortion. I am not proud of it, but I am grateful that I was able to go to a safe facility.

32-year-old woman

United States. About one-third of unwanted pregnancies in the United States end in abortion.[43]

Historical Overview

Women have ended unwanted pregnancies for thousands of years. The earliest methods used to induce an abortion were often either dangerous or used in ways to control women: 5,000 years ago, a Chinese emperor described how mercury could be used to induce an abortion; in the Western world, ancient Greeks and Romans considered abortion acceptable during the early stages of pregnancy, but they did not allow women an active role in family planning.[44] Later, women healers in western Europe and the United States provided abortions and trained other women to do so, until the late 1800s.

But by 1910, many states had passed legislation promoted by male physicians that prohibited abortion during all stages of pregnancy, with the exception of pregnancies that endangered the mother's health. During this time, the issue of equity emerged as an abortion public policy consideration. Women with greater personal financial resources were able to arrange for safer, more "legal" abortions by traveling to less rigid jurisdictions or by persuading physicians to make therapeutic exceptions. Women with fewer financial resources were more likely to suffer from unsafe abortions and incompetent abortionists. Legal prohibition did not have its intended effect of reducing the incidence of abortions, however. Estimates of the number of illegal abortions performed annually in the 1950s and 1960s range from 200,000 to 1.2 million.

The landmark Supreme Court decision *Roe v. Wade* legalized abortion in the United States on January 22, 1973. This decision declared unconstitutional all state laws that prohibited or restricted abortion during the first trimester of pregnancy. The decision stated that the "right of privacy . . . founded on the Fourteenth Amendment's concept of personal liberty . . . is broad enough to encompass a woman's decision whether or not to terminate her pregnancy." The ruling also limited state interventions in second-trimester abortions and left the issue of third-trimester abortions up to each individual state.

Socially conservative groups quickly rallied against the decision, organizing the "right to life" movement and working to enact laws restricting abortion at the state and federal levels.

In 1976, Congress introduced and passed the Hyde Amendment. This legislation banned Medicaid funding for abortion unless a woman's life was in danger. This amendment disproportionately affected low-income women, who were less likely than other women to be able to pay for abortion services or to receive contraception. A compromise version of the Hyde Amendment eventually added exceptions for promptly reported rape and incest cases in which two physicians would testify that the woman's health would be seriously impaired by maintaining the pregnancy. Although the Supreme Court reaffirmed the central holding of *Roe v. Wade* in 1986, a newly constituted Court agreed to hear the case *Webster v. Reproductive Health Services* in 1989. Its decision on the *Webster* case returned to the states the authority to limit a woman's right to a legal abortion.

The 1991 case of *Rust v. Sullivan* upheld the constitutionality of the "gag rule," which prohibited federally funded clinics from providing information about and referrals for abortion. In 1992, the Court's ruling in the case of *Planned Parenthood of Southeastern Pennsylvania v. Casey* reaffirmed the central holdings of *Roe v. Wade*, but allowed states to restrict abortion access. This decision prompted many states to require parental consent and waiting periods.

Laws have also limited antiabortion demonstrators' proximity to abortion clinics. These laws were instituted to ensure the safety and privacy of women seeking abortions after many attacks on abortion clinics, women seeking abortions, and abortion providers took place.

Legal Perspectives

During the presidency of George W. Bush, the appointments of Justices John Roberts and Samuel Alito made the Supreme Court significantly more conservative on social issues. This conservative slant was visible in the 2007 case of *Gonzales v. Carhart*, which upheld a federal ban on a rare abortion procedure known as dilatation and extraction, despite the fact that the law did not allow an exception to the ban when it was necessary to protect a woman's health. In 2000, a court without the Bush appointees had ruled against a Nebraska law that created a very similar "partial birth" abortion ban for this reason. Some political commentators believe the 2009 court could make a decision that would overthrow *Roe v. Wade*. President Barack Obama, who has voiced strong support for a woman's right

"I am on my own, financially and mentally. I can't stand it now, I think it's a sin to bring the child here and not be able to provide for it . . . . This is just in the best interest for me and the children—no, my children and this child."

19-year-old woman with three children, living below the poverty line

Source: Finer, L., et al. (2005). Reasons U.S. women have abortions: Quantitative and qualitative perspectives.

to end her pregnancy, will likely select at least one Supreme Court justice during his presidency. This nomination could tilt the balance of the current court away from the right.

With the shifting balance of the Supreme Court, socially conservative state governments have enacted stronger limitations on abortion. In South Dakota, for example, a law that went into effect in 2008 requires doctors to tell women that abortion "terminates the life of a whole, separate, unique human being" and to cite medically inaccurate information linking abortion to suicide and other risks.[45] **Figure 5.11** compares the relative strictness of abortion laws, as well as the comparative ease of access to abortion services, in the United States.

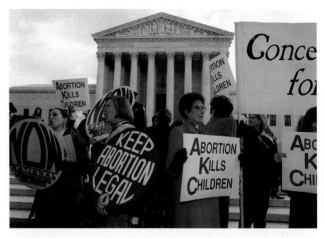

■ Abortion continues to be one of the greatest debates in American society.

Current Perspectives

Abortion is both one of the most common gynecological procedures women experience and among the most controversial and passionately debated topics in the United States. Generally, people who believe that abortion should be illegal describe themselves as "pro-life," whereas people who believe that women should be able to choose abortion to end their pregnancies describe themselves as "pro-choice." Journalists, who wish to appear neutral and not imply that either group is against life or choice, use the terms "antiabortion" and "abortion rights" to describe activists on either side.

Women choose to end their pregnancies for a variety of reasons. Women are most likely to choose abortion when facing an unwanted pregnancy. In a survey of more than 1,000 abortion patients, 74% of women said that having a child would reduce their ability to work, finish their education, or care for existing dependents; 73% said they could not afford to have a baby at the time; and 48% said they were either having relationship problems or did not want to be a single mother. Other commonly cited reasons were that the woman had completed her childbearing (38% of

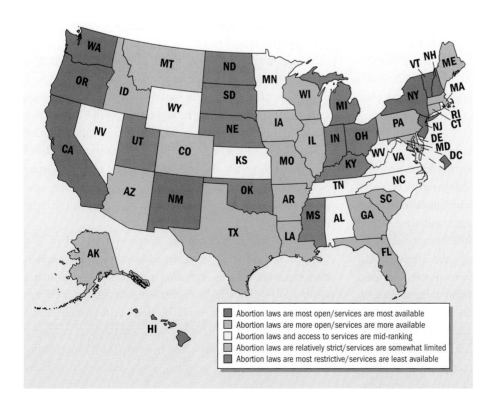

Figure 5.11

State-by-state comparison of abortion laws and access to services, 2006.

Source: Ipas, National Gay and Lesbian Taskforce, Sistersong Women of Color, Reproductive Health Collective, and Center for Reproductive Rights. (2008). Mapping our rights, www.mappingourrights.org.

■ Abortion laws are most open/services are most available
■ Abortion laws are more open/services are more available
□ Abortion laws and access to services are mid-ranking
■ Abortion laws are relatively strict/services are somewhat limited
■ Abortion laws are most restrictive/services are least available

women), was not ready for another child (32%), or did not want people to know she was pregnant or that she had had sex (25%).[46]

The Antiabortion Perspective

The antiabortion (or "pro-life") position is typically based on the belief that a fertilized ovum is a human being from the moment of conception onward. From this perspective, a fetus has a right to live, and a woman does not have the ability to override that right by choosing an abortion.

Antiabortion efforts to overturn abortion public policy have taken three major approaches: amendments to the U.S. and state constitutions that define human life beginning at conception; legislation and government action that defines human life beginning at conception; and efforts to slow or restrict access to abortion services. By defining a fetus as "human," antiabortion groups hope to afford fetuses the same legal rights and protection as adults and children and ultimately outlaw (or put severe legal restrictions on) all abortions.

The Abortion-Rights Perspective

Abortion-rights (or "pro-choice") advocates favor full legalization and ready availability of abortions. Abortion-rights advocates believe that women facing unwanted pregnancies will usually find a way to end them, and that legalizing abortion at least provides these women with safe services rather than putting their lives at risk. Additionally, abortion-rights activists typically do not believe that a fertilized ovum qualifies as "human life." Instead, they see abortion as part of a spectrum of a woman's reproductive health care. Abortion-rights advocates believe that a woman should be able to choose whether or not to end a pregnancy because the fetus is ultimately still part of her body.

Middle Ground

Most Americans' opinions about abortion have elements of both the antiabortion and the abortion-rights perspectives. A poll conducted by *Time* magazine in August 2008 found that 46% of respondents thought abortion should always be legal in the first trimester, 40% thought abortion should be legal in some circumstances, and 10% thought abortion should be illegal in all circumstances (4% said they had no answer). Finding a suitable compromise on such a divisive issue remains a political and personal challenge. For people who believe that human life begins at conception and that abortion ends that life, even the idea of compromise can be repugnant.

However, research has found some ways that abortions can be prevented without increasing or decreasing women's access to safe services. The easiest of these methods may be to increase access to contraception. Roughly half the pregnancies that occur in the United States are unintentional, and almost half of unintended pregnancies (or more than one in five total pregnancies in the United States) end in abortion.[46] Allowing women and their partners to control when and if they want to have children will prevent enormous psychological and financial burdens for families as well. Increasing public assistance may also reduce abortion levels, because funds and aid will allow women living in poverty to better care for unintended pregnancies that do occur.[46]

Epidemiology

Abortions have been legal throughout the United States since 1973 (state laws, however, make abortion services more difficult to obtain in some states than in others). **Figure 5.12** depicts the rate of abortions in the United States over the past three decades. After an initial rise in the 1970s following legislation, the number of induced abortions stabilized in the 1980s, at about 1.6 million per year.[5] This declining trend increased in the first years of the twenty-first century; from 2000 to 2005, the number of abortions dropped in the United States by 9%.[43] Possible reasons for this decline include increased contraceptive use, more women completing their pregnancies, fewer unintended pregnancies, and reduced access to abortion services in some areas.[43]

Several factors also appear to have played a part in this decline. Changes in U.S. demographics meant that a lower proportion of the female population was of childbearing age and at risk for having to consider abortion. The drive to educate girls about teen pregnancy and contraceptive options has also helped to reduce teen pregnancy. Other factors affecting the decline in abortions over time may include reduced access to abortion services, changing attitudes toward abortion, or continuation of unplanned pregnancies.

The profile of the typical abortion seeker has also changed in the last 20 years. In addition to young women who experience an unintended pregnancy, the growing number of women who get pregnant over the age of 35 has led to an increase in women who find out that their developing babies are at very high risk of birth defects or have a chromosomal abnormality like trisomy 18. Women living in poverty continue to be much more likely than wealthy

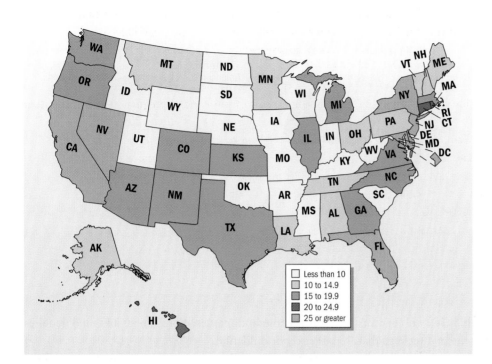

Figure 5.12

Rate of legal abortions per 1,000 women of reproductive age by state, 2005.

Source: Jones, R., Zolna, M., Henshaw, S., & Finer, L. (2008). Abortion in the United States: Incidence and access to service, 2005. *Perspectives on Reproductive Health* 40(1): 6–16.

women to have abortions, in large part because poor women are more likely to experience unwanted pregnancies. In 2005, the average cost of an abortion at 10 weeks was $413.[43]

More than half of women in the United States who receive abortions already have one or more children, seven out of 10 women who receive abortions have never been married. The average age of women receiving abortions has increased: in 1980, 64.7% of women who had abortions were 24 or younger; by 2005 this number had dropped to 50%.[5] **Figure 5.14** illustrates abortion rates by race/ethnicity and age.

Adolescent females are a special population of concern with abortions. Factors contributing to adolescent pregnancies and decisions about keeping or terminating the pregnancy depend on a variety of socioeconomic considerations. Girls age 19 and younger account for 20% of all abortions in the United States.[47] One study found that 61% of the adolescents indicated that one or both parents knew about the abortion.[48] Studies also have found that a

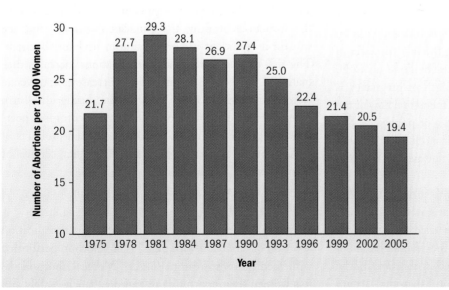

Figure 5.13

The number of abortions in the United States per 1,000 women ages 15–44, by year.

Source: Jones, R., Zolna, M., Henshaw, S., & Finer, L. (2008). Abortion in the United States: Incidence and access to service, 2005. *Perspectives on Reproductive Health* 40(1): 6–16.

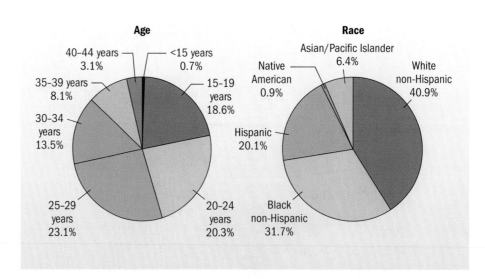

Figure 5.14

Percentage of total abortions in the United States, by age and race/ethnicity, 2000-2001.

Source: Jones, R.K., Darroch, J.E., and Henshaw, S.K. (2002). Patterns in the socioeconomic characteristics of women obtaining abortions in 2000-2001. *Perspectives on Sexual and Reproductive Health* 34(5): Table 1. Reprinted with permission from The Guttmacher Institute.

Abortion Procedures

Surgical Abortion

Vacuum curettage is the most widely used abortion technique in the United States. This procedure is performed while the woman is under local anesthesia. About 87% of all legal abortions done in the United States use vacuum curettage.[49] It involves dilating the cervix and then inserting a vacuum curette—an instrument consisting of a tube with a scoop attached for scraping away tissue—through the cervix into the uterus. The other end of the tube is attached to a suction-producing apparatus, and the contents of the uterus are aspirated into a collection vessel. Vacuum curettage is usually performed during the first trimester of pregnancy, or until 13 weeks, but can be done up to 20 weeks following conception. The length of pregnancy is determined from the onset of the last menstrual flow or the last missed period. Through 13 weeks of pregnancy, this procedure can be performed in a clinical office setting with appropriate backup facilities for unexpected medical problems.

Dilatation and curettage (D&C) is a technique used for many gynecological procedures but rarely in abortions. A sharp curette is used to scrape out the contents of the uterus. The procedure requires that the woman be under general anesthesia. D&C is rarely used in abortions in the United States because it is more painful than the vacuum

curettage method, causes more blood loss, and requires larger cervical dilation.

Dilatation and evacuation is a procedure that combines the D&C and vacuum curettage approaches. It is usually done between 13 and 15 weeks' gestation, but may be done through week 22. At this time, the cervix needs to be dilated to a greater extent because the products of conception are larger. This procedure is performed in the operating room of a clinic or hospital.

Oxytocin, a product produced in the posterior pituitary and also commercially manufactured, is often used to facilitate uterine contractions. It is commonly used with the D&C method and with hypertonic saline during second-trimester abortions.

As with all medical procedures, abortions carry some health risks. Abortion-related health risks are greatly reduced if the pregnancy is terminated as early as possible, the woman is healthy, the clinician is skilled, and the woman is confident in her decision to have an abortion.[8] The risk of death or serious complications increases dramatically as the gestation period increases; however, a woman is 11 times more likely to die during childbirth than from a legal abortion.[28] The most common post-abortion problems include infection, retained products of conception in the uterus, continuing pregnancy, cervical or uterine trauma, and bleeding.

Medical Abortion

A medical abortion (sometimes referred to as a medication abortion or "abortion with pills") is an abortion performed with medication instead of surgery. Medical abortion offers women the opportunity to end pregnancies safely and

teen's decision to have an abortion is based on concerns about how a baby would change her life and feelings that she is not mature enough or financially capable of raising a child.[48]

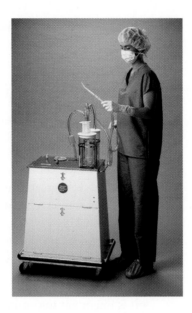

■ Most abortions in the United States are performed using vacuum curettage.

in a way that many women feel is less invasive and more private than surgical abortion procedures. Two drugs called mifepristone and misoprostol, used in succession, can end an early pregnancy. Since FDA approval of mifepristone, medical abortions have grown in popularity as a method of ending a pregnancy. About 13% of abortions performed in the United States in 2005 were performed with medical abortion.[43]

Mifepristone, formerly known as RU-486, is a hormone pill that blocks the action of progesterone, which is necessary for ending a pregnancy. The FDA approved mifepristone in 2000 as a safe and effective alternative to surgical abortion in the United States. A woman first takes mifepristone at a provider's office; this causes the uterine lining to break down. Days later, misoprostol is used to induce contractions and expel the fetal tissue. In some cases, a provider may use a medication called methotrexate instead of mifepristone.

Medical abortions must be administered by a woman's doctor. Heavy bleeding and cramping ensue as a result of the misoprostol. These symptoms may last from a few hours to two weeks. The entire abortion is therefore considered to take anywhere from a few days to a few weeks and requires several visits to the health-care provider's office. Possible side effects may include nausea, vomiting, diarrhea, headaches, hot flushes, and mouth sores.

Medical abortions may be performed as soon as a pregnancy is confirmed, and they must be performed within seven weeks after a woman's last menstrual period. Women who are older than 35 years of age or who smoke should not use methotrexate or mifepristone. Other conditions that may preclude a woman from having a medical abor-

tion include history of asthma, cardiovascular disease, uncontrolled hypertension, diabetes, ovarian cysts or tumors, and severe anemia.

Currently, lawmakers in many states are moving to restrict medical abortion. At both the federal and state levels, some have proposed legislation designed to curtail the availability of mifepristone and limit the number of doctors who can prescribe it.

Global Perspectives

Every year, problems caused by pregnancy or childbirth kill more than 500,000 women. Ninety-nine out of 100 of these deaths occur in the developing world.[50] Problems related to pregnancy and childbirth also cause serious health problems for 10 to 20 million women a year. Women in the developing world facing unplanned or unwanted pregnancies are especially vulnerable.

Despite the magnitude of this problem, the solutions to ending it are simple: provide women with skilled attendants (such as doctors or midwives) when they give birth, provide family planning so that women and their partners can choose when and if they want to have children, and allow women access to safe abortion services.[50] However, poor health systems, a lack of organized political willpower, and, in the case of abortion, legal restrictions and religious opposition have limited progress in this arena. Reduction in maternal mortality has been extremely slow over the past 20 years. Maternal deaths in sub-Saharan Africa, where the problem is the worst, have not lessened.[51]

Forty-two million women received abortions in 2003. Half of these abortions were performed under unsafe conditions or by people without the knowledge, training, or equipment to perform these abortions safely. There is a huge difference between abortions performed under safe and unsafe conditions. Abortions performed in safe conditions by qualified providers pose little risk to a woman's health. Abortions performed under unsafe conditions, or by people without enough training, equipment, or knowledge to perform these abortions safely, however, pose a grave risk to women's long-term health and survival.[52] Globally, about 13% of the deaths and 20% of the injuries developing from pregnancy and childbirth result from unsafe abortion. Almost all of these deaths and injuries occurred in countries with severe legal restrictions on abortion.[53] Laws that restrict abortion do not appear to affect its incidence: even though abortion is illegal under many circumstances in most countries in Africa and legal in most circumstances for most European countries, women in both Europe and Africa receive abortions at almost exactly the same rate.[53]

Informed Decision Making

Contraception

Many effective, yet imperfect, birth control methods are available to women today. The decision-making challenge is to determine which method or combination of methods best meets each woman's unique needs. Safety and reliability are always the first concern. Other factors, such as health status, lifestyle, financial considerations, and patterns in sexual activity, also determine which method is best suited to meet a woman's needs. Many women will decide to change to a different birth control method as factors change. Communication is an essential component of contraceptive decision making. It is important that couples talk about their feelings, needs, and fears.

Determining Personal Needs

Sexual urges and sexual activity are normal, but pregnancy is a very real possible consequence of heterosexual inter-course. Both homosexual and heterosexual relationships also carry the risk of sexually transmitted infections, including HIV. For both technological and sociological reasons, women have traditionally shouldered the major responsibility for contraception. This has been both unfair and unreasonable for women. Although most of the current contraceptives require primary use by women, couples can share the responsibility for contraception in many ways. Open and honest communication, sensitivity to each other's needs and feelings, and awareness of each method's strengths and weaknesses are essential components for effective decision making.

Specific strategies for informed contraceptive decision making include the following (**Self-Assessment 5.1**):

1. Review needs.

   ■ It is important to consider when or if pregnancy may be desired. If never, perhaps sterilization is a more logical option. If pregnancy is desired in a few years, the more effective hormonal methods may be preferable. If pregnancy is desired later within the year, one of the barrier methods may be a better choice. If a woman does not want to become pregnant and an abortion is out of the question, she may wish to consider a combina-

---

Self-Assessment 5.1

Strategies for Contraceptive Decision Making

Contraceptive decision making is a personal and private matter between a woman and her partner. The couple should consider several factors before deciding on what method to use. These factors include:

1. **Evaluate needs:**
   When/if a pregnancy will be desired
   How disruptive or difficult an unplanned pregnancy would be
   Frequency of intercourse
   Number of partners
   Risk of STIs
   Personal preferences for lovemaking
   Level of partner cooperation and interest
   Significance of spontaneity
   Comfort with touching one's own body or partner's
        comfort level of touching or being touched
   Manual dexterity for certain methods
   Financial considerations

2. **Review medical history:**
   Cardiovascular risk factors
   History of cancer
   Certain disabilities or chronic conditions
   Smoking status
   Allergies
   Circulatory disorders

3. **Review reproductive health history:**
   History of abortion or pregnancy scare
   Vaginal or cervical infections
   History of STIs
   Number of sexual partners or partner's number of partners
   Drug use (including alcohol)
   Past use of contraceptives

4. **Put risks and benefits of methods in perspective:**
   Weigh the advantages and disadvantages of each method in a personal perspective (see **Table 5.4**)

5. **Reevaluate decision periodically:**
   Each partner should assess level of compliance
   Each partner should assess level of satisfaction

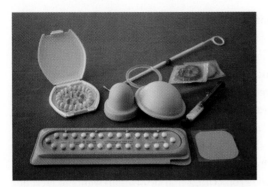

■ Several contraceptive choices are available today.

tion of two good birth control methods, such as foam and condoms, or pills and condoms.

- Frequency of intercourse is another major consideration to review. If intercourse occurs frequently, barrier methods may prove to be inconvenient.

- Number of partners should be considered. If a woman has more than one partner, or if her partner has another partner, she is at a greater risk for infection. In this case, a condom with spermicide in addition to birth control pills would provide the best protection against both sexually transmitted infections and pregnancy.

- Emotional, behavioral, and psychological needs should be considered. Even though a method may appear logical from a medical point of view, if it is distasteful or undesirable, chances are that compliance with that method will be poor. The degree of partner cooperation is another important consideration, because barrier methods are more likely to be successful if there is partner cooperation and support.

- Couples should be honest and realistic when deciding which kinds of contraception they will use. Couples who are unable or unwilling to use condoms every time they have sexual intercourse may wish to consider another form of contraception to supplement or replace condoms. Birth control pills will not be effective unless a woman remembers to take them every day.

- Perhaps one of the most important considerations is an evaluation of partner feelings and support. Ideally, the contraceptive choice will be a joint decision made by a couple following open, honest discussion of all the considerations and issues. In

a less than ideal situation, a woman would be unwise to depend on her partner for contraceptive decision making or use.

2. Consider medical factors. Risk factors for cardiovascular disease, smoking status, circulatory disorders, and other medical factors must be carefully reviewed before deciding on birth control pills. A history of vaginal or cervical infections may rule out the use of diaphragms or cervical caps.

3. Review failure rates. The higher the failure rate, the greater the risk of an unwanted pregnancy. The difference in failure rates between "typical" and "perfect" use provides an estimate of the role human error plays for most couples. Some contraceptive methods, such as sterilization, are effective for virtually all couples; for other methods, failure rates for the average couple may be several times higher than for a consistent and diligent couple. Remember that typical failure rates are only an average, and that failure rates for couples who are less than diligent may be even higher.

4. Put the risks and benefits of the various methods in perspective. It is important to weigh all dimensions and issues of the relationship carefully against the advantages and disadvantages of each birth control method. The risks and benefits of each method need to be carefully assessed in terms of the individuals involved and their relationship. Some couples find that they can use a numerical rating scheme to determine the best contraceptive that meets their unique needs.

5. Periodically reevaluate the decision. Regular gynecological check-ups are ideal opportunities to discuss contraceptive needs, options, and concerns with a clinician. At regular intervals, contracepting couples need to reexamine the level of effectiveness and their individual levels of satisfaction with the selected method. A couple may want to reconsider both partners' needs, feelings, and family planning goals.

When to See a Health-Care Provider

It is necessary to see a clinician for prescription of the diaphragm, cervical cap, any hormonal methods, IUD, or sterilization. Other forms of birth control do not require a clinician's prescription, but conditions associated with these forms may warrant a clinic visit. In general, a woman should consult a clinician any time she experiences pain during intercourse or any unusual bleeding, spotting, discharge, or odor. Any burning or itching associated with spermicide use may be an indication of an allergy to the agent.

With a diaphragm, it is wise to check with a clinician any time the diaphragm does not seem to be fitting properly or there is discomfort, pain, or recurring bladder infections. After having a baby, it may be necessary to be refitted for a different-sized diaphragm because vaginal depth and muscle tone are usually altered by full-term pregnancy.

Abortion

Decisions regarding an unwanted pregnancy are private, personal, and difficult. They should not be rushed, and all options should be carefully weighed. Being able to talk through the process with a trusted person is essential. Options include terminating the pregnancy, continuing the pregnancy and raising the child, or continuing the pregnancy and relinquishing the child for adoption. Many supportive services are available for each of these options.

If a woman elects to have an abortion and is confident in her decision, she can reduce her risk of medical complications from the procedure by making arrangements in a timely fashion. In selecting an abortion facility, a primary concern should be the availability of around-the-clock emergency care services. Infection, bleeding, and other complications can almost always be treated successfully if treatment begins promptly. Other ways to minimize risks from an abortion include making sure the surgeon who performs the procedure is well trained and experienced and verifying the facility provides comprehensive care including postoperative instructions, education, and supportive services. Abortion counseling services are perhaps one of the most important features of a comprehensive facility.

■■■■

Summary

Being able to control reproductive functioning is a necessary component of women's health, career preparation, and family growth management. Many methods of contraception are available today, and no method is perfect. **Table 5.4** compares the methods discussed in this chapter. Ulti-

mately, contraception is a shared responsibility. The best method is one that a woman and her partner feel comfortable using, and one that they will use correctly and consistently. Although ideally contraception is a shared responsibility between both partners, in today's world a woman is likely to bear the burden of an unexpected pregnancy. All women in relationships where there is the possibility of pregnancy should therefore make informed, well-thought-out decisions regarding contraception.

Abortion is something that no woman wants to face, but it is something that many women facing unwanted pregancies will have to consider. Whether a woman considers herself pro-life or pro-choice, she should be sensitive to the difficulties unwanted pregnancies bring. Abortion is not just an issue for young, unmarried women; many women who have planned a pregnancy turn to abortion when they discover their developing fetus has a serious birth defect or chromosomal abnormality. Questions around abortion continue to be a focus for much of the women's health and women's rights movements, as well as for conservative and religious political movements.

Preventing unwanted pregnancy is a primary responsibility of all sexually active couples. In the event of an unwanted pregnancy, understanding all options and risks is a critical prerequisite for effective decision making.

■■■■

Topics for Discussion

1. What are some explanations for the higher contraceptive failure rate among younger women compared with older women?

2. What are some of the common reasons for using birth control?

3. What are some reasons that couples fail to use contraceptives or fail to use them correctly?

4. How can couples share in the responsibilities associated with contraception?

5. When are contraceptive "risky" times likely to occur in a relationship?

6. How can a couple improve their communication about sexuality issues, including contraception?

7. How may sociocultural beliefs and practices influence contraceptive decision making?

Table 5.4 Comparisons: Contraceptive Options

Fertility Awareness Methods

"Perfect use" effectiveness	96%	**Disadvantages**	Requires considerable discipline and partner cooperation; does not reduce STI risk
Typical effectiveness	75%		
How it works	Prevents sperm from reaching egg	**Availability**	No purchase required
Advantages	No costs; causes no health problems; no side effects or contraindications; no supplies or advance preparation; partner shares responsibility; no delay or interference with spontaneity	**Comments**	Unreliable form of contraception

Withdrawal

"Perfect use" effectiveness	96%	**Disadvantages**	Requires consistent discipline and partner cooperation; compromises spontaneity; may decrease pleasure; does not reduce STI risk
Typical effectiveness	73%		
How it works	Prevents sperm from reaching egg	**Availability**	No purchase required
Advantages	No costs; causes no health problems; no side effects or contraindications; no supplies or advance preparation; partner shares responsibility	**Comments**	Unreliable form of contraception

Birth Control Pills

"Perfect use" effectiveness	99%	**Disadvantages**	No protection against STIs; may be contraindicated for women with cardiovascular risk problems or women who smoke; must be taken daily; inconsistent studies for breast cancer risk
Typical effectiveness	92%		
How it works	Prevents release of eggs from the ovaries; thickens cervical mucus; causes uterine lining changes	**Availability**	Requires clinical examination and prescription
Advantages	Fairly inexpensive; lighter and less painful periods; decreased PMS symptoms; improved skin conditions; protective for some chronic diseases; does not interfere with sexual activity; no delay or interference with spontaneity	**Comments**	Most effective form of temporary contraception; combination pills contain both synthetic estrogen and progesterone; minipill contains only progesterone and may cause some irregular bleeding

Hormonal Implants

"Perfect use" effectiveness	99%	**Disadvantages**	Must be removed by clinician; irregular menstrual bleeding may occur; no protection against STIs; may be contraindicated for women with cardiovascular risk problems or women who smoke
Typical effectiveness	99%		
How it works	Prevents release of eggs from the ovaries; thickens cervical mucus; causes uterine lining changes	**Availability**	Must be inserted by clinician; not all clinicians are trained for insertion and removal
Advantages	Fairly inexpensive; provides protection up to three years or until it is removed; highly convenient—nothing to remember; protective for some chronic diseases; no delay or interference with spontaneity	**Comments**	Highly effective contraceptive; reversible once implant is removed

(continues)

Table 5.4   Comparisons: Contraceptive Options *(continued)*

Injectable Contraceptives

"Perfect use" effectiveness	99%	**Disadvantages**	Must be prescribed by clinician; more weight gain and bleeding issues than with pill; no protection against STIs; may be contraindicated for women with cardiovascular risk problems or women who smoke
Typical effectiveness	97%		
How it works	Prevents release of eggs from the ovaries; thickens cervical mucus; causes uterine lining changes		
		Availability	Clinical exam required; must be injected by clinician; not as widely available as the pill
Advantages	Fairly inexpensive; lasts three to four months; less bloating and mood swings than with pill; convenient— nothing to remember; protective for some chronic diseases; no delay or interference with spontaneity	**Comments**	Highly effective contraceptive; reversible once injections wear off although there may be a waiting period; contains only progesterone so it is an option for women who cannot take estrogen

Hormonal Patches

"Perfect use" effectiveness	99%	**Disadvantages**	Less effective in women weighing more than 198 pounds; no protection against STIs; may be contraindicated for women with cardiovascular risk problems or women who smoke
Typical effectiveness	92%		
How it works	Prevents release of eggs from the ovaries; thickens cervical mucus; causes uterine lining changes		
		Availability	Requires clinical examination and prescription
Advantages	Fairly inexpensive; convenient; weekly schedule is easier than daily pill; similar side effects and benefits as pill; no delay or interference with spontaneity	**Comments**	Highly effective and convenient contraceptive

Vaginal Ring

"Perfect use" effectiveness	99%	**Disadvantages**	Requires clinical visit; women must learn to correctly insert and remove the ring; no protection against STIs; may be contraindicated for women with cardiovascular risk problems or women who smoke
Typical effectiveness	92%		
How it works	Prevents release of eggs from the ovaries; thickens cervical mucus; causes uterine lining changes		
		Availability	Relatively new form of contraception; not all clinicians may be prescribing it
Advantages	Inexpensive; convenient; requires removal every three weeks; weekly schedule is easier than daily pill; similar side effects and benefits as pill; no delay or interference with spontaneity	**Comments**	Highly effective and convenient contraceptive

Spermicide

"Perfect use" effectiveness	82%	**Disadvantages**	Required for each sex act; messy; must be applied just before intercourse; effective for 30–60 minutes; may be awkward, disruptive, or embarrassing to use
Typical effectiveness	71%		
How it works	Kills sperm; absorbs ejaculate; blocks sperm from entering vaginal tract		
		Availability	Easily available in drugstores and online pharmacies in creams, foams, gels, film, or suppositories
Advantages	Inexpensive; no clinical visit; able to use it only as needed; few side effects and contraindications; provides some protection against some STIs; provides additional lubrication; effective immediately	**Comments**	Best contraceptive results are achieved when spermicide is used with a barrier method such as a condom or diaphragm

Table 5.4	**Comparisons: Contraceptive Options** *(continued)*

Diaphragm			
"Perfect use" effectiveness	94%	Disadvantages	Fairly expensive one-time cost; clinical visit, fitting, and prescription required; must be used with a spermicide; may be awkward or inconvenient; may increase risk of urinary tract infections; dependent upon proper fit and diligent use
Typical effectiveness	84%		
How it works	Blocks sperms from reaching egg; spermicide inactivates sperm		
Advantages	Used only when needed; no side effects or contraindications (latex allergies are rare); can be inserted up to 6 hours ahead of time; reusable	Availability	Clinical visit and fitting required
		Comments	Spermicide must be used with each act of intercourse; diaphragm should be refitted when weight changes +/– 10 pounds

Contraceptive Sponge			
"Perfect use" effectiveness		Advantages	Easy to use; spermicide is contained in sponge; may be inserted up to 24 hours before sex; provides continuous protection for 24 hours; relatively inexpensive; available without a fitting or prescription; less messy than other forms of spermicides; may provide some protection against STIs; disposable
Parous women (women who have had children)	80%		
Nulliparous women (women who have not had children)	91%		
Typical effectiveness		Disadvantages	Less effective in women who have had children; requires some practice to insert and remove
Parous women	68%	Availability	Available in drugstores and online pharmacies
Nulliparous women	84%	Comments	Sponges should not be reused
How it works	Kills sperm; absorbs ejaculate; blocks sperm from entering cervix		

Cervical Cap			
"Perfect use" effectiveness	82%	Disadvantages	Fairly expensive one-time cost; clinical visit, filling, and prescription required; not all women can be fitted with a cap; due to smaller size it may be more difficult to insert and remove than a diaphragm; effectiveness is dependent upon proper fitting, proper placement, and spermicide use each time
Typical effectiveness	76%		
How it works	Blocks sperms from reaching egg; spermicide inactivates sperm		
Advantages	Easy to use once technique is mastered; may be inserted up to 48 hours before sex; some protection against STIs; few side effects (latex allergies are rare); resusable	Availability	Generally available, although not all clinicians are skilled in educating women about insertion and removal
		Comments	Should be replaced each year; should be refitted when weight changes +/– 10 pounds

Shield			
"Perfect use" effectiveness	94%	Disadvantages	Clinical visit required for prescription; must be used with a spermicide; may be awkward or inconvenient; dependent upon diligent use; may increase risk of urinary tract infections and toxic shock syndrome
Typical effectiveness	84%		
How it works	Blocks sperm from reaching egg; spermicide inactivates sperm		
Advantages	Used only when needed; no side effects or contraindications (latex allergies are rare); can be inserted up to 6 hours ahead of time; can be left in place for 48 hours; not sized or personally fitted; reusable	Availability	Not available over-the-counter or online
		Comments	Should remain in place 8 hours after last intercourse

(continues)

Table 5.4	Comparisons: Contraceptive Options *(continued)*		

Male Condom			
"Perfect use" effectiveness	98%	Disadvantages	Can be used for only one act of intercourse; can tear or slip during use; may decrease sexual pleasure; may interrupt lovemaking; requires cooperation of male partner; latex allergies may require use of polyurethane condoms
Typical effectiveness	85%		
How it works	Provides a physical barrier between the penis and vagina; prevents sperm and ejaculate from entering vagina		
		Availability	Widely available over-the-counter and from online sources; available with lubricants and spermicides, in a variety of colors, textures, and flavors
Advantages	Inexpensive; provides strong protection against most STIs; no clinical visit, fitting, or prescription required; can be used with other methods; can be used as a backup method for other contraception; no hormonal or systemic effects	Comments	More effective when used with a spermicide; can degrade with heat, light, and oxidation so should be stored in a cool, dry place

Female Condom			
"Perfect use" effectiveness	95%	Disadvantages	More expensive than male condom; may feel awkward; tendency to be noisy; requires partner cooperation; can be used for only one act of intercourse; requires attention to details for woman and her partner
Typical effectiveness	79%		
How it works	Prevents sperm from entering vagina; provides best level of protection for women from STIs by covering vagina and perineal area		
		Availability	Widely available over-the-counter and from online sources
Advantages	Used only when needed; no hormonal or systemic effects; empowering to women; clinical visit, fitting, or prescription not needed	Comments	More effective when used with a spermicide

Female Sterilization			
"Perfect use" effectiveness	99%	Disadvantages	Expensive one-time fee; no protection from STIs; surgical risks; not reliably reversible
Typical effectiveness	99%		
How it works	Prevents egg from traveling between ovaries and uterus	Availability	Widely available
		Comments	Even though actual risks with female sterilization are low, vasectomies pose far less risk to men; ideal option for women who do not desire more children
Advantages	Permanent—lifelong freedom from contraception after procedure for the woman; no interruption of lovemaking; highly effective; no need for partner compliance		

Male Sterilization			
"Perfect use" effectiveness	99%	Disadvantages	Expensive—one-time fee; not always reversible; surgical experience; no protection from STIs
Typical effectiveness	99%		
How it works	Prevents sperm from being in the ejaculate	Availability	Outpatient procedure
		Comments	
Advantages	Lifelong freedom from contraception worries for the male; no interruption of lovemaking; shared responsibility by the male		

Table 5.4 **Comparisons: Contraceptive Options** *(continued)*

Lactation Amenorrhea Method (LAM)			
"Perfect use" effectiveness	Uncertain	**Disadvantages**	Only effective with direct breastfeeding on demand, meeting all nutritional needs of baby; not effective when any menstrual bleeding returns or after 6 months postpartum
Typical effectiveness	80%		
How it works	Lactation suppresses ovulation		
Advantages	No clinical visit; no costs; easy for nursing mother	**Availability**	Only for nursing mothers
		Comments	Can be used with other forms of contraception

Intrauterine Device (IUD)			
"Perfect use" effectiveness	99%	**Disadvantages**	Clinical visit required; high insertion and removal costs; no STI protection; few days of mild cramping and light bleeding upon insertion
Typical effectiveness	99%		
How it works	Inhibits fertilization; thickens cervical mucus; inhibits sperm function; thins and suppresses the endometrium; copper ions may disrupt sperm motility	**Availability**	Dependent upon provider willingness and training for insertion; generally available
		Comments	IUDs are the most widely used reversible form of contraception in the world—used by 12% of women; are much less common in the United States
Advantages	Highly effective; does not interfere with sexual activity; no hormonal impact; long-acting; nothing to remember; decreased risk of endometrial cancer; reduced menstrual flow; reversible		

No Method			
"Perfect use" effectiveness	15%	**Disadvantages**	Risky for unwanted pregnancy; no protection against pregnancy or STIs
Typical effectiveness	15%		
How it works	Dependent upon good luck	**Availability**	
Advantages	No clinical visit; no costs	**Comments**	Couples using no method of contraception should plan on a pregnancy

■■■■
Web Sites

Association of Reproductive Health Professionals: http://www.arhp.org

Center for Reproductive Rights: http://www.crlp.org

The Emergency Contraception Website: http://ec.princeton.edu

EngenderHealth: http://www.engenderhealth.org

Guttmacher Institute: http://www.guttmacher.org

International Planned Parenthood Federation: http://www.ippf.org

The Henry J. Kaiser Family Foundation: http://www.kff.org

NARAL Pro-Choice America: http://www.naral.org

Planned Parenthood Federation of America: http://www.plannedparenthood.org

Public Agenda Issues Guide on Abortion: http://www.publicagenda.org

Profiles of Remarkable Women

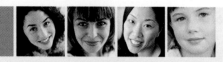

Margaret Sanger (1879–1966) and Mary Coffin Dennett (1872–1947)

Margaret Sanger and Mary Coffin Dennett were pioneers in the birth control movement.

Margaret Sanger began her career by attending the nursing program at White Plains Hospital in New York in 1900. She and her husband became involved in the pre-war radical bohemian culture in New York City and spent time with intellectuals, activists, and artists of the era. Sanger also joined the Women's Committee of the New York Socialist Party and took part in labor actions led by the Industrial Workers of the World.

As a nurse, Sanger focused on women's health and sex education. In 1912, she wrote a column on sex education for a New York publication, which was censored when she wrote about venereal disease. Upon seeing poor women suffering from miscarriages, abortions, and lack of effective birth control, Sanger began promoting the need to free women from unwanted pregnancies. Sanger published *Family Limitation*, a pamphlet that provided clear and frank descriptions of birth control methods and devices. The distribution of diaphragms and her publication were hampered by the Comstock Laws, which Congress enacted in 1873 to restrict the circulation of obscene materials—specifically birth control information—in the mail.

In 1916, Sanger opened the first birth control clinic in Brooklyn, New York. Although the clinic was raided and the staff was arrested shortly after its opening, the publicity brought supporters who helped to build a movement for birth control reform. Sanger founded the American Birth Control League (ABCL) in 1921 to promote the establishment of birth control clinics and the cause of fertility control. The ABCL set up its own clinic and dispensed diaphragms and lactic acid jelly for contraception. In 1942, the ABCL became the Planned Parenthood Federation of America.

Sanger continued fighting for the right to legally disseminate contraceptives. She met with much opposition due to her focus on radical feminism; in fact, she was even viewed as too radical for the birth control movement that she had launched. Ultimately, Sanger resigned from her position with ABCL and took respite from the birth control movement for many years.

After World War II, Sanger worked with family planning leaders in Europe and Asia to help establish the International Planned Parenthood Federation in 1952. She served as the organization's president until 1959. During this time, Sanger was instrumental in securing funding that helped make the development of birth control possible. Sanger died a few months after the Supreme Court decision *Griswold v. Connecticut* made birth control legal for married couples.

Mary Coffin Dennett attended the school of the Boston Museum of Fine Arts and taught design at Drexel University in Philadelphia from 1894 to 1897. Her interest in the suffrage movement began when Dennett worked first for the Massachusetts Woman Suffrage Association from 1903 to 1910 and then for the National American Woman Suffrage Association from 1910 to 1914. She advocated for pacifist beliefs and became a co-founder of the People's Council, an antiwar organization.

Dennett also became dedicated to reforming birth control laws. Opposing the radical, confrontational tactics espoused by Margaret Sanger, she focused on lobbying for legislative reform that would allow for the transmission of contraceptive information. Through her efforts to challenge the definition of legal obscenity, Dennett became one of the nation's most effective defenders of civil liberties. Along the way, she established the Voluntary Parenthood League. Unlike Sanger, who promoted the diaphragm, which only physicians could prescribe, Dennett stressed that ordinary people should be able to get birth control information without having to rely on medical experts.

Dennett was arrested during her career for mailing publications that were deemed obscene by the postal service. Throughout her life, she continued to press for women to become informed consumers and to gain direct access to birth control information. Dennett published a newspaper called the *Birth Control Herald* from 1922 to 1925 and several books, including *Birth Control Laws* (1926), *Who's Obscene* (1930), and *The Sex Education of Children* (1931).

■■■■

References

1. Guttmacher Institute. (n.d.). *Issues in Brief: U.S. policy can reduce cost barriers to contraception.* Avilable at http://www.guttmacher.org/pubs/ib_0799.html.

2. U.S. Department of Health and Human Services, Centers for Disease Control and Prevention, & National Center for Health Statistics. (2005). *Fertility, Family Planning, and Reproductive Health of US Women: Data from the 2002 National Survey of Family Growth.* Hyattsville, MD: U.S. Government Printing Office.

3. Mosher, W. D., Martinez, G. M., Chandra, A., Abma, J. C., & Wilson, S. J. (2004). Use of contraception and family planning services in the United States, 1982–2002. Advance data from Vital Health Statistics; no 350. Hyattsville, MD: National Center for Health Statistics.

4. Frost, J. E. (2004). The availability and use of publicly funded family planning clinics: U.S. trends, 1994–

2001. *Perspectives on Sexual and Reproductive Health* 36(5): 206–215.

5. Guttmacher Institute. (2008). *Facts on Contraceptive Use*. Available at http://www.guttmacher.org/pubs/fb_contr_use.html.

6. Guttmacher Institute. (2008, July 1). *State Level Contraception Resources*. Available at http://www.guttmacher.org/statecenter/contraception.html.

7. Kaiser Family Foundation. (2008). *Women's Health Policy*. Available at http://www.kff.org/womenshealth/index.cfm.

8. Guttmacher Institute. (2006). *Contraception Counts: State-by-State Comparative Data*. Available at http://www.guttmacher.org/statecenter/ccfs.html.

9. Grady, W. K.-W. (1999). Contraceptive characteristics: the perceptions and priorities of women and men. *Family Planning Perspectives* 31(4): 168–175.

10. Kost, K. S. (2008). Estimates of contraceptive failure from the 2002 National Survey of Family Growth. *Contraception* 77(1): 10–21.

11. Mohllajee, A. C. (2006). Does use of hormonal contraceptives among women with thrombogenic mutations increase their risk of venous thromboembolism? A systemic review. *Contraception* 73(2): 179–188.

12. Curtis, K. M., Mohllsjee, A. P., Martins, S. L., & Peterson, H. B. (2006). Combined oral contraceptive use among women with hypertension: a systemic review. *Contraception* 73(2): 179–188.

13. National Cancer Institute. (2006). *Oral Contraceptives and Cancer Risk: Questions and Answers*. Available at http://www.cancer.gov/cancertopics/factsheet/Risk/oral-contraceptives.

14. Burkman, R., Schlesselman, J. J., & Zieman, M. (2004). Safety concerns and health benefits associated with oral contraception. *American Journal of Obstetrics and Gynecology* 190(4 Suppl): S5–S22.

15. Marchbanks, P. A., McDonald, J. A. A., Wilson, H. G., et al. (2002). Oral contraceptives and the risk of breast cancer. *New England Journal of Medicine* 346(26): 2025–2032.

16. Guthman, R. A., Bang, J., & Nashelsky, J. (2005) Combined oral contraceptives for mothers who are breastfeeding. *American Family Physician* 72(7): 1303–1304.

17. Kwiecien, M., Edelman, A., Nichols, M. D., & Jensen, J. T. (2003). Bleeding patterns and patient acceptability of standard or continuous dosing regimes of a low-dose oral contraceptive: a randomized trial. *Contraception* 73(1): 41–45.

18. Nelson, A. (2007). Communicating with patients about extended-cycle and continuous use of oral contraception. *Journal of Women's Health* 16(4): 463–470.

19. Sulak, P. J., Buckley, T., & Kuehl, T. J. (2006). Attitudes and prescribing preferences of health care professionals in the United States regarding use of extended-cycle oral contraceptives. *Contraception* 73(1): 41–45.

20. Inal, M. M., Yildirim, Y., Ertopcu, K., Avci, M. E., Ozelmas, I., & Tinar, S. (2008). Effect of the subdermal contraceptive etonogestrel implant (Implanon®) on biochemical and hormonal parameters (three years follow-up). *Eur J Contraception and Reproductive Health Care* 13(3):238–242.

21. Merki-Feld, G. S., Imthurn, B., & Seifert, B. (2008). Effects of the progestagen-only contraceptive implant Implanon on cardiovascular risk factors. *Clinical Endocrinology (Oxford)* 68(3): 355–360.

22. Berenson, A. B., Odom, S. D., Breitkopf, C. R., & Rahman, M. (2008). Physiologic and psychologic symptoms associated with use of injectable contraception and 20 μg oral contraceptive pills. *American Journal of Obstetrics and Gynecology* 10(1016). Available at http://www.ajog.org/article/S0002-9378(08)00500-0/abstract.

23. Morrison, C. S., Bright, P., Wong, E. L., et al. (2004). Hormonal contraceptive use, cervical ectopy, and the acquisition of cervical infections. *Sexually Transmitted Diseases* 32(10): 644–645.

24. Burkman, R. T. (2002). The transdermal contraceptive patch: a new approach to hormonal contraception. *International Journal of Fertility and Women's Medicine* 47(2): 69–76.

25. Madden, T., & Blumenthal, P. (2007). Contraceptive vaginal ring. *Clinical Obstetrics and Gynecology* 50(4): 878–885.

26. Halpern, V., Roundtree, W., Raymond, E. G., & Law, M. (2008). The effects of spermicides containing nonoxynol-9 on cervical cytology. *Contraception* 77(3): 191–194.

27. Shane, D. (2006). The female condom: significant potential for STI and pregnancy protection. *Outlook* 22(2): 2.

28. Macaluso, M., Blackwell, R., Jamieson, D. J., et al. (2007). Efficacy of the male latex condom and of the female polyurethane condom as barriers to semen during intercourse: a randomized clinical trial. *American Journal of Epidemiology* 166(1): 88–96.

29. Therous, R. (2008). The hysteroscopic approach to sterilization. *Journal of Obstetrical and Gynecological Nursing* 37(3): 356–360.

30. Thiel, J. A., & Carson, G. D. (2008). Cost-effectiveness analysis comparing the Essure tubal sterilization procedure and laparoscopic tubal sterilization. *Journal of Obstetrics and Gynecology Canada* 30(7): 581–585.

31. Blenning, C. E., & Paladine, H. (2005). An approach to the postpartum office visit. *American Family Physician* 72(12): 2443–2444.

32. ESHRE Capri Workshop Group. (2008). Intrauterine devices and intrauterine systems. *Human Reproduction Update* 14(3): 197–208.

33. Harper, C. C., Blum, M., de Bocanegra, H. T., et al. (2008). Challenges in translating evidence into practice: the provision of intrauterine contraception. *Obstetrics and Gynecology* 111(6): 1359–1369.

34. Cheng, L., Guimezoglu, A. M., Piaggio, G., Ezcurra, E., & Van Look, P. F. (2008). Interventions for emergency contraception. *Cochrane Database System Review*. Apr. 16(2): CD001324.

35. The Kaiser Family Foundation. (2005). *Emergency Contraception*. Available at http://www.kff.org/womenshealth/3344-03.cfm.

36. Gee, R. E., Shacter, H. E., Kaufman, E. J., & Long, J. A. (2008). Behind-the-counter status and availability of emergency contraception. *American Journal of Obstetrics and Gynecology* 199(5): 478–480.

37. American College of Obstetricians and Gynecologists. (2005). Emergency contraception. *ACOG Practice Bulletin #69*. Washington, DC: American College of Obstetricians and Gynecologists.

38. Phipps, M. G., Matteson, K. A., Fernandez, G. E., Chiaverini, L., & Weitzen, S. (2008). Characteristics of women who seek emergency contraception and family planning services. *American Journal of Obstetrics and Gynecology*. Available at http://journals.elsevierhealth.com/periodicals/ymob/search/quick.

39. Jackson, R. A., Schwarz, E. B., Freedman, L., & Darney, P. (2003). Advance supply of emergency contraception: effect on use and usual contraception. *Obstetrics and Gynecology* 102(1): 1–2.

40. Polis, C. B., Schaffer, K., Blanchard, K., Glasier, A., Harper, C. C., & Grimes, D. A. (2007). Advance provision of emergency contraception for pregnancy prevention: a meta-analysis. *Obstetrics and Gynecology* 110(6): 1379–1388.

41. Page, S. T., Amory, J. K., & Bremmer, W. J. (2008). Advances in male contraception. *Endocrinology Review* 29(4): 465–493.

42. Mommers, E., et al. (2008). Male hormonal contraception: a double-blind placebo-controlled study. *Journal of Clinical Endocrinology and Metabolism* 93(7): 2572–2580.

43. Jones, R., Zolna, M., Henshaw, S., & Finer, L. (2008). Abortion in the United States: incidence and access to services, 2005. *Perspectives on Reproductive Health* 40(1): 6–16.

44. World Health Organization. (2007). Unsafe abortion: global and regional estimates of the incidence of unsafe abortion and associated mortality in 2003. Geneva: WHO.

45. Bazelon, E. (August 19, 2008). *Script Doctors: The Dilemma Facing South Dakota's Abortion Providers: Mislead Your Patients or Break the Law*. Slate. Available at http://www.slate.com/id/2198114/.

46. Finer, L., et al. (2005). Reasons U.S. women have abortions: quantitative and qualitative perspectives. *Perspectives on Sexual and Reproductive Health* 37(3): 110–118.

47. Jones, R., Darroch, J., & Henshaw, S. (2002). Patterns in the socioeconomic characteristics of women obtaining abortions in 2000–2001. *Perspectives on Sexual and Reproductive Health* 34(5): 226–235.

48. Koonin, L., et al. (1998). Abortion surveillance—United States, 1995. *Morbidity and Mortality Weekly Report* 47(SS-2): 31–68.

49. Strauss, L., et al. (2005) Abortion surveillance—United States, 2002. *Morbidity and Mortality Weekly Report* 54(SS07): 1–31.

50. Obaid, T. (2007). No woman should die giving life. *Lancet* 370(9595): 1287–1288.

51. Women: more than mothers (editorial). (2007). *Lancet* 370(9595): 1283–1284.

52. Sedgh, G., et al. (2007). Induced abortion: estimated rates and trends worldwide. *Lancet* 370(9595): 1338–1345.

53. Guttmacher Institute. (2007). *Facts on Induced Abortion Worldwide*. Available at http://www.guttmacher.org/pubs/fb_IAW.html.

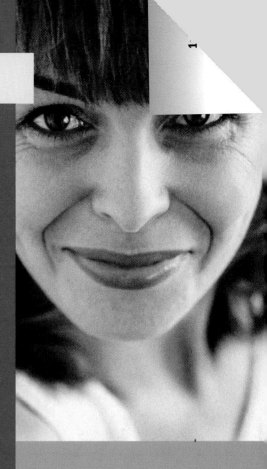

Chapter Six

Pregnancy and Childbirth

Chapter Objectives

On completion of this chapter, the student should be able to discuss:

1. Historical dimensions of pregnancy, childbirth, and breastfeeding.

2. Conception and the process of cell division after fertilization.

3. Hormonal changes and fetal changes during pregnancy.

4. Nutritional and weight gain recommendations for pregnancy and exercise concerns with pregnancy.

5. Detrimental effects of smoking, alcohol, drugs, and various environmental risks on pregnancy.

6. Techniques for prenatal testing and complications of pregnancy.

7. The significant issues surrounding childbirth preparation, labor and delivery, cesarean section, and vaginal birth after cesarean section.

8. Physiological changes of the breast for breastfeeding.

9. Benefits and complications associated with breastfeeding.

10. The concepts of fecundity and infertility.

11. Causes and diagnoses of infertility.

12. Treatment of infertility, including assisted reproductive technologies.

13. Emotional effects of infertility.

14. Trends in breastfeeding.

15. Prevalence of infertility, its major causes, and the types of treatments used.

womenshealth.jbpub.com

Women's Health Online is a great source for supplementary women's health information for both students and instructors. Visit

http://womenshealth.jbpub.com

to find a variety of useful tools for learning, thinking, and teaching.

Introduction

This chapter provides an overview of pregnancy, childbirth, breastfeeding, and infertility. In addition to the obvious biological aspects, pregnancy and childbirth are greatly influenced by social, cultural, historical, legal, and ethical dimensions.

Historical Dimensions

The academic examination of childbirth as a social phenomenon did not really begin until the 1960s. Before that time, knowledge about childbirth had been derived principally from the writings of medical historians who stressed the progressive history of scientific advances in obstetrics. This medical and historical account provided little insight into how the management of pregnancy or birthing affected women's experiences of birth or about women's reactions to and participation in such changes. The accounts also failed to document how the birth experience felt to the woman.

Today there is considerably more focus on the social, racial, economic, and ethnic aspects of childbirth. Childbirth history is now studied in a variety of contexts—medical, demographic, cultural, social, economic, professional, and symbolic, among others. In the United States, however, the medical perspective continues to dominate. The term *childbirth* generally evokes an image of a medical environment, with physicians and nurses, surgical drapes, intravenous poles, and fetal monitors. In contrast, in the early United States, childbirth did not have an association with medical personnel or equipment except when a woman's life was threatened. Both immigrant and native populations considered childbirth to be part of a woman's domestic responsibilities.[1] Although specific cultural and ethnic

variations existed in the management of the birthing process, all shared the tradition that only women attended other women. Women were the experts on birthing.[1]

During the mid-eighteenth century, the expertise of women in birthing began to be questioned. Women in France were beginning to deliver babies in hospitals under the watchful eyes of not only traditional midwives, but also physicians. Although physicians had previously witnessed or participated in abnormal deliveries, the hospitalization practices enabled them to study and understand the normal childbirth process. Through close observation, measurements, and recordings, French physicians attempted to explain what they saw as the mysterious process of childbirth.[2] During the same period, the English medical establishment became more oriented to surgical techniques—specifically, the development of instruments known as **forceps** to assist in the extraction of the fetus from the woman. The European obstetrical knowledge quickly crossed the Atlantic, and U.S. physicians began appearing at the births of middle- and upper-class urban women. At first, physicians attended along with traditional midwives, but soon physicians replaced midwives in the birthing process. Medical schools began to certify men as birth attendants, leading to a decline in traditional midwifery. By the end of the eighteenth century, physicians had established roles in managing childbirth experiences throughout urban areas, including those for poor women.

With the medical presence during childbirth came a widening array of interventions, including medications, anesthesia, and birthing instruments. Accompanying the

There is a realization that women's attitudes toward and behavior during birth are shaped and conditioned by the demands and expectations of family, peers, community, and often religion. What a woman expects from her childbirth experience, what she will do, what she will fear and not fear, how she will interpret what is happening to her, and what in fact will happen when she gives birth, depend in large measure upon how her society defines what birth should be and where she fits in the various hierarchies of that society.

Janet Carlisle Bogdan (1990). Childbirth in America, 1650 to 1990. In R. D. Apple (ed.), *Women, Health in Medicine in America.*

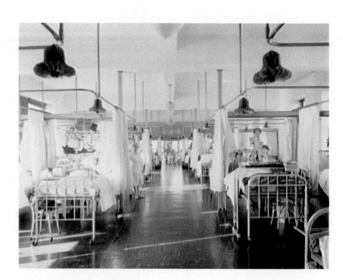

■ The twentieth century brought medicalization and hospitalization to the childbirth experience.

newly introduced technologies were additional problems of birth accidents, including tears and infections. Physician attitudes had changed from observing and learning to affecting and controlling. Women continued to actively participate in determining the terms of their childbirths only as long as the home was the birthing environment. Once birthing moved to the hospital, however, women lost this power.[3] The U.S. medical management of childbirth originated in urban northeastern areas. In the South and in some religious communities, childbirth retained much of its traditional aspects during the nineteenth and early twentieth centuries. Immigrant groups also were more likely to continue with traditional practices.

The twentieth century brought additional medicalization and hospitalization to the childbirth experience. Midwives remained in the more inaccessible portions of the United States. Despite the increased technology and promises of greater safety, women were exposed to greater mystification of childbirth than they had ever known.[3] This trend was in some ways ironic because women were electing to control their fertility and have fewer children, thereby increasing the significance of the childbirth experience. At the same time, they understood less about the process and were less in control of birthing than their grandmothers had been. This trend continued until the late 1950s and 1960s, when women began to openly express their dissatisfaction with medicalized births. Europe again was the leader in a new trend of childbirth experiences that suggested that childbirth should be anticipated with joy and knowledge, not fear and ignorance, and could be accomplished with less pain, less medication, and less of the medical and surgical control typical of U.S. births. These natural-birth relaxation techniques are the foundation of modern efforts toward "prepared childbirth."

Social scientists have studied many aspects of modern and traditional childbirth practices. Historically, the care pregnant women received focused on childbirth in the woman's home, and other women gave this support. But modern medical and hospital practices, while making childbirth safe in many regards, have also created situations where continuous support from physicians and nurses during labor has become more the exception rather than the routine. Some experts believe that childbirth has become an "over-medicalized" process, leading to excessive health costs, extensive stays for mothers, and a natural process becoming something to be feared and treated rather than experienced. A large meta-analysis of continuous support for women during childbirth found women who had medical

support were likely to have a slightly shorter labor, more likely to have a spontaneous vaginal birth, and less likely to report dissatisfaction with their childbirth experiences. The authors concluded that all women should have medical support throughout labor and birth.[4]

Other social scientists have examined the popular lay term of *natural childbirth*. These studies have found three practices common to natural childbirth: (1) activity during birth, (2) preparation before birth, and (3) social support, both in an individual and in a broader sociocultural sense.[5] For most considerations, the term *natural childbirth* does not exclude modern medical personnel or procedures, but rather attempts to create a more active and supportive experience for the mother during the birth of her baby.

Breastfeeding also has seen many changes over the years. The first variation on the practice of breastfeeding was the substitution of the mother's breast with that of a wet nurse—another woman who was able and willing to breastfeed for the mother. In the 1700s, "dry nursing," the mixing of flour, bread, or cereal with broth or water, became popular. This early form of infant formula was a cheaper option than "wet nursing." As women entered the workforce during the Industrial Revolution, substitutes for milk were produced, resulting in a decline in the practice of breastfeeding.[6] Formula substitutes remained popular for those women who could afford them, until reports surfaced on the benefits of breastfeeding in the 1970s. Since that time, breastfeeding rates have again fallen and risen as a result of various factors, ranging from a woman's place of employment to her personal finances, from her religious beliefs to her network of social support, and from her comfort with her own body to medical contraindications. Because breastfeeding has been shown to lower total healthcare costs by reducing sick care visits, prescriptions, and hospitalizations, the U.S. has identified breastfeeding as a major goal of the Healthy People 2010 National Health Objectives. As **Figure 6.1** shows, some progress has been made toward achieving these goals.

Pregnancy

Pregnancy lasts an average of 266 days from the time of fertilization or 280 days from the first day of the last menstrual period (often referred to as LMP). The gestational period is divided into three phases or trimesters of approximately three months each. Not all women have 28-day menstrual cycles, so due dates cannot be precisely determined (see **It's Your Health**).

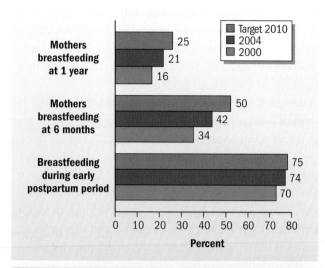

Figure 6.1

Healthy People 2010 breastfeeding objectives.

Source: U.S. Department of Health and Human Services. (2007). Progress Review, Maternal, Infant, and Child Health. *Healthy People 2010*. Downloaded August 21, 2008, from http://www.healthypeople.gov/data/2010prog/focus16.

■ Dizygotic twins (fraternal twins) have different genetic traits and therefore different physical appearances.

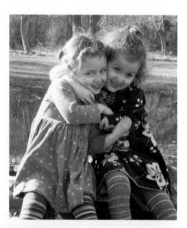

It's Your Health

Calculating a "Due Date"

To calculate the expected due date of a pregnancy:

1. Determine the first day of the last menstrual period.

2. Add one week to the first day of the last menstrual period.

3. Subtract three months.

4. Add one year.

For example, if the first day of the last menstrual period was April 2, 2009, add 1 week (which is April 9, 2009), subtract 3 months (which makes it January 9, 2009) and then add 1 year, which is January 9, 2010.

It is important to remember that this is an estimate, although approximately 60% of births occur within 5 days of the dates predicted in this manner.

Conception

Conception, also known as **fertilization**, is the union of the male sperm cell and the female egg cell. Before conception is possible, changes must take place within the sperm cells. They must mature in the male reproductive tract before ejaculation and undergo more biological changes in the female reproductive tract before they can fertilize the egg. The sperm cell is one of the smallest cells in the body and is produced in enormous quantities: approximately 50 million each day by a healthy male. Sperm production is a continuous, lifelong process. Sperm are produced in the testicles; they are then moved through the epididymis to the seminal vesicles, where the sperm mature into motile sperm and are stored until they are needed in the semen. Mature sperm cells swim like miniature tadpoles with an undulating movement of a threadlike tail. During the process of ejaculation, these cells are combined with secretions from the male reproductive tract to form semen. If ejaculation occurs into or around the entrance of the vagina, fertilization is possible. It has been estimated that as many as 300 million sperm are deposited with ejaculation, but fewer than 20 actually arrive anywhere near the unfertilized egg.[7]

The human egg, or ovum, is far rarer than the sperm. Each woman is born with a supply of approximately 1 million egg cells. Only about 300,000 eggs remain by the time a girl reaches puberty. One mature egg is released from a woman's ovaries each month during ovulation, usually resulting in 300 to 500 eggs being released during a woman's lifetime.

After the sperm separates from the seminal fluid, it becomes more mobile as it travels toward the egg. If the woman is in the early or middle segment of her menstrual cycle, the cervical mucus is of a consistency to allow the sperm to pass into the uterus. If progesterone is the dominant hormone, as in the late segment of the menstrual cycle, the cervical mucus inhibits sperm penetration past the cervix. Conception usually takes place in the upper third of the fallopian tube. In a process called the acrosome reaction, the sperm releases an enzyme called hyaluronidase, which works to dissolve the outer layer of the egg cell and allows the sperm cell to advance toward the center of the egg to join with its nucleus. Only one sperm is able to penetrate the protective coating of the egg.

Two offspring born of the same pregnancy are called twins.

■ **Dizygotic twins** (also known as fraternal twins) result when two eggs are released from the ovary in one

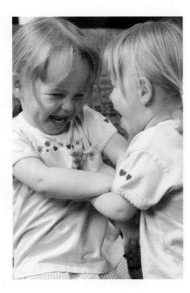

■ Monozygotic twins (identical twins) result from a single fertilized egg splitting into equal halves. As a result, these babies have identical genetic information.

Table 6.1	Selected Sex Chromosome Abnormalities

Chromosomal Arrangement for Girls	Description
Turner syndrome (monosomy X; XO)	■ Short stature and may have certain physical features such as a webbed neck ■ Lack ovarian development and are infertile ■ May be born with heart or kidney abnormalities ■ Intelligence may be impaired
Triple X (XXX)	■ Girls tend to be taller than expected but otherwise normal in appearance ■ Normal fertility ■ At risk for language and motor delay

Chromosomal Arrangement for Boys	Description
Klinefelter syndrome (trisomy XXY)	■ Boys tend to be taller than expected and effeminate but otherwise normal in appearance ■ Decreased testicular size, normal sex function, but usually infertile ■ May have slight breast development during adolescence ■ At risk for learning disabilities
XYY male	■ Boys tend to be taller than expected but otherwise normal in appearance ■ Sexual function, genitalia, and fertility are normal ■ Increased risk for motor delay, developmental delay, and learning disabilities

menstrual cycle and fertilized at the same time. Fraternal twins may be of the same or opposite sex and have different genetic traits and therefore different physical appearances. They are sustained through separate placentas and membranes.

■ **Monozygotic twins**, also referred to as identical twins, result from a single fertilized egg splitting into equal halves. If both eggs become implanted within the uterus, two babies with identical genetic information will develop. Identical twins may share or have separate placentas and membranes.

At fertilization, the 23 **chromosomes** from the sperm combine with the 23 chromosomes of the egg to form the **zygote**. The zygote, or fertilized egg, contains the full complement of 46 chromosomes. This genetic information determines the unique characteristics of the individual, including eye and hair color, height, and all the other physical characteristics that are passed from one generation to the next. One pair of chromosomes determines the sex of the individual, with the usual arrangement of males having one X and one Y chromosome and females having two X chromosomes; however, chromosomal abnormalities can occur. Among the most common chromosomal abnormalities are those that involve missing or extra sex chromosomes. Abnormalities involving the X or Y chromosome can affect sexual development and may cause infertility, growth abnormalities, and other problems. (See **Table 6.1**.)

Cell division of the zygote usually occurs within 36 hours of fertilization and continues as it propels the dividing cell mass in the fallopian tubes toward the uterus. It generally takes three to five days to reach the uterus; at this stage, the cell mass is known as a **blastocyst**. The blasto-

cyst freely floats within the uterus for one to two days before implanting itself into the lining of the uterus. **Implantation** is often the marker for the beginning of a pregnancy. The products of conception are generally referred to as the **conceptus**. For the first eight weeks of gestation, the material is known as an **embryo**; from week nine until birth, it is known as a **fetus**.

My niece was very short and she had some unique characteristics. It took a while for the doctors to diagnose her as having Turner syndrome. We have learned that this affects about one in every 2,500 females.

27-year-old woman

Confirming Pregnancy

The benefits of early diagnosis of pregnancy are immeasurable. When pregnancy is desired, good prenatal care can begin immediately, and efforts can be made to protect the vulnerable embryo from chemical and physical agents. When pregnancy is not desired, early detection permits early decision making; if the woman elects to have an abortion, risks of complications are reduced at this stage.

Several symptoms often occur in the first six weeks of pregnancy (see **It's Your Health**). Most women begin to have symptoms two or three weeks after conception. An overdue period is usually the first definitive sign of pregnancy, although it is important to note that there are many reasons for missed periods other than pregnancy. Some women do not always miss periods when they are pregnant, and missed periods do not always signal a pregnancy.

Confirming a pregnancy involves a pregnancy test and a pelvic examination. **Human chorionic gonadotropin (hCG)**, a hormone specific to pregnancy, is easily detectable in blood and urine throughout the first three months of pregnancy. All pregnancy tests use chemical procedures to detect its presence.

Home pregnancy tests can be purchased without a prescription. Such tests are fairly expensive but quite simple to use. It is important to follow the directions carefully to ensure accurate results. If an initial test is negative and the menstrual period has still not started, it is often a good idea to repeat the test in a week or so. Tests give the most reliable results when the urine is highly concentrated; hence, women are advised to use early morning urine as the testing sample. Some studies have also found that digital over-the-counter home pregnancy tests offer significant advantages over the more traditional nondigital methods.[8]

Although home pregnancy tests are valuable sources of information, they are merely the beginning. If the findings are

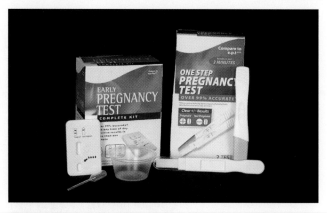

■ Home pregnancy tests are fairly expensive but quite simple to use.

positive, it is important to set up an appointment for a pelvic examination. If the findings are negative, there is a need to determine why the menstrual period is late or missed. Urine or blood tests performed in a doctor's office are virtually 100% accurate and can be used to validate the pregnancy.

Hormonal Changes During Pregnancy

During pregnancy, a woman's hormone levels and physical characteristics change dramatically. The secretion of certain hormones, such as follicle-stimulating hormone (FSH) and luteinizing hormone (LH) produced by the anterior pituitary gland, is suppressed throughout pregnancy. Pregnancy-specific hormones, such as hCG and human placental lactogen (HPL), are responsible for influencing the course of the pregnancy. Likewise, the production of estrogen and progesterone is important for pregnancy.

Shortly after implantation, specific cells in the outer portion of the developing embryo secrete hCG. The presence of this hormone in the woman's system produces a positive pregnancy test result because, as noted earlier, hCG can be detected in the woman's blood and urine. The body produces large amounts of hCG during the first trimester to stimulate the **corpus luteum**, a structure formed on the wall of the ovary that secretes estrogen and progesterone to prepare the body for pregnancy. The corpus luteum is essential for the maintenance of early pregnancy. If it regresses, a spontaneous abortion, or miscarriage, results.

After the first three months of pregnancy, the corpus luteum is no longer essential to maintain the pregnancy and hCG levels drop off. This change occurs because the placenta begins producing large amounts of estrogen and progesterone. The fetus also plays a role in maintaining the pregnancy. The fetal adrenal glands produce a precursor hormone during the first three months of pregnancy that is

It's Your Health

Early Signs of Pregnancy

Symptoms of pregnancy that often occur in the first six weeks:

Missed period(s)

Breast swelling and tenderness

Fatigue

Queasiness or nausea, vomiting

Slightly elevated body temperature

Mood swings

Need to urinate frequently

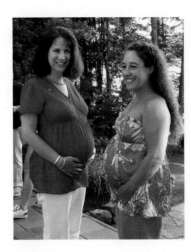

■ A woman's body experiences significant changes throughout pregnancy.

converted to estrogen in the placenta. The growing fetus and placenta contribute increasing quantities of estrogen and progesterone to the maternal blood system as the pregnancy progresses; the levels of both hormones rapidly decline at birth. Estrogen helps to regulate progesterone, thereby protecting the pregnancy, and initiates one of the major processes of fetal maturation; without estrogen, fetal lungs, liver, and other organs and tissues cannot mature. Estrogen also promotes the growth of ducts in the breast to prepare for lactation. Progesterone suppresses uterine contractions during pregnancy and stimulates the alveoli of the breasts.

Another hormone unique to pregnancy is human placental lactogen (HPL). It is also called human chorionic somatomammotropin. The structure and function of HPL are similar to that of human growth hormone. HPL modifies the metabolic state of the mother during pregnancy to facilitate the energy supply of the fetus. It is believed to stimulate breast growth during pregnancy and to prepare the breasts for lactation. HPL levels rise throughout pregnancy. As birth approaches, the levels decline.

Physical and Emotional Symptoms

A woman's body experiences significant changes throughout pregnancy, with each trimester bringing new physical and emotional symptoms. **Figure 6.2** shows many of the physical changes that occur during pregnancy. The first trimester is characterized by enlarged and tender breasts and, for many women, nausea and vomiting (commonly referred to as morning sickness). Women also may experience extreme fatigue, decreased interest in sex, moodiness and irritability, and skin changes such as darkening of the nipple and areola.

During the second trimester, morning sickness usually subsides, but is replaced for many women with other gastrointestinal problems such as heartburn, gas, and constipation. The second trimester also is the period in which women gain most of their weight, usually between 12 and 14 pounds. The growing fetus can lead to breathing problems, due to pressure of the uterus and fetus on the bottom of the rib cage, and backache, caused by changes in posture to accommodate the growing fetus. Some women experience muscle and leg cramps, numbness and tingling of the hands, swollen or bleeding gums, and **Braxton-Hicks contractions** (false labor). Swelling of the feet, ankles, and hands is common and is caused by the increased weight of the uterus slowing down blood and fluid circulation. Many women have significant changes in their skin's appearance during the second trimester. Striae gravidarum (known as stretch marks) begin to appear on the abdomen, breasts, and thighs; for some women, varicose veins appear in the legs. Other skin changes may include chloasma (brown patches on the face or neck) and linea nigra (a dark line from the belly to the pubic area) due to increases in

I didn't need a pregnancy test to tell me I was pregnant. I just knew it. My breasts were tender and I had some vague queasiness. Sure enough—my home pregnancy test confirmed what I knew. I realize that some women aren't as sure, but I was totally positive that I was pregnant.

25-year-old mother

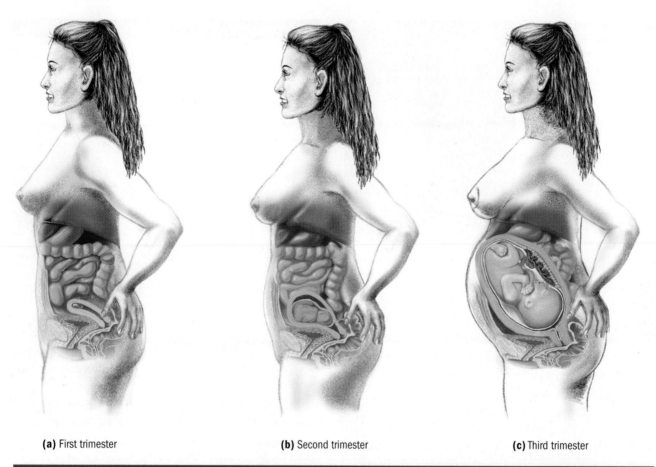

(a) First trimester   **(b)** Second trimester   **(c)** Third trimester

Figure 6.2

Changes in a woman's body during pregnancy. Through the three trimesters, the shape of the pregnant woman's body changes dramatically.

melanocyte-stimulating hormone. Changes in estrogen levels may cause redness of palms and red spots on the upper body. The second trimester also may be a time of renewed interest in sex.

In the third trimester, many of these symptoms—for example, heartburn and constipation, leg cramps, backache, breathlessness, and Braxton-Hicks contractions—continue. Women often experience an increase in leukorrhea (a whitish vaginal discharge) and colostrum (pre-milk) leaking from the breasts. Hemorrhoids, pelvic and buttock discomfort, and an itchy abdomen also are common complaints. A woman's interest in sex may decrease.

Fetal Development

The process of development for the fertilized egg is both fascinating and complex. When the cluster of cells reaches the uterus, it is smaller than the head of a pin. Once the cells become embedded into the uterine lining, they are collectively known as an embryo. The embryo soon takes on an elongated shape that is rounded at one end. A sac known as

the **amnion** or fetal sac envelops the embryo. As water and other small molecules cross the amniotic membrane, the embryo floats freely. The **amniotic fluid** protects the embryo from shocks and bumps and helps maintain a homeostatic, or constant, environment for the developing embryo. A primitive placenta soon forms. The **placenta** is an organ that supplies the growing fetus with oxygen and nutrients from the maternal bloodstream and serves as a conduit for the return of waste products back to the mother for disposal.

Major changes occur with the developing embryo as it evolves into a fetus (**Figure 6.3**).

First Month   The embryo grows to about one-tenth to one-fourth of an inch in length and one-seventh of an ounce in weight. Foundations form for the nervous system, genito-urinary system, circulatory system, digestive system, skin, bones, and lungs. The embryo has a two-lobed brain and a spinal cord. The arm and leg buds start to appear. The heartbeat appears on the twenty-fifth day. Rudiments of the eyes, ears, and nose appear. The head is disproportionately large because of the early brain development.

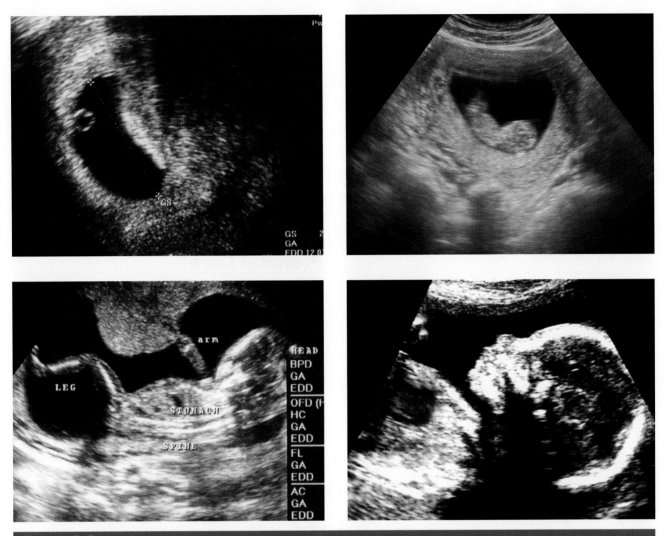

Figure 6.3

Fetal development. Top left, human embryo between four and five weeks of development. Top right, human fetus about 11 to 12 weeks of development. Bottom left, human fetus about five months (20 weeks) of development. Bottom right, human fetus nearly full term—eight to nine months.

Second Month The embryo's length is about one to two inches, and it weighs about one-sixth of an ounce. Ears, eyelids, fingers, and toes are distinct. At eight weeks, all the major organs are formed. The circulatory system is closed, and the placenta starts working. The neural tube closes. After eight weeks the embryo is called a fetus.

Third Month The length of the fetus is two to three inches and it weighs about an ounce. The sex of the fetus is defined, and it starts growing fuzzy hair, buds for future teeth, and soft fingernails and toenails. Kidneys begin to excrete urine. Other organs further develop. The nose and palate take shape, and the ears and earlobes are developed. At this time, the fetal heartbeat can be heard with a Doppler device.

Fourth Month The fetal length is five to six inches, and the weight is two to five ounces. The mother will start to discern fetal movements. The fetus can hear, move, kick, swim, sleep, and swallow. At this point, ultrasound can recognize external genitalia. The skin is pink and transparent, and eyebrows have formed.

Fifth Month Fetal length is 7 to 11 inches. It may weigh up to 1.5 pounds. The skin is loose and wrinkled. Vernix, a white, greasy substance, and lanugo, a soft fine hair, cover the skin for protection. Ultrasound can examine the baby's anatomy in detail.

Sixth Month The fetus weighs about two pounds. The skin is red and eyelids remain sealed. The fetus becomes active by kicking, punching, stretching, and turning over. It also coughs, hiccups, and responds to sudden noise. If born, the infant will cry and breathe, and it can survive with intensive neonatal care.

Seventh Month The fetal length is about 15 inches, and it weighs about three pounds. The eyes open and close, and the baby sucks its thumb. If born, the infant can usually survive. Eyelids are open, and fingerprints are set.

Eighth Month The fetus now gains about one-half pound per week and will most likely settle into position for birth. It is now about 17 inches long and weighs 4 to 5.5 pounds. The face and body have a loose and wrinkled appearance. Bones harden.

Ninth Month By the end of 37 weeks, the fetus is considered mature and ready to breathe. By 38 to 40 weeks, the baby weighs six to nine pounds and is 19–21 inches in length. In the final month, the fetus gains about an ounce per day. The skin is filled out and smooth. The skull bones have hardened, and the baby is ready for survival outside the womb. The lanugo hair and most of the vernix have disappeared.

Preconception Care

Preconception care is the collective name for the steps a woman can take before she decides to become pregnant to ensure she is in good health when conception occurs. Many health-care providers recommend that a woman see a clinician before getting pregnant and take a few basic steps to reduce the risk of certain problems during pregnancy. These steps include:

1. *Ensuring an adequate intake of folic acid.* The U.S. Public Health Service recommends that women of childbearing age get at least 400 micrograms of folic acid daily, through food or dietary supplements. Many health-care providers suggest supplementing the diet with folic acid for the three months before getting pregnant.

2. *Proper immunizations.* Women who are thinking of getting pregnant should be immunized against the communicable diseases that can harm a developing fetus, such as chicken pox and rubella before conceiving.

3. *Healthy behaviors.* The preconception period is a good time for a woman to assess her health behaviors—smoking, alcohol use, caffeine intake, drug use, and medications. Items that should be avoided or limited during pregnancy should be minimized or eliminated in the preconception period.

4. *Nutrition.* Scientific research has shown that good nutrition is important for male and female fertility. A balanced diet including regular servings of fruits, vegetables, whole grains, lean meats, and dairy products will optimize the preconception period. Women should also get at least 1,000 mg of calcium daily (three eight-ounce glasses of milk) in the preconception period. (See Chapter 9 for more information.)

Prenatal Care

A pregnant woman should to take good care of herself to ensure proper development of her unborn child. Good prenatal care encompasses a spectrum of topics from proper nutrition to regular prenatal health care.

Nutrition

Good nutrition is an integral part of both preconception and prenatal care. Throughout pregnancy, a well-balanced diet is critical. Pregnancy increases a woman's need for nutrients and calories, making a balanced diet essential for women of childbearing age (**Table 6.2**). Sensible eating during pregnancy includes the basic concepts discussed in Chapter 9. Pregnant women should consume approximately an additional 100 calories per day in the first trimester and an additional 300 calories per day during the second and third trimesters. It is important not to diet during pregnancy but rather to eat sensibly. Pregnant women do not need to eat twice as much food or calories, but rather consume the essential nutrients required for healthy development of the fetus.

Although it is recommended that a woman try to meet her vitamin and mineral requirements by eating a balanced diet, many health-care providers recommend prenatal supplements to ensure adequate intake in addition to this diet. **Folate** is a B vitamin that is essential for the healthy development of the fetus; it is found naturally in green, leafy vegetables, nuts, beans, citrus fruits, and some fortified cereals. **Folic acid**, the synthetic form of the B vitamin folate, appears to help prevent **neural tube defects** such as spina bifida. As a result of folic acid's role in preventing neural tube defects, the FDA has required enriched grain products, such as breads, pasta, and bagels, to be fortified with folic acid. Childbearing women should include 400–600 micrograms (0.4–0.6 milligram) of folic acid in their daily

Table 6.2 | Healthy Food Choices for a Pregnant Woman

Eating foods from a variety of sources will provide the best combination of nutrients needed for the pregnant or breastfeeding woman. (For more information on nutrition, see Chapter 9.)

Vegetable Group (choose fresh, frozen, canned, or dried)

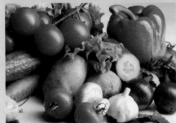

- Carrots
- Sweet potatoes
- Pumpkins
- Spinach
- Cooked greens (such as kale, collards, turnip greens, and beet greens)
- Winter squashes
- Tomatoes and tomato sauces
- Red sweet peppers

Fruit Group (choose fresh, frozen, canned, or dried)

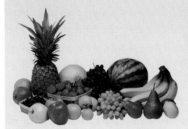

- Cantaloupes
- Honeydew melons
- Mangoes
- Prunes or prune juice
- Bananas
- Apricots
- Oranges and orange juice
- Red or pink grapefruit
- Avocados

Milk Group

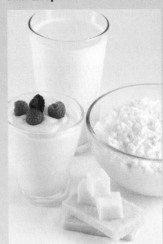

- Fat-free or low-fat yogurt
- Fat-free milk (skim milk)
- Low-fat milk (1% milk)

Grain Group

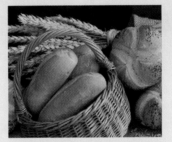

- Fortified ready-to-eat cereals
- Fortified cooked cereals
- Wheat germ

Meat and Beans Group

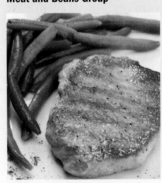

- Cooked dry beans and peas (such as pinto beans, soybeans, white beans, lentils, kidney beans, and chickpeas)
- Nuts and seeds (such as sunflower seeds, almonds, hazelnuts, pine nuts, peanuts, and peanut butter)
- Lean beef, lamb, pork, and poultry
- Shrimp, clams, oysters, and crab

Source: U.S. Department of Agriculture. MyPyramid for Pregnancy and Breastfeeding. Modified from http://www.mypyramid.gov/mypyramidmoms/index/html, retrieved September 1, 2008.

diet before and during pregnancy. Since 1998, the Food and Drug Administration (FDA) has required grain products to be fortified with folic acid to reduce the occurrence of neural-tube defects. This fortification has prevented many cases of neural-tube defects, but the effects have not been equally seen across all racial and ethnic groups. Non-Hispanic white and Hispanic births have shown significant decreases in neural-tube defects. Researchers emphasize that efforts to increase folic acid consumption should be continued for all racial and ethnic groups.[9]

Calcium and iron are important minerals for all women, including pregnant women. Calcium is essential to the formation of bone and teeth in the fetus, and it prevents the pregnant woman from losing her own bone density while providing for the growing fetus. Iron helps carry oxygen in the blood and reduces the risk of pregnancy-induced hypertension. Women often require iron supplements, because most female iron stores are not adequate to supply both mother and unborn child given the large demand for iron throughout the pregnancy. Iron supplements should be taken with vitamin C to facilitate their absorption.

Women should drink plenty of fluids throughout pregnancy. A woman's blood volume and blood fluids increase significantly during pregnancy, and drinking enough fluids will help to prevent dehydration and constipation. Pregnant women should also avoid certain foods during pregnancy, to help prevent infections that may harm the fetus (see **It's Your Health**).

It's Your Health

Foods to Avoid During Pregnancy

Sushi and other raw fish, especially shellfish (oysters, clams).

Hot dogs or luncheon meats (such as ham, turkey, salami, and bologna) unless they are reheated until steaming hot.

Unpasteurized milk, unpasteurized fruit and vegetable juices, or foods made from unpasteurized milk, including soft cheese (feta, brie, Camembert, Roquefort, queso blanco, queso fresco). Soft cheeses may be eaten if they are made with pasteurized milk.

Refrigerated pates, meat spreads, or smoked seafood. Canned versions of these products are safe to eat.

Raw vegetable sprouts (alfalfa, clover, and radish), which can carry *Salmonella* or *E. coli.*

Raw or undercooked meat, poultry, and eggs, as well as products made with raw or partially cooked eggs (such as eggnog, hollandaise sauce, and some Caesar salad dressings).

Some herbal supplements and teas.

Swordfish, shark, king mackerel, and tilefish, which have high levels of mercury.

■ According to the FDA/EPA, women who are pregnant can eat up to 12 ounces (two average-sized fish meals) per week of fish or shellfish that are lower in mercury, such as shrimp, salmon, catfish, and canned light tuna. White (albacore) tuna contains more mercury than canned light tuna, so women should limit their consumption of canned white tuna and tuna steaks to no more than 6 ounces per week.

■ Women should check for local advisories about any fish caught in waters by family and friends. If no advice is available, women should limit their consumption to less than 6 ounces per week of this type of fish and not eat any other fish during the week.

■ Folic acid appears to be a protective factor against neural tube defects, which develop in the first month of pregnancy. It is important for a woman to begin increasing her folic acid intake before she becomes pregnant.

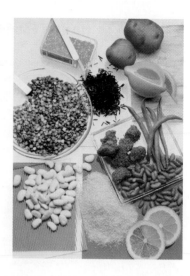

Weight gain is another important prenatal nutritional issue. It is important that the mother gain the right amount of weight. It is not necessary to "eat for two," but extra nutrients and calories are needed in the prenatal period. A woman should consult with her health-care provider about how much weight to gain during her pregnancy. Her weight before pregnancy will be a factor. A woman of average weight is generally advised to gain 25 to 35 pounds during her pregnancy. As shown in **Table 6.3**, pregnancy weight gain is distributed throughout a woman's body. An underweight woman should gain more than the 25–35 pounds and overweight women may need to gain only 15–25 pounds. Women who are expecting multiple births will need to gain more weight than a single pregnancy. Failure to gain adequate weight is associated with higher infant morbidity, lower birth weight, and preterm deliveries.[10]

Steady weight gain is important. Erratic weight gains may be symptomatic of an underlying problem such as

Table 6.3 Pregnancy Weight Gain Distribution

	Pounds
Baby	8
Placenta	2-3
Breasts	2-3
Amniotic fluid	2-3
Blood supply	4
Fat stores	5-9
Uterus	2-5
Total	25-35 pounds

toxemia (also known as **preeclampsia**), in which fluid is retained and toxic substances end up in the blood. Most of a woman's weight gain should occur at the end of the second trimester and the beginning of the third trimester. Women often average a weight gain of four to six pounds in the first trimester and one pound per week in the second and third trimesters.

Exercise

Proper exercise during pregnancy can have many benefits. Studies show that women who exercised in the three months before pregnancy felt better during the first trimester than did those who did not exercise; similarly, women who exercised in the first and second trimesters felt better in the third trimester than those who did not exercise. Well-conditioned women often have shorter labor, less need for obstetric intervention during pregnancy and childbirth, and speedier recovery after childbirth. The American College of Obstetricians and Gynecologists (ACOG) recommends at least 30 minutes of daily active exercise during pregnancy to reduce backaches, constipation, bloating, and swelling. Exercise also helps prevent or treat gestational diabetes; improves energy and mood; improves posture; promotes muscle tone, strength, and endurance; and helps the pregnant woman sleep better. The ACOG, however, does not recommend exercise for weight reduction while a woman is pregnant.[11]

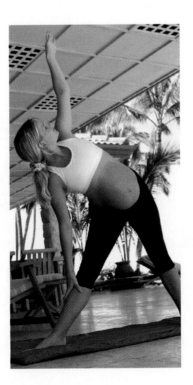

■ Proper exercise during pregnancy can have many benefits. Walking, swimming, and low-impact aerobics are particularly good choices for pregnant women.

The exercise program of a pregnant woman must be geared to her current level of fitness, medical history, past pregnancies, stage of fetal development, and maternal complicating factors. Generally, women are advised not to take up a new exercise program during pregnancy. It is better to stay with usual routines. Pregnancy places extra demand on the lungs and heart. In particular, oxygen consumption and heart rate increase during pregnancy. As pregnancy advances, breathing becomes more difficult because of the displacement of the enlarging uterus downward with each inhalation. Walking, swimming, and low-impact aerobics are particularly good exercise choices for pregnant women. Classes or exercise videos made specifically for pregnant women are also good options.

Activities that involve bouncing, jarring, or twisting and any activity that places the abdomen in jeopardy should be avoided during pregnancy. Examples of activities that should be avoided include horseback riding, scuba diving, and downhill skiing. Contact sports are too risky, as is any activity that requires rapid stops and starts or an extreme range of motion. The center of gravity for the body changes during pregnancy, increasing the risk of loss of balance. Laying on the back, particularly after the fourth month, can be dangerous because it can block the blood supply to the uterus and depress fetal heart rate. A resting position on the side does not compromise fetal blood supply.

Many questions regarding the safety and benefits of exercise during pregnancy remain unanswered. Although women with medical or obstetric complications should avoid rigorous physical activity, healthy women should continue exercising under their health-care provider's supervision. Because both pregnancy and exercise require an increase in caloric intake, a woman and her health-care provider should monitor her weight gain closely throughout the pregnancy.

Another form of exercise, known as pelvic muscle or Kegel exercises, is important during pregnancy. Increasing the strength of the pelvic muscles decreases urine loss during late pregnancy and may speed up the rehabilitation of the pelvic floor after vaginal delivery.

Avoiding Toxic Substances

Maternal exposure to many substances during pregnancy has been shown to have detrimental effects on the developing fetus. Many of these topics are discussed in detail elsewhere in this book. Note, however, that cigarettes, alcohol, and drugs have specific detrimental effects on the fetus.

Not smoking is essential to a healthy pregnancy and birth. The Centers for Disease Control and Prevention

(CDC) reports that smoking before and during pregnancy is the single most preventable cause of illness and death among mothers and infants.[12] Women who smoke before pregnancy are twice as likely to experience a delay in conception and have a 30% increased risk of being infertile compared to nonsmoking women. Women who smoke during pregnancy are also twice as likely to experience complications including premature rupture of membranes, early separation of the placenta from the uterus, and blockage of the cervix by the placenta. The CDC also reports that babies born to women who smoke during pregnancy have a 30% increased risk of being born premature, of low birth weight, and of being more likely to die of sudden infant death syndrome (SIDS). Unfortunately, about 13% of women still smoke during pregnancy. As **Figure 6.4** shows, younger, less educated, non-Hispanic white, and American Indian women are more likely to smoke during pregnancy.

Alcohol also is detrimental for both the mother and her developing baby. Alcohol consumption during pregnancy is known to cause alcohol-related defects among infants and **fetal alcohol syndrome (FAS)**, which is characterized by growth retardation, facial malformations, and central nervous system dysfunctions, including mental retardation. Alcohol appears to act in concert with several other factors to promote the development of FAS in infants:

- Differences in the degree of prenatal exposure to alcohol
- Maternal drinking patterns

- Possible genetic susceptibility to FAS
- Differences in maternal metabolism of alcohol
- Time of gestation during heavy alcohol consumption
- Interactions of alcohol use with other drugs and medications
- Maternal nutritional status

The fetus is especially vulnerable to the effects of alcohol during the first trimester of pregnancy, when the development of the central nervous system occurs. Recent research also links maternal drinking during pregnancy with an increased risk of early stillbirth.[13] In spite of campaigns to reduce alcohol consumption during pregnancy, usage levels still remain fairly high. About 1 in 12 pregnant women in the United States reports alcohol use, and about 1 in 30 pregnant women reports binge drinking (having five or more drinks at one time).[14]

Recently, alcohol use during pregnancy has become a controversial topic. Some medical experts have stated that women can probably safely consume small amounts of alcohol during pregnancy without harm to the fetus. ACOG, fearing that this message was potentially dangerous to pregnant women, released an official statement saying, "The bottom line according to ACOG: Women should avoid alcohol entirely while pregnant or trying to conceive because damage can occur in the earliest weeks of pregnancy, even before a woman knows that she is pregnant."[15]

Figure 6.4

Prevalence of smoking during the last three months of pregnancy by race/ethnicity, education, and age.

Source: Adapted from: Centers for Disease Control and Prevention. (2007). Preventing Smoking and Exposure to Secondhand Smoke Before, During, and After Pregnancy Fact Sheet. Downloaded September 12, 2008 from http://www.cdc.gov/nccdphp/publications/factsheets/Prevention/smoking.htm.

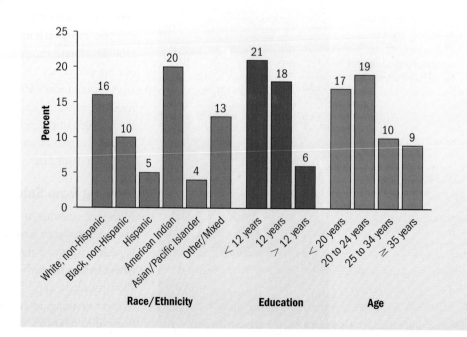

Consumption of other drugs also can adversely affect a developing fetus. No medications or over-the-counter preparations should be taken during pregnancy without first consulting with a clinician. Illicit drug use—most notably the use of cocaine—is associated with fetal distress, lower birthweight, and impaired fetal growth. The consequences of drug use during pregnancy include severe damage to the baby's brain and nervous system as well as other birth defects. Compared with mothers who did not smoke marijuana, smokers had smaller, sicker babies and a higher risk of stillbirths. Also, babies may be prone to excessive crying and trembling. Drug use may lead to neurochemical birth defects by disrupting normal development of the brain, and, in turn, cause long-term effects on intelligence, mental development, and learning.

Data indicate that nearly 4% of pregnant women use illicit drugs such as marijuana, cocaine, Ecstasy and other amphetamines, and heroin.[16] These and other illicit drugs may pose various risks for pregnant women and their babies. It is difficult for scientists to ascertain which birth defects are attributable to which illicit substance. Because many pregnant women who use illicit drugs also use alcohol and tobacco, which also pose risks to unborn babies, it often is difficult to determine which substance causes the adverse outcomes. Additionally, illicit drugs may be prepared with impurities that may be harmful to a pregnancy. What is known is that some of these drugs can cause a baby to be born too small or too soon, or to have withdrawal symptoms, birth defects, or learning and behavioral problems. Women who are pregnant and using heroin should work with a physician to quit using. Abruptly stopping use of the drug can cause miscarriage.[17]

Many over-the-counter prescription medications can prove dangerous during pregnancy as well. The antibiotic streptomycin can cause deafness, and the antibiotic tetracycline can lead to bone abnormalities and discolored teeth. Even aspirin and acetaminophen may affect a developing fetus. Clearly, it is important for pregnant women to consult their physicians before taking any type of medication.

Environmental Risks

Although not all environmental hazards can be avoided, a pregnant woman should take some precautions to protect herself and her baby. Although data are scarce, it is believed that the rapidly developing fetus is especially vulnerable to pollutants, toxic wastes, heavy metals, pesticides, gasses, and other hazardous compounds. For example, the element lead can cross the placenta and has been associated with intrauterine death, prematurity, and low birthweight.[18] Air pollution, such as secondhand smoke, can be detrimental to both a woman's health and the developing fetus. Scientists also have concluded that prenatal exposure to tobacco and environmental lead is a risk factor for attention deficit hyperactivity disorder (ADHD) in children.[19]

In addition, high levels of the type of radiation used for cancer therapy have been associated with birth defects. Diagnostic X rays should be avoided if possible throughout the pregnancy or if there is the possibility of pregnancy. X-ray exposure is associated with respiratory diseases and blood disorders in the fetus, as well as miscarriage.

Another environmental risk to consider during pregnancy is heat exposure. Women who use hot tubs and saunas or who have high fevers early in pregnancy have been found to be at greater risk of having children with neural tube defects such as spina bifida. Although more research is needed on this subject, it appears that the greatest risk arises early in the pregnancy when the fetal central nervous system is developing.

A woman who knows that she is pregnant or has a good likelihood of being pregnant should be advised of the limits of heat exposure. She should also be aware of the possible variability in hot tub or spa temperature readings and be able to accurately monitor maximum water temperature so that her body temperature can be maintained below 38.9 degrees C (102 degrees F).[20]

Prenatal Testing

Prospective parents often worry whether their baby will be born normal and healthy. Most of the time, these worries are unfounded: Almost all children born in the United States are healthy. However, the CDC reports that 1 of every 33 babies is born with a birth defect.[21] A birth defect can affect almost any part of the body. The well-being of the child depends mostly on which organ or body part is involved and how much it is affected. Most birth defects occur during the first three months of pregnancy. Birth defects can be genetic in origin, or they can be caused by exposure to harmful agents.

Risk factors that increase the likelihood of birth defects include family or personal history of birth defects, a previous child with a birth defect, certain medications used around the time of conception, diabetes before pregnancy, and women being age 35 years or older when the baby is due.

Screening tests are performed during pregnancy to assess the risk of certain birth defects. Screening tests simply show if a fetus is at risk of having a birth defect. If a screening test shows an increased risk for a certain defect, further diagnostic tests can confirm whether it actually exists. In

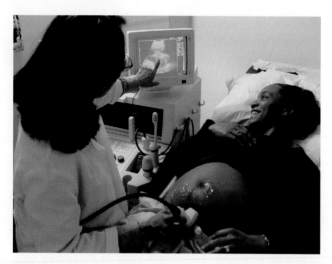 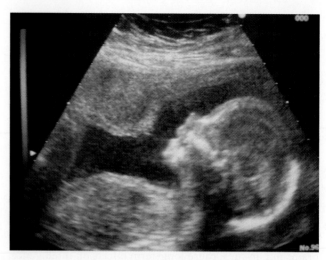

■ Performed at various times during pregnancy, ultrasound uses sound waves to show a picture of the baby. Ultrasound can check the age, growth, and size of a fetus; identify multiple pregnancies; and diagnose complications or birth defects.

most cases, the baby is healthy even if there is an abnormal result from a screening test. Screening tests include:

- *First-trimester screening tests* combine the result of special **ultrasound** tests and blood tests to detect **Down syndrome** and trisomy 18. Ultrasound is a noninvasive procedure that uses high-frequency sound waves to project an image or sonogram of the fetus. It is most accurate between the sixth and twentieth weeks of pregnancy.

- *Maternal serum screening tests* examine blood for abnormal levels of substances linked with certain birth defects such as Down syndrome and neural-tube defects. This group of tests includes **maternal serum alpha-fetoprotein (MSAFP)** screening, which measures a substance the fetal kidneys produce between the thirteenth and twentieth weeks of pregnancy.

- *Detailed ultrasound exams* are usually done after 18 weeks of pregnancy and allow for a more extensive view of the baby's organs and features.

Diagnostic tests try to detect a genetic disorder or birth defect. They are offered to women at risk of genetic disorder based on family history or the results of screening tests. Diagnostic tests include:

- **Chorionic villus sampling (CVS) (Figure 6.5A)** detects some of the same chromosomal abnormalities as **amniocentesis**. It can be performed earlier, though, at 10 to 12 weeks of pregnancy. The doctor guides either a small tube through the vagina and cervix or a thin needle through the abdomen and uterine wall to take a small sample of tissue from the placenta. The chorionic villa contain cells with the same genetic makeup

as the fetus. The results may be inconclusive and require a follow-up amniocentesis. The sample is studied for chromosomal or other defects. This procedure can be performed during the first trimester, permitting a greater range of options for the pregnancy. Complications from CVS are rare. One large study found that the procedure-related fetal loss rate after mid-trimester amniocentesis performed on patients in a contemporary prospective clinical trial was 0.06%. There was no significant difference in loss rates between those undergoing amniocentesis and those not undergoing amniocentesis.[22]

- *Amniocentesis* (**Figure 6.5B**) is usually performed at 15 to 20 weeks of pregnancy. The doctor guides a thin needle through the abdomen and uterus and withdraws a small amount of amniotic fluid. Cells from the fluid are analyzed for chromosomal defects. The alpha-fetoprotein (AFP) level can be tested for neural-tube defects. Complications from the procedure are rare.

- *Fetal blood sampling*, also known as cordocentesis, tests fetal blood for chromosomal defects and other problems. This procedure involves the insertion of a needle through the abdomen and uterine wall to take blood from a vein in the umbilical cord. This procedure is usually performed when amniocentesis or CVS is not possible because results are needed quickly. There is a small chance of fetal loss after fetal blood sampling.

Most of the time, the results will confirm that a baby is healthy. If the results are abnormal, counseling and supportive services can help the parents make decisions that best meet their needs.

Prenatal Testing

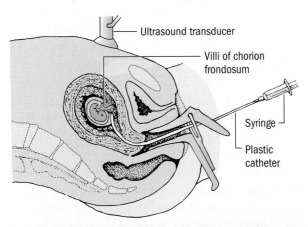

Figure 6.5A

In chorionic villus sampling, fetal cells from the chorionic villi (fingerlike projections on the developing placenta) are suctioned out through the cervix.

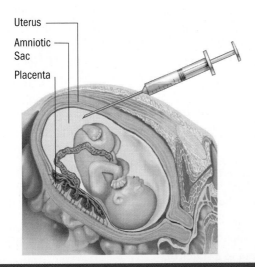

Figure 6.5B

Amniocentesis is a test for fetal abnormalities that involves withdrawing amniotic fluid and inspecting the cells contained within it.

Women also should be tested for **Rh incompatibility** through a simple blood test. Most people produce Rh factor, a protein located on the surface of a red blood cell. A person who does not produce Rh factor has Rh-negative blood. Rh incompatibility occurs when an Rh-negative mother and an Rh-positive father conceive a baby who inherits the father's Rh-positive blood type. This situation may present problems during pregnancy and in labor and delivery if the fetal Rh-positive blood cells enter the mother's bloodstream. The mother forms antibodies against the fetal blood cells in a process called maternal sensitization. This situation often occurs in a first pregnancy with an Rh-positive fetus, but because of the small amount of antibodies produced, it does not cause problems with the fetus. Future pregnancies, however, are at greater risk of antibodies crossing the placenta and causing Rh disease in the fetus. Rh-negative mothers should receive an injection of Rh immune globulin after delivery, during pregnancy, after a miscarriage, and after certain procedures such as amniocentesis. Without treatment, the most severely affected fetuses will be stillborn. In the newborn, Rh disease can result in jaundice, anemia, brain damage, heart failure, and death. Rh disease does not affect the mother's health.

Complications of Pregnancy

Most pregnancies progress without complications to the mother or the fetus. However, complications can occur, and regular prenatal visits and close medical coordination are important to find and treat these complications quickly and effectively. Five common complications of pregnancy—ectopic pregnancy, gestational diabetes, preterm delivery, stillbirth, and preeclampsia—are responsible for one-quarter of maternal and neonatal morbidity and mortality.[23]

Ectopic Pregnancy

Ectopic pregnancy occurs when the fertilized egg implants outside the uterus, usually in the fallopian tube. The egg begins to grow outside the uterine cavity and presents a risk for rupture and hemorrhage. This problem occurs in about 2% of pregnancies.[24] Increased awareness and improved technologies that identify early ectopic pregnancies have greatly decreased maternal deaths; however, ectopic pregnancy remains the leading cause of pregnancy-related death during the first trimester. National data indicate that ectopic pregnancy–related deaths account for 9% of all pregnancy-related deaths.[25]

Several factors increase the risk of an ectopic pregnancy by causing disruption of fallopian tube function (see **Table 6.4**). Pelvic inflammatory disease (PID), commonly caused by gonorrhea or chlamydia, is the most common risk

I had some rather severe abdominal pain and some bleeding. I knew my period was late, but I was shocked to learn from my doctor that I had had a miscarriage. I didn't even know that I was pregnant.

24-year-old woman

Table 6.4   Ectopic Pregnancy Risk Factors

- Pelvic inflammatory disease (PID)
- Previous ectopic pregnancy
- Previous tubal or pelvic surgery
- Endometriosis
- Infertility or infertility treatments
- Utero or tubal abnormalities
- DES (a drug once prescribed to prevent miscarriage) exposure
- Cigarette smoking

factor. (See Chapter 7 for more information.) Symptoms of ectopic pregnancy usually begin in the seventh or eighth week of gestation. The most common symptoms are abdominal pain and tenderness and a missed menstrual period. The abdominal pain can be subtle at first, sometimes localized on one side, and increase in severity if tearing of the fallopian tube causes internal bleeding. Abnormal vaginal bleeding or spotting occurs in most ectopic pregnancies. Blood tests and vaginal or abdominal ultrasound tests can effectively diagnose an ectopic pregnancy. In some cases, an ectopic pregnancy may degenerate and require no intervention. In most cases, however, laparoscopic surgery may be performed to remove the fertilized egg that cannot survive outside the uterus.

Gestational Diabetes

Gestational diabetes usually occurs in the second half of pregnancy. Three to eight out of every 100 pregnant women in the United States will develop gestational diabetes.[26] Most women can control their blood sugar levels with diet and exercise. Some women with gestational diabetes or women who had diabetes before pregnancy need insulin injections to control their blood sugar levels. A woman is considered to be at high risk for gestational diabetes if she is very overweight, previously had gestational diabetes, has a strong family history of diabetes, or has glucose in her urine. The baby of a mother with gestational diabetes is at risk of being born very large and with extra fat, making delivery difficult and more dangerous, with an increased risk of cesarean section. The baby is also at greater risk of having breathing problems and low blood glucose after birth. Gestational diabetes may increase the mother's risk of high blood pressure during pregnancy. For most women, glucose levels return to normal after pregnancy, but they are at increased risk for acquiring type 2 diabetes later in life.

Preterm Delivery

Pregnancy usually lasts from 38 to 42 weeks. Labor that starts before week 37 of a pregnancy is called **premature labor**. Babies born prematurely may have problems with breathing, eating, and temperature control, and they are more likely to die within the first month of life than a full-term baby. Approximately 12% of babies in the United States are born preterm, an increase of 3% over the last 20 years.[27] Women are at higher risk of preterm birth if they have had a previous preterm birth, are pregnant with twins or more, have certain uterine or cervical abnormalities, or have certain medical conditions. Women who seek late prenatal care or no care at all, as well as women who smoke, drink alcohol, use drugs, or experience stress, are also at greater risk. Women can decrease their risk of premature birth by recognizing the warning signs of preterm labor (see **It's Your Health**).

Stillbirth

Stillbirth is a common term for death of a fetus in the middle of the second trimester or later, while the fetus is still in the uterus. It is also called intrauterine fetal death or demise. There are multiple causes of stillbirth including mother with diabetes or high blood pressure, infection in the mother or in the fetal tissue, congenital abnormalities, and Rh disease (a blood incompatibility problem between the mother and fetus). In addition, umbilical cord problems including knots, tightened cord, cord wrapped around fetal body or neck, cord prolapse (the cord falling down through the open cervix during labor), and placental problems including poor circulation, and twin-to-twin transfusion (when twin circulations connect in a shared placenta) can lead to a stillbirth.

It's Your Health

Warning Signs of Preterm Labor

A health-care provider should be contacted immediately if any of the following symptoms develop during pregnancy:

- Contractions every 10 minutes or more frequently
- Vaginal bleeding
- Vaginal fluid leakage
- Pelvic pressure
- Low, dull backache
- Cramps that feel like menstrual cramps
- Abdominal pain or vomiting

Symptoms of a stillbirth vary but they may include the following common conditions: stopping of fetal movement and kicks, spotting or bleeding, no fetal heartbeat heard with stethoscope or Doppler, and no fetal movement or heartbeat seen on ultrasound. Treatment of a stillbirth depends on many factors such as the number of weeks gestation, the size of the fetus, and how long since the fetal heartbeat stopped. Treatment of a stillbirth may include waiting until the mother goes into labor on her own, dilating the cervix and using instruments to deliver the fetus and tissues, or inducing labor using medications to open the cervix and make the uterus contract and push out the fetus and tissues. Stillbirth is often very difficult for parents and other family members. It is sometimes harder than an earlier miscarriage because it happens later in pregnancy when the fetus has developed and the mother has felt movement. Often, the fetus is fully formed and is delivered just as any baby. It may be very hard emotionally for a woman to go through labor, yet not have a baby to take home. Counseling is important for all parents with a stillbirth to help them understand their feelings and begin the work of grieving.

Miscarriage

A **miscarriage**, or spontaneous abortion, is defined as a pregnancy that ends before the twentieth week of gestation. An estimated 10–15% of clinically recognized pregnancies end in spontaneous abortion.[28] Experts acknowledge challenges in estimating rates. Miscarriages often occur early in the pregnancy, and before women are aware of the pregnancy. Factors associated with miscarriage include advanced maternal age, chromosomal abnormalities, single gene mutations, structural uterine abnormalities, endocrine abnormalities, immunologic factors, genital infections, cigarette smoking, alcohol use, and various environmental and occupational exposures. Some of these, such as chromosomal abnormalities, are clearly related to the embryo and others, such as uterine abnormalities, are clearly related to the mother host. Karyotyping of the products of conception after miscarriage indicates that about two-thirds are chromosomally abnormal.[29]

A miscarriage is usually characterized by bleeding and cramping. Generally, when a woman experiences bleeding or cramping early in the pregnancy, bed rest is recommended. In some cases, the symptoms subside and the pregnancy proceeds normally. In other cases, the bleeding increases, the cervix dilates, and the embryo is released from the body. If the miscarriage is complete, the bleeding stops, and the uterus returns to its normal shape and size.

If the miscarriage is incomplete, any remaining fragments must be removed in a procedure known as a dilatation and curettage (D&C). The risk for miscarriage decreases after the first trimester of pregnancy.

The causes of miscarriage vary and are not always clear. This uncertainty is a source of frustration for many couples that feel the need to understand why the miscarriage happened. Grief associated with miscarriage is often underestimated, so many affected women find themselves with inadequate support from their partners, friends, family, and health-care providers.[30] Most women experience grief after their loss, as well as feelings of guilt, self-blame, and abandonment. The intensity of a woman's emotional distress may be related to the desirability of the pregnancy, late gestational age of the fetus, lack of social support, a lengthy period of trying to get pregnant, and use of infertility treatments. Women also may feel that they have disappointed their partners or families.

Preeclampsia

Preeclampsia is pregnancy-related high blood pressure. It can also be called toxemia. Preeclampsia usually occurs after about 30 weeks of pregnancy. In addition to having high blood pressure, mothers with preeclampsia often experience protein in their urine, swelling of the hands and face, sudden weight gain (a pound a day or more), blurred vision, severe headaches, dizziness, and intense stomach pain. The only real cure for preeclampsia is delivery, which may not be best for the baby. Labor is usually induced if the condition is mild and the woman is near term (37 to 40 weeks gestation). If a woman is not ready for labor, she and the baby will be monitored, often in a hospital setting, until her blood pressure stabilizes or the baby is born.

Genetic Disorders and Congenital Abnormalities

Genetic disorders are diseases caused in whole or in part by a variation or mutation of a gene. Scientists are learning that thousands of diseases have genetic components. Genetic disorders are responsible for a significant number of miscarriages, often without being diagnosed, so calculating the total number of disorders is a complicated process. Today more than 6,000 abnormalities have been identified, ranging from mild differences (as in certain hemoglobin abnormalities) to fatal or overwhelmingly disabling conditions, such as trisomy 18 (Edwards') syndrome and trisomy 13 (Patau's) syndrome. The risk of a single gene disorder is estimated at 1 in 200 births.

Genetic diseases result from single-gene alterations, chromosomal abnormalities, or multifactorial errors. Single-gene disorders are caused by a mutation in a single gene. The mutation may be present on one or both chromosomes (one chromosome inherited from each parent). Sickle cell disease, cystic fibrosis, and Tay-Sachs disease are single-gene disorders. Chromosome disorders are caused by extra or missing chromosomes or chromosome parts. (Each chromosome contains thousands of individual genes.) Down syndrome, for example, is caused by an extra copy of chromosome 21, but no individual gene on the chromosome is abnormal. Multifactorial inheritance disorders are caused by a combination of small variations in genes, often in concert with environmental factors. Heart disease and most cancers are examples of these disorders. Another multifactorial example is albinism, an inherited inability to generate the protective pigment melanin. Albinism greatly increases susceptibility to skin cancer after excessive exposure to sunlight. Behaviors are also considered to be multifactorial. Behaviors are complex traits involving multiple genes that are affected by many other factors. Researchers are learning more about the genetic contribution to behavioral disorders such as alcoholism, obesity, certain mental illnesses, and Alzheimer's disease.

Because early detection of these conditions is essential, state-based newborn screening programs began over 40 years ago. States and territories mandate newborn screening of all infants born within their jurisdiction for certain disorders that may not otherwise be detected before developmental disability or death occurs. Newborns with these disorders typically appear normal at birth. A recent expert panel has identified 29 conditions for which screening should be mandated.[31]

Infections

Any infection in the mother can potentially cause harm to an unborn fetus. Sexually transmitted infections, including HIV, can be particularly dangerous during a pregnancy. (For more information, see Chapter 7.)

- Gonorrhea, chlamydia, and syphilis can cause preterm delivery and miscarriage.

- **Bacterial vaginosis (BV)**, an infection of the vaginal area that is usually benign and asymptomatic, can lead to preterm delivery as well as low-birthweight babies. The presence of BV also is associated with an increased risk of HIV infection.

- Perinatal transmission of HIV can occur during pregnancy, labor and delivery, or via breastfeeding. Since medications can reduce the risk of perinatal HIV transmission, testing of pregnant women and subse-

quent treatment of those who are infected have dramatically reduced transmission rates. Perinatal transmission is the most common route of HIV infection in children, and it is now the source of almost all AIDS cases in children in the United States.[32] The actual number of AIDS cases associated with perinatal transmission has decreased dramatically in recent years, though the disease burden remains disproportionately high for racial and ethnic minorities (**Figure 6.6**).

The CDC recommends that all pregnant women be tested for HIV as early in pregnancy as possible. Pregnant women should also be screened for chlamydia, gonorrhea, hepatitis B, and syphilis.[33]

The most common prenatal infection today is **cytomegalovirus (CMV)**, a viral infection. CMV causes mild flulike symptoms in adults, but in newborns, it can cause small birth size, brain damage, developmental problems, enlarged liver, hearing and vision impairment, and other malformations. Each year in the United States, about 1 in 750 children are born with or develop disabilities as a result of CMV infection.[34] A blood test can ascertain if a woman already had a CMV infection. More invasive tests, such as amniocentesis, can help determine if the fetus is infected. Because CMV is found in body fluids, including urine, saliva, breast milk, blood, tears, semen, and vaginal fluids, a woman can become infected with CMV when she comes in contact with them. Good hygiene by pregnant women is still the best way to protect unborn babies against CMV infection.

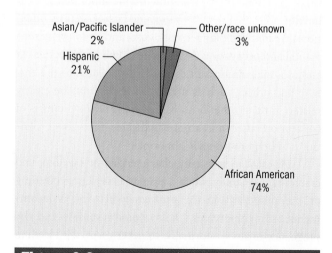

Figure 6.6
Race/ethnicity of children with AIDS.

Rubella is also linked with birth defects. A rubella infection is usually mild and often asymptomatic. The biggest danger of rubella is if a woman gets it during the first 20 weeks of pregnancy. She may lose the pregnancy, or the virus could cause problems to her unborn baby such as cataracts, deafness, or damage to the heart or brain. There is no treatment for rubella, but the measles-mumps-rubella (MMR) vaccine can prevent it. All women of reproductive age should be immunized against rubella if they have not had this formerly common childhood illness.

Group B streptococcus (GBS) is a bacterium that can cause illness in newborn babies and pregnant women. It is the most common cause of life-threatening infections in newborns. It is a frequent cause of newborn pneumonia. In 2001 there were about 1,700 babies less than one week old who had early-onset group B strep disease.[35] In most cases, this disease can be prevented in newborns by administering IV antibiotics to women in labor who had a baby with group B strep disease in the past, or who now have a urinary tract infection caused by group B strep. Pregnant women who carry the bacterium, as confirmed with a positive test during pregnancy, should also be given antibiotics during labor.

Other Considerations

Women should be aware of postpartum issues, such as depression. Many women will experience postpartum "blues," mood swings, and slight depression for several days after a baby's birth. These feelings are normal and will go away in the first few weeks. Some women experience more severe symptoms, however, which will warrant treatment. Women who are more susceptible to postpartum depression include those women who suffer from depression, have experienced postpartum depression in a previous pregnancy, have severe PMS or PMDD, and/or are experiencing other stressors in their family, marriage, or life at the time of the birth. (See Chapter 12 on mental health.)

Women with disabilities and chronic conditions who want to become pregnant may have special considerations to discuss with their health-care providers. Certain conditions that are common in pregnant women, such as vaginal and urinary tract infections, fluid retention, and decreased mobility, may create even more significant problems for women with preexisting conditions or disorders. Other difficulties may also impair the mobility of women with physical disabilities. As her body changes with pregnancy, a woman with impaired mobility may experience balance problems and new pressure points if she is in a wheelchair. Each disability or condition may present with different is-

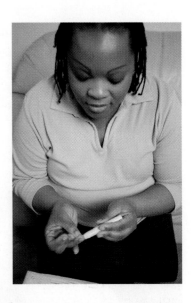

■ Women with diabetes are at an increased risk for complications with pregnancy.

sues, just as each pregnant woman may present with different complications and issues. Throughout the pregnancy, from preconception to postpartum, women with disabilities or chronic conditions should work with a team of health-care providers to ensure favorable pregnancy and postpregnancy outcomes.

Childbirth

Many women have special concerns about their childbirth experience. Experts agree that interfering with the normal physiological process of labor and birth in the absence of medical necessity increases the risk of complications for the mother and baby. Unfortunately, hospital routines and procedures have often taken priority over the needs of the laboring mother and her baby. Some experts argue that many modern medical interventions, including cesarean surgery, labor induction, electronic fetal monitoring, ultrasound examinations, episiotomies, unphysiological positions, pubic shaving, enemas, IV lines, drugs, and forced mother and baby separations are too normative, and often do not improve birth outcome or the labor and delivery

I knew that having a baby would be difficult, but I was not prepared to feel so numb, miserable, hopeless, and worried. I learned that I was one of the 10-15% of mothers who experience postpartum depression. Fortunately my doctor was really helpful. I would encourage any new mom to talk to her doctor if she is feeling really sad or "down." Sometimes it is just normal "baby blues." But sometimes it can be serious. Getting help early can make a huge difference.
30-year-old mother

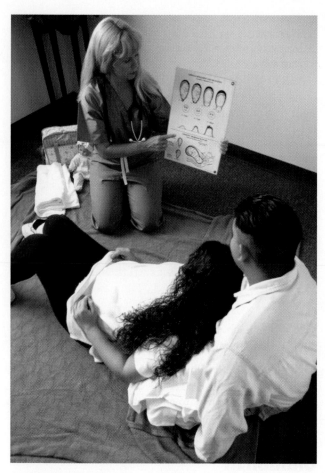

■ Childbirth education classes help a couple prepare for delivery by teaching relaxation and pain management techniques. The classes also provide the opportunity for the couples to discuss their concerns and excitement.

process.[36] Today, many birthing centers encourage the following practices to promote an optimal physiological birth experience for the mother and her baby[37]:

- Avoiding medically unnecessary induction of labor
- Allowing freedom of movement for the laboring woman
- Providing continuous labor support
- Avoiding routine interventions and restrictions
- Encouraging spontaneous pushing in nonsupine positions
- Keeping mothers and babies together after birth without restrictions on breastfeeding

In many areas, women can decide what type of health-care provider they want for the birth of their baby. High-risk mothers or mothers with high-risk infants have fewer options because they may require options for more sophisticated specialties. The preferences of the mother and her partner are important considerations for making many childbirth decisions. Self-Assessment 6.1 provides a checklist for childbirth considerations. The list can serve as a basis for further questions and decision making between a woman and her childbirth health-care providers.

Preparation for Childbirth

Preparation for childbirth is a concept that has been popular in the United States for the last 40 years. "Preparation" usually entails attending organized classes to prepare a woman and her partner for labor and delivery. Some individuals anticipate or desire having a "natural childbirth" experience (meaning childbirth without use of medications for pain relief and with minimal mechanical monitoring), and others wish to learn more about the birthing events. Regardless of the plans for childbirth, organized classes provide an opportunity to learn about local birthing options and to discuss personal issues and concerns. They also provide an opportunity to learn about pregnancy and childbirth, and to develop pain management skills. Strategies that are taught may include breathing techniques, such as **Lamaze**, relaxation techniques, muscle-strengthening exercises, and different positions that facilitate labor, thereby promoting an uncomplicated birth. Perhaps the greatest advantage of childbirth education is the opportunity to prepare for a more satisfying birth experience.

Labor and Delivery

Labor and delivery can be rewarding and satisfying when a woman anticipates the sequence of events and is prepared for the process. Long before actual labor begins, the uterus changes to prepare itself to function efficiently during labor and delivery. By the end of the pregnancy, the uterus measures about 10 to 14 inches. Its capacity has increased nearly 500 times during the pregnancy, and it increases in weight from 1.5 ounces to 30 ounces. The uterine muscle fibers grow to 10 times their original thickness. The uterus is one of the strongest muscles in a woman's body, and it contracts powerfully during labor. Throughout pregnancy, the uterus contracts at slightly irregular intervals. These irregular contractions, known as Braxton-Hicks contractions, differ from "real" labor contractions in that they do

Childbirth Considerations

Birthing issues	Very Important	Not Important	Don't Want
Hospital delivery room	_____	_____	_____
Hospital birthing room	_____	_____	_____
Birthing center	_____	_____	_____
Home	_____	_____	_____
Obstetrician	_____	_____	_____
Family practitioner	_____	_____	_____
Certified nurse-midwife	_____	_____	_____

Partner/coach			
Present during labor	_____	_____	_____
Present during delivery	_____	_____	_____
Present for all procedures	_____	_____	_____
Present during cesarean	_____	_____	_____
Present during recovery	_____	_____	_____

Early labor			
Stay home as long as possible	_____	_____	_____
Arrive early and settle in	_____	_____	_____
Wear own clothes	_____	_____	_____
Perineal shave	_____	_____	_____
Enema	_____	_____	_____
Intravenous tube	_____	_____	_____

First-stage labor			
Labor room	_____	_____	_____
Birthing room	_____	_____	_____
External fetal monitor	_____	_____	_____
Internal fetal monitor	_____	_____	_____

Second-stage labor			
Labor room	_____	_____	_____
Delivery room	_____	_____	_____
Birthing room	_____	_____	_____
Family present	_____	_____	_____
Delivery position flexibility	_____	_____	_____
Episiotomy	_____	_____	_____

After delivery			
Prolonged holding of baby	_____	_____	_____
Warm-water bath for baby	_____	_____	_____
Breastfeeding in birthing area	_____	_____	_____

Postpartum			
Private room	_____	_____	_____
Baby rooming in with mother	_____	_____	_____
Breastfeeding	_____	_____	_____
Bottle-feeding	_____	_____	_____
Length of stay in facility	_____	_____	_____
Sibling/family visitation	_____	_____	_____
Postpartum depression concerns	_____	_____	_____

Decisions on places of birth, birthing positions, pain relief, and breastfeeding can be made based on this checklist. After completing the assessment, women should discuss their issues of concern with their partner and their health-care provider.

not gradually increase in frequency, intensity, or duration. Instead, they serve to increase the blood circulation and help the uterus to accommodate the growing baby.

Three distinctive signs indicate that labor is beginning:

- Regular, progressive uterine contractions that occur every five minutes or so and last from 45 seconds to a minute. The contractions gradually become longer, stronger, and closer together.
- Rupture of the membranes, or "bag of waters." This rupture may be a "slow leak" or a gush. The fluid is usually clear.
- The "bloody show." It involves the passage of a small amount of bloodstained mucus, which served as a plug in the cervix to protect the fetus from infection. As the cervix begins to dilate, this plug is released.

Other less distinctive signs of approaching labor include diarrhea, backache, and an increase in Braxton-Hicks contractions. The only confirmation that labor has begun is a pelvic examination that reveals a softening, thinned-out, and dilating cervix.

Many factors affect the progress of labor, including the position of the baby and the shape of the mother's pelvis. Although all experiences are different, each labor progresses through three distinct stages (**Figure 6.7**).

Stage I is from the onset of labor to full dilation of the cervix. Before labor begins, the wall of the uterus is thin, the cervix is long and thick, the birth canal is narrow, and the membranes may still be intact. As labor begins, the bands of longitudinal muscle fiber in the upper part of the uterus contract and thus gradually draw up, thin, and open the mouth of the cervix. The cervical canal shortens until the cervix is as thick as the uterine wall. This process, in which the cervix is "taken up" into the uterus, is known as **effacement**. Once the cervix is effaced, the force of the uterine contractions begins to dilate the cervix, although effacement and dilation may occur simultaneously. Dilation refers to the size of the round opening of the cervix. It

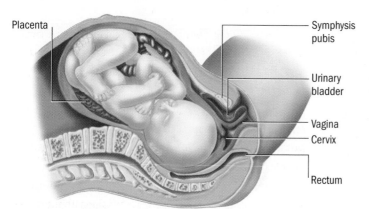

(a) Early first-stage labor

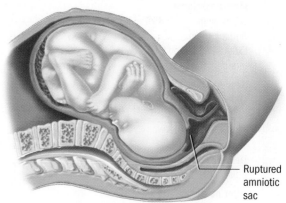

(b) Later first-stage labor: the transition

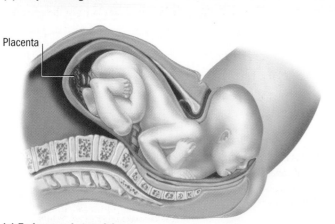

(c) Early second-stage labor

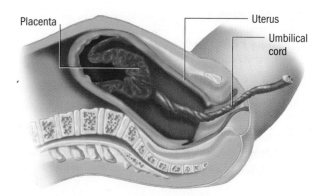

(d) Third-stage labor: delivery of afterbirth

Figure 6.7

Labor and delivery. Stage I: the cervix becomes fully dilated; stage II: the infant is born; stage III: the afterbirth is delivered.

is measured in centimeters or finger widths. Full dilation is 10 centimeters or five finger widths (**Figure 6.8**).

Stage II of labor begins when the cervix is completely dilated and ends with the birth of the baby. The presentation of the baby—the part of the body positioned to emerge first—is usually by the top of the head, known as a vertex presentation. When the feet or buttocks present first, it is known as a **breech** presentation. The breech position occurs in about 3% of deliveries. A breech presentation usually results in a longer labor. Because a breech delivery presents greater risks to the mother and baby, a cesarean delivery is often performed.

As the baby's head appears, or crowns, an episiotomy may be performed. An episiotomy is an incision in the perineum that enlarges the vaginal opening for birth. The traditional argument for performing this procedure is that a surgical incision heals better and faster than a jagged tear. Once routine with vaginal deliveries, the practice of episiotomies has been seriously questioned as to its necessity and benefits for all pregnancies. Recent studies show that episiotomies were linked with more pain, more difficulty healing, and a longer wait for resuming sex after childbirth, with no obvious benefits for most women. Only women requiring a quick delivery for babies in distress should receive an episiotomy. An estimated 1 million women have unnecessary episiotomies every year.[38,39]

Some mothers find that a sitting or squatting position facilitates the second stage of labor. Such positions permit gravity to help with the birth. Squatting specifically enlarges the pelvic opening. Under usual circumstances, the birth of the baby is a gradual process with head first, then shoulders, and then the body.

Stage III lasts from the completion of delivery of the baby to completion of delivery of the **afterbirth**, or placenta. In this final stage of labor, the uterus contracts firmly after the delivery of the baby. The placenta separates from the uterine wall and is expelled. If an episiotomy has been performed, it is sutured at this time.

Pain Relief in Childbirth

Women experience different levels of pain during childbirth. The reality of childbirth is that it usually involves some physical hurt. The physical and psychological techniques promoted in childbirth preparation classes can dramatically influence the perception of pain and the confidence in dealing with labor difficulties. These pain relief measures have the inherent advantage of not producing any chemical disruption in the mother's body, which could then affect the baby or the birthing process.

Good labor support helps a woman throughout labor. Physical and emotional comfort, information, guidance, and communication with the health-care staff are invaluable to the laboring woman and can greatly reduce her anxiety and need for pharmacological interventions. Nondrug options include:

- *Comfort measures:* These are things that a woman can do for herself, that her companion can do for her, or that can be done to the laboring environment to increase her personal comfort level.

- *Mental strategies:* Many women employ a variety of techniques including special breathing, meditation, prayer, music, focal points, and singing to reduce anxiety and create a sense of calm during labor.

- *Medications:* A variety of pain-relieving medications are available for childbirth. Most decisions about medications are actually personal choices, not medical decisions. For this reason, it is important for the pregnant

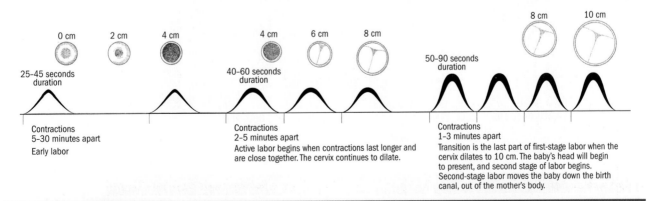

Figure 6.8

Dilation through stages of labor.

woman to learn about possible medications before she goes into labor. Tranquilizers and analgesics are often used together for general relaxation and to take the edge off of contractions.

Anesthetics used during labor and delivery may be given in different forms. **Epidural anesthesia** is the most popular choice among pregnant women. It allows the mother to be awake during the delivery. The anesthetic is injected through a catheter that is placed in a space adjacent to the spinal cord. Spinal anesthesia is injected directly into the spinal canal. Like the epidural, it prevents a woman from being able to move around in labor and often inhibits a woman from pushing. Pudendal anesthesia is injected into the area around the vagina and perineum. This method is least likely to affect the baby.

Cesarean Delivery

A **cesarean delivery** (also known as a cesarean section) is the birth of a baby through surgical incisions made in both the wall of the mother's abdomen and her uterus. Anesthesia is required for the procedure. Clearly, a cesarean birth is sometimes necessary for the safety of the mother or the baby—for example, when there are problems with the baby, problems with the woman's passage area, or problems with the delivery process. However, considerable contro-

versy exists today over whether this type of delivery is being performed too often. The rate of cesarean sections had increased dramatically between 1970 and 1988, rising from 5.5% of all births in 1970 to a high of 24.7% in 1988. Between 1991 and 1996, however, the U.S. cesarean rate dropped by 8%, but then increased again between 1996 and 2003 to the highest percentage ever recorded in the United States (**Figure 6.9**).[40]

One cause for cesarean section is **fetal distress**, a condition in which some aspect of labor or the baby's environment places the baby at risk. For example, the baby's oxygen supply might be cut off owing to **abruptio placentae**, in which the placenta separates prematurely from the wall of the uterus. This event threatens not only the baby, but also the mother with a risk of hemorrhage. A **prolapsed cord** is another risky situation in which the umbilical cord comes through the pelvis before the baby and can disrupt the flow of oxygen to the baby due to a compressed cord.

Problems with the birth passage also influence the decision for a cesarean delivery. **Cephalopelvic disproportion**, in which the baby is too large for the pelvis, is a common reason for choosing this type of delivery. Often a fetus indicates that the pelvis may not be a comfortable "fit" by assuming a position other than the normal head-first position for birth. A woman in labor whose baby is in a transverse lie, a crosswise position in the uterus, will need

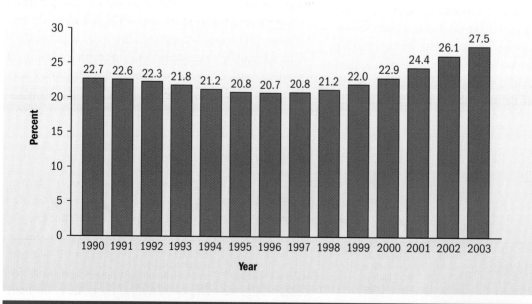

Figure 6.9

Total cesarean rates for first births, United States, 1990–2003.

Source: Adapted from: Menacker, F. (2005). Trends in cesarean rates for first births and repeat cesarean rates for low-risk women: United States, 1990–2003. *National Vital Statistics Reports.* 54(4). Downloaded September 14, 2008 from http://www.cdc.gov/nchs/data/nvsr/nvsr54/nvsr54_04.pdf.

a cesarean delivery because neither the head nor the buttocks are in the pelvis. When a baby is in a breech position, the buttocks emerge before the head. The head has a larger diameter than the buttocks, and the risk is that it will not fit well through the passage because it has not had the opportunity to mold and nestle into the pelvis throughout the labor process. Multiple births are also more likely to require cesarean delivery. A relatively rare complication of the passageway is obstruction by a fibroid, a benign tumor, or even the placenta (**placenta previa**). Usually these obstructions or other problems with fetal passage can be diagnosed before labor and delivery, which permits time to discuss various options with the health-care provider.

Other conditions may also indicate the need for cesarean delivery. For example, the term "failure to progress" describes cervical failure to dilate adequately despite regular uterine contractions. To avoid prolonged distress to mother and baby in this situation, a cesarean delivery may be performed. Herpes is another reason for a cesarean delivery. If a woman has active lesions in the birth canal, a cesarean delivery is indicated to avoid infecting the baby.

Vaginal Birth After Cesarean Delivery

For many years, a widely held philosophy about childbirth was "once a cesarean, always a cesarean." This philosophy may be partially responsible for the overall increase in cesarean birth rates in the United States during recent years. National data indicate a steady decline in cesarean sections through 1996, owing in part to the movement encouraging vaginal birth after cesarean delivery (VBAC). By the late 1990s, however, studies revealed that some women should not attempt VBAC for fear of uterine rupture or the need for an emergency cesarean section. Many smaller hospitals stopped offering VBAC out of medical liability concerns.[41]

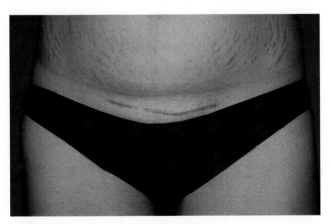

■ Many women with a prior history of cesarean birth are able to deliver their subsequent pregnancies vaginally.

The American College of Obstetricians and Gynecologists (ACOG), as well as many hospital boards, has taken a strong position on VBAC to help control the morbidity associated with major abdominal surgical procedures and to help reduce the spiraling costs of health care. A trial of labor is recommended for most women who underwent a previous cesarean section and have no unusual circumstances or conditions. ACOG has found that the mother usually experiences fewer complications with VBAC than with cesarean birth in terms of infection, bleeding, and anesthesia. Other advantages of VBAC include a shorter hospital stay and recovery period as well as significant cost savings. Women giving birth in hospitals that are not equipped for emergency cesarean sections and women with certain medical contraindications should not undergo VBAC.[41]

Breastfeeding

The practice of breastfeeding varied greatly throughout the second half of the twentieth century. As formula became popular in the 1950s and 1960s, many women who had the money to purchase formula, bottles, and nipples as well as the time to sterilize the bottles and nipples stopped breastfeeding. Reports in the 1970s on the benefits of breastfeeding resulted in a return to breastfeeding, especially for educated women and women of higher socioeconomic status. This trend continued until the 1980s, when many women again returned to formula feeding. Breastfeeding rates have increased since 1999, but room for improvement remains. Among children born in 2005, 74% initiated breastfeeding, whereas 43% were breastfeeding at six months and 21% at 12 months of age. Approximately 32% of infants born in 2005 were exclusively breastfed through three months of age, and 12% were exclusively breastfed for six months.[42]

Physiological Changes of the Breast

Hormones during pregnancy change the breasts to prepare them for **lactation** (milk production). The breasts enlarge as the cells that produce milk increase in number and the ducts that carry milk develop (**Figure 6.10**). The nipple and areola become more elastic and are protected by a natural lubricant secreted from tiny glands under the skin. After delivery, levels of estrogen and progesterone in the body rapidly decrease, triggering the production of milk. Two hormones are released in response to a baby's suckling:

- *Prolactin* stimulates lactation.
- *Oxytocin* is responsible for the transportation of milk from the producing cells to the milk ducts to the nipple.

Figure 6.10

The female breast.

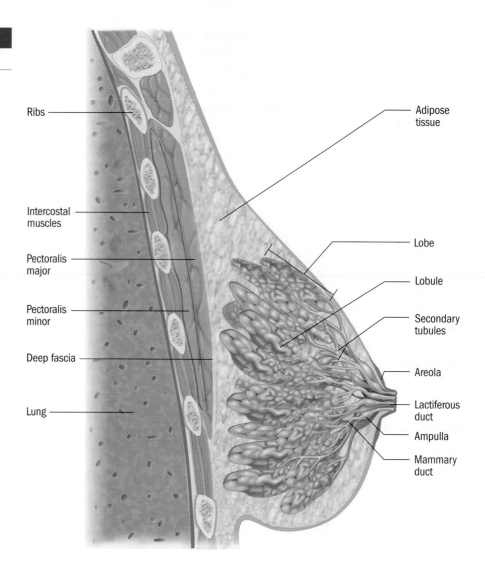

The composition of breast milk varies depending on the stage of lactation, the stage of feeding, and the mother's diet. Early milk, or milk produced during the pregnancy and for 3 to 5 days after birth, is called **colostrum**. Colostrum is yellowish in color, thicker than milk, and rich with protective antibodies and protein. Transitional milk leads to regular mature milk after about 10 days. During feedings, low-fat, thirst-quenching milk is released first, followed by higher-fat, more nourishing milk. The milk's vitamin content is representative of the mother's vitamin intake.

Benefits of Breastfeeding

Breastfeeding provides many benefits, including protection against many acute and chronic diseases as well as advantages for general health, growth, and development (see **It's Your Health**). Breast milk is highly nutritious, providing all of the nutrients that a growing baby needs. It is ideal as a baby's sole source of nutrients for the first six months of life. In addition, breast milk contains enzymes to aid the infant's digestion as well as antibodies to protect against infection. Evidence has shown that breastfed infants have fewer and less severe episodes of diarrhea; fewer cases of upper respiratory, ear, and even urinary infections; and fewer hospitalizations and doctor's visits. Many studies show the possibilities of breast milk protecting against type 1 diabetes mellitus (childhood-onset diabetes), Crohn's disease, SIDS, chronic digestive disease, and childhood cancers, such as lymphoma and leukemia. Breastfeeding is also believed to bestow cognitive benefits.[43]

New mothers may also reap benefits from breastfeeding. Due to the increased levels of oxytocin from breastfeeding, the uterus returns to its normal size more quickly and the woman experiences less postpartum bleeding. Breastfeeding also helps a woman to return to her pre-pregnancy weight more quickly, although she is less likely to lose her

Benefits of Breastfeeding

Infant's Benefits

- Fewer episodes and decreased severity of diarrhea and gastrointestinal difficulties

- Decreased incidence of ear infections, urinary tract infections, and upper respiratory infections

- Fewer hospitalizations and visits to the doctor's office

- Fewer food allergies

- Possible protection against diabetes, Crohn's disease, SIDS, chronic digestive disease, and childhood cancers

- Possible benefits of cognitive development

Mother's Benefits

- Less postpartum bleeding

- Faster return to pre-pregnancy weight

- Possible decreased incidence of ovarian cancer, breast cancer, and osteoporosis

Benefits for Both

- Special bond between mother and infant

Table 6.5	Economic Benefits of Breastfeeding

- Families spend $2.5 billion a year on breast milk substitutes such as infant formula.

- The U.S. Department of Agriculture's Special Supplemental Nutrition Program for Women, Infants and Children (WIC) spends $740 million per year to buy formula for babies who are not breastfeeding.

- Every 10% increase in the breastfeeding rate among WIC recipients would save WIC almost $1 million per year.

- Insurers, including Medicaid, spend $1.6 billion a year to cover sick-child office visits and prescriptions to treat the three most common illnesses—respiratory infections, otitis media (ear infections), and diarrhea—in the first year of life for formula-fed infants versus breastfed infants.

- From $4.6 to 9 billion excess dollars are spent every year on conditions and diseases that are preventable by breastfeeding.

Source: Health Resources and Services Administration (HRSA) Maternal and Child Health Bureau, and the Centers for Disease Control and Prevention (CDC). (2002). *[Adjusted for inflation for 2009 dollars]*

last five pounds of weight. Women who breastfeed may have a lower incidence of ovarian and premenopausal breast cancer, as well as improved bone mass leading to reduced fractures and risk of osteoporosis in the postmenopausal years.[43] Besides all of the physical health benefits, breastfeeding can create a special bond between mother and infant. Additionally, breastfeeding has the economic benefit of saving money that would otherwise be spent on formula and medical conditions that breastfeeding can prevent (**Table 6.5**).

Although any length of breastfeeding is better than no breastfeeding, research indicates that exclusive and prolonged breastfeeding has a greater protective effect than short-term nursing or nursing along with supplemental formula feeding. Experts recommend that mothers breastfeed their babies exclusively for six months, and that they continue to breastfeed while supplementing with solid foods until the baby's first birthday.

Optimizing Breastfeeding

Even though breastfeeding offers many advantages for children and mothers, society, and the environment, nursing mothers still must face social and cultural barriers. Education is a primary challenge, especially for first-time mothers, who benefit from antenatal and postpartum breastfeed-

ing instruction and support.[44] Breastfeeding is not always easy, especially for first-time mothers, but experienced guidance and care can solve problems in many cases.

Worksite support for working nursing mothers is an important challenge for many women. In one national study, the availability of employer-sponsored child care was found to increase the likelihood of breastfeeding six months after birth by 47%. In addition, on average, working an additional eight hours at home per week increased

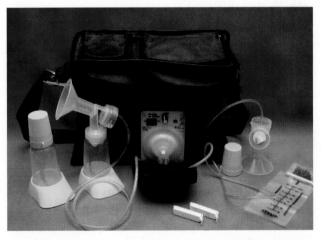

■ Breast pumps are useful to mothers who work or who have difficulty breastfeeding.

the probability of breastfeeding initiation by 8% and breastfeeding six months after birth by 16.8%.[45]

Studies on breastfeeding in the United States have historically shown substantial racial/ethnic and socioeconomic disparities. In a recent national study, immigrant women in each racial/ethnic group had higher breastfeeding initiation and longer duration rates than native women of the same racial/ethnic group. Acculturation was associated with lower breastfeeding rates among both Hispanic and non-Hispanic women.[46] In another study, researchers found that immigration status was strongly associated with increased breastfeeding initiation, suggesting that cultural factors are important in the decision to breastfeed.[47]

Geographical variance is also a factor in U.S. breastfeeding. There are wide state variations in breastfeeding initiation and duration, with the western and northwestern states having the highest rates.[48] Additional research is needed to ascertain the influence of state legislation and local programs designed to promote breastfeeding practices.

Complications of Breastfeeding

Breastfeeding is not always the best option for some infants. Women who are infected with HIV; have untreated active tuberculosis; are users of alcohol, tobacco, or other recreational drugs; are undergoing cancer chemotherapy or radiation treatment; or are using certain necessary medications that may not be healthy for the developing infant should not breastfeed. Infants with **galactosemia** (an inherited disease caused by a lack of enzyme for processing galactose that can lead to organ enlargement, cataracts, and mental retardation) should not be breastfed.

Women may experience difficulties with feeding, including the following problems:

- Inverted or flat nipples
- Raw or cracked nipples
- Severely swollen breasts
- Problems with the infant latching on
- Pain during latch-on

These problems often can be resolved by changing positions, massaging the breasts, or using a nipple shield to protect the breast. Other complications may require medical attention, such as **mastitis** (bacterial infection of the breast) or **thrush** (yeast infection that affects the mouth of the baby). Women should talk to their health-care provider or a nursing lactation specialist if they experience problems with breastfeeding.

Diet, Drugs, and Alcohol During Breastfeeding

Women who choose to breastfeed should consume a healthy diet to ensure adequate intake of the necessary vitamins and minerals. Caloric intake should be increased by 500 calories per day relative to a woman's pre-pregnancy diet. Women should maintain a sufficient calcium intake (1,000 mg per day) to rule out any possibility of long-term effects of breastfeeding on the mother's bone density. Note that any substance taken in by the mother can be passed to the infant through the breast milk, including harmful substances such as caffeine, alcohol, and certain drugs. For this reason, breastfeeding women should consult their health-care providers before taking any medications.

Infertility

Fecundity refers to a woman's physical ability to have a child. Women with impaired fecundity include those who find it physically difficult or medically inadvisable to conceive or deliver a child. The term *impaired fecundity* is also used to describe women who, although having sexual intercourse on a regular basis without contraception for 36 months or more, fail to become pregnant. This definition of reduced ability to bear children differs from the medical definition of infertility, which is the inability of couples who are not surgically sterile to conceive after 12 months of regular intercourse without contraception.[49]

Causes

Fertility-related difficulties can arise at many points, including the process of ovulation in women, sperm produc-

It's Your Health

Pregnancy requires the following:

- A woman must effectively release an egg from one of her ovaries. This is known as *ovulation*.
- The egg must effectively travel from the ovary through the fallopian tube toward the uterus.
- A man's sperm must join with the egg, *fertilization*, en route to the uterus.
- The fertilized egg must effectively attach to the lining of the uterus, *implantation*.

Infertility can result from problems that arise from any of these requirements.

tion in men, or the maintenance of the embryo once the egg has been fertilized by the sperm.

- In 25% to 35% of couples, the fertility problem is in the male.
- In 25% to 35% of couples, the fertility problem is in the female.
- For the remaining couples, infertility is a result of both a male and a female factor or unknown causes.

Many factors contribute to infertility. Problems with ovulation are responsible for most cases in women. Without ovulation, eggs are not present for fertilization. Symptoms that might indicate a woman is not ovulating include irregular or absent menstrual periods. Blocked or scarred fallopian tubes due to pelvic inflammatory disease (PID), endometriosis, or previous surgery for an ectopic pregnancy can all cause infertility in women. Physical or anatomical problems with a woman's uterus or uterine fibroids may also contribute to infertility.

Age and other factors can affect a woman's ability to conceive. Because more women are delaying childbirth until their 30s and 40s, age is becoming a more common infertility consideration. In addition to age, poor diet, smoking, alcohol, sexually transmitted infections (STIs), and health problems that cause hormonal changes can also contribute to infertility. Depression and stress may have a direct effect on hormonal regulation and ovulation. Weight is another important factor in infertility. Women who are overweight or obese often have irregular or infrequent menstrual cycles and are at increased risk of infertility. Underweight women also have infertility issues due to low body fat levels.

Diagnosis

Various tests can often determine the cause of infertility and thus the appropriate treatment method. A simple method of determining whether ovulation is occurring, for example, is to monitor a woman's basal body temperature to see whether a slight increase in her temperature occurs midway through her menstrual cycle.

Tests can also examine the quality of the mucus. The ferning test involves collecting mucus near the time of ovulation to see if, when smeared, it resembles the fronds of a fern. If so, the woman's estrogen levels are normal, and the mucus is creating a desirable environment for the sperm to travel.

A postcoital test may also be performed before ovulation. Mucus is collected within six hours after intercourse

Gender Dimensions

MALE INFERTILITY

Problems with male fertility contribute to about one-third of cases of infertility. Many of the same factors that reduce fertility in women also affect male fertility. In most cases, male infertility is caused by producing too few sperm, **oligospermia**, or none at all, **azoospermia**. Other sperm production problems include issues with sperm motility or sperm ability to fertilize the egg. Abnormal sperm shape or structure that prevents sperm from moving correctly may also contribute to male infertility. Age and health problems are also factors in male infertility.

Alcohol or drugs, anabolic steroids, and pollutants and other chemicals in the environment can reduce fertility in men. Smoking can also affect male infertility. Studies have shown that smokers' sperm are less likely to bind tightly to an egg—a necessary step for fertilization.

Environmental factors such as prolonged exposure to high temperatures, radiation, or heavy electromagnetic or microwave emissions can decrease sperm count or affect the viability of the sperm. Medical treatments such as medicines, chemotherapy, or radiation therapy can also contribute to male infertility. Emotional factors such as high levels of stress can also play a role.

Unprotected sex, having multiple sex partners, and not using condoms may increase the risk of sexually transmitted infections (STIs). As with women, STIs are also an important cause of male infertility.

and is viewed under a microscope to see whether it contains multiple, active sperm.

Other tests used to diagnose infertility include the following:

- Blood tests for measuring hormone levels
- Radiograph studies such as a hysterosalpingogram, which outlines obstructions or abnormal growths in the uterus or fallopian tubes
- Laparoscopic surgery to view the uterus, fallopian tubes, and ovaries

A common test used to diagnose male infertility is semen analysis. Semen is evaluated for the number of sperm present, the volume of ejaculate, the motility of the sperm, and the size and shape of the sperm. If a man has a low sperm count, blood tests may be performed to measure various hormones and proteins. A physical examination and an ultrasound of the scrotum also may be performed to detect varicose veins that may need repair.

For a couple dealing with infertility, finding the cause can be a long, complicated, and trying process. It can take months. And for couples without health insurance that covers therapy, the process can be quite expensive.

Treatment

A variety of treatment approaches can be employed depending on the cause of the infertility. The most basic form of treatment relies on a change in sexual activity. By using a basal body temperature chart, for example, women can monitor their temperature changes and better determine their exact time of ovulation. About 85% to 90% of infertility cases are treated with drug therapy or surgical repair of reproductive organs. Medical approaches to infertility may involve hormones to treat cervical mucus problems or difficulties in ovulation, while ultrasound is used to monitor the response of the ovaries during treatment.

- Estrogen and prednisone may be given to improve the quality of cervical mucus, thereby allowing sperm to penetrate the mucus.

- To stimulate ovulation, a medication called clomiphene citrate (trade name Clomid) is often prescribed. It stimulates the release of luteinizing hormone and causes an increase in estradiol, thereby triggering ovulation.

- Gonadotropin-releasing hormone (GnRH) may be administered to improve a woman's response to ovulation stimulants.

Microsurgery is a useful technique for male and female problems that require surgical intervention. Using a laparoscope, doctors can open blockages in a woman's fallopian tubes or correct structural abnormalities of the uterus or ovary. Surgery may also be used in males to open blocked sperm ducts or to repair a **varicocele** (a mesh of varicose veins in and around the testicle), which is often associated with infertility.

Other techniques that have shown success to date include **artificial insemination** and **assisted reproductive technologies (ART)**. Artificial insemination is the process of implanting sperm from a donor into a woman near the time of her ovulation. Sperm donors are screened for HIV infection and various genetic disorders, as well as categorized by certain features to create as optimal a match as possible between the woman and the donor. Artificial insemination is often used when the infertility problem is based on a male factor.

Any treatment or procedure that involves the handling of human eggs and sperm for the purpose of helping a woman become pregnant qualifies as a type of ART. All ART procedures involve stimulating the ovary to produce eggs, harvesting the eggs with a microscopic needle, and then removing the eggs from the woman's body. The CDC estimates that ART accounts for slightly more than 1% of total U.S. births. In 2004, 82% of the pregnancies resulting from ART cycles were live births, with 55% resulting in a single birth and 27% in multiple-infant birth. Seventeen percent of pregnancies resulted in an adverse outcome of miscarriage, induced abortion, or stillbirth.[50] ART methods are listed below.

- **In vitro fertilization (IVF)** involves removing the ova from a woman's ovary just before normal ovulation would occur. The woman's egg and her partner's sperm are placed in a special fertilization medium for a specific period of time and are then transferred to another medium for continued development. If the fertilized egg cell shows signs of development, it is returned to the woman's uterus within several days by means of a hollow tube placed through the vagina and cervix. The egg cell implants itself in the lining of the uterus, and the pregnancy continues as normal.

- **Gamete intrafallopian transfer (GIFT)** involves placing sperm and eggs into the fallopian tubes. This procedure is less time-consuming and less expensive than IVF. GIFT mimics nature by permitting fertilized eggs to divide in the fallopian tubes. It has a success rate similar to that seen with IVF, but is more invasive than IVF.

- **Zygote intrafallopian transfer (ZIFT)** is a similar process that involves adding the fertilized egg to the fallopian tube at an earlier point than GIFT.

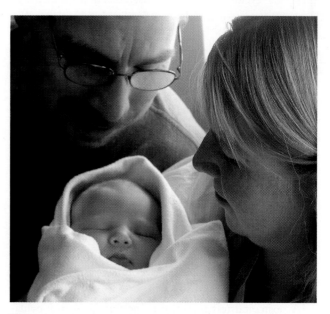

■ Many couples who have had trouble conceiving use assisted reproductive technologies to assist them in getting pregnant.

- **Intracytoplasmic sperm injection (ICSI)** involves injecting sperm directly into the egg with a microscopic needle.

- **Egg donation** is used when a woman is unable to produce eggs or she has a genetic disorder that will be passed on to the child. Egg donors must be willing to dedicate an enormous amount of time to this process because of the amount of drug treatment and monitoring that they must undergo. It is not a simple procedure for either the donor or the recipient of the egg.

- **Embryo transfer** is a procedure in which the sperm of the infertile woman's partner is placed in another woman's uterus during ovulation. Approximately five days later, the fertilized egg is transferred to the uterus of the infertile woman, who then carries the developing embryo.

- **Host uterus** is a procedure in which the sperm from a man and the egg from a woman are combined in a laboratory. The fertilized egg is then implanted into the uterus of a second woman who agrees to bear the child, which is not genetically related to her.

- **Surrogacy** occurs when a woman is artificially inseminated with the sperm of an infertile woman's partner. She carries the baby to term, usually for an established fee and the provision of her health care. After delivery, the baby is turned over to the couple.

Each of these procedures, while offering hope to infertile couples, can raise ethical and legal questions.

Emotional Effects of Infertility

Infertility and the procedures used to treat it are extremely stressful for most couples. In some cases, women who undergo the often arduous tests experience anger and resentment toward their partners, especially if their partners do not provide adequate support and share in their experiences. If the cause of infertility is determined, the man or woman who is experiencing the medical problem may feel guilty and blame himself or herself for failing to become pregnant. The experience of becoming pregnant and miscarrying can also lead to excitement and anticipation followed by depression and frustration. Once involved in testing, couples may become hopeful again but hesitant. The mix of emotions often leads to confusion and miscommunication between the couple.

As a couple prepares to undergo an ART procedure such as IVF, more grief may be experienced. In addition to fearing that it is the last option available, couples must

We had been trying to have a baby for several years. It was so frustrating because all of our friends were having babies. We felt so many things—guilt, embarrassment, fear, and anger. Finally, after a lot of testing, we tried IVF and it worked! We have a little girl. It was a long and difficult journey to have her, but we are so pleased.

35-year-old woman

shoulder the exorbitant costs of infertility treatment and face the possibility that it may be unsuccessful. Women who fail to become pregnant following any type of fertility therapy experience grief and depression before, during, and after treatment. Women may feel despair, anger, and a loss of control as their hopes of becoming pregnant faded. Effective coping behaviors and a strong network of family and friends appear to reduce a couple's emotional stress. If treatment fails, some couples accept happiness without their own children in their lives, whereas other couples may opt for adoption.

Epidemiology

Traditional epidemiological data on pregnancy and childbirth have focused on issues of maternal and child morbidity and mortality. In recent years, an expanded focus has provided insight into other important considerations of pregnancy, childbirth, breastfeeding, and infertility.

Pregnancy

In 2004, the U.S. birth rate was 14 per 1,000 persons. Teenage birth rates fell to a new record low, continuing a decline that began in 1991. The birth rate fell to 41.2 births per 1,000 females 15–19 years of age in 2004. Significant variations exist in the birth rates for teenagers among racial groups; **Figure 6.11** compares 1991 and 2004 birth rates for white, black, Hispanic, American Indian, and Asian/Pacific Islander teenagers, ages 15–19. Birth rates for women in their twenties were generally down, while births to older mothers (30–49) were still on the rise.[51]

Pregnancy and childbirth are safe experiences for many women; however, any medical or obstetric complication is one too many. In the early 1900s, 1 in 150 women died from causes related to pregnancy, with the death rate among women of color being nearly double that of white women.[52] These deaths were typically caused by infection, toxemia, abortion, and hemorrhage. Today, the leading

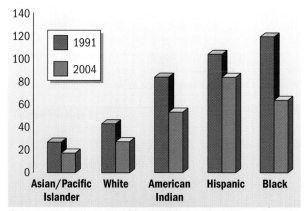

Rates are live births per 1,000 women in specific group.

Figure 6.11

Birth rates for teenagers 15–19 years of age by race and Hispanic origin.

Source: Hamilton, B. E., Martin, J. A., Ventura S. J., Sutton, P. D., and Menacker, F. (2005). Births: preliminary data for 2004. *National Vital Statistics Reports* 54(8). Hyattsville, MD: National Center for Health Statistics.

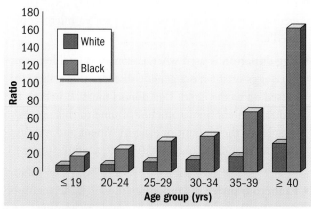

Deaths per 100,000 live births.

Figure 6.12

Pregnancy-mortality ratios, by age and race, United States, 1991–1999.

Source: Chang, J., et al. (2003). Pregnancy-related mortality surveillance— United States, 1991-1999. *Morbidity and Mortality Weekly Report* 52(SS02): 1-8.

causes of pregnancy-related deaths are embolism, hemorrhage, and pregnancy-related hypertension. In 1900, there were approximately 850 maternal deaths per 100,000 live births in the United States, about 1% of what it is today. Although this reduction in maternal mortality is impressive, data indicate that women of color are still three to four times more likely than white women to die of pregnancy-related causes, and the risk for black women is the highest among all racial groups (**Figure 6.12**). Women 35 years of age and older also are at increased risk for maternal mortality.[53]

The **infant mortality rate** (also called the infant death rate) is the number of children dying under a year of age divided by the number of live births that year. This rate is an important measure of the well-being of infants, children, and pregnant women because it is associated with factors such as maternal health, quality of and access to medical care, socioeconomic conditions, and public health practices. In 2005, the U.S. infant mortality rate was 6.86 infant deaths per 1,000 live births.[54] As **Figure 6.13** shows, the rates range from 4.42 deaths per 1,000 live births for Cuban mothers to 13.63 for non-Hispanic black mothers. Infant mortality rates were higher for infants who were born in multiple deliveries or whose mothers were unmarried. Infant mortality was also higher for male infants and infants born preterm or at low birthweight. Con-

genital malformations, low birthweight, and sudden infant death syndrome (SIDS) accounted for 44% of the infant deaths.

Low birthweight is defined as a birthweight of less than 2,500 grams (5.5 pounds); this and the period of gestation are the most important predictors of an infant's subsequent health and survival. Because of their much greater risk of death, infants born at the lowest birthweights and gestational ages have a large impact on overall U.S. infant mortality. As **Figure 6.14** shows, infants weighing less than 1,000 grams accounted for only 0.8% of births but nearly one-half of all infant deaths in the United States. A similar pattern is seen with infant gestation data. Only 0.8% of births occurred at less than 28 weeks of gestation, but they account for nearly one-half of all infant deaths in the United States (**Figure 6.15**).

I cannot remember much about the birth of my first baby. I was young and scared, and I only wanted to be "knocked out." Afterwards, I realized that I had missed one of the most important events of my life. With my second baby, we went to classes and I read everything I could. I really was prepared. I felt so much more in control of what was happening to me. Birth is something too wonderful to miss.

30-year-old woman

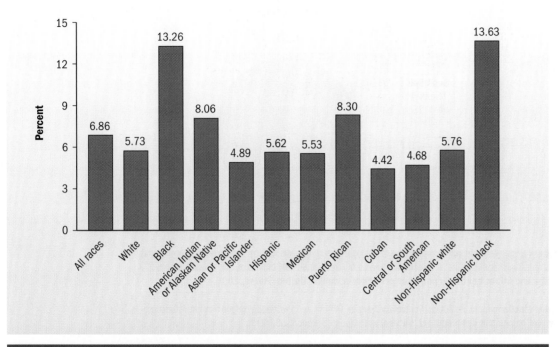

Figure 6.13

Infant mortality rates by race and ethnicity of mother: United States, 2005.

Source: Mathews, T. J., and MacDorman, M. F. (2008). Centers for Disease Control and Prevention. Infant mortality statistics from the 2005 period linked birth/infant death data set. *National Vital Statistics Reports.* 57(2).

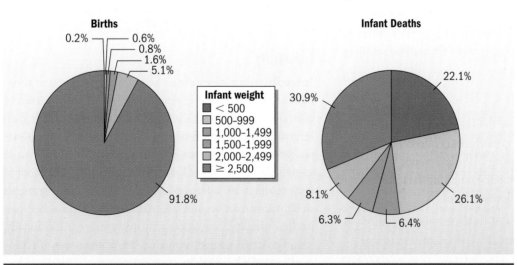

Figure 6.14

Percentage of live births and infant deaths by birthweight in grams: United States, 2005.

Source: Mathews, T. J., and MacDorman, M. F. (2008). Centers for Disease Control and Prevention. Infant mortality statistics from the 2005 period linked birth/infant death data set. *National Vital Statistics Reports.* 57(2).

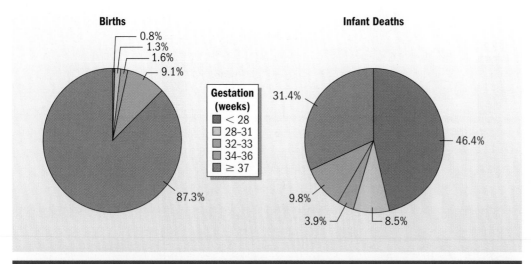

Figure 6.15

Percentage of live births and infant deaths by period of gestation in weeks: United States, 2005.

Source: Mathews, T. J., and MacDorman, M. F. (2008). Centers for Disease Control and Prevention. Infant mortality statistics from the 2005 period linked birth/infant death data set. *National Vital Statistics Reports*. 57(2).

Breastfeeding

Breastfeeding rates in the United States have increased every year since 1999, but they continue to fall short of Healthy People 2010 objectives for duration and exclusivity (not relying on formula). Among children born in 2005, 74% initiated breastfeeding, 43% were breastfeeding at six months, and 21% were breastfeeding at 12 months of age (**Figure 6.16**).[55] Nearly half of U.S. states have achieved their specific objectives for breastfeeding for initiation, but fewer have achieved their objectives for duration and exclusive breastfeeding.

Fertility

Technically, fertility simply denotes successful production of offspring. The U.S. Census Bureau collects fertility data and provides reports showing historical trends with childbearing and associated sociodemographic data. Recent fertility data indicate the following trends[55]:

- More women in their early 40s are childless, and those who are having children are having fewer than ever before. In the last 30 years, the number of women ages 40 to 44 with no children has doubled.

- Women 40 to 44 years old will end their childbearing years with an average of 1.9 children each, a number below replacement-level fertility. Hispanic women will have an average of 2.3 children each, higher than that of white non-Hispanic, black, or Asian women.

- About 36% of women who gave birth in the previous 12 months were separated, divorced, widowed, or unmarried.

- Unemployed women had about twice as many babies as working women, although women in the labor force accounted for the majority (57%) of recent births.

- A quarter of all women who had a child in the past year were living below the poverty level.

Infertility

Infertility is usually defined as not being able to get pregnant after trying for one year. Of the 62 million women of reproductive age in 2002, about 1.2 million, or 2%, had an infertility-related medical appointment within the previous year, and 8% had an infertility-related medical visit at some point in the past. Infertility services include medical tests to diagnose infertility, medical advice and treatments to help a woman become pregnant, and services other than routine prenatal care to prevent miscarriage. Additionally, 7% of married couples in which the woman was of reproductive age (2.1 million couples) reported that they had not used contraception for 12 months and the woman had not become pregnant.[56] Assisted reproductive technology (ART) is associated with a substantial risk for multiple births. **Figure 6.17** shows the number of ART cycles performed, live-birth delivery, and infants born using ART from 1996 to 2005.

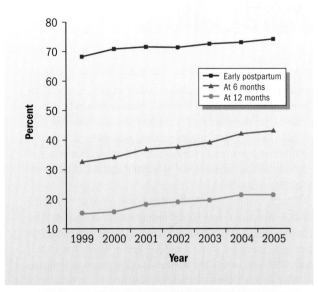

Figure 6.16

Percentage of U.S. children who were breastfed by birth year, United States.

Source: Centers for Disease Control and Prevention. (2008). Breastfeeding among U.S. children born 1999-2005. *CDC National Immunization Survey.* Downloaded September 16, 2008 from: http://www.cdc.gov/breastfeeding/data/NIS_data/index.htm.

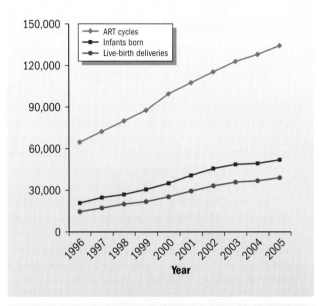

Figure 6.17

Numbers of ART cycles performed, live-birth deliveries, and infants born using ART, 1996-2005.

Source: Centers for Disease Control and Prevention. (2008). Assisted reproductive technology (ART) report: section 5–ART Trends, 1996-2005. Downloaded September 15, 2008 from http://www.cdc.gov/ART/2005/sect5_fig46-60.htm#f49.

Informed Decision Making

Informed decision making about pregnancy should begin before conception. The newly conceived offspring depends on its mother for nutrition and well-being weeks before the mother may know that she is pregnant. If the mother is a smoker or is abusing alcohol or drugs during this critical early period of development, her child is at a decided disadvantage.

Pregnancy

A pregnant woman has to take good care of herself to provide the best care for her unborn child. Regular prenatal care that begins early in the pregnancy is essential and is associated with reduced infant morbidity and mortality. Most women see their clinician once a month during the pregnancy until week 28. In the last trimester, this frequency increases to every other week until week 36, when weekly visits until delivery are indicated. Proper nutrition, adequate and appropriate exercise, and avoidance of alcohol, tobacco, caffeine, and illegal drugs are all essential components of good prenatal care.

Childbirth

Childbirth is a personal, special, and an irreplaceable event. Preparation for birthing helps to ensure the best possible experience. Childbirth education classes provide many valuable opportunities for learning, practical preparation, and building skills for a rewarding and facilitated childbirth experience. They also provide an opportunity to share concerns and discuss plans. Local resources for childbirth options, such as birthing centers or home deliveries, can be evaluated. Classes provide motivation to learn relaxation and pain management techniques.

Resources in childbirth preparation vary. Some communities offer many resources; in other communities, resources are rather few and far between. To maximize the benefits from a childbirth education class, the qualifications of the instructor, class size, and class focus should be carefully evaluated.

Instructors in childbirth education should be certified. The most prestigious certification program for childbirth educators is conducted by Lamaze International. Educators with this certification use the credential LCCE (Lamaze Certified Childbirth Educator). Those who have

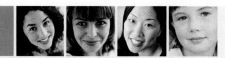

Profiles of Remarkable Women

Martha May Eliot, M.D. (1891–1978)

Martha May Eliot, a pioneer in maternal and child health, graduated from Radcliffe College and the medical school at Johns Hopkins University. She taught at Yale University's Department of Pediatrics until 1935, while also directing the National Children's Bureau Division of Child and Maternal Health. As Bureau Chief, Eliot conducted community studies, exploring issues of social medicine and ways that public health measures could prevent disease. She also drafted most of the Social Security Act's language dealing with maternal and child health in 1934. During World War II, Eliot provided care for more than 1 million servicemen's wives through the Emergency Maternity and Infant Care program. She continued her involvement with women's and children's health after the war by working with the World Health Organization (WHO) and the United Nations Children's Fund (UNICEF) in significant capacities.

After leaving her position at the National Children's Bureau Division of Maternal and Child Health, Eliot became Department Chair of Child and Maternal Health at Harvard University's School of Public Health. She received many honors throughout her lifetime that recognized her work as a leading pediatrician and the force behind many maternal and child health programs. She was one of the first women admitted into the American Pediatric Society, the first woman elected president of the American Public Health Association (APHA), and the first woman to receive APHA's Sedgwick Memorial Medal. APHA now awards the Martha May Eliot Award to recognize others' achievements in maternal and child health.

made significant contributions to the field may use the credential FLCCE (Fellows of the College).

The most appropriate class size is eight to twelve couples. This number allows for individual attention, time for discussion, and adequate floor space for practice. In addition to providing the basic information on pregnancy and childbirth, classes should discuss birthing options and developing personal plans for birth based on personal medical requirements and resources.

Breastfeeding

Breastfeeding can be a very rewarding experience. Women who have difficulty beginning the process are encouraged to "stick with it" as both the mother and the infant learn how to work with each other. Although suckling is instinctual for the infant, feeding from the breast is a learned behavior for the mother. Adjusting positions, anticipating the infant's hunger, and relaxing during the feeding are ways to make breastfeeding more pleasurable for both mother and infant. Breastfeeding assistance is usually offered postpartum at the hospital, and lactation specialists also are available for women when they return home with the baby. Aside from the bond created between mother and child, breastfeeding offers significant health benefits to both parties.

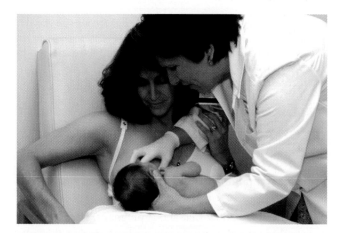

■ Hospitals and birthing centers often have lactation specialists on staff to help new mothers learn the ropes of breastfeeding.

Infertility

Infertility should be recognized as a problem of a couple, not the woman or her partner. Because the factors that reduce fertility are shared, both partners must be evaluated when initiating an infertility workup. Infertility services are widely available today, and evolving technologies have enabled many couples to have a child. Infertility clinics can offer couples information, support, and procedures to address their specific needs. Identification of infertility services is often facilitated through referral from a gynecologist.

Summary

Pregnancy, childbirth, and breastfeeding are exciting, yet complex, dimensions of women's health. Cultural, historical, legal, and ethical factors all influence how women deal with pregnancy, give birth, and care for their infants. Understanding the physiological causes for the physical and emotional changes that occur in a pregnant woman can often help make the pregnancy process more manageable. Prenatal care is a vital component of a healthy pregnancy, and usually includes nutritional counseling, genetic testing, ultrasounds, and ongoing monitoring of the mother and baby. Many women experience the changes of pregnancy and the birth of their child without complications. Others learn firsthand the emotional hardships of infertility, miscarriage, diagnosis of abnormalities in the fetus, premature delivery, or complications during the delivery. For couples who have difficulty conceiving, a host of medical and surgical options exist to achieve a pregnancy; however, these methods are imperfect and often carry a high financial (as well as emotional) cost. As with other areas of women's health, informed decision making is critical throughout the prenatal to postnatal periods.

Topics for Discussion

1. What are the possible advantages and disadvantages of treating childbirth as a "medical" condition (i.e., constant medical care led by doctors and health-care providers, hospitalization, etc.)?

2. Should pregnant women be restricted in their access to tobacco, alcohol, or drugs?

3. What should you do, if anything, if you see a young mother smoking? If she is drinking? Or if she is not wearing a seatbelt?

4. Should preparation for childbirth be required for all women?

5. Discuss the rights of pregnant teenagers as parents. What rights do a teen's parents have in regard to her pregnancy?

6. Does the father of the child have any say in pregnancy decisions if the mother and father are not married?

7. What are possible ethical and legal dilemmas associated with infertility techniques and treatments?

Web Sites

American Academy of Pediatrics: http://www.aap.org

Centers for Disease Control and Prevention: Breastfeeding: http://www.cdc.gov/breastfeeding

Centers for Disease Control and Prevention: Reproductive Health Information Source: http://www.cdc.gov/reproductivehealth

La Leche League International: http://www.lalecheleague.org

March of Dimes: http://www.marchofdimes.com

National Campaign to Prevent Teen Pregnancy: http://www.teenpregnancy.org

Resolve: The National Infertility Association: http://www.resolve.org

References

1. Bogda, J. C. (1990). Childbirth in America, 1650 to 1990. In R. D. Apple (ed.). *Women, Health, and Medicine in America*. New York: Garland Publishers.

2. Wertz, R. W., & Wertz, D. C. (1977). *Lying-In: A History of Childbirth in America*. New York: Free Press.

3. Leavitt, J. W. (1986). *Brought to Bed: Childbirthing in America, 1750–1950*. New York: Oxford University Press.

4. Hodnett, E. D., Gates, S., Hofmeyr, G. J., & Sakala, C. (2007). Continuous support for women during childbirth. *Cochrane Database of Systematic Reviews*. Jul 18;(3):CD003766.

5. Mansfield, B. (2008). The social nature of natural childbirth. *Social Science Medicine* 66(5): 1084–1094.

6. Barness, L. A. (1991). Brief history of infant nutrition and view to the future. *Pediatrics* 88: 1054–1056.

7. Ansley, D. (1992). Spermtales. *Discover* 13(6): 66–69.

8. Tomlinson, C., Marshall, J., & Ellis, J. E. (2008). Comparison of accuracy and certainty of results of six home pregnancy tests available over-the-counter. *Current Medical Research Opinion* 24(6): 1645–1649.

9. Williams, L. J., Rasmussen, S. A., Flores, A., Kirby, R. S., & Edmonds, L. D. (2005). Decline in the prevalence of spina bifida and anencephaly by race/ethnicity: 1995–2002. *Pediatrics* 116(3): 580–586.

10. Cox, J. T., & Phelan, S. T. (2008). Nutrition during pregnancy. *Obstetrics and Gynecology Clinics of North America* 35(3): 369–383.

11. American College of Obstetricians and Gynecologists. (2008). *Exercise During Pregnancy.* Available at: http://www.acog.org/publications/patient_education/bp119.cfm.

12. Centers for Disease Control and Prevention (CDC). (2007). *Preventing Smoking and Exposure to Secondhand Smoke Before, During, and After Pregnancy Fact Sheet.* Available at: http://www.cdc.gov/nccdphp/publications/factsheets/Prevention/smoking.htm.

13. Aliyu, M. H., et al. (2008). Alcohol consumption during pregnancy and the risk of early stillbirth among singletons. *Alcohol* 42(5): 369–374.

14. Centers for Disease Control and Prevention (CDC). (2005). *Alcohol Use and Pregnancy.* Available at: http://www.cdc.gov/ncbddd/factsheets/FAS_alcoholuse.pdf.

15. American College of Obstetricians and Gynecologists. (2008). *Alcohol and Pregnancy: Know the Facts.* Available at: http://www.acog.org/from_home/publications/press_releases/nr02-06-08-1.cfm.

16. Substance Abuse and Mental Health Services Administration. (2006). *Results from the 2005 National Survey on Drug Use and Health: National Findings.* Rockville, MD: Office of Applied Studies. NSDUH Series H-30, DHHS, Publication No. SMA 06-4194.

17. March of Dimes. (2006). Illicit drug use during pregnancy. *Quick Reference Fact Sheets for Professionals.* Available at: http://www.marchofdimes.com/professionals/14332_1169.asp.

18. Papanikolaou, N. C., et al. (2005). Lead toxicity update. A brief review. *Medical Science Monitor* 11(10): RA329–RA336.

19. Braun, J. M., et al. (2006). Exposures to environmental toxicants and attention deficit hyperactivity disorder in US children. *Environmental Health Perspectives* 114(12): 1904–1909.

20. Chambers, C. D. (2006). Risks of hypothermia associated with hot tub or spa use by pregnant women. *Birth Defects Research. Part A. Clinical and Molecular Teratology* 76(8): 569–573.

21. Centers for Disease Control and Prevention (CDC). (2007). *Birth Defects: Frequently Asked Questions (FAQs).* National Center on Birth Defects and Developmental Disabilities. Available at: http://www.cdc.gov/ncbddd/bd/faq1.htm#CommonBD.

22. Eddleman, K. A., First and Second Trimester Evaluation of Risk (FASTER) Trial Research Consortium. (2006). Pregnancy loss rates after midtrimester amniocentesis. *Obstetrics and Gynecology* 108(5): 1067–1072.

23. Moore, L. E. (2008). Recurrent risk of adverse pregnancy outcome. *Obstetrics and Gynecology Clinics of North America* 35(3): 459–471.

24. Tenore, J. L. (2000). Ectopic pregnancy. Problem-oriented diagnosis. *American Family Physician* 61(4): 1080–1088.

25. Centers for Disease Control and Prevention (CDC). (1995). Current trends ectopic pregnancy—United States, 1990–1992. *Morbidity and Mortality Weekly Report* 44(3): 46–48.

26. National Institute of Diabetes and Digestive and Kidney Diseases (NIDDK), National Institutes of Health. (2006). *What I Need to Know About Gestational Diabetes.* National Diabetes Information Clearing House. Available at: http://diabetes.niddk.nih.gov/dm/pubs/gestational/.

27. Martin, J. A., Hamilton, B. E., Sutton, P. D., Ventura, S. J., Menacker, F., & Munson, M. L. (2005). Births: final data for 2003. *National Vital Statistics Reports* 54(2): 1–116.

28. Schieve, L. A., Tatham, L., Peterson, H. B., Toner, J., & Jeng, G. (2003). Spontaneous abortion among pregnancies conceived using assisted reproductive technology in the United States. *Obstetrics and Gynecology* 101(5): 959.

29. Heffner, L. J. (2004). Advanced maternal age—how old is too old? *New England Journal of Medicine* 351(19): 1927–1929.

30. Côté-Arsenault, D. (2007). Threat appraisal, coping, and emotions across pregnancy subsequent to perinatal loss. *Nursing Research* 56(2): 108–116.

31. Watson, M. S., Mann, M. Y., Lloyd-Puryear, M. A., Rinaldo, P., & Howell, R. R. (2006). Newborn screening: toward a uniform screening panel and system. *Genetics in Medicine* 8(Suppl 5): 1S–11S.

32. Centers for Disease Control and Prevention (CDC). (2007). *Mother-to-Child (Perinatal) HIV Transmission and Prevention*. Available at: http://www.cdc.gov/hiv/topics//perinatal/resources/factsheets/pdf/perinatal.pdf.

33. Centers for Disease Control and Prevention (CDC). (2006). *Sexually Transmitted Diseases Treatment Guidelines 2006*. Available at: http://www.cdc.gov/std/treatment/2006/specialpops.htm#specialpops1.

34. Centers for Disease Control and Prevention (CDC). (2006). *Frequently Asked Questions About Cytomegalovirus (CMV)*. Available at: http://www.cdc.gov/cmv/.

35. Centers for Disease Control and Prevention (CDC). (2008). *General Public—Frequently Asked Questions About Group B Strep Prevention*. Available at: http://www.cdc.gov/GroupBStrep/general/gen_public_faq.htm.

36. Klein, M. C., et al. (2006). Why do women go along with this stuff? *Birth* 33(3): 245–250.

37. Romano, A. M., & Lothian, J. A. (2008). Promoting, protecting, and supporting normal birth: a look at the evidence. *Obstetric, Gynecologic, and Neonatal Nursing* 37(1): 94–105.

38. Hartmann, K., et al. (2005). Outcomes of routine episiotomy: a systematic review. *Journal of the American Medical Association* 293(17): 2141–2148.

39. Agency for Healthcare Research and Quality (AHRQ). (2005). *The Use of Episiotomy in Obstetrical Care: A Systematic Review*. Evidence Report/Technology Assessment No. 112 (AHRQ Publication No. 05-E009-2). Available at: http://www.ahrq.gov/downloads/pub/evidence/pdf/episiotomy/episob.pdf.

40. Centers for Disease Control and Prevention (CDC). (2005). Quickstats: total and primary cesarean rate and vaginal birth after previous cesarean (VBAC) rate—United States, 1989–2003. *National Statistics Vital Reports* 54(2): 1–5.

41. American College of Obstetricians and Gynecologists. (2004). Vaginal birth after previous cesarean section. *ACOG Practice Bulletin 54*.

42. Centers for Disease Control and Prevention (CDC). (2008). *Breastfeeding Among U.S. Children Born 1999–2005, CDC National Immunization Survey*. Available at: http://www.cdc.gov/breastfeeding/data/NIS_data/index.htm.

43. United States Breastfeeding Committee. (2002). *Benefits of Breastfeeding*. Available at: http://www.usbreastfeeding.org/Issue-Papers/Benefits.pdf.

44. Keister, D., Roberts, K. T., & Werner, S. L. (2008). Strategies for breastfeeding success. *American Family Physician* 78(2): 225–232.

45. Jacknowitz, A. (2008). The role of workplace characteristics in breastfeeding practices. *Women's Health* 47(2): 87–111.

46. Singh, G. K., Kogan, M. D., & Dee, D. L. (2007). Nativity/immigration status, race/ethnicity, and sociodemographic determinants of breastfeeding initiation and duration in the United States, 2003. *Pediatrics* 119(Suppl 1): S38–S46.

47. Celi, A. C., et al. (2005). Immigration, race/ethnicity, and social and economic factors as predictors of breastfeeding initiation. *Archives of Pediatrics and Adolescent Medicine* 159(3): 255–260.

48. Kogan, M. D., et al. (2008). Multivariate analysis of state variation in breastfeeding rates in the United States. *American Journal of Public Health* 98(10): 1872–1880.

49. Stephen, E. H., & Chandra, A. (2000). Use of infertility services in the United States. *Family Planning Perspectives* 32(3): 132–137.

50. Centers for Disease Control and Prevention (CDC), & American Society for Reproductive Medicine. (2006). *Assisted Reproductive Technology Success Rates: National Summary and Fertility Clinic Reports*. Available at: http://www.cdc.gov/ART/ART2004/508PDF/2004ART_Intro-NationalSum_t508.pdf.

51. Hamilton, B. E., Martin, J. A., Ventura, S. J., Sutton, P. D., & Menaker, F. (2005). Births: preliminary data for 2004. *National Vital Statistics Reports* 54(8): 1–17.

52. Rochat, R. W., Koonin, L. M., Atrash, H. K., Jewett, J. F., & Maternal Mortality Collaborative. (1988). Maternal mortality in the United States: report from the Maternal Mortality Collaborative. *Obstetrics and Gynecology* 72(1): 91–97.

53. Centers for Disease Control and Prevention (CDC). (2003). Pregnancy-related mortality surveillance—

United States, 1991–1999. *Morbidity and Mortality Weekly Report* 52(SS02): 1–8.

54. Mathews, T. J., & MacDorman, M. F. (2008). Infant mortality statistics from the 2005 period linked birth/infant death data set. *National Vital Statistics Reports* 57(2): 1–26.

55. Dye, J. L. (2008). Fertility of American women. *Current Population Reports*. U.S. Census Bureau. Washington, D.C. Available at: http://www.census.gov/prod/2008pubs/p20-558.pdf.

56. Centers for Disease Control and Prevention (CDC). (2008). *Assisted Reproductive Technology*. Available at: http://www.cdc.gov/ART/.

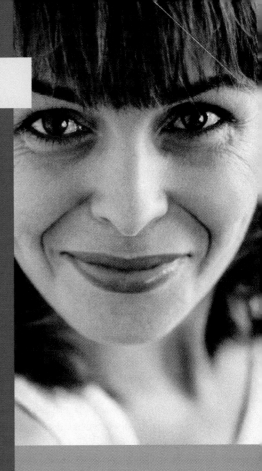

Chapter Seven

Reproductive Tract Infections and HIV/AIDS

Chapter Objectives

On completion of this chapter, the student should be able to discuss:

1. Basic information about sexually transmitted infections (STIs) and how they differ from other reproductive tract infections.

2. Relative prevalence and infection rates of STIs in women, the United States as a whole, and different ethnic groups.

3. Biological and cultural reasons why STIs disproportionately affect and infect women.

4. The diagnosis process, transmission, symptoms, and course of infection of each of the major reproductive tract infections in the United States.

5. The stigma associated with many STIs and how it both hurts people who are infected and slows prevention and treatment efforts.

6. The role of open communication, both with clinicians and with partners, in regard to STIs.

7. The course of HIV/AIDS infection and how treatment works.

8. National and global trends related to the AIDS epidemic.

9. The importance of personal responsibility and risk reduction in making decisions about one's sexual life.

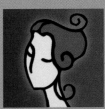

womenshealth.jbpub.com

Women's Health Online is a great source for supplementary women's health information for both students and instructors. Visit

http://womenshealth.jbpub.com

to find a variety of useful tools for learning, thinking, and teaching.

Introduction

Reproductive tract infections (RTIs) are caused by a variety of organisms that affect the upper reproductive tract, the lower reproductive tract, or both. Most women experience at least one—and often several—reproductive tract infections in their lifetimes. Reproductive tract infections pose a significant health risk for women. Women are not only at higher risk for acquiring RTIs than men, but also suffer more significant sequelae from these conditions. Most infections are transmitted by sexual intimacy and, therefore, are referred to as **sexually transmitted infections (STIs)**. STIs include chlamydia, gonorrhea, herpes, hepatitis, and human immunodeficiency virus (HIV) infections. Human papillomavirus (HPV), a virus that can lead to cervical cancer in women, also is sexually transmitted. Sexually associated infections include vaginitis, trichomoniasis, yeast infections, and bacterial vaginosis.

The consequences of an STI depend on the organism causing the infection. Gonorrhea and chlamydia can cause permanent damage to the reproductive system, even in the absence of symptoms. Herpes is an incurable disease with painful and often emotionally devastating symptoms, but the disease generally does not pose a long-term health risk. AIDS, and in some cases syphilis and hepatitis, can threaten life itself. Although some infections attack a single structure, such as the labia or cervix, others ascend upward from the vagina, through the cervical canal, and into the uterus, where further invasion into the fallopian tubes, ovaries, and entire pelvis can occur.

Having one STI increases a person's risk of acquiring another STI and may make that individual up to seven times more likely than an uninfected person to acquire HIV through sexual contact.[1] STIs also increase a person's infectiousness: An HIV-positive individual infected with another STI is more likely to transmit HIV through sexual contact and to acquire other STIs if exposed.[2] Some bacteria and viruses may enter the bloodstream and result in systemic effects. Other infections, such as bacterial vaginosis or yeast infections, may be major annoyances, but they do not have serious life-threatening sequelae.

Sexually transmitted organisms know no class, racial, ethnic, or social barriers. All individuals are vulnerable if exposed to the infectious organism. Society, however, has a tendency to look on STIs as punishment for immoral activity. In addition, women have been viewed as the source of disease. Thus, when a woman learns that she has an STI, her reaction may include disbelief, hurt, a feeling of victimization, guilt, embarrassment, anger, fear, shame, and

■ Historically, society has looked on STIs as punishment for immoral activity. In addition, women have been viewed as the source of disease.

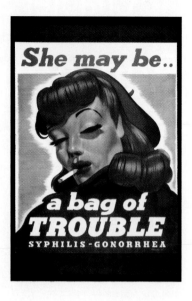

a feeling of loss of control over her sexuality and health. With viral diseases, there is often the added pressure of worry over how the lingering virus will affect present and future relationships. The emotional effects for women are often as serious or worse than the physical effects of reproductive tract infections. Clearly, knowledge and prevention are the best defenses against STIs, followed by early diagnosis and treatment to reduce or eliminate the consequences of infection.

Perspectives on STIs

Historical Overview

Although STIs are a modern epidemic, they are not modern infections. STIs have been referenced in medical literature for hundreds and, in some cases, thousands of years. The oldest books in the Bible describe diseases that probably were gonorrhea and syphilis. Some Biblical descriptions of leprosy more accurately fit the conditions of diseases now called syphilis or scabies. Ancient Greek and Roman physicians identified genital warts and syphilis chancres in their writings. The term *condyloma*, once defined as meaning "fig" and now solely used to refer to genital warts, is of Greek origin. Hippocrates described the mechanism for gonorrhea transmission as "excesses of the pleasures of the Venus." Susruta, an ancient Hindu, also described gonorrhea. In ancient Rome, Tiberius issued a decree outlawing public kissing to curb a herpes epidemic. Spanish explorers may have brought syphilis to Europe from the New World; Falstaff, a character in Shakespeare's *Henry IV*, appears to be suffering the disease. Between

1495 and 1500, syphilis ravaged Europe, killing hundreds of thousands of people. The HIV/AIDS epidemic today has been likened to these historical STI epidemics.

Epidemiological Data and Trends

STIs are a major public health problem: One of every four women in the United States between the ages of 14 and 19—3.2 million adolescents—has a common sexually transmitted infection.[3] STIs are also at epidemic proportions among Americans of reproductive age and present serious threats, especially to young women. In 2000, there were 9.1 million new cases of STIs among U.S. youth from the ages of 15 to 24 alone.[4] Adolescents have a greater biological risk of infection, and their risk of exposure is higher because of difficulties accessing appropriate health care, the increased risk of multiple short-term sexual relationships, and inconsistent use of barrier contraception.[2] The United States has the highest rate of STI infection in the industrialized world. More than 65 million Americans are now living with an incurable STI.[4]

Although antibiotics work effectively against several of the pathogens, STI rates continue to climb. More than 20 organisms and numerous syndromes are currently recognized as being transmitted sexually.

Measuring the scope of the STI epidemic is a difficult task. Some STIs are reportable conditions (diseases required by federal law to be reported to prevent and control their spread), and national data on them are available (**Figure 7.1**). Other STIs are not reportable, and actual incidence rates can only be estimated (**Figure 7.2**). Health-care providers are required to report cases of chlamydia, gonorrhea, and syphilis, but health-care facilities vary widely in the manner that they report these diseases. Chlamydia, the reportable disease with the highest incidence, is spreading at a rate of 3 million new cases each year in the United States.[5] Many STIs are asymptomatic, so many infected individuals are not diagnosed.

Prevalence rates provide an even more startling picture of the STI epidemic. For example, 18% of women between the ages of 15 and 19 have HPV, and 4% have chlamydia.[3] About one in five Americans has genital herpes. In 2006, infections of chlamydia were more than seven times higher among African American females than among white females, and 69% of the recorded cases of gonorrhea in the United States occurred among African Americans.[5] STIs also affect Hispanics at higher rates than non-Hispanic whites (**Figure 7.3**). Native American/Alaska Native and Asian/Pacific Islander women have rates of chlamydia consistently higher than whites.[5] Although rates appear to be consistently higher among minorities, some reporting bias may affect the data collected. Minorities are more likely than Caucasians to visit public clinics, which are often the main source of STI estimates, accounting for some increased reporting of disease among these groups.

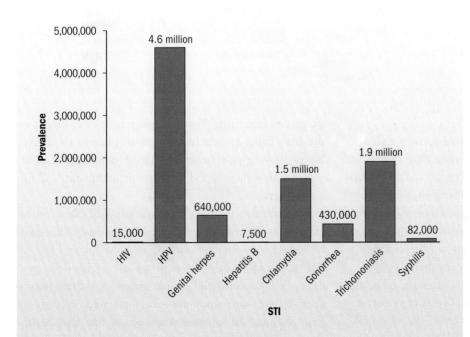

Figure 7.1

Estimated incidence (new cases) of major STIs in the United States among American youth (ages 15–24) in 2000.

Source: Weinstock, H., Berman, S., and Cates, W. Jr. (2004). Sexually transmitted diseases among American youth: incidence and prevalence estimates, 2004. *Perspectives on Sexual and Reproductive Health* 36(1): Table 2. Reprinted with permission from The Guttmacher Institute.

Figure 7.2

Estimated prevalence (existing cases) of selected common STIs in the United States among American youth (ages 15–24) in 2000.

Source: Weinstock, H., Berman, S., and Cates, W. Jr. (2004). Sexually transmitted diseases among American youth: incidence and prevalence estimates, 2004. *Perspectives on Sexual and Reproductive Health* 36(1): Table 2. Reprinted with permission from The Guttmacher Institute.

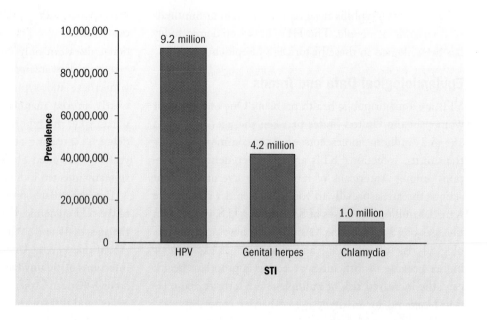

Figure 7.3

Race/ethnicity differences in rates of gonorrhea, syphilis, and chlamydia, 2006.

Source: Centers for Disease Control and Prevention. (2008). Sexually Transmitted Disease Surveillance 2006.

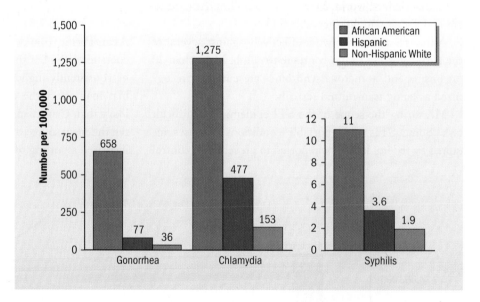

Social Issues and Dimensions

STIs are biologically sexist, presenting greater risk and causing more complications for women than for men. Women experience most of the STI burden and complications, including infertility, perinatal infections, genital tract neoplasia, and death. In women, these diseases are often silent, presenting as asymptomatic but remaining damaging and infectious. STIs in pregnant women frequently place unborn babies at risk of illness, congenital anomalies, developmental disabilities, and death. Because STIs are most prevalent among women 15 to 24 years of age,[2] these women experience the greatest burden of chronic pelvic pain, pelvic inflammatory disease (PID), ectopic preg-

nancy, and infertility. Women constitute the majority of individuals living at or below the poverty line in the United States, and the poor bear the added burden of limited access to comprehensive STI diagnostic, treatment, and follow-up services.

Considerable stigma accompanies an STI diagnosis, regardless of the culprit organism. Many people still equate STIs with immorality, promiscuous behavior, and low social status. All sexually active people are at risk for acquiring an STI, especially if they have unprotected sex. Reproductive tract infections may be perceived as dirty or shameful, and an infected woman may fear that healthcare providers will not care for her or will be offended by doing so. Women are more vulnerable than men to the STI stigma owing to society's double standard that requires women to be "pure" or virginal, while men are often expected to "sow their wild oats," or engage in sexual activity with multiple partners. Some women may view an STI as punishment for previous behavior. Public health education efforts need to counter these false perceptions.

Cultural dimensions often complicate public health and education efforts. Although STI educational and behavioral issues cut across all racial and ethnic groups, the situation is far worse in poor African American communities due to other social problems complicating the STI epidemic. Men in cultures or regions that are intolerant of homosexuality may have high-risk encounters with other men while keeping these behaviors secret, identifying themselves as "straight," and ultimately infecting their girlfriends or wives. Many women are not in charge of contraceptive decision making and may unknowingly put themselves at risk by engaging in sexual activities with philandering or infected partners. Crack-related sexual behaviors (selling or trading sex for crack), as well as risky sexual activity while under the influence of various drugs including alcohol, compound STI transmission. Emotions often dominate logical behavior and rational thinking—for example, among prostitutes who wear condoms

with clients but not with boyfriends, and among teenage girls who believe that condoms are unnecessary when a boyfriend declares his love.

Health-care providers may also neglect certain populations of women when it comes to screening for these diseases. Women whose sexual partners are exclusively women appear to have a lower prevalence of some STIs, but they are still at risk for infection and therefore should be advised on prevention guidelines. Latex barriers, such as dental dams, can be used for oral–genital or oral–anal contact, as well as for direct skin-to-skin contact, so as to prevent STI transmission among people of all sexual orientations. Health-care providers also may not screen women with disabilities for STIs. To complicate matters, a woman with a disabling condition may have sensory impairments that limit self-diagnosis or may manifest altered symptoms of common STIs. It is important that women's health-care providers always test sexually active women for STIs.

Economic Dimensions

The medical costs of STIs among young people in the United States are more than $10 billion each year. The entire economic burden of STIs on all age groups would undoubtedly be significantly higher.[6] This estimate does not include costs like lost wages, loss of productivity due to

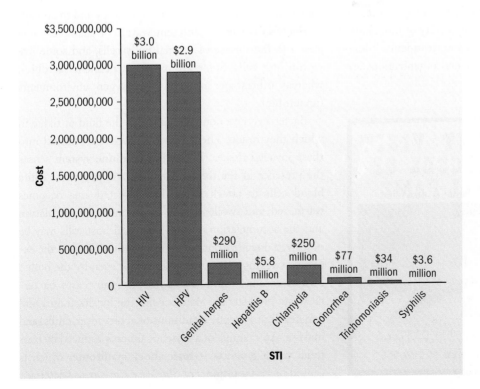

Figure 7.4

Estimated cost of major STIs among U.S. youth, 2000.

Source: Chesson, H. W., Blandford, J. M., Gift, T. L., Tao, G., and Irwin, K. L. (2004). The estimated direct medical cost of sexually transmitted disease among youth, 2000. *Perspectives on Sexual and Reproductive Health* 36(1): Table 1. Reprinted with permission from The Guttmacher Institute.

STI-related illness, out-of-pocket costs, or costs incurred by the transmission of STIs to infants, which can result in significant lifelong expenditures.

For bacterial STIs, the greatest costs result from complications of untreated chlamydia and gonorrhea. Without medical attention, these STIs can lead to PID and future fertility problems, leading to even more significant costs.

Because viral STIs cannot be cured and may require treatment for years, they tend to cost more than bacterial STIs. The greatest costs associated with viral STIs result from treatment of precancerous cervical lesions caused by HPV infection and treatment of sexually transmitted HIV infection (**Figure 7.4**). In addition to their economic dimensions, STIs carry a high human cost of pain, suffering, and grief. Chlamydia and gonorrhea complications can lead to chronic pain, infertility, and tubal pregnancies, which can affect a woman's health and well-being throughout her lifetime.

HIV/AIDS creates enormous costs at both the societal and individual levels. The devastating effects of the disease on entire communities in many parts of the world, especially sub-Saharan Africa, have brought catastrophic economic consequences. In the United States, many families' primary wage earners are sick with the disease, leading to significant economic hardship. In addition, the cost of the drugs required to keep HIV infection in check can approach $15,000 per year. People living with HIV/AIDS in the United States are thus a population with special needs for health insurance and prescription drug coverage, as the costs of the disease far exceed the ability of most individuals to pay for necessary services and treatments. Globally, governments and nongovernmental organizations are working together to fund programs that provide access to diagnostic and treatment services for people living with HIV/AIDS.

In 2007, global spending on AIDS reached $10 billion, six times the money spent in 2001. The mobilization of this money as well as the accompanying resources represent a major global achievement. Yet it is not enough: UNAIDS, the department within the United Nations that addresses AIDS-related issues, estimated that $22 billion would be needed to fight this disease in 2010.[7] UNAIDS recommends that half of this money be spent on prevention. As this global realization continues, care will have to be taken to make sure that these funds are spent strategically and effectively.[7]

Clinical Dimensions and Treatment Issues of Sexually Transmitted Infections

A spectrum of organisms cause STIs, so considerable variation exists in the manifestation of symptoms and in treatment options. This section reviews the clinical and treatment perspectives of each major STI.

Infection Process

Reproductive tract infections can be caused by a variety of organisms, including bacteria, viruses, or parasites. Each organism requires a unique diagnostic strategy and treatment.

Bacteria behave in different ways. For example, some attach to the surface of normal body cells, and some live within host cells. Some are oxygen dependent (**aerobic**), whereas others are intolerant of oxygen environments (**anaerobic**).

Bacteria receive nourishment from the fluid or tissue in which they reside. Their waste products are released into these invaded tissues. The body's **immune system** senses the presence of the foreign bacteria, and mobilizes white blood cells to attack them. The infected area becomes warm, red, and swollen owing to the increased circulation and the accumulation of **pus**. The local host cells may be destroyed directly from the bacteria, indirectly from the excessive swelling and waste products, or even by the body's own overzealous immune response. In many cases, bacterial waste products are toxic beyond the localized area and may result in systemic conditions of aches, fever, chills, and malaise. An example of a systemic illness produced by bacterial waste products is **toxic shock syndrome**, which is caused by certain strains of *Staphylococcus aureus* bacteria.

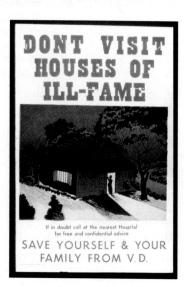

■ Although this public service announcement is many decades old, people still equate STIs with immorality, promiscuous behavior, and low social status.

Although normal infection defenses routinely fight off invading organisms throughout the body, reproductive tract infections are particularly challenging. The pelvis contains ideal media for bacterial growth and proliferation, especially during menstruation and after a miscarriage or abortion. Bleeding seems to facilitate bacterial invasion, and blood enhances bacterial growth. In addition, many kinds of bacteria normally live in the intestine and vaginal area. Thus the normal ecosystem of these areas involves a delicate balance of organisms. Harmful bacteria that upset this balance can be killed by antibiotics, but taking such drugs to kill one organism often results in the "killing off" of the normal bacteria and may produce a domino effect. When bacteria levels are reduced, yeast colonies may proliferate, and additional treatment may be necessary.

Viruses follow unique invasion patterns. These tiny organisms are made of DNA or RNA and are hundreds to thousands of times smaller than bacteria. Their attack mechanism also differs from that of bacteria. Viruses invade normal cells and take over the metabolic functions, fueling themselves on the cells' resources. In the process, the viruses often destroy their host cells. The body's immune system eventually recognizes invading viruses and mobilizes responses to them, creating an immune response with symptoms of pain, swelling, heat, redness, and/or fever. Unfortunately, a compromised immune system is ineffective against viral invaders. Viral STIs, especially HIV, present difficult challenges to medical researchers. HIV weakens and even subverts the host immune system, allowing **opportunistic infections** that the body normally fights off easily to invade and proliferate. Because antibiotics are ineffective against viral organisms, researchers are constantly looking to develop effective antiviral drugs that are not too toxic to use. Herpes, genital warts, hepatitis, and AIDS are all reproductive tract infections caused by viruses.

Ectoparasitic infections are caused by tiny parasites that reside on the skin and survive on human blood and tissue. Infections include scabies and pubic lice ("crabs"). Parasites cause itching and may cause bumps or a rash, but are easily treated with a topical cream. Parasitic infections are not considered major STIs; although they affect many people, they are more an annoyance than a serious health threat.

Gonorrhea

Despite a national public health effort, **gonorrhea** remains prevalent in the United States. In 2006, there were 358,366 reported cases of gonorrhea in the United States. Women, adolescents, and young adults bear the highest burden of this disease.[5] Many women do not experience any symptoms with gonorrhea, especially in the early stages. Instead, gonorrhea in women is often detected at routine gynecological screenings or when their male partners develop symptoms that lead to clinical treatment. When symptoms do present in women, they may include unusual vaginal discharge or bleeding, painful urination, painful intercourse or bleeding after intercourse, pelvic pain or tenderness, or fever. The gonococcus bacterium thrives in moist warm cavities, such as the mouth, throat, rectum, cervix, and urinary tract. As a consequence, gonococcal infections may present in the reproductive tract, throat, eyes, and rectum. Accurate diagnosis of gonorrhea requires a culture taken from the cervix and urethra, and from the throat and anal area if those areas may have been exposed.

There are several treatment options for gonorrhea, but treatment is complicated by the frequent coexistence of unrecognized chlamydial infection and the increasing incidence of gonorrheal antibiotic–resistant strains. Because neither gonorrhea nor chlamydia may be apparent upon physical examination, gonorrhea treatment usually includes screening for resistant strains of gonorrhea and prescribing additional antibiotics to treat chlamydia effectively. The sequelae of gonorrhea are so severe and threatening to general health and reproductive capability that any woman exposed to a partner with gonorrhea, even in the absence of symptoms, should be treated. Symptoms may indicate gonorrhea has spread, so longer and more intensive antibiotic treatment is indicated. This often means hospital admission for intravenous antibiotic therapy. About a week after antibiotic treatment for gonorrhea, reculture is necessary for a woman and her partner(s). This follow-up is especially important because gonorrhea is now

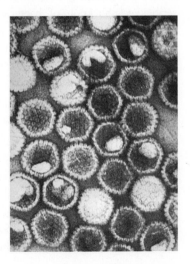
Magnified view of herpes simplex virus. Viral STIs such as herpes are incredibly common among young populations.

often resistant to certain antibiotics, and further treatment may be necessary to eliminate the disease.

Reinfection with gonorrhea is common, so sexual intercourse should be avoided until cultures on both partners confirm that treatment was successful. Untreated or unsuccessful treatment of gonorrhea may result in PID or a syndrome caused by disseminated gonococcal infection, which can include septicemia (blood poisoning), joint infection, skin problems, and heart and brain infections.

Chlamydia

Chlamydia is the most commonly reported infectious disease in the United States (**Figure 7.5**). Young women are most likely to be infected. More than 1 in 35 women between 15 and 24 years old in the United States is infected.[5] Chlamydia is also becoming even more common: The percentage of Americans infected with chlamydia in 2002 was six times the percentage of Americans infected in 1987.[8] Chlamydia infections, which are caused by a bacterium that is transmitted sexually, are the leading cause of preventable infertility and ectopic pregnancy. Symptoms of chlamydia are often similar to symptoms of gonorrhea. Most women and about half of men with this STI do not have any symptoms. If symptoms are present, women usually experience a yellowish vaginal discharge, burning with urination, or general pain in the lower abdomen. Chlamydia can invade the uterus, fallopian tubes, cervix, urethra, and even liver, without symptoms ever manifesting themselves. When the chlamydia infection moves into the upper reproductive tract, the condition is known as pelvic inflammatory disease (PID).

Chlamydia screening remains one of the most important national efforts to maintain and improve fertility. It is estimated that routine chlamydia screening could prevent 60% of the new cases of PID in the United States.[5] To screen for chlamydia, a culture may be obtained, although this bacterium is difficult to grow in solution and inaccurate results sometimes occur. Newer, more accurate urine-based tests that identify the genetic makeup of the chlamydia bacteria are being used more often; these tests also make screening easier for men. Clinician suspicion of chlamydia is heightened in a woman with a reddened, swollen cervix and a yellowish cervical discharge. Because gonorrhea and chlamydia often coexist, culture for gonorrhea is a standard procedure when chlamydia is suspected.

A woman may be treated for chlamydia, even without a confirmed diagnosis, based on symptoms and physical examination. The affected woman's partner(s) should be treated at the same time, and a follow-up examination is

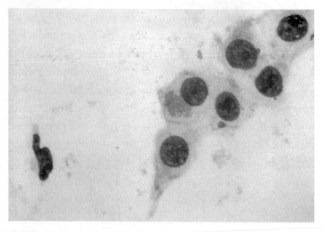

■ Magnified view of the bacteria that cause chlamydia. Bacterial sexually transmitted infections can be treated with antibiotics, but they often appear without symptoms.

usually performed about four weeks after treatment to ensure that the therapy was successful. Sexual intercourse should be avoided until after treatment is successful.

Aggressive treatment is necessary with chlamydia because uterine invasion occurs fairly rapidly, and the invasion process may be asymptomatic. Full PID treatment is undertaken if any evidence indicates that the organism has invaded the uterus. Treatment delay may result in the organism reaching the fallopian tubes with resultant scarring, tubal obstruction, infertility, and ectopic pregnancy. Pregnant women infected with chlamydia may be at increased risk for spontaneous abortions, stillbirth, preterm delivery, and delivery of low-birthweight infants. Transmission of the organism to the baby may result in eye infections and pneumonia in the infant.

Pelvic Inflammatory Disease

Pelvic inflammatory disease (PID) is the most frequent serious complication of bacterial infections, particularly chlamydia and gonorrhea. Each year more than 1 million women experience an episode of PID, causing more than 100,000 cases of infertility and 150 deaths in women.[5] PID from chlamydia is a leading cause of ectopic pregnancies. In 2005, 40,000 women were hospitalized in the United States for ectopic pregnancy.[5] PID also may result in infertility. The Centers for Disease Control and Prevention (CDC) has estimated that 12% of those affected become infertile after the first episode of PID.[5] PID costs to society remain high—about $1.3 billion a year.[9] Recent emphasis on national screening seems to be producing a downward trend of overall PID, with documented decreases in hospital and ambulatory settings from 1993 through 2006.[5]

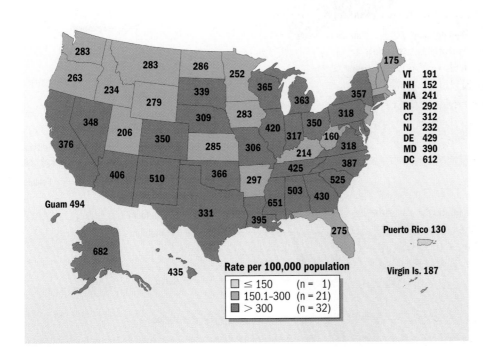

Figure 7.5A

Chlamydia—rates by state: United States and outlying areas, 2006.

Note: The total rate of chlamydia for the United States and outlying areas (Guam, Puerto Rico, and Virgin Islands) was 345.0 per 100,000 population.

Source: CDC. (2008). Sexually Transmitted Disease Surveillance, 2006.

VT	191	
NH	152	
MA	241	
RI	292	
CT	312	
NJ	232	
DE	429	
MD	390	
DC	612	

Rate per 100,000 population

☐ ≤ 150 (n = 1)
▨ 150.1–300 (n = 21)
▧ > 300 (n = 32)

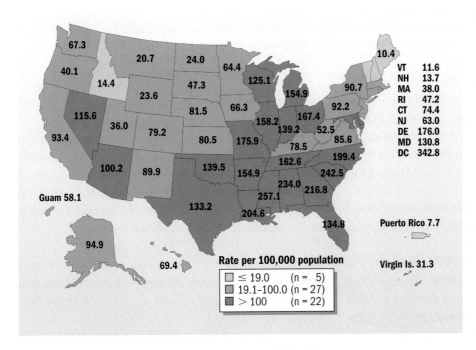

Figure 7.5B

Gonorrhea—rates by state: United States and outlying areas, 2006.

Note: The total rate of gonorrhea for the United States and outlying areas (Guam, Puerto Rico, and Virgin Islands) was 119.4 per 100,000 female population. The Healthy People 2010 target is 19.0 cases per 100,000 population.

Source: CDC. (2008). Sexually Transmitted Disease Surveillance, 2006.

VT	11.6
NH	13.7
MA	38.0
RI	47.2
CT	74.4
NJ	63.0
DE	176.0
MD	130.8
DC	342.8

Rate per 100,000 population

☐ ≤ 19.0 (n = 5)
▨ 19.1–100.0 (n = 27)
▧ > 100 (n = 22)

Chlamydia and gonorrhea are responsible for the majority of cases of PID. *Pelvic infection* and *PID* are both general terms for an infectious process that occurs anywhere in a woman's pelvic organs (**Figure 7.6**). The infection process may be diffuse—that is, spread out throughout the pelvic cavity—or it may be localized in specific areas. Terms for localized infections include the following:

- Endometritis—infection of the lining of the uterus
- Myometritis—infection of the muscular layers of the uterus
- Salpingitis—infection of the fallopian tubes
- Oophoritis—infection of the ovaries
- Peritonitis—infection of the lining of the abdominal cavity

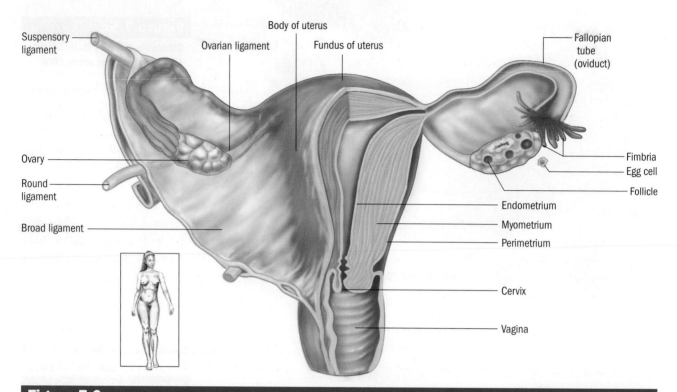

Suspensory ligament

Body of uterus

Ovarian ligament

Fundus of uterus

Fallopian tube (oviduct)

Ovary

Round ligament

Broad ligament

Fimbria

Egg cell

Follicle

Endometrium

Myometrium

Perimetrium

Cervix

Vagina

Figure 7.6

Pelvic inflammatory disease can affect any or all of a woman's reproductive organs.

There is considerable variability with PID symptoms. Some women experience very insidious symptoms, including vaginal discharge, mild but persistent abdominal or back pain, or pain during intercourse. Other women experience sudden and severe pelvic pain, fever, shaking chills, or heavy vaginal discharge or bleeding. Chlamydial PID is more likely to present with the former, more subtle symptoms, and gonorrheal PID is more likely to present with the latter, more severe set of symptoms.

Clinical evaluation is necessary for PID diagnosis. The first step in confirming the presence of PID is eliminating the possibility of other serious conditions that may manifest themselves in a similar manner. Although uterine tenderness and discharge indicate possible infection, bacterial culture is necessary to identify the causative bacterium and to determine the most appropriate treatment course.

If PID is limited to the uterus, antibiotic treatment usually is sufficient to resolve the problem with little likelihood of permanent damage or future complications. In contrast, infection in the fallopian tubes, ovaries, or abdominal cavity is a cause for significant concern. Permanent damage from PID is more likely if the infection has invaded the fallopian tubes, because the tubes are fragile and easily damaged by an infectious process. Infection causes swelling and scarring of the tubes, which can lead to blockage and distortion, impairing future fertility.

Pelvic abscess is another serious PID complication. Pus and live bacteria may leak from the open end of a fallopian tube and result in peritonitis and an abdominal abscess. A sonogram may be performed if an abscess is suspected; if one is present, the sonogram can help determine whether laparoscopy is indicated to drain the abscess.

Women who have had PID must take elaborate precautions to avoid reinfection. Present and previous sexual partners must be treated with the same antimicrobial regimen as the infected woman, whether or not the partners have symptoms.

Syphilis

After falling for 59 years, **syphilis** rates in the United States started to rise in the year 2000.[5] Public health officials had hopes of completely eliminating syphilis in the United States. Since then, the incidence of syphilis cases has increased every year, mostly among men, but also among women and infants. Although minorities are still more likely than their white counterparts to be infected with syphilis, these differences have shrunk over the past decade.[5]

Syphilis is caused by the bacterial organism *Treponema pallidum*. Syphilis is highly infectious and has a long, varied clinical course. If untreated, it may result in serious consequences, including cardiac and neurological damage and ultimately death. Although the syphilis bacterium can be killed with antibiotics, the damage caused by long-term infection is permanent.

There are three major stages of syphilis: primary, secondary, and tertiary.

Primary syphilis, the first disease stage, usually occurs in about three weeks but can occur as long as 12 weeks after sexual contact with an infected individual. The first symptom is an open sore, called a chancre, at the site of sexual contact. Only a small number of women who develop a chancre know it because this sore is often located deep inside the vagina. The chancre is usually painless despite its appearance. The chancre heals and disappears without scarring within two to six weeks, whether or not the individual receives treatment.

The course of *secondary syphilis* is also variable and occurs within one week to six months after primary syphilis. There are a variety of secondary-stage symptoms, most notably a rash on the palms of the hands and soles of the feet. This rash often appears on the external genitals as well and may develop into open sores. Individuals are highly infectious in the secondary stage of syphilis. Symptoms usually last three to six months but may reappear and then disappear again for several years. This latent phase of syphilis may be temporary or permanent.

A few people progress to the most dangerous phase, *tertiary syphilis*. Tertiary syphilis symptoms appear 10 to 20 years after initial exposure if the individual has not received treatment. They may include heart disease, nerve and brain damage, spinal cord damage, blindness, and death.

Syphilis can pass from an infected woman to her developing fetus. Early screening and treatment of pregnant women are essential to prevent congenital syphilis. Untreated syphilis infection during pregnancy often results in miscarriage, stillbirth, or severe birth defects. Babies born with syphilis who survive may suffer from skin sores, rashes, swollen liver and spleen, jaundice, and anemia, and if they are untreated after birth, damage to the heart, brain, and eyes.

A diagnosis of syphilis is confirmed by identification of antibodies in a blood test, although the antibodies do not appear until six to seven weeks after exposure. Syphilis sores may be recognized during a physical examination and may help in identifying the stage of the disease.

High doses of antibiotics are prescribed for early-stage syphilis. More prolonged, intensive treatment is indicated if the individual has been infected for a year or longer. For all stages of syphilis, sexual partners must be concurrently treated.

Special Precautions

Syphilis is a highly infectious, destructive disease. Preventive measures for this STI are similar to those for other STIs (see "Informed Decision Making: Reproductive Tract Infections"). A woman infected with syphilis and her sexual partner(s) should be treated at the same time. Both should avoid intercourse and all sexual intimacy for at least a month until repeat blood tests indicate that the treatments have been effective. Effective treatment and follow-up in the primary and secondary stages of the disease can prevent further serious, permanent damage.

Vaginitis

Several kinds of vaginal infections can be transmitted through sexual interaction. Because they may be frequently transmitted through nonsexual means, however, they are not generally referred to as STIs. *Trichomonas* infection, yeast infections, and bacterial vaginosis are fairly common reproductive tract infections. Although they are responsible for physical and emotional discomfort, they do not pose long-term health problems among otherwise healthy women.

Trichomoniasis

Trichomonas infection is caused by a one-celled protozoan and is usually transmitted via sexual contact. The infectious organism is, however, capable of surviving outside a human host in a wet environment, such as on a swimsuit or wet towel, and transmission between individuals can occur via these objects.

Some women do not experience any symptoms with **trichomoniasis**. When symptoms do occur, they typically include a frothy, thin, grayish or greenish vaginal discharge; intense vaginal itching; an objectionable odor; pain during urination and intercourse; and urinary frequency. Diagnosis of *Trichomonas* infection is confirmed with a wet smear of vaginal secretions.

Metronidazole (Flagyl, Metryl, Protostat, Satric) is the most effective antibiotic treatment for *Trichomonas* infection and is available in either a single-dose or multiple-dose format. Because many women and most men infected with *Trichomonas* do not experience symptoms, sexual partners should be treated at the same time, and condoms should be used for the first four to six weeks after treatment to avoid reinfection. Recurrent infections are common with trichomoniasis in pregnant women. This disease may result in premature rupture of membranes, preterm delivery, low birthweight, or a genital or lung infection in the newborn.

Yeast Infections

Yeast organisms (also known as *Candida albicans*, fungus infection, monilia, and candidiasis) normally exist in the microscopic ecosystem of a woman's body. Yeast is usually not sexually transmitted. When yeast overgrows, however, the symptoms are quite annoying. A thick, white, cottage cheese–type vaginal discharge; redness; swelling; and itching are common symptoms. Diagnosis is generally made by microscopic examination of a sample of the vaginal discharge. If yeast is not apparent but symptoms point to a yeast infection, a culture may be performed.

Yeast infections are usually treated with antibiotic vaginal cream (Monistat, Gyne-Lotrimin, Vagistat, Femstat) with dosage regimens of one, three, or seven days, depending on the medication. Treatment of partners is usually unnecessary. FDA approval has made these medications available in over-the-counter forms. For women with chronic and recurrent infections, this has facilitated treatment by reducing the waiting time for a prescription and the expense of a clinical visit. For women who are not sure what type or kind of vaginal infection they may have, self-treatment is not a good idea. Although some groups advocate treatments such as yogurt douches, commercial douches, *Lactobacillus* capsules, and cranberry juice, these regimens have not been subjected to clinical trials, and their efficacy is unknown.

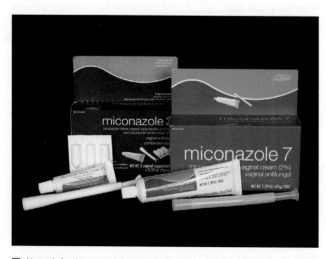

■ Yeast infections can be treated with many products that are available over the counter.

Although yeast infections do not usually invade the pelvis and affect fertility, reinfection is common and annoying. Recurrent attacks may occur shortly after treatment or be delayed for a considerable period of time. What causes yeast to grow out of control is unknown. Yeast is a ubiquitous inhabitant of intestinal and vaginal tracts. Persistent yeast problems often present during pregnancy and in women who take oral contraceptives. Women with diabetes and women who are overweight also report higher frequencies of such infections. For women with recurrent infections, prolonged or intermittent treatment is often recommended to keep yeast growth under control. Concurrent treatment for yeast whenever antibiotics are prescribed may also help women with chronic yeast infections.

Bacterial Vaginosis

Bacterial vaginosis (BV) is known by many terms, including nonspecific vaginitis, *Gardnerella vaginalis*, bacterial vaginitis, *Haemophilus vaginalis*, *Corynebacterium vaginalis*, and anaerobic vaginosis. This condition is caused by an overgrowth of several species of vaginal organisms, which may be transmitted by sexual activity.[10] Bacterial vaginosis is considered a sexually associated condition but not necessarily a sexually transmitted infection. Although BV does not usually cause complications on its own, it is considered to be a co-factor in the acquisition of other sexually transmitted diseases, including HIV.[11] BV is more prevalent among women with more than one sexual partner, intrauterine device (IUD) users, and women who have cervicitis.

The most common cause of abnormal vaginal discharge, BV is very common, usually detected in 10% to 40% of women worldwide.[12] Symptoms include a gray or white frothy discharge that may be thick or watery and that may have an objectionable odor. Painful urination, vaginal pain or burning during intercourse, redness, and itching may also be present.

While many women complain of vaginal odor, discharge, or irritation, as many as 50% of women with BV may be asymptomatic; thus, routine screening is recommended whenever STI testing is indicated.[2] Identifying bacterial vaginosis is relatively straightforward. Diagnosis may be made with microscopic examination of a discharge sample or a wet mount of vaginal cells. Recent studies have shown that pregnant women with bacterial vaginosis have an increased risk of delivering preterm, low-birthweight infants. Bacterial vaginosis may coexist with other STIs and has been identified as a possible factor in HIV transmission. Because BV also may be associated with PID, definitive diagnosis is important to ensure adequate treatment.

Recommended treatment regimens consist of antibiotics, usually either oral or vaginal metronidazole or vaginal clindamycin. The vaginal treatment regimen is associated with fewer gastrointestinal side effects than the oral regimen.[2] Treatment of sexual partners is not standard procedure, although it may be indicated if reinfection occurs after treatment or if sexual transmission is suspected as the mode of acquisition.

Regular douching can increase a woman's risk of bacterial vaginosis. Douching may harm the vaginal flora and can increase the risk for bacterial vaginosis as well as other infections.[13]

Human Papillomavirus

Human papillomavirus (HPV) is an extremely common sexually transmitted virus spread by genital-skin-to-genital-skin contact. Each year, more than 6 million people in the United States, most of them in their teens or early 20s, are infected with HPV. Most people who are sexually active will acquire HPV at some point in their lives; most of these people will never know it.[1] There are many strains or types of HPV, but they all manifest themselves in one of two distinct forms. "High-risk" HPV can cause cervical dysplasia, a form of abnormal cell growth that can lead to cervical cancer. "Low-risk" HPV can cause warts on or around the genital area. Because HPV is so prevalent, it is easily possible to be infected with both HPV types; however, low-risk HPV cannot turn into high-risk HPV, and vice versa.

Fortunately, although cervical cancer is a relatively common cancer for women, almost all cases of cervical cancer are preventable. A screening program that includes Pap smears and HPV DNA testing (see **It's Your Health** on page 186) can almost always find cervical dysplasia before it becomes cancerous. Additionally, there is now an FDA-approved vaccine that can provide protection against two high-risk and two low-risk strains of HPV. Together, these four strains are responsible for 70% of cases of cervical cancer and 90% of cases of genital warts.[2] Used together, vaccination and screening to find and prevent the remaining 30% of cervical cancer cases could virtually eliminate cervical cancer. The technology to end this disease is here; however, a considerable challenge remains with educating the public about cervical cancer and expanding women's access to care.

There is no "cure" for HPV, but symptoms of both high-risk and low-risk HPV can be treated. Additionally, the body's immune system is often effective at ridding the body of the virus. HPV infections are often asymptomatic, and a person can have HPV for years without the virus causing harm to the body. Left untreated, however, cervical dysplasia caused by high-risk HPV can cause serious harm or death, so prevention and screening efforts are extremely important for women's health.

For many women, the first indication of a high-risk HPV infection is a routine Pap smear that identifies cervical cellular changes consistent with HPV infection. For a woman with an inconclusive Pap test, HPV DNA testing conducted on the residual material collected from a Pap can help identify the presence of HPV to determine if she is at risk for cervical dysplasia. Women who are 30 or older can get an HPV test along with their Pap tests. Women who are negative on both tests can be reassured that they do not have HPV and they are not at risk for developing cervical cancer in the near future. If the HPV DNA test is positive, a gynecologist may look for evidence of warts in the cervix or vagina.

Women who have cervical dysplasia may need to seek aggressive treatment to prevent possible cancer development. Colposcopic examination and biopsy of suspicious areas are indicated. It is also important to be diligent about personal care, medical follow-up care, and annual Pap smears and pelvic examinations.

HPV infection with low-risk HPV is usually characterized by single or multiple lesions or warts, which may first appear as small wens (round elevations in the skin) but may grow in size and number and blend together in a cauliflower-like growth. Genital warts vary in size, may exist in single or multiple units, and may be raised or flat. In women, these painless lesions may occur on the buttocks, anus, inner thighs, vulva, vagina, and cervix; depending on their location, symptoms can be present without a woman knowing about them.

When warts regress, HPV may still be present, just not readily apparent. Once contracted, the virus has a variable incubation period during which no symptoms are visible and the person is not yet infectious. Warts usually appear one to eight months after exposure, may not manifest themselves for years, or may not appear at all. A **prodrome** period follows the incubation period, during which there are still no symptoms but the disease is contagious.

Diagnosis of low-risk HPV is usually based on visual detection during clinical examination.

Although warts may regress spontaneously, they are frequently symptomatic or psychologically distressing, so treatment is often indicated to remove visible warts for psychological and aesthetic reasons, as well as to reduce (but not eliminate) the likelihood of transmission. HPV infections can be quite persistent and can recur regardless of which treatment method is selected. Treatment is easier and less painful in earlier stages. Although no treatment can "cure" HPV, evidence suggests that most individuals' immune systems will eventually clear the virus even with-

Gender Dimensions

HPV

HPV may be the most biologically sexist of all sexually transmitted infections. Low-risk HPV can cause genital warts in both men and women. Both men and women can get or receive high-risk HPV, but men are almost never affected by it. (Some strains of HPV have been linked to penile or anal cancer in men, but these cancers are extremely rare.) It is not yet known whether the vaccine for HPV is effective in men.[1]

These gender differences raise interesting philosophical and epidemiological questions about who should be vaccinated. The CDC currently recommends that only females receive the vaccine. But if the vaccine turns out to be as effective in preventing infection in men as it is in women, some people may want men to be vaccinated to reduce their risk of transmitting HPV to their partners and to possibly reduce their chances of getting those obscure types of penile and anal cancer. However, vaccinating men for HPV would cost hundreds of millions of dollars. Leaving men (as well as women over 26, who are at substantially greater risk for acquiring HPV) unvaccinated and investing those funds in other forms of STI prevention could have a dramatically larger impact on the health of men and women.

[1]**Source:** CDC Fact Sheet: HPV Vaccine Information for Young Women.

It's Your Health

HPV Testing and Vaccination

Pap Tests (Pap Smears)

The Pap test is an examination that looks for signs of abnormal cell growth in the cervix. In the five decades they have been in use, Pap smears have helped to dramatically reduce deaths from cervical cancer.

Strengths: A national screening program based on Pap tests is already in place. Pap tests find most cases of abnormal cell growth before they become cancerous.

Limitations: Pap tests sometimes produce positive results in the absence of dysplasia; because the tests look for abnormal cell growth, not the actual virus, frequent screenings are required. Because so many screenings are necessary, the Pap test is not an especially cost-effective solution.

HPV Testing

Instead of looking for cervical dysplasia, an early sign of disease, the HPV test looks for the DNA of the actual virus.

Strengths: Studies consistently show that HPV tests outperform Pap testing. A combined program of HPV testing and Pap tests is nearly 100% effective at identifying women at risk.

Limitations: The current screening infrastructure in the United States is based on Pap testing; implementing a new system will require political will and financial investment. The presence of high-risk HPV does not guarantee that cancer will develop.

HPV Vaccination

The Gardasil vaccine, approved by the FDA in 2006, provides protection from four strains of HPV. The vaccine is given as a series of three injections over a six-month period. The CDC currently recommends vaccination for 11- and 12-year-old girls, and women from the ages of 13 to 26 who have not received the full vaccination.

Strengths: The low-risk HPV strains 6 and 11 are responsible for 90% of current cases of genital warts; the high-risk strains 16 and 18 are responsible for 70% of current cases of cervical cancer. Studies have shown the vaccine to be safe and effective.

Limitations: Screening programs still need to be in place to find the other 30% of cervical cancers caused by high-risk strains of HPV not covered by the vaccine. The vaccine does not protect women who have already been infected, and it requires three doses to be effective. The vaccine is relatively expensive (about $400) to complete.

out treatment. At this point, a person would no longer have HPV, though he or she could be reinfected with a new exposure. The particular treatment depends on the extent of HPV infection and its location. Options include topical agents applied by the patient or provider, cryotherapy (freezing of warts), laser surgery, electrosurgery, and surgical removal.

There is risk of recurrence after any therapy for external genital warts; however, recurrence rates may be the lowest with patient-applied topical therapies.

HPV can present problems in pregnancy, though this is relatively rare. A pregnant woman with low-risk HPV has a small chance of passing the virus to her child during vaginal delivery. In these cases, a doctor may treat warts before childbirth to reduce these risks.

Only a small percentage of the millions of women who contract high-risk HPV every year will ever develop cervical cancer. Instead, most women will clear the infection based on their bodies' own immune response. The strength of the immune system appears to affect the course of infection: Conditions that alter or slow the immune response may encourage dysplasia. Men infected with these strains of HPV are still capable of transmitting the virus, even if the virus never affects them or causes symptoms. HPV DNA testing is more sensitive and the results more easily reproducible than Pap testing and colposcopy for the detection of existent and incipient cervical precancerous conditions and cancer. A negative HPV test provides a degree and duration of reassurance not achievable by any other diagnostic method[14] (**Table 7.1**).

Special Precautions

Although latex condoms may reduce the likelihood of HPV transmission, they probably do not provide as reliable protection from HPV as they do against some other STIs, such as HIV. HPV is spread by genital skin-to-skin contact, not by bodily fluids. Because a latex condom does not cover all of the genital skin, it cannot guarantee prevention of transmission, even if no visible symptoms are present. A female condom may provide more protection than a traditional condom that covers the penis, but there are no guarantees with either type of condom use.

Herpes Simplex Virus

Herpes simplex virus (HSV) is a very common sexually transmitted infection. Herpes can be caused by two distinct, closely related viruses: HSV-1 and HSV-2. HSV-1 is the main cause of recurring sores in the mouth known as cold sores or fever blisters. HSV-2 typically causes similar symptoms that appear in the genital area. However, if HSV-1 is exposed to the genital area of an uninfected person (for example, through oral sex), HSV-1 can infect the genital area of that person; similarly, exposure to HSV-2 can infect the oral area of a person as well.

Herpes is incredibly common; an estimated 58% of the U.S. population has an infection of HSV-1 and 17.2% is infected with HSV-2.[1] **Figure 7.7** shows the number of

My husband of 22 years and I divorced recently, and so I'm new to the dating scene. I've started seeing a very sweet guy who later told me that he has herpes. I was very shocked at first, but now that I know about the disease, it's not nearly as bad as I first thought. My daughter, who's in college now, and I had a real heart-to-heart conversation about safer-sex practices afterward. She actually knew more than I did!

50-year-old mother of two

Table 7.1 **Understanding Cervical Cancer Screening: Pap and HPV Test Results and What They Mean**

Normal and Abnormal Pap Test Result	What It Means
Normal Pap smear (Pap test)	Your cervical cells appear to be healthy.
Abnormal Pap smear (Pap test)	There appear to be changes in your cervical cells that need to be evaluated further.
Borderline or inconclusive Pap test result (officially called "ASC-US," which stands for atypical squamous cells of undetermined significance)	Your cervical cells are not obviously normal, but they are not clearly abnormal either. Having an HPV test can help determine whether you need further evaluation.

Figure 7.7

Genital herpes—initial visits to physicians' offices, United States, 1966–2006.

Source: Centers for Disease Control and Prevention. (2008). *Sexually Transmitted Diseases Surveillance, 2006.*

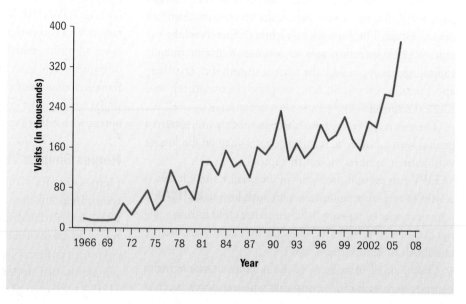

visits to a physician's office for primary herpes outbreak over the past 40 years. Most of these people do not know they are infected.[16] Herpes is incurable, and it can be extremely painful and psychologically devastating. Yet for the vast majority of cases, herpes is not a serious medical condition.

Symptoms of HSV are usually most severe just after acquiring the infection. Symptoms may appear as soon as one day or as long as three to four weeks after exposure. Lasting about 12 days, herpes generally presents as single or multiple small, painful blisters that appear in the vulva or buttocks of women. If they are present on the cervix, they usually go unnoticed. The blisters evolve into painful ulcers in a couple of days. These symptoms may be accompanied by vulvar swelling, fever, and enlarged and tender lymph nodes. Sores usually heal in one to four weeks with little or no scarring. The time between outbreaks is referred to as the latent or inactive phase. During this time, genital sores have healed but the infection remains. A prodrome or warning phase often precedes a herpes outbreak. The warnings may consist of tingling or itching sensations in

the area where sores later appear. It is not known what causes repeat outbreaks of herpes. Some people find that irritating stimuli to the infected area, such as tight clothing, menstrual changes, or exposure to sunlight or extreme heat or cold, can trigger an outbreak whereas others do not notice any such effects.

The human body can never rid itself of the herpes virus. Between outbreaks, the virus evades the immune system by lying dormant within host nerve cells, where the immune system cannot reach it; however, in most cases the immune system does get better at fighting the virus. Recurrent outbreaks are usually milder in severity and shorter in duration than the original outbreaks. People with herpes generally have fewer outbreaks as time goes by. Although there is no surefire way to prevent all outbreaks, maintaining a healthy lifestyle helps the immune system keep the virus in check. Any stress on the body can also stress the immune system; indeed, many people report that outbreaks begin when they are already sick with a cold or flu, have gone a long time without getting enough sleep, or are experiencing stressful times in their lives—all things that can burden the immune system. Ironically, refraining from obsessing or worrying excessively about a herpes infection, while still remaining knowledgeable about the disease, may help prevent outbreaks.

Herpes outbreaks show considerable variability from person to person. Some herpes outbreaks last as long as three weeks; others are as short as a few days. Some outbreaks are characterized by multiple blisters; others involve only a single blister. Some individuals experience outbreaks

I don't sleep around a lot. I have been with only three guys. But I have herpes. I can't tell where I got it . . . I mean, it's like I have slept with not only those guys, but everyone else they have had sex with. How can a person really trust someone not to have an STD these days?

21-year-old woman

every few months; others have one or more each month. Some individuals never experience recurrent outbreak symptoms after the initial event, though this is an uncommon occurrence. Infectiousness remains an important concern, even for individuals who are unaware of their herpes symptoms.

Active herpes sores are very contagious during both the initial attack and the recurrences. Both HSV-1 and HSV-2 can be spread from sores to the eye, where serious infection is possible. An oral infection can be spread to infants and children via kissing or casual contact. People infected with herpes undergo periods of **asymptomatic viral shedding**. During these periods, active herpes virus is present on a person's infected area and may be infectious, whether or not symptoms are present. Viral shedding typically lasts for 2 to 20 days during an initial outbreak and for 2 to 5 days during recurrent outbreaks. Researchers have not been able to determine exactly how infectious an individual is when asymptomatic shedding occurs. However, the risk of transmission is highest when active sores are present. Active sores contain hundreds of times more virus than viral sheddings from genital secretions.

Diagnosing herpes may be based on the person's history or a recurrent pattern of illness. Because clinical diagnosis is often inaccurate, viral culture and type-specific serology are used to confirm a diagnosis.

There is no cure for herpes. Prescribed antiviral medications may reduce or suppress symptoms, and antibiotic ointment may help prevent a secondary bacterial infection of the sores. Taking herpes medication may also reduce, but not eliminate, the chance of transmission between outbreaks.[16] Acyclovir, valacyclovir, and famciclovir are the current treatments of choice for herpes; although they do not cure the condition, they can relieve symptoms and shorten healing time. All three medications work by inhibiting the ability of the virus to use proteins, thereby interfering with its ability to replicate. Clinicians may prescribe acyclovir to women who acquire herpes during pregnancy or who have severe outbreaks around the time of delivery.[2] The FDA has approved three different treatment regimens for herpes: (1) therapy for an initial outbreak, (2) episodic therapy to speed healing and relieve discomfort during recurrences, and (3) suppressive therapy on a daily basis to attempt to prevent outbreaks. Because the effects of a herpes transmission are usually limited to symptoms and transmission, a woman with herpes should take an active role in deciding the treatment regimen, if any, that is right for her. Women with severe symptoms may wish to take suppressive therapy, whereas women who

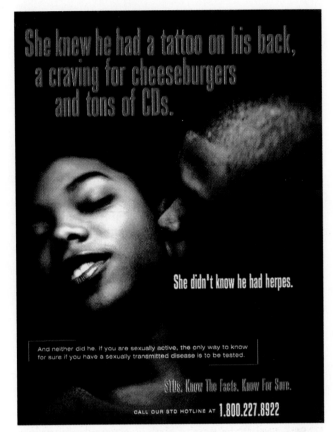

■ Many people with HSV are asymptomatic but can still transmit the herpes virus. The only way a person can know if he or she has an STI is to get tested. Reprinted with permission from the American Social Health Association.

have outbreaks that are mild or not noticeable may opt for episodic therapy or seek to manage the virus without medication.

Special Precautions

Good personal hygiene is essential during a herpes outbreak. The infected individual should wash his or her hands thoroughly after touching a herpes sore to avoid possible transmission to another mucous membrane, such as the eyes or mouth. Care should be taken to avoid spreading the virus to others, including infants and children. If active herpes is present in or near the mouth, kissing should be avoided. As a precautionary measure, personal objects such as washcloths, toothbrushes, drinking cups, and towels should not be shared. Although clinical studies have not demonstrated effective indirect transmission, the virus can remain alive outside the body for several hours in a moist environment.

There are no guarantees of "safe sex" with herpes, but there are ways to reduce risk. At a minimum, sexual intercourse, including oral sex, should be avoided when active herpes sores are present. Because viral populations are so high in sores, individuals should wait until the sores are completely healed before resuming sexual activity. Because it is difficult to tell when a herpes outbreak is beginning, open communication about risks and feelings is essential. Condoms appear to provide some protection, with female condoms providing better coverage than male condoms.[18] Because herpes sores can be present in areas not covered by either condom, however, there are no guarantees against transmission. Condoms are especially important in a situation in which the male partner has herpes and the female partner does not and is pregnant. An initial attack of herpes during pregnancy presents serious risks to the developing fetus, including possible pregnancy loss or preterm delivery.

Women with herpes should be diligent about protecting themselves from further infection by other STIs. Such women are at increased risk for acquiring HIV and HPV because of the open sores associated with the herpes virus.

Pregnant women with herpes should begin prenatal care early. The risk is greatest for women who contract herpes during their pregnancy. If active lesions are present in the vaginal canal at the time of birth, a cesarean delivery may be undertaken to avoid exposing the infant to the virus. Infant exposure to the virus may cause infections of the eyes, skin, mucous membranes, and central nervous system, and even death. However, most pregnant women with herpes deliver vaginally and give birth to healthy babies.[16]

Although no one wants to get genital herpes, in most cases the stigma of the disease vastly outweighs its physiological effects. Herpes is closely related to the viruses that cause chickenpox and mononucleosis (mono), yet because herpes is sexually transmitted, people with herpes may describe themselves as "dirty" or "tainted" or feel that they will never be lovable or able to enter a sexual relationship again. The truth is that many people with herpes have strong relationships and healthy sex lives. Although there is no way to guarantee prevention of sexual transmission, there are many ways to reduce risk, from avoiding sex or wearing condoms between outbreaks, to taking suppressive therapy to reduce outbreaks and asymptomatic shedding. Some people decide to enter relationships with other people who have herpes, although other STIs would still be a potential concern. Because the symptoms of herpes infections are transient and often ultimately quite mild, some couples with one infected partner decide that the benefits of a healthy, unique loving relationship outweigh the drawbacks of possible herpes transmission.

Comfort Measures

Keeping the genital area clean and dry minimizes discomfort during a herpes flare-up. A hair dryer on a cool setting may be used to dry the area thoroughly without irritation or discomfort. Genital cleansing must be gentle because rubbing can cause lesions to break and bleed. Many women find **sitz baths** comforting during outbreaks of herpes. Domeboro solution or baking soda may be added to the sitz bath. Cold, wet compresses or individually wrapped cleansing pads containing glycerol and witch hazel applied to the sores may also provide temporary relief of discomfort, especially during oozing. In addition, some women find icepacks helpful in reducing discomfort during outbreaks.

Hepatitis

Hepatitis, an inflammation of the liver, is caused by infection with one of several viruses—type A, B, C, D, E, F, or G. Although hepatitis A, B, and C may be transmitted via sexual intimacy, hepatitis B is the only infection transmitted primarily through sexual contact.

Hepatitis A is usually a mild illness that resolves within a few weeks. It primarily affects young adults and children and usually spreads through consumption of contaminated food or water. It also may be spread through exposure to fecal matter of an infected person. A common source of hepatitis A is uncooked shellfish from contaminated waters. Sexual oral–anal contact is another mode of transmission. A two-shot vaccine can provide lifetime immunity to hepatitis A.

Hepatitis B is spread mainly by sexual contact, although it is also transmitted via needle sharing among intravenous drug users and accidental needlesticks or contaminated

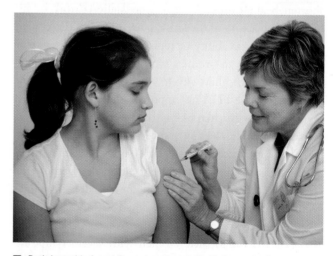

■ Both hepatitis A and B can be prevented with immunization.

surgical instruments among health-care workers. Hepatitis B has the distinction of being the one STI that is entirely preventable; a three-shot series can provide lifetime immunity to heptatis B.

Hepatitis B symptoms range from nonexistent to severe incapacitation. Those who do have symptoms often experience low-grade fever, fatigue, headache, generalized aches, loss of appetite, nausea and vomiting, abdominal pain, and **jaundice**. Liver failure is a severe complication of hepatitis B. Another serious complication is persistent infection, which can occur with no apparent symptoms (called a carrier state) and can lead to chronic liver disease, resulting in permanent liver scarring and liver failure. Hepatitis B infected approximately 46,000 individuals in the United States in 2006, a decline of 80% since 1991.[19] It is also a common infection in Africa and Southeast Asia.

Hepatitis C is both the most common cause of chronic liver disease and the most common bloodborne disease in the United States.[20] It is mostly transmitted through contact with infected blood, intravenous drug use, or contaminated blood transfusion. Sexual transmission accounts for 10% to 15% of hepatitis C infections, but this route is most likely to occur when there is possible exposure to blood in addition to sexual fluids.[20] Transmission rates from mother to child during pregnancy are about 4%.[21] Most people with hepatitis C will go on to have chronic infections, and some may die from severe liver complications.

Diagnosis of hepatitis is based on clinical symptoms and laboratory blood tests, which confirm the type of virus involved. Diagnosis is often difficult because any form of hepatitis can be present without symptoms. There is no cure for hepatitis. Symptoms are treated, and rest and supportive care are recommended. A healthy diet is important, and alcohol should be avoided until liver function tests indicate that the liver is functioning normally. Women on estrogen therapy, either birth control pills or replacement therapy, should discontinue these medications until normal liver function returns.

Although most individuals with hepatitis recover within a few weeks, 10% to 30% of infected individuals develop a persistent hepatitis infection, either with or without symptoms. Chronic hepatitis may lead to severe liver impairment and is associated with the later development of liver cancer. Chronic infections may be treated with alpha-interferon to relieve symptoms and improve liver function; unfortunately, this treatment regime is expensive, may cause severe side effects, and in the majority of cases is not effective in eliminating infection.

Special Precautions

Under most circumstances, B is the only type of hepatitis that is transmitted sexually. Individuals need to take the same precautions against infection with hepatitis as other viral STIs.

Hepatitis A and B may be prevented by vaccination or treatment with immune globulin within two weeks of exposure. The vaccine actually prevents infection from three forms of hepatitis, since hepatitis D is a defective virus that requires co-infection of heptatitis B to survive. The vaccination consists of a three-injection series that must be given in a six-month period and provides long-term immunity. Vaccination is expensive but is recommended for groups who are at higher risk for exposure to the virus.

Sexual partners of infected individuals, pregnant women with hepatitis B (to prevent transmission to the fetus), a newborn baby of an infected mother, and household contacts of an individual with hepatitis A or B should receive immune globulin for hepatitis A and B. If the

---

It's Your Health

Individuals Who Should Be Vaccinated for Hepatitis A

People traveling to certain countries where hepatitis A is common (e.g., Africa, Asia)

People engaging in anal-oral sex

Intravenous drug users

Daycare and institutional workers

People with chronic liver problems

It's Your Health

Individuals Who Should Be Vaccinated for Hepatitis B

Health-care workers who come in contact with blood or other bodily fluids

Household contacts of a person infected with hepatitis B

Sexual partner(s) of a person infected with hepatitis B

Individuals with multiple sexual partners

Staff and clients of residential institutions, including prisons

Individuals receiving hemodialysis or blood products

Intravenous drug users

Individuals with recent sexually transmitted diseases

Infants born in the United States

infected person is a member of an institutional facility, such as a daycare center, prison, or nursing home, staff and fellow clients should also receive immune globulin.

AIDS

AIDS (acquired immune deficiency syndrome), a progressive disease caused by **HIV (human immunodeficiency virus)**, is characterized by the destruction of the immune system. There are no constant, specific symptoms associated with this condition, and no effective cure or vaccine is available. The best way to stop HIV is to prevent infection. Recent therapeutic advances have allowed people living with HIV to live longer, fuller lives; however, HIV remains a serious life-threatening infection.

HIV is a **retrovirus**, a virus that incorporates its genetic material into the genome of the cell it attacks. When HIV, also known as the AIDS virus, enters the bloodstream, it attacks specific white blood cells called CD4 or T lymphocytes. The virus also replicates. The CD4 cells are no longer able to stimulate a cellular defense response, and the body's systemic immune system is compromised. The number of CD4 cells in an infected person's body decreases as the number of HIV-infected cells increases. AIDS is the final stage of HIV; it is diagnosed when the person has a positive test for antibodies to HIV and a low T-lymphocyte count. An HIV-positive person also may be diagnosed with AIDS when one of 26 known infections, called opportunistic infections, is present. Opportunistic infections present a potentially fatal risk to individuals with AIDS.

HIV is transmitted from one person to another through sexual intercourse, shared intravenous needle use, or contaminated blood or blood products. HIV is not spread by casual, social, or family contact. Although HIV is a sophisticated and elusive killer within the body, the virus quickly dies when exposed to the open air; unbroken human skin provides excellent protection from HIV. An individual with HIV may have no physical symptoms, so it is impossible to tell whether a person is infected just by looking at him or her. In fact, one out of four people living with HIV does not know that he or she is infected.[21] HIV-infected individuals are capable of transmitting the virus to others, however, even in the absence of symptoms. The HIV incubation period ranges from months to years. No individual or groups of individuals are immune to HIV/AIDS.

Perspectives on AIDS

Historical Overview

Although the history of AIDS is relatively short, the human toll exacted by the disease cannot be calculated. It is now believed that HIV is a mutated descendant of SIV, a virus in wild African chimpanzees. Genetic analyses of the oldest known specimens of HIV indicate that the virus probably first began spreading among humans between 1884 and 1924 in what is now the Democratic Republic of the Congo.[23] These cases went unnoticed because they spread at low levels among relatively unexamined populations, and because technology to identify the virus was nonexistent. AIDS was first diagnosed in the United States in 1981.

About 56,300 people are infected with HIV in the United States each year, and 1.3 million people in the United States are living with HIV.[24] Three-quarters of U.S. women with HIV acquire their infections through heterosexual intercourse; almost all of the rest acquire it through intravenous drug use. African American women bear a heavy burden of the disease and are more than 12 times more likely than white women to have HIV.[23]

Men who have sex with men still constitute a disproportionate percentage of people infected with HIV. However, anyone who engages in risky sexual behavior or intravenous drug use is at risk for HIV. HIV epidemics in other countries have been spread primarily by intravenous drug users or heterosexual sex. A complicating factor is that, like many intravenous drug users, many men who have sex with men hide or deny their risky behaviors and pose as non-injecting, straight men.[21]

Advances in antiretroviral treatment mean that people are living longer with HIV and therefore dying less rapidly. But at the same time, prevention efforts have not been nearly as effective as they were in the 1980s and early 1990s. The number of people newly infected with HIV has remained stable for more than a decade.

It's Your Health

AIDS Facts: Dispelling AIDS Myths

AIDS is not a disease of homosexual men.

Women are susceptible to AIDS.

AIDS may not be spread by casual contact.

AIDS cannot be transmitted to humans from insects.

There is no risk of acquiring AIDS by donating blood.

Information and education are the best weapons against AIDS.

Confidential, anonymous testing for AIDS is available.

Global Perspective

More than 33 million people—95% of whom live in developing countries—are living with HIV. Half of all people currently living with HIV are women. In 2007, 2.7 million people were infected, and 2 million people died of HIV-related causes.[24]

This worldwide epidemic has hit sub-Saharan Africa the hardest. Even though sub-Saharan Africa contains only 10% of the world's population, in 2007, it was home to two-thirds of the total number of people living with HIV and three-fourths of AIDS-related deaths. Estimates of deaths and infections reveal only part of this grim picture: More than 12 million children in sub-Saharan Africa have lost their parents to AIDS, and sickness and deaths among the current generation of young adults may cripple many local economies for decades.[24]

The global community has launched a massive, coordinated response to this epidemic. The chief goal of this combination of people, money, and political will is to stop and reverse the growth of this epidemic by 2015.[24] This work has shown promising results, particularly in expanding access to treatment and improving estimations of infections. Clearly, however, much work needs to be done, particularly in prevention efforts in the developing world. The global fight to control this catastrophic disease is only getting started.

Epidemiological Data and Trends

AIDS presents different epidemiological patterns by sex. Women did not constitute a sizable proportion of the total number of HIV cases in the United States until several years into the AIDS epidemic, but this number has since then grown. In 1992, women accounted for 13.8% of people infected with HIV; by 1998, they represented 20% of this total. Recently this proportion appears to have stabilized at about 26%.[21] Women infected with AIDS are more likely to be living in the Northeast or the South.[21] **Figure 7.8** shows AIDS cases by region and race/ethnicity in the United States. Most HIV-infected women acquire the virus through heterosexual transmission, as shown in **Figure 7.9**. Nearly 20% of newly reported women's HIV cases are the result of injection drug use.

I knew that there was no way I could be positive for HIV. I am not a virgin, but I don't sleep around a lot, and I don't use drugs. I wasn't worried. I guess I should have been because here I am, 27 years old, and I have HIV. I keep thinking, why me? I don't deserve this.

27-year-old woman

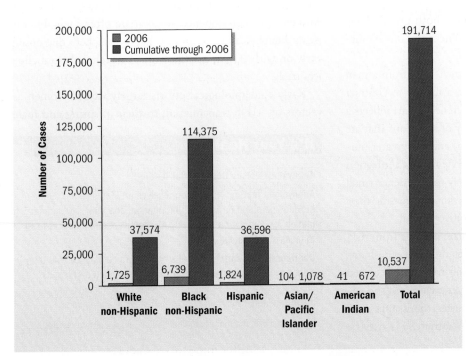

Figure 7.8

Reported AIDS cases in female adults and adolescents, United States.

Source: Centers for Disease Control and Prevention. (2008). *HIV/AIDS Surveillance Report, 2006.*

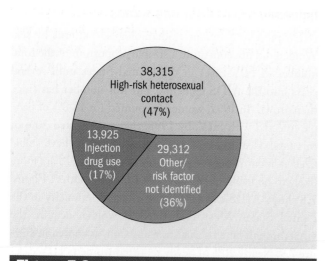

38,315
High-risk heterosexual
contact
(47%)

13,925
Injection
drug use
(17%)

29,312
Other/
risk factor
not identified
(36%)

Figure 7.9

Reported cases of HIV infection among U.S. female adults and adolescents.

Source: Centers for Disease Control and Prevention. (2008). *HIV/AIDS Surveillance Report, 2006.*

Special Concerns for Women

Women are an at-risk, HIV-susceptible population. A focus on male homosexuality as a risk factor slowed the initial acknowledgment of this vulnerability. Failure to focus on women as a unique high-risk group for HIV has created significant obstacles in diagnosis, prevention, and treatment. As a consequence, women may be subject to delayed recognition of symptoms, diagnosis, and treatment. In the United States, women are more likely to die from AIDS than men; however, when both groups have equal access to health care, no differences in rates of survival are expected.

Women are far more likely to contract HIV from a man through heterosexual intercourse than a man is to contract the infection from a woman. This difference in part reflects a woman's exposure to a greater quantity of secretions that are possibly carrying the virus (i.e., semen) and the greater mucosal surface area of the vagina and cervix in which infection can occur. In addition, women are likely to experience small tears in the vaginal lining during intercourse, increasing their susceptibility to infection by HIV-positive semen.

Women who partner with women are not free from risk, however. Many women who consider themselves lesbians have had heterosexual intercourse and may have received HIV through that avenue without knowing it. And although woman-to-woman sexual contact does appear to be less risky for transmission of HIV, other STIs may be spread that way.

Since 1985, the proportion of all AIDS cases involving adult and adolescent women has almost quadrupled, from 7% in 1985 to 26% in 2006.[21] The epidemic has increased most dramatically among women of color. African American women are 12 times more likely than white women to be infected with HIV. Hispanic women are also disproportionately more likely to be infected, albeit not as dramatically.[21] In 2004, HIV infection was the leading cause of death for African American women ages 25–34 years and was among the four leading causes of death for African American women ages 20–24 and 35–44 years, as well as Hispanic women ages 35–44 years.[25]

Social Issues

African American women with HIV face the dual stigma of being neither white nor male. African American women who have HIV are less likely to recieve treatment than other ethnic groups and are more likely to die early. About half the people in the United States who die from AIDS are African American.[21] Class undoubtedly plays a large role in this disparity. Women who are economically deprived often have inadequate access to health-care facilities and are more likely to be unhealthy in general. Many do not have health insurance, or are chronically uninsured or underinsured, or lack information on how to access and use scarce public health-care facilities.

Early limitations with the male-based CDC diagnostic criteria for AIDS prevented many women with AIDS from being correctly diagnosed. Even with the revised criteria, few studies have provided clear diagnostic criteria for women. As a consequence, women are often ineligible for many benefits and services available to others diagnosed early on with AIDS, and they may be excluded from clinical trials.

Early epidemiological efforts largely viewed women as vectors of AIDS transmission to their offspring and male

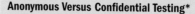

It's Your Health

Anonymous Versus Confidential Testing*

Anonymous testing: The person receives an identification number, provides no name or personal information, and may provide information for demographic use only. An identification number is used to receive test results.

Confidential testing: Test results are kept in confidence (not disclosed to others); however, the patient is identified and results are part of the patient's medical records. These records may be made available to certain people under certain conditions.

*Some facilities may offer both confidential and anonymous testing.

sexual partners. Early studies were limited to perinatal assessment efforts and surveys of prostitutes. As a consequence, women were not considered as victims of transmission from their male partners. The identification of "high-risk groups" (homosexual and bisexual men, intravenous drug users, hemophiliacs, prostitutes, inmates, and people from specific geographical areas) both stigmatized the members of these groups and denied risk among non-group members. Women are often unaware of the risks to themselves or others because they do not belong to these high-risk groups, even if they practice high-risk behaviors. Likewise, some women may not be aware of the high-risk behaviors or behavioral histories of their partners.

In recent years, HIV/AIDS research and program efforts have attempted to address the many social issues associated with the disease. Some public health research and service efforts are attempting to provide culturally competent HIV/AIDS prevention, information, and services. They face a formidable challenge; however, properly providing and tailoring resources for people who have been hit the hardest by HIV may be essential to reducing the burden of this disease.

Clinical Dimensions and Treatment Issues of AIDS

Transmission of HIV can occur through several routes:

- Sexual intercourse with an exchange of bodily fluids
- Injection with HIV-contaminated needles, syringes, blood, or other substances
- An HIV-positive woman infecting her fetus during pregnancy or childbirth
- An HIV-infected mother infecting her infant during breastfeeding

Diagnosis of HIV is extremely important both for early treatment and for prevention of further transmission. Persons with HIV are contagious whether or not they have symptoms. In fact, the month just after infection is generally one of the most infectious periods in the course of infection. Many tests attempt to detect HIV antibodies, which are found in blood and other bodily fluids of an infected person. The **enzyme-linked immunosorbent assay (ELISA)** is an HIV screening test that determines whether a person's serum contains antibodies to one or more HIV antigens. It is used for screening large samples of blood and as a preliminary screening test for individuals because of its low cost and fast results. The ELISA test is repeated if positive results are found. If a repeat ELISA also gives positive results, a confirmatory **Western blot test** should be performed. When used together, the two tests are highly accurate. Other tests, such as fluorescent antibody tests, polymerase chain reaction (PCR), the Single-Use Diagnostic System (rapid testing), and saliva and urine tests, may be used by some clinicians as well.

The ELISA test does not look for HIV itself, but rather for HIV antibodies—the body's unique immune response to HIV. The longer a woman waits after a risk to get tested, the more confidence she can place in a negative result. It takes about 25 days for the average person with HIV to develop detectable antibodies. An early negative HIV antibody test is not a guarantee against infection. Those at risk of HIV should have a repeat test at least three months after the initial test to confirm their results. HIV tests are available at local blood banks, AIDS research programs, and alternative test sites that have mechanisms in place to provide anonymous testing, confidential results, and pre-testing and post-testing counseling services. The FDA has approved four different rapid antibody tests for HIV. These tests have the advantages of offering testing at a lower cost and provide a patient with results on the same visit she got tested.[26]

Home testing kits purchased at drugstores are available for people who are reluctant to visit a health-care provider or have limited access to health-care facilities. A woman can collect her own blood sample through a finger prick; the sample is then mailed to a laboratory. She can then use an identification number to obtain anonymous results over the phone. After hearing her results, the caller can be connected to a counselor to discuss the meaning of the test.

Once infected with HIV, symptoms vary. Some women experience a temporary flulike illness one to two months

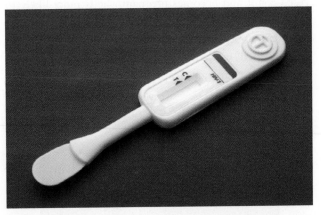

■ Home testing is an important option for those women who wish to be anonymous.

after exposure to the virus; these symptoms typically disappear on their own without treatment. A person may begin to experience symptoms 2 to 10 years after diagnosis depending on when during the course of infection diagnosis is made. These symptoms may include swollen lymph nodes, fatigue, recurring yeast infections, weight loss, and chronic diarrhea. Although studies suggest that gynecological symptoms are often the first signs of HIV infection in women, symptoms in women have only recently been included in the CDC criteria for diagnosis. When women seek treatment for these gynecological conditions, HIV testing may be delayed or avoided because it is not suspected. Potential indicators of HIV infection in women include gynecological infections such as candidiasis (yeast infection), PID, HPV, genital ulcers, HSV, pneumonia, and sepsis. When AIDS develops, opportunistic infections often begin to further break down the immune system.

Early treatment of HIV delays the onset of AIDS and can even reduce the virus to unmeasurable levels in the blood. Combination drug therapy has improved the quality of life for many people. AZT, also known as zidovudine, was the first anti-HIV drug approved in 1987. New types of drugs, including nucleoside analogs and protease inhibitors, are now used together as part of the "AIDS cocktail" or HAART (highly active antiretroviral therapy). HAART therapy usually consists of three medications that attack HIV in distinct ways and that are taken at the same time; this simultaneous "triple attack" helps prevent HIV, which mutates rapidly, from developing resistance to any one type of medication. These drugs still have significant limitations and side effects, however, and the search continues for more effective and more affordable treatment regimens.

Perinatal transmission of AIDS is a special concern for women because the majority of HIV-infected women are of reproductive age. If an HIV-infected woman has a low T-cell count and becomes pregnant, she is more likely to develop HIV-associated illness during pregnancy. Without treatment, approximately one-fourth of all babies born to HIV-infected mothers will be infected with the virus. Prompt treatment can greatly reduce the chance of trans-

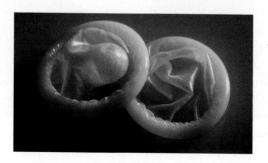

Joe had a long-term relationship with this girl, and they broke up last year. I used to worry about that relationship, but now I am more worried about the insignificant encounters he had after they broke up. He doesn't know anything about them, and neither do I. How do I evaluate my risk?

23-year-old woman

mission; perinatal transmission of HIV has decreased over the past 20 years, but unfortunately it continues to exist (**Figure 7.10**). In one study of HIV-infected women, HAART therapy regimens prevented perinatal HIV transmission among all women who were compliant with their treatment regimens.[27]

Informed Decision Making: Reproductive Tract Infections

When a woman elects to become sexually active, she assumes responsibility for her decision. This responsibility extends beyond the pregnancy protection arena to include STI protection. A strong knowledge base is the first step in STI protection. Every woman should have a thorough understanding of STI risk, symptoms to watch for, and prevention strategies. Prevention is especially important because many STIs are incurable.

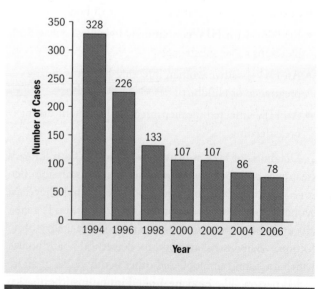

Figure 7.10

Reported HIV/AIDS cases in infants born to HIV-infected mothers, United States.

Source: Centers for Disease Control and Prevention. (2008). *HIV/AIDS Surveillance Report, 2006.*

Table 7.2 Some Sexual Activities and Their Relative Risk Levels

Activity	Level of Risk	Ways to Reduce Risk
Anal intercourse without a condom	High	Use a latex condom; only have sex with a mutually monogamous, tested partner
Vaginal intercourse without a condom	High	Use a latex condom; only have sex with a mutually monogamous, tested partner
Oral sex	High, though less risky than vaginal or anal intercourse for several STIs, including HIV	Use a latex condom for oral sex with a man or a dental dam or other moisture barrier for oral sex with a woman; only have sex with a mutually monogamous, tested partner
Mutual masturbation (hand-to-genital contact)	Very low, assuming no visible symptoms or cuts in the skin are present	Refrain from activity when there are symptoms or cuts in the skin
Kissing, no sores or broken skin	Very low; slight risk of oral herpes or syphilis infection	Refrain from kissing when possible symptoms are present
All sexual activities with a mutually monogamous partner who is free from infection	None, assuming partner is truly negative	Make sure partner has been tested for *all* STIs and is trustworthy
Abstaining from all sexual contact	None	

Apart from abstinence, the most reliable prevention strategy for reproductive tract infections is long-term mutual monogamy with a single partner. The most significant risk factor for any STI is the woman's partner(s). The risk of contracting an STI increases when a woman has more than one sex partner and when her partner has more than one sex partner. STIs should be considered a possibility whenever a woman is not in a strictly exclusive monogamous long-term relationship.

If there is any doubt about a partner's or one's own monogamy or HIV status, safer sex practices are important for any sexual relationship. Safer sex entails any form of sex in which semen, blood, or vaginal secretions are not passed from one person to another. Latex condoms with spermicide are the key ingredient of safer sex practices. Latex condoms must be used correctly each time a person has oral, anal, or vaginal intercourse. If a condom breaks or falls off, its protective effect is lost. Data consistently show that latex condoms, when used consistently and correctly, greatly reduce the chances of transmission of HIV and many other STIs. The risk of acquiring an STI increases with the number of partners a person has, but a person only needs to be exposed once to acquire an STI.

STIs are transmitted by sexual intimacy. Intimacy includes "traditional" sex (penis in vagina) and other forms of intimate skin-to-skin and mucous membrane-to-mucous membrane contact. These diseases can, therefore, be transmitted with oral or anal sex. STIs can be transmitted in both homosexual and heterosexual encounters, although many STIs are less common among lesbian women. Although the notion of safe sex is misleading, safer sex practices do exist that reduce the overall risk of acquiring an STI. **Table 7.2** provides a comparison of safer, risky, and dangerous sex practices.

Birth control choice influences STI risk. Consistent and correct use of latex condoms can reduce the risk of STI transmission.[17]

HIV and many other STIs are spread when blood or sexual fluids from one person get into the mucous membranes (areas of the body not covered by skin, such as the

It's Your Health

Questions for Women to Ask Potential Sex Partners

- What do you know about STIs, including HIV/AIDS?
- Have you ever suspected that you had an STI?
- Have any of your partners (or their partners) suspected that they were infected?
- Have you ever been tested for STIs? If so, when were you tested and what tests did you receive?
- Have you or a sex partner ever shared needles to inject drugs, even once?
- How many sex partners have you had?
- What kind of sexual activities did you engage in with previous partners?
- What do you know about your partner's (partners') sexual history?

interior of the vagina, the tip of the penis, or even cuts or nicks in the skin) of another person. Although latex condoms are effective at preventing fluid exchange, they probably provide less protection for STIs that have other modes of transmission. Herpes and HPV, for example, are spread by contact with symptoms or infected genital skin. Because a condom covers some but not all of the potentially infectious area, it is not a reliable means of protection against these STIs. Some practices are more risky for contracting some STIs than for others. A person is extremely unlikely to get HIV from receiving oral sex even without a condom, for example, but could easily get syphilis, an oral gonorrhea infection, or herpes in this way.

Consistent condom use can greatly reduce risk, but there are no guarantees; viruses located at sites other than the penis, such as the scrotum, anal region, vulva, or inner thighs, are not covered by condoms, and transmission from these sites can still occur.

Frank, honest communication before sexual intimacy is essential. Although it may be difficult to have an honest discussion about infections and previous risk behaviors, the price of not communicating can be high. Honest communication is a mark of personal maturity. If a potential partner is unable or unwilling to discuss infections and intimacy concerns, it may be an indication of other issues that merit evaluation before proceeding with sexual closeness. Sexual closeness should be avoided if either partner has any symptoms of infection or if there are any suspicions of infection. Delaying activity for a few days and having symptoms evaluated may prevent lifelong consequences. Because many people with STIs honestly do not know they are infected, many couples now see a clinician together for examination and STI testing before initiating a sexual relationship.

Talking about incurable STIs such as herpes and HPV is especially difficult. The timing of communication is im-

It's Your Health

Symptoms That May Suggest a Sexually Transmitted Infection and Warrant Clinical Evaluation

Unusual vaginal discharge or bleeding

Pain or burning with urination or bowel movements

Genital itching

Sores, warts, blisters, or growths in the genital area

Pain or bleeding associated with intercourse

Abdominal or back pain or tenderness

Severe menstrual cramping

Chills, fever, aches, malaise

portant—waiting until after sex to tell someone about a herpes infection may understandably upset a partner. But because of the stigma of the disease, a person with herpes may want to wait until some level of trust has been established before informing a potential sex partner. Being calm and knowledgeable about an infection also aids in communication. Many people are ignorant about the course of infection of STIs or the means by which they are spread. Open and frank discussion benefits both partners; studies have found that sharing a herpes diagnosis with a supportive spouse or lover and avoiding denial as a coping mechanism help people with herpes come to better and healthier terms with their infections.

I felt weird when Karen insisted that we go to the doctor together before we had sex. I guess I was afraid that one of us would have something. But we didn't and, you know, I think that our relationship is stronger because she insisted. I respect her for having the courage it took to do that. I wish that it had been my idea.

22-year-old man

■ Honest communication before sexual intimacy is essential for assessing risk behaviors and avoiding transmission of disease. Reprinted with permission from the American Social Health Association.

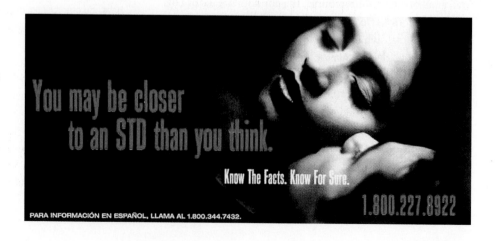

You may be closer to an STD than you think.

Know The Facts. Know For Sure.

1.800.227.8922

PARA INFORMACIÓN EN ESPAÑOL, LLAMA AL 1.800.344.7432.

Assessing Sexual Practices—Safety First for Sexual Health

Answer each of the following questions:

1. I avoid having multiple sex partners.   yes   no

2. I avoid having anonymous sex partners.   yes   no

3. I avoid having sex with someone who has symptoms of AIDS, is infected with HIV, or is at high risk of HIV.   yes   no

4. I avoid exchanging sex for money or drugs.   yes   no

5. Male partners use a latex condom with a spermicide.   yes   no

6. I avoid anal sex.   yes   no

7. I avoid sex with someone whom I don't know well.   yes   no

8. I avoid using intravenous drugs.   yes   no

9. I avoid sex with anyone who has genital sores or lesions.   yes   no

10. I take precautions to prevent unwanted pregnancy.   yes   no

If you answered any of these questions with a "no," it is important to reconsider the risks involved with your personal sex behaviors. You should also be tested for STIs and HIV/AIDS.

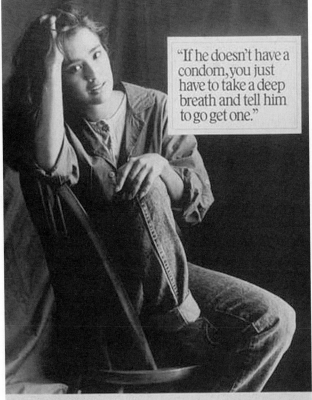

"If he doesn't have a condom, you just have to take a deep breath and tell him to go get one."

It's not the easiest thing in the world to say. But these days, you have to. If you're dating someone who doesn't like condoms, talk before having sex. Explain how you feel. Offer to help during the awkward moments. And if this doesn't work, ask yourself, is it worth the risk?

For more information on condoms and AIDS, call 1-800-342-AIDS for answers you can count on.

AMERICA RESPONDS TO AIDS

■ Latex condoms, although not a guarantee against HIV infection, are a key consideration in prevention of HIV transmission.

When to See a Clinician

STIs present special clinical challenges for women. As noted earlier, symptoms may be present, absent, or mistaken for other conditions. There are several critical times when a woman should seek assistance in evaluating a possible reproductive tract infection. If a woman suspects that she *may* have an infection, she should be evaluated. STIs can be accompanied by a spectrum of symptoms or no symptoms. Waiting for symptoms to go away is an exercise in futility, because although some symptoms may temporarily disappear, the disease may still be present, transmissible, and damaging.

If a partner has an infection or is suspicious of an infection, it is important to curtail sexual activity, and both individuals should seek clinical evaluation. Treating one partner and not the other often results in a "ping-pong" reinfection process. In addition, sharing one antibiotic prescription between two people usually means that neither partner receives adequate treatment and can contribute to

It's Your Health

If you or someone you know would like to get tested for STIs, but do not have a clinician or are embarrassed to meet with your current provider, you can contact your local health department or Planned Parenthood clinic. (Planned Parenthood's Web site [http://www.plannedparenthood.org] has a national database of testing facilities.) Be sure to ask what tests are included: Not all facilities test for all STIs.

antibiotic resistance. Using leftover antibiotics from previous infections is equally foolhardy because supplies are usually inappropriate and inadequate, and may serve merely to mask the symptoms, complicating an accurate diagnosis later. Sexual activity should be curtailed or condoms diligently used until both partners are certain of an STI cure.

Women are often embarrassed to mention their fears about STIs to a clinician. If there is a risk of infection, it is important to discuss this possibility. Although no woman wants to find out that she has an STI, it is always better to know than not to know: STIs can be spread and do serious biological damage even in the absence of symptoms, and all STIs are treatable, if not curable. Clinicians may not routinely test for STIs or look for them in a routine gynecological examination. If a woman knows she has an infectious condition such as HSV or HPV, she should disclose this to her clinician to reduce the likelihood of accidental transmission to the clinician. If oral or anal sex has been part of a woman's sexual experience, the clinician should be advised so that a comprehensive examination may be conducted for an accurate diagnosis. A clean bill of health from a gynecologist is not of much value if an undiagnosed gonococcal throat infection is present. Finally, it helps to be prepared. Writing down a list of questions to ask a clinician and practicing questions to ask with a friend beforehand are two strategies women can use to make sure they get all the information they need without making additional visits.

A physical examination for STIs is often like a routine gynecological examination, but it is not limited to the genital area. An examination of the mouth, throat, and lymph nodes usually precedes the genital examination. The genital examination is conducted in a lithotomy position, which requires that the woman lie on her back with her legs spread and positioned in stirrups. This position enables the health-care provider to examine the perineal area. The examination begins with a careful visual inspection by the clinician. A speculum is inserted into the vagina for an internal examination. The clinician then examines the vagina for discharge, odor, ulcerations, or in-

flammation. If a woman has douched before the visit, the clinician may not be able to diagnose the condition accurately. A bimanual examination follows the internal examination. (See Chapter 4 for details of the gynecological examination.) Any suspicious lesion in the perineal area is cultured, and a rectal culture is obtained if the woman has had anal intercourse.

Treatment Concerns

Treatment regimens for STIs vary according to the specific pathogen involved, severity of infection, location of infection, previous infections, and personal medical history. A woman should inform her clinician if she is taking any prescriptions or over-the-counter medications. Previous drug reactions also constitute important information, because any previous reaction to a drug ending in "cillin" is a contraindication to any other "cillin" drug. If a woman suspects that she may be pregnant, it is important to advise the clinician of that possibility as well. Some antibiotics should not be taken by pregnant women because they produce severe staining of the permanent teeth of the developing fetus or other side effects.

It is of paramount importance that prescribed medications be taken as recommended. If antibiotics are prescribed for 10 days, then they need to be taken for 10 days, even if symptoms dissipate earlier.

Several STIs require follow-up examinations to ensure that the treatment regimen was successful. Failure to comply with follow-up guidelines may result in unsuccessful treatment and continued disease transmission and damage. Because reproductive tract infections may cause abnormal Pap test findings, after an infection has cleared up, it is a good idea to have a Pap test repeated in 6 to 12 weeks. A reading at that time will give a more accurate report of the cervical status than one conducted during a period of inflammation.

■■■■

Summary

Reproductive tract infections, including STIs and HIV, can pose serious health threats to women. By understanding these conditions (**Table 7.3**) and making informed decisions about personal behaviors and health-seeking behaviors, women can significantly reduce their risk of exposure and the effects of disease sequelae. Personal responsibility and informed decision making are essential to the prevention and management of reproductive tract infections.

I don't know if I should be upset or not. Over spring break my boyfriend went skiing and he said he "slept around a little." So what should I do about protecting myself? I'm on the pill, but should we get tested or use a condom? I really am confused.

22-year-old woman

Table 7.3   Basic Information About the Major Sexually Transmitted Infections

AIDS (Acquired Immune Deficiency Syndrome)

Organism:	Viral—HIV (human immunodeficiency virus)
Transmission:	Blood or sexual fluids entering the body, usually through sexual intercourse, sharing needles, or from mother to child before or during birth
Symptoms:	Flu-like symptoms such as fever, weight loss, fatigue, and enlarged lymph nodes may appear and disappear shortly after infection; identifiable opportunistic infections may take years to appear.
Diagnosis:	AIDS diagnoses are made based on T-cell counts or the presence of opportunistic infections. HIV can be easily identified with antibody tests.
Treatment:	No treatment will cure AIDS or prevent HIV infection; antiviral medications, when used properly, can delay the onset of AIDS and improve quality of life.
Special Concerns for Women:	Increased reproductive health problems; risk to babies before and during birth can be dramatically reduced with treatment.
Potential Long-Term Consequences:	If AIDS goes untreated, opportunistic infections can cause grave illness or death.

Chlamydia

Organism:	Bacteria—*Chlamydia trachomatis*
Transmission:	Direct contact with infected mucosal membrane or sexual fluids
Symptoms:	Most women are asymptomatic; symptoms may include vaginal discharge and excessive urination, pelvic pain, fever, and nausea.
Diagnosis:	Urine tests or culture of symptoms or discharge; alternatively, a diagnosis may be made by examining symptoms and ruling out gonorrhea.
Treatment:	Antibiotics will stop infection but may not be able to repair damage from long-term infection.
Special Concerns for Women:	Pelvic inflammatory disease (*see PID*), possible co-infection with gonorrhea, reinfection with an untreated partner, perinatal (mother-to-child) transmission
Potential Long-Term Consequences:	Infertility, ectopic pregnancy, chronic pelvic pain, possibility of systemic infection

Gonorrhea

Organism:	Bacteria—*Neisseria gonorrhoeae*
Transmission:	Direct contact with infected mucosal membrane or sexual fluids
Symptoms:	Most women are asymptomatic; symptoms may include vaginal discharge and excessive urination, pelvic pain, fever, and nausea.
Diagnosis:	Urine tests or culture of discharge or the infected area
Treatment:	Antibiotics will stop infection but may not be able to repair damage from long-term infection.
Special Concerns for Women:	Pelvic inflammatory disease (*see PID*), possible co-infection with chlamydia, reinfection with an untreated partner, perinatal (mother-to-child) transmission
Potential Long-Term Consequences:	Infertility, ectopic pregnancy, chronic pelvic pain, possibility of systemic infection

Hepatitis B (HBV)

Organism:	Virus—hepatitis B virus
Transmission:	Entrance of blood or sexual fluids into the body; most cases occur through unprotected sexual contact or shared needles.

(continues)

Table 7.3   Basic Information About the Major Sexually Transmitted Infections (continued)

Hepatitis B (HBV) (continued)

Symptoms:	Often asymptomatic; symptoms include nausea, fever, dark urine, jaundice (yellowing of the skin and eyes), and abdominal discomfort.
Diagnosis:	Blood tests to identify virus or antibodies; liver tests and symptoms may also be used in diagnosis.
Treatment:	No cure for hepatitis B exists, but antiviral medications may help in some chronic cases; a three-shot vaccine will prevent hepatitis B infection.
Special Concerns for Women:	Perinatal transmission
Possible Long-Term Consequences:	Possible liver disease or liver cancer in chronic cases; most infections eventually resolve on their own.

Herpes Simplex Virus (HSV)

Organism:	Virus—herpes simplex (two types—1 and 2)
Transmission:	Direct contact with symptoms; contact with the infected area carries a low but real risk even without symptoms.
Symptoms:	Possibly painful sores, blisters, or rashes on the genital area, rectum, or mouth that appear and disappear periodically; women are often asymptomatic or have symptoms in the cervical area that go unnoticed.
Diagnosis:	Examination or culture of symptoms; blood tests can identify herpes antibodies.
Treatment:	No cure or vaccine available; three antiviral medications (acyclovir, Famvir, and valacyclovir) can reduce duration or number of outbreaks.
Special Concerns for Women:	Possible perinatal transmission, especially if herpes infection takes place during pregnancy; herpes sores may increase the likelihood of receiving HIV if exposed.
Possible Long-Term Consequences:	Rare in otherwise healthy adults; severity, duration, and frequency of symptoms usually diminish over time.

HPV (Human Papillomavirus)

Organism:	Virus—human papillomavirus (almost 100 strains, about a dozen of which are sexually transmitted)
Transmission:	Genital skin-to-genital skin contact
Symptoms:	Some kinds of HPV can cause warts to appear on the external genital or anal areas; others may cause abnormal cell growth in the cervix.
Diagnosis:	Warts may be diagnosed by physical examination; cervical dysplasia may be diagnosed with biopsy; DNA testing of the virus can identify the presence of HPV.
Treatment:	Treatment for genital warts revolves around removing symptoms, not eliminating the virus, and consists of topical caustic agents, electrocautery, cryotherapy, and laser surgery; abnormal cell changes in the cervix may be treated by cryotherapy, loop electrosurgical excision (LEEP), cone biopsy, or laser surgery.
Special Concerns for Women:	Cervical changes, if untreated, may develop into cervical cancer; warts may interfere with pregnancy in rare cases.
Possible Long-Term Consequences:	Cervical growths can lead to cervical cancer if undiagnosed or untreated; most cases of HPV go away on their own eventually.

Table 7.3 Basic Information About the Major Sexually Transmitted Infections (continued)

Pelvic Inflammatory Disease (PID)

Organism:	Bacteria—usually *Chlamydia trachomatis* (chlamydia) or *Neisseria gonorrhoeae* (gonorrhea)
Transmission:	PID itself is not transmitted but usually develops as a complication of gonorrhea or chlamydia.
Symptoms:	Cases may be asymptomatic; abdominal pain or pain during intercourse, unusual vaginal discharge or bleeding, fever, and nausea.
Diagnosis:	Clinical evaluation based on symptoms and possible presence of a causative bacterial agent
Treatment:	Antibiotics; surgery may be necessary in advanced cases.
Special Concerns for Women:	Reinfection of bacterial infection from untreated or undertreated partners; possible perinatal transmission of bacterial agent
Possible Long-Term Consequences:	Infertility, ectopic pregnancy, recurrent infection, chronic pelvic pain

Syphilis

Organism:	Bacteria—*Treponema pallidum*
Transmission:	Skin-to-skin contact with infected area or symptoms; perinatal (mother-to-child)
Symptoms:	Primary stage: painless sore (chancre)
	Secondary stage: rash, hair loss, enlarged lymph nodes
	Tertiary stage: systemic damage
Diagnosis:	Blood tests; microscopic verification of organism; examination of symptoms
Treatment:	Antibiotics will stop infection but cannot undo systemic damage.
Special Concerns for Women:	Perinatal transmission, possible reinfection from untreated or undertreated partners, sores may increase likelihood of receiving HIV if exposed.
Potential Long-Term Consequences:	Untreated infections can cause permanent damage to all major body systems or even death.

Trichomoniasis

Organism:	Single-celled protozoan—*Trichomonas vaginalis*
Transmission:	Direct sexual contact, less likely through contaminated wet objects (towels, swimming suits)
Symptoms:	Many women and most men are asymptomatic; symptoms may include white or greenish yellow discharge, vaginal itching, or painful urination.
Diagnosis:	Examination of symptoms or culture of infected area
Treatment:	Oral antibiotics
Special Concerns for Women:	Reinfection from untreated or undertreated partners
Possible Long-Term Consequences:	Rare for otherwise healthy women

■■■■
Topics for Discussion

1. STIs are biologically "sexist." What does this mean?
2. How do cultural and emotional dimensions complicate STI public health and educational efforts?
3. Why is reinfection so common with some bacterial STIs?
4. Imagine that you are in a relationship and that you have an infection with HSV or HPV. How and when would you begin discussing your infection? How would you feel if the situation were reversed?
5. Describe three productive and three nonproductive ways to inquire about a person's past.
6. In spite of the knowledge base about AIDS, people still report a strong fear of AIDS. Why? What are some of the myths associated with AIDS?
7. What should a woman do upon learning of a positive AIDS antibody test?
8. HIV is similar to HSV and HPV in that it is a sexually transmitted virus that has no cure. How is it different?
9. What would you tell a friend or loved one who suspected that she might have an STI but was afraid to get tested?
10. Balancing STI risk reduction with flexibility and intimacy in sexual relationships is a difficult task for many people. How do you balance these two needs? Are these two needs always in opposition to each other?

■■■■
Web Sites

AIDS Education Global Information System:
http://www.aegis.com

American Social Health Association:
http://www.ashastd.org

Centers for Disease Control, Division of STIs:
http://www.cdc.gov/STI

EngenderHealth: http://www.engenderhealth.org

Hepatitis Foundation International: http://www.hepfi.org

HIVandHepatitis.com: http://www.hepatitisandhiv.com

International Herpes Alliance:
http://www.herpesalliance.org

Planned Parenthood: http://www.plannedparenthood.org

Sexuality Information and Education Council of the
United States: http://www.siecus.org

The Body: The Complete HIV/AIDS Resource:
http://www.thebody.com

UNAIDS: http://www.unaids.org

Profiles of Remarkable Women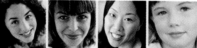

Felicia Hance Stewart, M.D. (1943–2006)

Felicia Hance Stewart was an obstetrician/gynecologist who was also a distinguished clinician and researcher.

Following her time as a practicing physician, Stewart served as Deputy Assistant Secretary for Population Affairs in the Department of Health and Human Services, making her the most senior official in the United States responsible for domestic and international policies on family planning and population issues. In this position, she had direct responsibility for management of the National Family Planning Program (Title X) and the Adolescent Family Life Program (Title XX).

In 1996, Stewart was appointed the Director of Reproductive Health Programs for the Henry J. Kaiser Family Foundation, where she focused on improving services for low-income women and preventing unintended pregnancy. In 1999, she joined the Center for Reproductive Health Research and Policy at the University of California, San Francisco. As a Co-Director of the Center, Stewart conducted a wide range of U.S. and international projects that spanned the disciplines of contraception, abortion, and sexually transmitted diseases.

Stewart served as the principal investigator on many research projects and published numerous articles and textbooks on contraception and family planning. She contributed greatly to issues concerning reproductive health and, consequently, served on many national scientific and professional advisory and review committees. Stewart authored *Understanding Your Body: The Concerned Woman's Guide to Gynecology and Health*, a nontechnical reference book, and co-authored *Contraceptive Technology*, a professional reference for family planning. Stewart may be most remembered for her leading role in the research establishing that the emergency contraceptive known as Plan B is both safe and effective when sold without a physician's prescription. Her published research led to the availability of over-the-counter Plan B in a number of states, including California.

References

1. Hanson, J., Ponser, S., Hassig, S., & Farley, T. (2005). Assessment of sexually transmitted diseases as risk factor for HIV seroconversion in a New Orleans sexually transmitted disease clinic, 1990–1998. *Annals of Epidemiology* 15(1): 13–20.

2. Centers for Disease Control and Prevention. (2002). Sexually transmitted disease treatment guidelines. *Morbidity and Mortality Weekly Report* 51: 1–80.

3. Centers for Disease Control and Prevention. (2008). *National Representative CDC Study Finds 1 in 4 Teenage Girls Has a Sexually Transmitted Disease*. Available at: http://www.cdc.gov/stdconference/2008/media/release-11march2008.htm.

4. Rietmejer, C., Van Bemmelen, R., Judson, F., & Douglas, J. (2002). Incidence and repeat infection rates of *Chlamydia trachomatis* infections among male and female patients in an STD clinic: implications for screening and rescreening. *Sexually Transmitted Diseases* 29: 65–72.

5. Centers for Disease Control and Prevention. (2008). *Sexually Transmitted Disease Surveillance, 2006*. Available at: http://www.cdc.gov/std/stats/toc2006.htm.

6. Chesson, H., Blandford, J., Thomas, L., Gifte, G., & Irwin, K. (2004). The estimated direct medical costs of sexually transmitted disease among American youth, 2000. *Perspectives on Sexual and Reproductive Health* 36(1): 11–19.

7. Joint U.N. Programme on HIV/AIDS. (2007). *Call to Intensify Prevention*. Available at: http://www.unaids.org/en/KnowledgeCentre/Resources/FeatureStories/archive/2007/20070702_HIVPrevention.asp.

8. Adderley-Kelly, B., & Stephens, E. (2005). Chlamydia—a major threat to adolescents and young adults. *Association of Black Nursing Faculty* May/June: 52–55.

9. Rein, D., Kassler, W., Irwin, K., & Rabiee, L. (2000). Direct medical cost of pelvic inflammatory disease and its sequelae: decreasing but still substantial. *Obstetrics and Gynecology* 95: 397–402.

10. Schwebke, J., & Desmond, R. (2005). Risk factors for bacterial vaginosis in women at high risk for sexually transmitted diseases. *Sexually Transmitted Diseases* 32(11): 654–658.

11. Myer, L., Kuhn, L., Stein, Z., Wright, T., & Denny, L. (2005). Intravaginal practices, bacterial vaginosis, and women's susceptibility to HIV infection: epidemiological evidence and biological mechanisms. *Lancet Infectious Diseases* 5(12): 786–794.

12. Klebanoff, M., Schwebke, J., Zhang, J., et al. (2004). Vulvo-vaginal symptoms in women with bacterial vaginosis. *Obstetrics and Gynecology* 104: 267.

13. Zhang, J., Hatch, M., Zhang, D., et al. (2004). Frequency of douching and risk of bacterial vaginosis in African-American women. *Obstetrics and Gynecology* 104: 756–760.

14. Schiffman, M., & Castle, P. (2005). The promise of global cervical-cancer prevention. *New England Journal of Medicine* 353(20): 2101–2104.

15. Ellison, R. (2006). Prevalence of herpes simplex decreasing in the U.S. *Journal Watch Infectious Diseases.*

16. Corey, L., Wald, A., Patel, R., et al. (2004). Once-daily valacyclovir to reduce the risk of transmission of genital herpes. *New England Journal of Medicine* 350: 11–20.

17. Holmes, K., Levine, R., & Weaver, M. (2004). Effectiveness of condoms in preventing sexually transmitted diseases. *Bulletin of the World Health Organization* 82(6): 454–461.

18. Wasley, A., Grytdal, S., & Gallagher, K. (2008). *Surveillance for Acute Viral Hepatitis—United States, 2006*. Atlanta: CDC.

19. Centers for Disease Control and Prevention. (2008). *National Hepatitis C Prevention Strategy*. Available at: http://www.cdc.gov/hepatitis/HCV/strategy/NathepCprevStrategy.htm.

20. Centers for Disease Control and Prevention. (2008). *Hepatitis C Fact Sheet*. Available at: http://www.cdc.gov/hepatitis/HepatitisC.htm.

21. Centers for Disease Control and Prevention. (2008). *HIV/AIDS Surveillance Report, 2006*. Available at: http://www.cdc.gov/hiv/topics/surveillance/resources/reports/index.htm.

22. Centers for Disease Control and Prevention. (2008). *New Technology Reveals Higher Number of New HIV Infections in the United States Than Previously Known*. Available at: http://www.cdc.gov/media/pressrel/2008/r080803.htm.

23. HIV outbreak began decades earlier than thought. (October 1, 2008). *Washington Post*. Available at: http://www.washingtonpost.com/wp-dyn/content/article/2008/10/01/AR2008100101660.html.

24. Joint U.N. Programme on AIDS. (2008). *2008 Report on the Global AIDS Epidemic*. Available at: http://

www.unaids.org/en/KnowledgeCentre/HIVData/ GlobalReport/2008/2008_Global_report.asp.

25. Centers for Disease Control and Prevention. (2007). Deaths: Leading causes for 2004. *National Vital Statistics Reports* 56(5).

26. Greenwald, J., Burstein, G., Pincus, J., & Branson, B. (2006). A rapid review of rapid HIV antibody test. *Current Infectious Disease Reports* 8: 125–131.

27. Bunders, M., Bekker, V., Scherpbier, H., et al. (2005). Haematological parameters of HIV-1 uninfected infants born to HIV-1 infected mothers. *Acta Paediatrica* 94(11): 1571–1577.

28. Centers for Disease Control and Prevention. (2001). *Fact Sheet for Public Health Personnel: Male Latex Condoms*. Available at: http://www.cdc.gov/nchstp/od/ condoms.pdf.

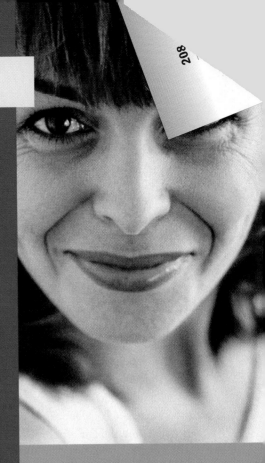

Chapter Eight

Menopause and Hormone Replacement Therapy

Chapter Objectives

On completion of this chapter, the student should be able to discuss:

1. The basic demographic aging trends in the United States.

2. The definition of menopause and the different stages that women go through before, during, and after menopause.

3. The ways in which cultural and societal attitudes about aging have influenced attitudes about menopause.

4. The positive effects that menopause can have in women's lives.

5. The basic biological sequence of events associated with menopause.

6. Health effects associated with menopause.

7. Hormone replacement therapy (HRT) as an option for menopause management.

8. Benefits of HRT for relieving symptoms associated with menopause.

9. Cardiovascular, osteoporotic, and neurological issues associated with HRT.

10. Other methods for managing menopause.

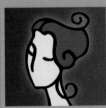

womenshealth.jbpub.com

Women's Health Online is a great source for supplementary women's health information for both students and instructors. Visit

http://womenshealth.jbpub.com

to find a variety of useful tools for learning, thinking, and teaching.

Introduction

Women, as they reach midlife, experience menopause, the end of their menstrual cycles. This natural life event brings both physical and emotional changes. Menopause, a topic that was once not discussed in public, is now recognized as an important topic of research and an issue of women's health. Nevertheless, millions of women continue to lack basic information about menopause, its effects on the body, and the potential benefits and drawbacks to hormone replacement therapy (HRT) and other forms of treatment.

As the average age of the population in the United States continues to increase (see **Figure 8.1**), a growing proportion of women will have experienced, or will be experiencing, menopause. In 2007, more than 22 million women were between the ages of 45 and 54, the age group at which menopause most often occurs.[1] This chapter reviews naturally and surgically induced menopause, the health effects of menopause, options for managing menopause, and the latest information about HRT.

Perspectives on Menopause

It was not until the twentieth century that the life expectancy of U.S. women reached a point where most women lived much beyond menopause; today most women will live a third or more of their lives postmenopausally. The medical and public health communities have begun to study menopause, but media coverage and public discussion of the emerging research have often been misunderstood or exaggerated.

In the United States, where society values youthful behaviors and appearance in women, menopause has often been viewed as a negative event. This trend is not universal: In many Asian countries, for example, women traditionally gain respect and influence, often becoming the head of the household, as they reach middle age. Menopause has been perceived in the United States as a difficult time for women, during which they experience uncontrollable moodiness, irritability, and depression. In the 1800s and early 1900s, popular myths and stereotypes, often encouraged by the medical community in the United States, portrayed menopause as a tragedy that resulted in hypochondria, hysteria, and irritability. This view implied that solace to these conditions could be found only in a physician's office with pharmacological remedies or surgical intervention. In the 1940s and 1950s, treatment for menopause often focused on psychiatric conditions of depression and melancholy. The menopausal woman was

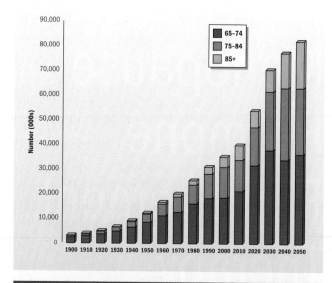

Figure 8.1

Older population by age: 1900–2050.

Source: U.S. Bureau of the Census. Tables 42 and 45; Data for 1990 from 1990 Census of Population and Housing, Series CPH-L-74, Modified and Actual Age, Sex, Race, and Hispanic Origin Data. The 2000 data are from the 2000 Census. The figures for 2010 to 2050 are from NP-D1-A Census Projections issued January 13, 2000.

portrayed as a burden to herself, to her family, and if she was married, to her suffering husband. In subsequent decades, menopause was examined as a "disease" because clinical concern focused on women reporting symptoms and seeking medical intervention.

Now menopause is understood as a process of normal change. Open discussions about sexuality and life issues have allowed women to talk about menopause and aging without fear, embarrassment, or stigmatization. Many women, in contrast to the myths, either welcome or do not fear menopause. The cessation of menses frees them from contraception concerns, in some cases leading to increased sexual satisfaction. Others appreciate the freedom from menstrual periods, which may have been inconvenient or uncomfortable. Menopause may be a time of fewer obligations accompanied by increased opportunities in the workforce. This experience can be inviting and invigorating for women who are seeking added dimensions in their personal and professional lives. For some, this life stage is often more flexible in terms of leisure time and financial resources, increasing the opportunities for new forms of activity and self-expression. For others, it is merely the continuation of intense work, with many women taking on additional childcare responsibilities for grandchildren. In a study by the North American Menopause Society, more

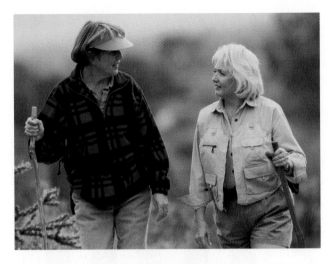

■ Women today are more open in their discussions about all aspects of their sexual well-being, including menopause.

I was well into my menopause before I realized what was happening. My symptoms were so minor and rather vague. I didn't understand all the hype about symptoms.

50-year-old woman

than half of postmenopausal women reported being happier and more fulfilled in their postmenopausal years as compared with earlier years.[2]

Menopause

Also known as the climacterium or "change of life," menopause marks the end of menstruation and childbearing capability. **Perimenopause** is the stage immediately before menopause, in which physical changes begin to accelerate and women are most likely to experience perceptible physical changes due to drops in hormone production. A woman is considered to be in menopause when she has gone through 12 months without menstruation. **Postmenopause** refers to life after the final menstrual period.

Most women enter and complete menopause between the ages of 45 and 55. Like the age of onset of a girl's first period, the age of onset of menopause varies widely. The average age of natural menopause—defined as one year without a menstrual period—is 51, and by age 58, 99% of women are postmenopausal.[3] Many factors influence the age at which a woman has her last period. Family history is one such factor. Increased body mass index and history of more than one pregnancy are linked to later menopause, whereas smoking and never being pregnant are related to earlier onset. Smokers generally experience menopause about two years earlier than nonsmoking women.

Natural Menopause

Natural menopause occurs when the ovaries begin to fail to respond to the luteinizing and follicle-stimulating hormones that are produced in the anterior pituitary, which is under the control of the hypothalamus. Although these hormones are still secreted into the bloodstream, the ovaries do not produce **estrogen** and **progesterone** in response. As a result, ovulation becomes somewhat erratic. The mechanisms underlying these changes are not well understood. Whatever the reasons, a woman beginning menopause will have more luteinizing and follicle-stimulating hormones present in the bloodstream and less estrogen and progesterone than she had during her regular cycling. For most women, menopause lasts from a few months to two or three years. Pregnancy remains a possibility because ovulation may occur in sporadic intervals during this time. Menopause is considered complete once monthly periods have ceased altogether for at least 12 months.

Generally in a woman's early to mid-forties—two to eight years before actual menopause—her menstrual cycle begins changing. The level of estrogen produced by the ovaries decreases, ovulation stops or becomes irregular, and the pattern of menstrual cycling changes. Although the pattern is not consistent for all women, initially the change may be characterized by heavier, more frequent periods, which later become less heavy and less frequent. Lack of ovulation may cause some light bleeding or spotting between periods.

After menopause, women continue to produce estrogen, but far less is manufactured in the ovaries. Most postmenopausal estrogen is produced through a process in which the adrenal gland makes precursors of estrogen that are converted by stored fat to estrogen. Far less estrogen, however, is produced in this manner than was produced in the ovaries before menopause.

Surgically Induced Menopause

Hysterectomies, or the surgical removal of the uterus, are the second most frequently performed procedure, after cesarean sections, on women of reproductive age in the United States.[4] Hysterectomies are performed for certain reproductive cancers and for other conditions. Hysterectomy performed with the removal of both ovaries and the fallopian tubes, known as a **total hysterectomy** and **bilateral salpingo-oophorectomy**, has become increasingly common (**Figure 8.2**). When a woman's ovaries are surgically removed, a more abrupt and earlier menopause results. The pituitary gland continues to produce luteinizing and follicle-stimulating hormones, but the ovaries are not present to respond with ovulation. Estrogen and progesterone are no longer produced at the same level as prior to surgery because of the absence of the ovaries. Although the adrenal glands still produce these hormones, the levels are considerably lower without the ovarian production. Studies have found that women who have had both ovaries removed before the onset of menopause experience more severe menopausal symptoms, and possibly an increased incidence of cardiovascular morbidity and mortality, than women who experience a natural menopause.[5–7]

Approximately 600,000 hysterectomies are performed annually in the country, and approximately 20 million U.S. women have had a hysterectomy.[8] More than 25% of all women will have undergone a hysterectomy before they reach the age of 60.[9] This high prevalence has generated significant controversy regarding the risks and benefits of the procedure. The hysterectomy controversy is further fueled, as shown in **Figure 8.3**, by the national geographical variance that is present in the distribution of hysterectomy procedures.

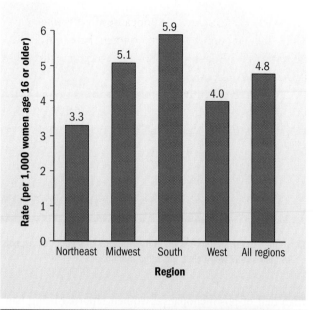

Figure 8.3

Hysterectomy rates, by geographic region: United States.

Source: Wu, J. et al. (2007). Hysterectomy rates in the United States, 2003.

Figure 8.2

Four types of hysterectomy.

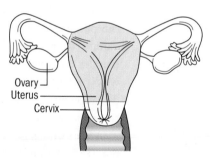

Partial hysterectomy: only the uterus is removed.

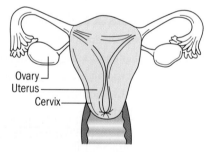

Total hysterectomy: both the uterus and cervix are removed.

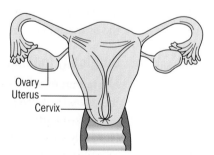

Total hysterectomy with bilateral salpingo-oophorectomy: both ovaries, the fallopian tubes, the uterus, and the cervix are removed.

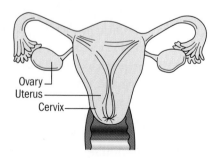

Radical hysterectomy: both ovaries, the fallopian tubes, the uterus, the cervix, and the lymph nodes are removed.

Health Effects of Menopause

Hormonal changes during menopause affect women physically and emotionally. Many women have only a few symptoms, while others experience everything from hot flashes to depression.

The most frequently reported physical symptom is the vascular response or instability known as **hot flashes** or hot flushes. Hot flashes are generally described as uncomfortable sensations of internally generated heat, beginning in the chest and moving to the neck and head, or spreading throughout the body. Increased heart rate and finger temperature, shallow breathing, and sweating followed by chills are all common during hot flashes. Hot flashes may begin during perimenopause, before a woman has stopped menstruating, and they may continue for several years after menopause. Hot flashes can be an early and acute sign of estrogen deficiency.

Despite some commonalities, menopause-related symptoms vary greatly among women.[10]

- Roughly 85% of women have at least one or more symptoms. Of these women, about 10% will have symptoms severe enough to warrant a visit to their physician.

- At least 40% of women complain of hot flashes.

- As many as 29% of women experience some depression.

- As many as 45% of women experience some sleep disturbances, with more disturbances occurring in the later stages of menopause.

- Many women appear to suffer from some sexual dysfunction, although this seems to be correlated with hormonal changes throughout the stages of menopause.

- Vaginal dryness, which increases as menopause progresses, is a common complaint among women.[10]

I was only 42 when I had my hysterectomy. Within two days, I discovered what "night sweats" were and I thought I would never survive the hot flashes. Thank goodness for hormone replacement therapy. As soon as I was put on estrogen, life became wonderful again. I am now 57, and every day I thank that little pill.

57-year-old woman

The symptoms also vary depending on the woman's cultural background. African American women often present with menopausal symptoms earlier than do white women, while Asian American women seem to have the fewest symptoms. Hispanic women appear to have more mood changes, fatigue, and vaginal dryness compared to white women.[11]

However, it is often difficult for women to directly associate any or all of these symptoms with menopause. Often, factors such as aging, family life, health issues, work and home stresses, and others contribute to the process.

Hot flashes often occur at night, resulting in sleep disruption, and therefore they are often credited with much of the insomnia associated with menopause. Sleep disturbances increase for many women in their forties and plateau during a woman's late fifties.[12] Many women find relief from hot flashes by changing their diets, reducing room temperatures, and wearing light layered clothing; 25% of women experience enough discomfort to seek medical attention.[13]

Thinning of the vaginal lining, known as **vaginal atrophy**, is another physical symptom that occurs with some frequency following menopause. As estrogen levels decline, layers of the vaginal surface become drier and more sensitive. The vaginal wall becomes thinner, less elastic, and more vulnerable to infection. Some women experience pain or burning during intercourse, vaginal discharge, and more frequent vaginal infections. In addition, some may experience atrophy of the urinary tract. Diminished muscle tone may result in urinary incontinence. Some women also experience an increase in urinary tract infections. As many as one-third of women age 50 or older experience vaginal or urinary tract problems.[14] Physiological changes that affect the vaginal tract may affect a woman's sexual response as well. For example, lack of vaginal lubricant may affect sexual arousal. A change in hormone levels—specifically androgen production—may diminish libido.

Psychiatric syndromes have been linked to reproductive endocrine system changes at various stages of life. These include postpartum psychosis and depression, premenstrual syndrome, post-hysterectomy depression, and menopausal psychiatric syndromes. Much of the current information on these conditions is based on myths, unwarranted assumptions, and conclusions derived from methodically flawed studies. Perimenopausal changes in mental wellness and cognitive function are not well defined and remain an area of extensive research and debate. As with the physical symptoms associated with menopause, most women have few, if any, symptoms of psychological disturbances; most of the women who do experience these problems feel that these symptoms are manageable.[14]

Some women report irritability, mood swings, depression, and anxiety during menopause. These emotional changes may be due to the physical changes occurring in the body, but they also may be highly influenced by traditional, cultural, and social expectations of a woman's worth expressed in relation to her reproductive capabilities. Significant psychosocial changes often happen during the midlife transition, such as children leaving home, which eliminates some women's view of their primary role as mother and forces them to reevaluate their positions in life. Medication or counseling may help women who experience severe symptoms. Estrogen has been correlated with a positive effect on mood and overall sense of well-being, and is believed to be important for memory and mental functioning. As with all hormone-related issues, sensitivity and validation by a woman's physician is an important component of any treatment.

Other changes associated with menopause include increased weight, breast changes, changes in hair growth, and changes in skin. As estrogen levels decrease during menopause, a rapid loss of collagen occurs, causing the skin to become thinner and less elastic. The cycling levels of hormones also may cause a change in the prevalence or intensity of headaches. Women with a history of migraines during the menstrual period may find that their headaches worsen during perimenopause.

Long-Term Effects

Cardiovascular disease is the leading cause of death in women (see Chapter 10). Its incidence, which begins to rise in the perimenopausal years, continues to increase after menopause. Evidence shows that high levels of **HDL (high-density lipoprotein) cholesterol** and low levels of **LDL (low-density lipoprotein) cholesterol** are protective against the development of atherosclerosis. Research has also shown that the decrease in estrogen as a result of natural and surgical menopause is associated with changes in serum lipid profiles (blood cholesterol levels), such as a decline in HDL levels and an increase in LDL levels. These serum cholesterol changes may be factors in a woman's increased risk of developing postmenopausal cardiovascular disease.[15]

Another serious concern of many postmenopausal women is the development of **osteoporosis**, the loss of bone mass or bone density in which bones become brittle and more likely to fracture, or **osteopenia**, a related but less severe condition (see Chapter 11). The spine may also lose flexibility and begin to curve. Osteoporosis is a major problem for many elderly women, and falls resulting from or leading to bone fractures constitute a leading health problem. Osteoporosis affects more than 30 million U.S. women and causes approximately 300,000 hip fractures every year.[16] Estrogen deficiency is an important factor in bone loss, with approximately 20% of bone loss occurring within five to seven years of a woman reaching menopause.[15]

The prevalence of reduced bone density in older women varies by race and ethnicity. Low bone density is most common among non-Hispanic white women (17% with osteoporosis and 42% with osteopenia), less common among Mexican American women (12% with osteoporosis and 37% with osteopenia), and least common in non-Hispanic black women (8% with osteoporosis and 28% with osteopenia).[17] White and Asian American women have the highest incidence of low bone density, while women who smoke in all races have higher than average incidence and prevalence.

Estrogen loss that occurs with menopause may be a factor in the development of **Alzheimer's disease**, another disease associated with aging. Alzheimer's disease involves a slow, progressive loss of mental function caused by a neurodegenerative process in the brain (see Chapter 11). As the leading cause of lost independence and institutionalization, it is a major issue for older women for two reasons. First, women live longer than men and are therefore more likely to suffer from the disease. Second, Alzheimer's disease presents itself earlier in women than in men.

Menopause Management

The question of whether menopause should be treated, and if so, how, is one of the most controversial and poorly understood topics in modern women's health. Some experts are concerned that menopause, a natural life process, is often viewed as a condition to be "fixed" with medical treatment. Many of these experts correctly point out that lifestyle factors can be at least as effective for reducing unwanted symptoms of menopause, while also improving overall health. Regular exercise; avoiding smoking; a balanced, healthful diet; a thorough, honest examination of one's position in life; and, if warranted, counseling, allow women to take an active role in maintaining health, rather than relying on prescribed medications. Women can also take actions to avoid specific symptoms; for example, wearing less or lowering the temperature to deal with hot flashes, or reducing stress and eliminating caffeine to cope with insomnia.

Despite these objections, hormone replacement therapy (HRT) undeniably provides relief for millions of women. HRT comes in many different forms. It provides relief from many symptoms, yet can cause side effects of its own. Media coverage of HRT has often been one-sided one way or another, but the reality is that for most women, HRT plays only a small role in preventing or promoting disease. Learning about the advantages and disadvantages of HRT from unbiased sources and one's own health-care provider are two key steps women can take to decide if or in what way HRT is right for them.

Hormone Replacement Therapy

Hormone replacement therapy (HRT), also sometimes called hormone therapy, consists of medications that boost the levels of specific **hormones** in the body. HRT does not "cure" any disease; rather, HRT is usually used to reduce symptoms associated with hormone changes that result from menopause. Women most often take HRT during menopause and perimenopause. Physicians began prescribing HRT in the 1960s to treat symptoms of menopause such as hot flashes and vaginal dryness. Despite recent controversies, the HRT market continues to grow. From 1998 to 2007, the global market for HRT grew from $2.5 billion to $9 billion a year.[18,19] Women spend $2 billion each year on HRT in the United States.[19]

During perimenopause and menopause the ovaries shrink, and their production of estrogen and progesterone becomes lower and then stops altogether. This drop causes many of the symptoms associated with menopause. HRT increases hormones to their premenopausal levels. Early data indicated that HRT might not only make menopausal women feel better, but also improve death and disability from heart disease, osteoporosis, and certain cancers. Over the last decade, however, several large-scale studies have found that HRT can actually increase the risk for some diseases for some women, but fear and sensational coverage of these studies have often exaggerated these risks. HRT typically consists of one of three hormone combinations[3]:

- *Estrogen alone (ERT)*, which is currently prescribed to women who have had a hysterectomy.

- *Estrogen together with progesterone or progestin*, a synthetic version of progesterone. Early research found that estrogen alone could increase the risk of uterine cancer. Progesterone and progestin protect against the overgrowth of cells in the uterus that can occur if estrogen is given alone. This is the most common form of HRT used today.

- *Estrogen, progesterone, and testosterone together* is usually prescribed for women who experience a reduced sexual drive after menopause.[20]

Hormones can be taken in a variety of preparations, routes of administration, and dosages (see **Table 8.1**). HRT can be given orally, as a vaginal cream or ring inserted into the vagina, or through skin patches (transdermally). Oral preparations are prescribed most frequently. Women can take HRT daily, or only on certain days of the month.[3] The ideal regimen for every woman will depend on her own symptoms, risks, and feelings, so flexibility and discussion with a health-care provider are key to determining the correct dose and form of HRT for each individual. Vaginal creams containing estrogen, for example, can help women whose only symptom is vaginal dryness, but they do not appear to provide other benefits, such as relief from hot flashes. Transdermal application of HRT can be beneficial for women whose livers respond to oral doses of estrogen by deactivating it with enzymes that raise triglycerides, which contribute to heart disease, but oral doses of estrogen increase levels of HDL cholesterol, the "good" cholesterol, for some women.

A class of drugs called **selective estrogen receptor modulators (SERMs)**, which are often used to treat breast cancer, is also being investigated for use in managing menopause. Sometimes called "designer estrogens," SERMs were made to provide the beneficial effects of estrogen while eliminating the hormone's undesirable effects. Trial results of one new SERM drug indicate that it may be able to provide relief from hot flashes and insomnia without increasing breast tenderness, a common complaint associated with traditional HRT.[19] The results of the Women's Health Initiative, which will end in 2010, will provide

Table 8.1	**Types of HRT**

Oral preparation
- Natural estrogen
- Synthetic
- Progestin
- Combination therapy
- Selective estrogen receptor modulators
- Natural dietary supplement

Vaginal cream

Vaginal ring

Transdermal patch

additional information about the potential advantages and disadvantages of SERMs as a treatment for symptoms of menopause.[3]

Known Benefits of HRT

HRT provides relief from many symptoms of menopause, including hot flashes, night sweats, and related symptoms, as well as vaginal atrophy and dryness. HRT can sometimes prevent changes to the vagina that occur with menopause, making a woman less likely to experience urinary tract infections or incontinence. HRT that includes testosterone may be effective for some women who experience a reduced sex drive, but HRT that includes testosterone is generally not recommended for other menopausal-related symptoms.[20]

HRT also appears to reduce a woman's risk for certain diseases. HRT can help prevent bone fractures by slowing bone loss; it can also help prevent tooth loss.[21] For women who begin taking HRT during or shortly after menopause, it may reduce their risk of coronary heart disease. HRT may also help to prevent diabetes in some women.[22]

Known Disadvantages of HRT

Although HRT can provide relief from symptoms of menopause, it can also cause side effects, most often breast tenderness and vaginal discharge. However, the most controversial negative effects of HRT are the increased risk for several diseases (see **Table 8.2**).

Estrogen therapy alone can increase the risk of endometrial cancer, or cancer of the uterus. However, researchers have found that the addition of a progestin (a related type of hormone) to estrogen therapy protects women against endometrial cancer by opposing the negative effects of estrogen. Progestin appears to cause shedding of the estrogen-thickened endometrium, which reduces the chance of cancer development. Women who have had a hysterectomy and who choose hormone replacement therapy, however, usually receive estrogen alone, because they do not have a uterus.

For other diseases, the greatest dangers associated with HRT are for women already at risk for those diseases (stroke, venous thromboembolism, and dementia) or for women who begin HRT 10 years or more after menopause (cardiovascular disease). Continued use of HRT for more than three to five years may also slightly increase the risk of breast cancer.

Table 8.2   HRT's Known Effects on the Body

Symptoms:

- **Hot flashes, night sweats, and related symptoms:** HRT can reduce or eliminate these symptoms. HRT is most often prescribed for this set of symptoms.

- **Vaginal changes:** HRT can relieve vaginal dryness and atrophy associated with menopause. If these are the only symptoms a woman is experiencing, local hormone therapy or estrogen therapy is usually recommended. Local HRT treatments may also benefit some women with incontinence that results from changes in the vagina induced by menopause. HRT can be prescribed for pain during intercourse, but the North American Menopause Society recommends that other treatment options be considered as well.

- **Weight loss/gain:** There is currently no evidence to show a relationship between HRT and weight loss or weight gain.

Disease Risk:

- **Osteoporosis and fractures:** HRT reduces the risk of bone fractures for menopausal women with or without osteoporosis. HRT also appears to reduce the rate of bone loss in women with osteoporosis.

- **Heart disease and stroke:** HRT appears to slightly reduce the risk of coronary heart disease (CHD) in women who begin to take HRT at a relatively young age (usually around menopause), and to slightly increase the risk for women who begin HRT 10 years or more after menopause. For stroke, data are inconsistent, but HRT may slightly increase the risk of stroke for some women. HRT appears to increase the risk for venous thromboembolism (VTE), or blood clots forming in the veins, for women who already have VTE. (See Chapter 10 for more information about these diseases.)

- **Diabetes:** HRT may reduce a woman's risk for developing type 2 diabetes.

- **Endometrial (uterine) cancer:** Estrogen therapy alone increases the risk for endometrial cancer. Therefore, for women who have not had a hysterectomy, the recommended form of HRT would be combined HRT with estrogen and progestogen.

- **Breast cancer:** Extended use of HRT (more than three to five years) appears to increase women's risk for breast cancer; continued HRT use may also make reading mammograms more difficult.

- **Mood and depression:** HRT may help improve mood for some women; however, evidence for this effect is limited, and other more specific treatments should be considered to treat depression.

- **Dementia and cognitive decline:** HRT appears to slightly increase the risk of dementia and cognitive decline for women who begin taking it 10 or more years after menopause.

Source: North American Menopause Society, July 2008 position statement.

I am very frustrated with the lack of clear information about menopause and hormone replacement therapies. First, hormone replacement was supposed to be a cure-all; now, everyone seems to think you're risking your life if you choose to take it. Haven't we been using this stuff for decades? Why is there so much we still don't know?

46-year-old lawyer

Controversial Issues

From the 1960s until 2000, HRT was believed to be an important medication in the fight against heart disease in menopausal women. Because animal and human observational studies showed that estrogen can slow the atherosclerotic process, physicians began prescribing estrogen replacement therapy (ERT) for their perimenopausal and postmenopausal patients. The original purpose of ERT was for the short-term treatment of perimenopausal symptoms, such as hot flashes and vaginal dryness. As more observational studies' findings were released, however, ERT became an important tool in the fight against heart disease. At the same time, studies showed that prescribing estrogen alone was not safe for women with a uterus—unopposed estrogen increases the risk of uterine cancer. Therefore, scientists began prescribing progestin, a counteractive medication, along with the ERT in women with a uterus. In this way, the combination of estrogen and progestin (HRT) came into use.[23]

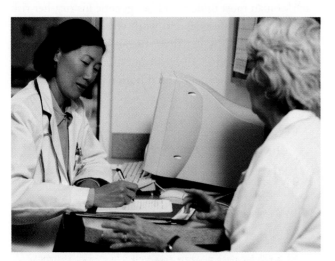

■ Replacement hormones can be taken in a variety of different preparations, by various routes of administration, and in different dosages. A woman should speak to her health-care provider to determine what type of HRT will work for her.

Scientists understood that although observational studies were important, they did not have the power of clinical trials in which the experimental medication was tested against a placebo (a pill that looks like the test medication, but that contains no medicine). The National Institutes of Health therefore began to fund clinical trials that examined the role of ERT and HRT as prevention against heart disease and stroke. Some of the first data released publicly came from ERT/HRT studies done in women who already had heart disease—the Estrogen Replacement and Atherosclerosis (ERA) Trial and the Heart and Estrogen Replacement Study (HERS). Both studies showed no significant difference in coronary heart disease risk reduction between users and nonusers. Furthermore, some women experienced an increase in coronary events in the first year of use and a modest decline thereafter. [24,25]

During the 1990s, the first female director of the National Institutes of Health, Bernadine Healy, a cardiologist, initiated the Women's Health Initiative (WHI). This three-part study examined the role of ERT/HRT in several health areas in postmenopausal women: heart disease, stroke, dementia, breast and colon cancer, and osteoporosis. The study, which began in 1994, involved more than 67,000 postmenopausal women of all racial and ethnic groups across the United States. The ages of the participants ranged from those who had just entered the menopausal state to women who had been postmenopausal for more than 20 years. In 2002, the HRT portion of the study was stopped because of the apparent dangers of HRT use. The women taking HRT had higher rates of heart disease, strokes, blood clots, dementia, and breast cancer.[23] The ERT-alone portion of the study was stopped a year later with somewhat similar findings.

The release of these findings set off a storm of anxiety, distress, and action. The U.S. Food and Drug Administration officially declared that ERT/HRT was not to be used for cardiovascular disease (CVD) prevention and should be prescribed only for short periods in women suffering from perimenopausal symptoms. A number of other prestigious medical organizations agreed with the FDA's position. The press covered the findings with vigor. The end result was that the thousands of women who had been on ERT or HRT now had to make a decision about what to do. They were encouraged to discuss their next steps with their physicians. The only difficulty was that often the physicians were not entirely certain either. The observational

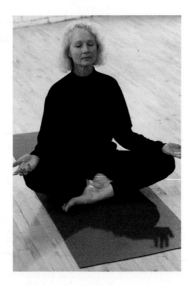

■ Symptoms associated with hormonal changes of menopause, such as hot flashes, may improve with regular exercise.

studies had been so positive and now the clinical trials appeared so negative. Ultimately, a substantial number of women stopped taking ERT or HRT.

In 2003, a study was released comparing the findings from the observational studies and two of the clinical trials, HERS and WHI (**Figure 8.4**).[26] Clearly, there is both risk and benefit from taking HRT. Yet some scientists were not satisfied and so, early in 2006, some of the WHI investigators published a more in-depth examination of another long-term observational study, the Nurses' Health Study.[27] This latest analysis provided additional information regarding the WHI findings. Basically, it appears that women who began taking ERT or HRT during the perimenopausal period—as many of the women in the earlier observational studies did—did not have as many negative effects from ERT/HRT as women who had been post-

menopausal for five years or more when they started the therapy. The latest findings suggest that estrogen may have a positive effect when used continuously. In contrast, those women who had a break in estrogen exposure over time appear to be at increased risk for CVD. The reasons for this discrepancy are not entirely clear.

Another question also emerged: Might the study findings have differed if other forms of the medication had been used and/or administered? The medication given to the experimental group was the same as had been generally prescribed for the majority of women during the last several decades; however, it was administered in a manner that does not mimic the usual hormonal cycling. The same dosages of both estrogen and progesterone were taken every day throughout each month. In addition, it is not entirely clear what effect particular types of estrogen and progestin have on CVD as opposed to other formulas of those hormones.

This reexamination of the evidence has not changed the latest recommendations on ERT/HRT use. Further examination of current data and additional studies are required. All of these studies—both observational and clinical trials—have shed light on the importance of conducting studies, knowing how to interpret their results, and understanding what clinical applications should occur. This example also strongly underscores the importance of a woman's partnership with her physician. All women are not the same, and each should be treated as an individual. Each woman must understand her genetic history, her risk factors, and her lifestyle, and work with her physician to find the best healthy practices. Regarding ERT or HRT, women should consider several questions when deciding whether to take postmenopausal hormone therapy:

Figure 8.4

Observational versus clinical trial data on hormone replacement therapy's effect on risk for certain diseases.

Source: Grodstein, F., Clarkson, T. B., Manson, J. E. (2003). Understanding the divergent data on postmenopausal hormone therapy. *New England Journal of Medicine* 348: 645–650.

		Amount of Risk	
Disease	WHI	HERS	Observational
Coronary heart disease	29% greater	No difference	49% less
Stroke	41% greater	20% greater	45% greater
Pulmonary embolism	113% greater	180% greater	110% greater
Breast cancer	26% greater	30% greater	115% greater
Colorectal cancer	37% less	N/A	54% less
Hip fracture	34% less	No difference	39% less

> *It can take a while to find a regimen that is right for you. The major responsibility of this task is yours. HRT affects your mood and energy level, as well as your mental and physical well-being. I'm seven years into menopause and had six HRT regimens (and several gynecologists!) before finding the "right" dosage and delivery mode. Be assertive with your doctor. Don't be afraid to change health-care providers until you find one who truly listens and responds to you. Do not settle for a regimen unless it is one that is totally comfortable for your mind and body.*
>
> **57-year-old woman**

1. What are my risk factors for the particular diseases studied?
2. Am I more susceptible to the negative effects of ERT or HRT?
3. What type of ERT or HRT should I take?
4. In my case, do the benefits outweigh the risks?

Other Methods of Menopause Management

Good nutrition and regular exercise are important factors in maintaining well-being throughout premenopause and postmenopause. A diet rich in fruits, vegetables, and whole grains, and low in saturated fat and cholesterol, will improve health through most stages of life. Adequate calcium, vitamin D, and antioxidants such as vitamins E and C are also important for bone health and possibly prevention of CVD and cancer.

Exercise is critical in the menopausal years, a time when a woman is at increased risk for osteoporosis and osteoporosis-related fractures, heart disease, and chronic diseases such as diabetes. Weight-bearing exercise can increase bone density and improve balance and flexibility to decrease falls, thereby reducing fractures. Aerobic exercise can reduce a woman's risk for CVD by improving cardiac function, decreasing high body weight, and lowering LDL cholesterol levels. Regular exercise also may reduce the incidence and severity of hot flashes. Other symptoms associated with hormonal changes of menopause, such as insomnia, depression, other mood changes, weight gain, and headache, all may improve with exercise.[28]

Traditional herbal medicine has long offered a variety of treatments to address some of the symptoms of menopause. Proponents of herbal supplements such as black co-

hosh, vitex, and dong quai say these treatments can relieve many symptoms of menopause. However, further work is needed to determine how effective these herbal remedies are.

Informed Decision Making

Although it is commonly believed that health problems are inevitable as women age, many can actually be prevented or controlled. Clearly, it is best to have a full lifetime of healthy behaviors, but changing unhealthy behaviors, even in later years, can improve both the quality and the quantity of life. Health-promoting behaviors include cessation of cigarette smoking (it is best to never start), maintenance of good nutrition, loss of excess weight, and participation in regular physical exercise. For some women, menopause is a time of reflection and renewed determination to engage in healthier living. Protecting the body from heart disease and osteoporosis means not smoking, exercising throughout the life span, eating a healthy diet, and knowing one's body.

As they age, many women remain uninformed about their health and about how they can take steps to become and remain healthy. In a study looking at racial differences regarding menopause, 40% of African American women listed family members as their primary source of information about menopause, while one-third of white women

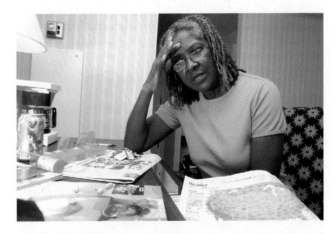

■ Rapidly changing information about the safety and effectiveness of HRT can be confusing for women deciding whether to use it to alleviate symptoms of menopause.

I tried HRT but with all the contradictory news I decided that I preferred to not take "medicine" to get through a normal transition. Yes, I do have hot flashes, but they are manageable. It really is an individual decision.

61-year-old woman

cited television and magazines as their most common sources of information. Only 11% of African American women and 12% of white women listed health professionals as their primary source of information.[29] This study provides strong evidence that health-care providers need to communicate better with their patients about menopause and provide helpful, practical, and informative advice to help women in their decision making regarding menopause.

The decision whether to take HRT is a personal one. No two women respond exactly the same way to the same therapy. Dosages, products, and regimens may require readjusting more than once to find an appropriate balance. Women with difficult menopause symptoms, who have thin bones as measured by a bone density test, or who are at high risk of heart disease are possible candidates for HRT. Women who have a history of liver disease, who are prone to blood clots, or who have had breast cancer are generally considered to be at too high a risk to begin HRT (**Table 8.3**).

As with any form of medication, treatment, or procedure, the benefits must be carefully weighed and considered against the spectrum of associated risks before a decision is made (see **Self-Assessment 8.1**). Improving women's access to accurate, relevant information in this re-

Table 8.3	**Conditions That May Preclude the Use of Hormone Replacement Therapy**

Personal history of breast cancer

History of blood clots in legs, lungs, or eyes

Undiagnosed or abnormal vaginal bleeding

Preexisting cardiovascular conditions, such as blood clots, stroke, or uncontrolled hypertension

History of liver, gallbladder, or pancreatic disease; impaired liver function

Self-Assessment 8.1

Strategies for HRT Decision Making

The decision to use HRT is a personal and private one. Several factors should be carefully considered when making the decision:

1. Medical history
   - History of breast cancer
   - Blood clots in the legs, lungs, or eyes
   - Abnormal vaginal bleeding
   - Preexisting cardiovascular conditions, such as blood clots, stroke, or uncontrolled high blood pressure
   - Liver, gallbladder, or pancreatic disease
2. Menopausal symptoms and their severity
   - Hot flashes
   - Vaginal irritation and discomfort
   - Urinary tract problems
   - Emotional and mood changes
3. Review risks and benefits
4. Reevaluate decision periodically

gard will be necessary to help them better make these important health decisions.

Summary

Today menopause is no longer seen as the beginning of the end of life, but rather as the beginning of a second life, no longer confined or defined by procreative abilities. Fears about aging and the myths and misconceptions about the aging process need to be replaced with better knowledge and insight into the myriad opportunities that exist in the second half of a woman's life. For some women, menopause brings physical symptoms; for others, it inspires questions about changing roles. Menopause management—especially hormone replacement therapy—remains a controversial area that deserves ongoing research and requires individual choices by women and their physicians. For some women, this therapy is the ideal solution to their health issues associated with menopause. For other women, HRT may cause more health problems than it solves and leaves many women confused about their options. As a result, women must actively work with their physicians to understand the best course of action for themselves as it relates to menopause and their individual process of aging.

Profiles of Remarkable Women

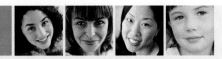

Gail Sheehy (1937–)

Gail Sheehy, the author of 15 books, has been tracking the stages of adult development for more than 20 years. In 1976, Sheehy published the book *Passages*, which offered the perspective that adult life proceeds through predictable stages. *Passages* was eventually published in 28 languages and remained on the *New York Times* bestseller list for three years.

Sheehy's next bestseller, *The Silent Passage: Menopause*, broke the silence around the previously taboo subject of menopause. Its author demystified issues surrounding menopause by presenting the facts, the myths, and the fears of women. The sequel to *Passages*, titled *New Passages: Mapping Your Life Across Time*, discusses Sheehy's discovery of a shifting in all of the stages of adulthood. Through extensive research and surveys, Sheehy created a book that helps women to make sense of their lives by understanding other women's experiences.

Sheehy's other books have covered a wide range of topics. For example, *Pathfinders* was created from a study of 60,000 American men and women; *Spirit of Survival*, a story of healing, is an account of a survivor of the Cambodian genocide. *Understanding Men's Passages: Discovering the New Map of Men's Lives* focuses on the fears and self-doubts of men over 40.

Sheehy was one of the original contributors to *New York Magazine* and has revolutionized political writing through her role as contributing editor of *Vanity Fair*. Through her in-depth character portraits of national and world leaders, Sheehy has explored the psyches of Saddam Hussein, George Bush, Mikhail Gorbachev, Margaret Thatcher, Jesse Jackson, Gary Hart, Dan Quayle, Hillary Clinton, and Newt Gingrich.

In her newest book, *Sex and the Seasoned Woman: Pursuing the Passionate Life*, Sheehy reports on Baby Boomer women, covering topics such as sex, dating, divorce, remarriage, and living more passionately in the second half of life.

Topics for Discussion

1. Why has medical research been slower to understand the physiological dimensions of menopause than those of other reproductive health matters?

2. What can be done to continue to change societal images of menopause, aging, and older women?

3. How can women understand menopause as a stage of life?

4. What can a woman do to maximize the effectiveness of her decision making about hormone replacement therapy?

5. What are some of the physical, emotional, and social dimensions of menopause?

Web Sites

American College of Obstetricians and Gynecologists: http://www.acog.org

American Heart Association—Women and Cardiovascular Disease: http://www.goredforwomen.org

The Hormone Foundation: http://www.hormone.org

National Institute on Aging Information Center: http://www.nia.nih.gov

National Women's Health Information Center: http://www.womenshealth.gov

National Women's Health Resource Center: http://www.healthywomen.org

North American Menopause Society: http://www.menopause.org

Power Surge (an online community for menopausal women): http://www.power-surge.com

Society for Women's Health Research: http://www.womenshealthresearch.org

References

1. U.S. Census Bureau. (2008). *Annual Estimates of the Population by Sex and Five-Year Age Groups for the United States: April 1, 2000 to July 1, 2007*. Available at: http://www.census.gov/popest/national/asrh/NCEST2003/NC-EST2003-01.pdf.

2. Utian, W. H., & Boggs, P. P. (1999). *The North American Menopause Society 1998 Menopause Survey. Part 1: Postmenopausal Women's Perceptions about Menopause and Midlife*. New York: North American Menopause Society.

3. U.S. Department of Health and Human Services. (2005). *Facts about Menopausal Hormone Therapy*. Washington, DC: U.S. Department of Health and Human Services, National Institutes of Health.

4. Wu, J. M., Wechter, M., Geller, E., Nguyen, T., & Visco, A. (2007). *Hysterectomy Rates in the United States, 2003*. Chapel Hill, NC: Department of Obstetrics, University of North Carolina.

5. Bachmann, G. A. (1999). Vasomotor flushes in postmenopausal women. *American Journal of Obstetrics and Gynecology* 180: 312–316.

6. Bush, T. (1990). The epidemiology of cardiovascular disease in postmenopausal women. *Annals of the New York Academy of Science* 592: 263–271.

7. Stampfer, M. J., Colditz, G. A., & Willett, W. C. (1990). Menopause and heart disease: a review. *Annals of the New York Academy of Science* 392: 193–203.

8. Keshavarz, M. D., Hillis, S. D., Kiekel, B. A., & Marchanks, P. A. (2002). *Hysterectomy Surveillance—United States, 1994–1999*. Washington, DC: Division of Reproductive Health, National Center for Chronic Disease Prevention and Health Promotion, Epidemic Intelligence Service Program, Epidemiology Program Office.

9. Lepine, L. A., et al. (1997). Hysterectomy surveillance—United States, 1980–1993. *Morbidity and Mortality Weekly Report* 46(SS-4): 1–15.

10. Woods, N. F., & Mitchell, E. S. (2005). Symptoms during the menopause: prevalence, severity, trajectory, and significance in women's lives. *Journal of American Medicine* 118(12B): 14S–24S.

11. Ice, V. M. (2005). Strategies and issues for managing menopause-related symptoms in diverse populations: ethnic and racial diversity. *Journal of American Medicine* 118(12B): 142S–147S.

12. Owens, J. F., & Matthews, K. A. (1998). Sleep disturbance in healthy middle-aged women. *Maturitas* 30: 41–50.

13. Hammond, C. B. (1999). Confronting aging and disease: the role of HRT. *Medscape Women's Health*. Available at: http://www.medscape.com/viewprogram/696.

14. Samsoie, G. (1998). Urogenital aging: a hidden problem. *American Journal of Obstetrics and Gynecology* 178: S245–S249.

15. Stampfer, M. J., Colditz, G. A., Willett, W. C., et al. (1991). Postmenopausal estrogen therapy and cardiovascular disease: 10 year follow-up from the Nurses' Health Study. *New England Journal of Medicine* 325: 756.

16. National Osteoporosis Foundation. (2006). *Fast Facts on Osteoporosis*. Washington, DC: National Osteoporosis Foundation. Available at: http://www.nof.org/osteoporosis/diseasefacts.htm.

17. Centers for Disease Control and Prevention. (1996). *National Health and Nutrition Examination Survey III*. Available at: http://www.cdc.gov/nchs/products/elec_prods/subject/nhanes3.htm.

18. International Menopause Society. (2002). *The International Menopause Society Report on the 10th World Congress on the Menopause Climacteric* 5: 219–228.

19. Johnson, L. (September 25, 2008). Wyeth: menopause drug reduces multiple symptoms. *Washington Post*.

20. North American Menopause Society. (2005). The role of testosterone therapy in postmenopausal women: position statement of the North American Menopause Society. *Menopause* 12(5): 497–511.

21. Krall, E. A. (2006). Osteoporosis and risk of tooth loss. *Clinical Calcium* 16(2): 287–290.

22. North American Menopause Society. (2008). Estrogen and progestogen use in postmenopausal women: July 2008 position statement of the North American Menopause Society. *Menopause* 15(4): 584–602.

23. Writing Group for the Women's Health Initiative Randomized Controlled Trial. (2002). Risks and benefits of estrogen plus progestin in healthy postmenopausal women. *Journal of the American Medical Association* 288(3): 321–333.

24. Herrington, D., et al. (2000). Effects of estrogen replacement on the progression of coronary-artery atherosclerosis. *New England Journal of Medicine* 343(8): 522–529.

25. Hulley, S., et al. (1998). Randomized trial of estrogen plus progestin for secondary prevention of coronary heart disease in postmenopausal women. Heart and Estrogen/Progestin Replacement Study (HERS) Research Group. *Journal of the American Medical Association* 280: 605–613.

26. Grodstein, F., Clarkson, T. B., & Manson, J. E. (2003). Understanding the divergent data on postmenopausal hormone therapy. *New England Journal of Medicine* 348(7): 645–650.

27. Grodstein, F., Manson, J. E., & Stampfer, M. E. (2006). Hormone therapy and coronary heart disease: the role of time since menopause and age at hormone initiation. *Journal of Women's Health* 15(1): 35–44.

28. Burghardt, M. (1999). Exercise at menopause: a critical difference. *Medscape Women's Health* 4(1).

29. Grisso, J. A., et al. (1999). Racial differences in menopause information and the experience of hot flashes. *General Internal Medicine* 14: 98–103.

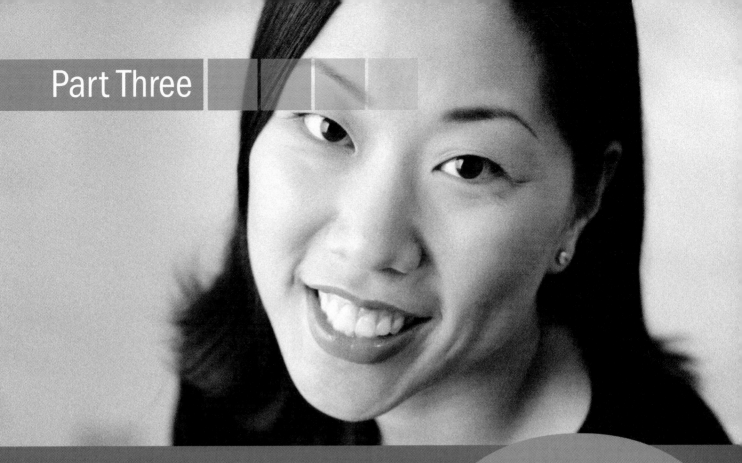

Part Three

Physical and Lifespan Dimensions of Women's Health

3

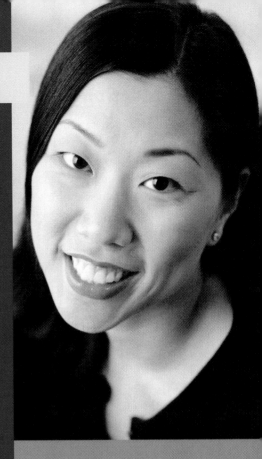

Chapter Nine

Nutrition, Exercise, and Weight Management

Chapter Objectives

On completion of this chapter, the student should be able to discuss:

1. The importance of a healthful diet and an active lifestyle for disease prevention and health promotion.

2. The way in which nutrients fit into a balanced diet.

3. The building blocks of nutrition.

4. The concept of physical fitness and how it relates to health.

5. The physiological and psychological benefits of exercise.

6. The major components of physical fitness and total fitness, and their benefits.

7. Maximum and target-range heart rate.

8. Physical fitness concerns that are specific to women.

9. Myths and facts about exercise and fitness.

10. The ability of exercise to counter some of the natural conditions of the aging process.

11. Causes of athletic amenorrhea.

12. Reasons why women should maintain a healthy weight.

13. The cause of weight gain.

14. The effects of obesity and overweight on health.

15. Economic consequences of obesity and overweight.

16. Ways that women can achieve their weight-loss goals.

17. How body images of women have changed over time.

18. Sociocultural influences on body image.

19. Probable causes and health consequences of extreme underweight.

20. The effects of world hunger and malnutrition.

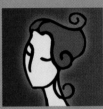

womenshealth.jbpub.com

Women's Health Online is a great source for supplementary women's health information for both students and instructors. Visit

http://womenshealth.jbpub.com

to find a variety of useful tools for learning, thinking, and teaching.

Introduction

Despite scientific research documenting that healthful eating and regular exercise help people live longer, healthier, happier lives, many women continue to follow unhealthy eating patterns and lead sedentary lives. Together, these two behaviors are responsible for 400,000 deaths each year. These behaviors are the second leading preventable cause of death in the United States, just behind tobacco.[1]

A well-balanced diet—one that is low in fat and high in fruits, vegetables, and fiber—can play a significant role in the prevention of cardiovascular disease, various cancers, diabetes, and other diet-related chronic conditions. It also makes the body stronger and more capable in every aspect of life. Physical fitness greatly reduces the risk of developing heart disease, hypertension, colon cancer, and diabetes. Exercise promotes psychological well-being, controls body fat and fat distribution, and fosters healthy muscle, bones, and joints. Exercise also helps older adults maintain function and preserve independence. This chapter describes the components of a healthful diet, discusses different types of physical activity and how it is important, discusses healthful and non-healthful ways to maintain a healthful weight, provides different perspectives about body image, and discusses hunger from a global and national perspective.

It's Your Health

Definition of Common Nutritional Claims

Enriched: The replacement of nutrients in a product that may have been lost during processing; for example, bread may be enriched with iron, niacin, thiamin, and riboflavin.

Fortified: The addition of vitamins and minerals that were not originally present in a food product; for example, orange juice may be fortified with calcium.

Light or lite: A relatively meaningless descriptor that may refer to reduced calories, fat, or sodium, or even a "light" taste or fluffy texture.

Low-calorie: Term used for a food that has less than 40 calories per serving and less than 0.4 calorie per gram.

Low-fat: Term used for a food that has 3 grams or less of fat per serving. Be careful: food manufacturers sometimes add large amounts of sugar to low-fat foods to compensate for the taste.

Low-sodium: Term used for food that has 140 mg or less of sodium per serving.

Natural: A relatively meaningless descriptor that may refer to minimal processing or a product that is free of artificial ingredients. Many foods labeled as natural are highly processed, high in fat or sugar, or loaded with preservatives.

Organic: Term used for food that is produced using renewable resources and without traditional pesticides or artificial fertilizers. Animals that produce organic products, meat, and eggs receive no antibiotics or growth hormones.

RDA: Recommended Dietary Allowance, the estimated amount of various nutrients needed each day to maintain good health. The guidelines were developed to address population-based dietary needs such as for pregnant women; individual needs may vary owing to genetic, personal, and demographic factors.

Reduced-calorie: Term used for a food that has at least 25% fewer calories than regular preparations. The nutritional comparison must be displayed on the product label.

Sugarless and sugar-free: Another misleading descriptor because the current FDA definition of "sugar" means sucrose but does not include other forms of sugar such as glucose, fructose, or sorbitol, which contain as many calories.

It's Your Health

Dietary Guidelines for Americans

The USDA recommends the following for the five food groups as part of a healthy, 2,000-calorie per day diet:

Grains

Eat 6 ounces every day.

Make half of the grains you eat whole.

Vegetables

Vary the vegetables you eat.

Eat 2½ cups every day.

Vegetables to eat more of:

    Dark green vegetables like spinach and broccoli.

    Orange vegetables like carrots and sweet potatoes.

    Dry beans and peas like kidney beans, pinto beans, and lentils.

Fruits

Eat a variety of fruit.

Eat 2 cups of fruit every day.

Try to consume whole fruits rather than fruit juices.

Dairy Products

Try to consume 3 cups of dairy products or other calcium-rich foods every day.

Try to consume low-fat dairy products when possible.

Consume fortified food or other sources of calcium if dairy products are unavailable or unpalatable.

Meat and Beans

Eat 5½ ounces of meat or beans every day.

Consume baked, broiled, or grilled meat products when possible.

Vary sources of protein, emphasizing fish, peas, beans, nuts, and seeds.

Nutrition and Healthful Eating

Nutrition is the science that explores the need for food and the role of food in nourishing the body and fostering good health. Nutritional needs change during different stages of a woman's life.

There are six groups of **nutrients**, which are categorized into three types:

- *Macronutrients*, which include carbohydrates, proteins, and fats, are needed in large amounts.

- *Micronutrients*, which include vitamins and minerals, are needed in smaller amounts.

- *Water*, a substance often overlooked as a nutrient, is indispensable for virtually every bodily function.

To achieve healthful eating, a woman should choose a diet that provides the right balance of carbohydrates, proteins, and fats; the necessary amounts of essential vitamins and minerals; and a constant supply of water.

Dietary Guidelines

The U.S. Department of Agriculture (USDA) has revised its dietary guidelines for Americans every five years since the guidelines' introduction in 1980. Based on current nutritional research, the 2005 guidelines identify unhealthy eating habits and a sedentary lifestyle as major causes of death and injury in the United States. To promote health and prevent disease, the guidelines encourage Americans to participate in regular physical activity, consume adequate nutrient requirements within a healthy caloric intake, reach and maintain a healthy weight, and adopt fats and sodium as a necessary but limited portion of their diets. The guidelines also highlight food choices that can help people meet their **Recommended Dietary Allowances**.[2] (See **It's Your Health:** Dietary Guidelines for Americans.)

Food Guide Pyramids

The 2005 dietary guidelines use a pyramid to symbolize the proportion of different foods that make up a healthy diet (see **Figure 9.1**). The 2005 pyramid is divided into vertical slices. It replaces the traditional "four food groups" (breads and grains, fruits and vegetables, dairy products and meats) with six food groups: (1) grains; (2) vegetables; (3) fruits; (4) fats, sugars, and sodium; (5) meat and beans; and (6) dairy products. A figure climbing a flight of stairs along the side of the pyramid represents the importance that physical activity plays in a healthy lifestyle.[2] The different sizes of the food group "slices" in the pyramid represent

the nutritional concept of **proportionality**—eating different amounts from each of the food groups on a daily basis. Unfortunately, Americans "gobble huge amounts of added fats and sugars . . . and heaping plates of pasta and other refined grains [but] . . . are sorely lacking in the vegetables, fruits, low-fat milk products, and other nutritious foods in the middle of the pyramid."[2,3] More than 60% of young people eat too much fat, and fewer than 20% eat the recommended five or more servings of fruits and vegetables each day. Poor eating habits are often established during childhood and carry into adulthood.[4] Only one-third of U.S. adults eats fruit two or more times per day, and only one-quarter of adults eat vegetables three or more times per day, according to a CDC study.[5]

Other food guide pyramids challenge or complement the USDA's food guide pyramid. In addition, food guides exist for special populations, such as people older than 70 years of age and vegetarians. Culture-specific food guidelines, including ones for Arabic, Chinese, Indian, Russian, and Mexican populations, also offer guidance for a balanced, healthful diet.

The Mediterranean food guide, based on the dietary traditions of Crete, much of the rest of Greece, and southern Italy, has received much attention of late. Rates of chronic disease are among the lowest in the world and life expectancy is among the highest for populations in this region. The food guide highlights the following characteristics of the Mediterranean diet:

- An abundance of food from plant sources, including fruits and vegetables, bread and grains, beans, nuts, and seeds

- Emphasis on fresh, locally grown foods

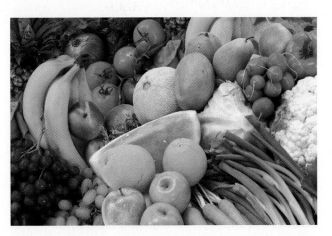

■ Fruits and vegetables contain numerous substances that could help prevent disease and promote good health.

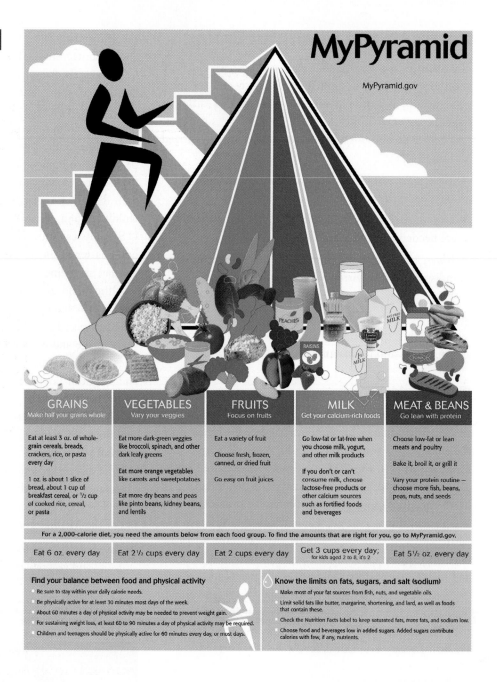

Figure 9.1

MyPyramid: The 2005 food guide pyramid.

Source: U.S. Department of Agriculture. www.MyPyramid.gov.

- Olive oil as the principal fat
- Moderate amounts of fish, poultry, cheese, and yogurt
- Moderate consumption of wine

Nutrition Facts Label

The Nutrition Facts label is designed to help people make healthful food choices and compare the nutritional quality of foods. The food label lists information on serving size, calories, nutrients, and vitamins and minerals, as well as other important facts relevant to a healthful diet (**Figure 9.2**). The Daily Value (%DV) section indicates how the nutrients in a serving of food contribute to satisfying one's total daily requirements for each nutrient. These values are based on recommendations for a 2,000-calorie diet. A woman under doctor's orders to eat a higher- or lower-calorie diet will need to recalculate these numbers to fit her own needs.[2]

Carbohydrates

Carbohydrates provide the basic fuel for the body and are available in two forms: simple carbohydrates (sugars) and complex carbohydrates (starches). Sugars provide little more than a quick spurt of energy, whereas starches are rich in vitamins, minerals, and other nutrients that provide

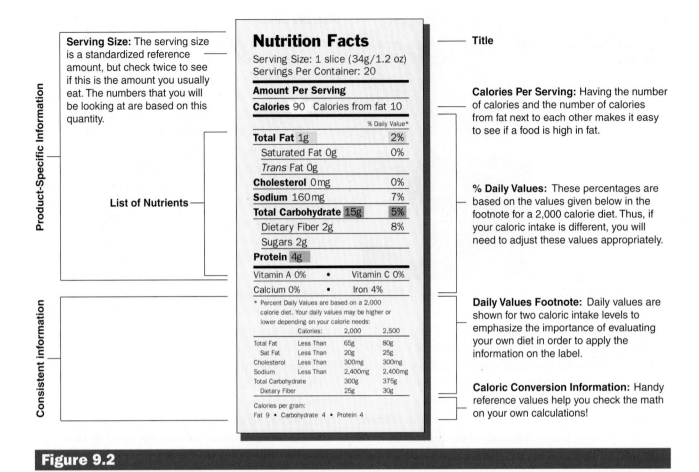

Serving Size: The serving size is a standardized reference amount, but check twice to see if this is the amount you usually eat. The numbers that you will be looking at are based on this quantity.

Product-Specific Information

List of Nutrients

Consistent Information

Nutrition Facts

Serving Size: 1 slice (34g/1.2 oz)
Servings Per Container: 20

Amount Per Serving

Calories 90   Calories from fat 10

% Daily Value*

Total Fat 1g	2%
Saturated Fat 0g	0%
Trans Fat 0g	
Cholesterol 0mg	0%
Sodium 160mg	7%
Total Carbohydrate 15g	5%
Dietary Fiber 2g	8%
Sugars 2g	
Protein 4g	

Vitamin A 0%	•	Vitamin C 0%
Calcium 0%	•	Iron 4%

* Percent Daily Values are based on a 2,000 calorie diet. Your daily values may be higher or lower depending on your calorie needs:

	Calories:	2,000	2,500
Total Fat	Less Than	65g	80g
Sat Fat	Less Than	20g	25g
Cholesterol	Less Than	300mg	300mg
Sodium	Less Than	2,400mg	2,400mg
Total Carbohydrate		300g	375g
Dietary Fiber		25g	30g

Calories per gram:
Fat 9 • Carbohydrate 4 • Protein 4

Title

Calories Per Serving: Having the number of calories and the number of calories from fat next to each other makes it easy to see if a food is high in fat.

% Daily Values: These percentages are based on the values given below in the footnote for a 2,000 calorie diet. Thus, if your caloric intake is different, you will need to adjust these values appropriately.

Daily Values Footnote: Daily values are shown for two caloric intake levels to emphasize the importance of evaluating your own diet in order to apply the information on the label.

Caloric Conversion Information: Handy reference values help you check the math on your own calculations!

Figure 9.2

Example of the Nutrition Facts label.

more sustained fuel for the body. During digestion, all carbohydrates are broken down into sugar. The sugar enters the blood, increasing blood sugar levels. The body's normal response is to increase the production of insulin, which in turn uses the sugar for energy.

Simple Carbohydrates

Simple carbohydrates, or sugars, are consumed in four virtually identical forms: sucrose, glucose, fructose, and lactose. They are present in many foods, from fruit to milk to ice cream and ketchup. Processed foods often have much more sugar than their natural counterparts. A typical 12-ounce soft drink contains the equivalent of eight teaspoons of sugar, and a typical chocolate bar contains about three teaspoons of sugar per ounce. Foods high in sugar are often high in fat, and a high-fat diet is a major culprit in cardiovascular disease, obesity, and other chronic diseases. Sugar provides "empty calories"—that is, energy in the form of calories but with no other significant nutritional value. In addition, consumption of a sugared product, such

as a soft drink, usually occurs in lieu of something else that may be nutritious, such as a glass of skim milk or water.

Foods high in sugar can be particularly harmful to dental health because sugar nourishes cavity-causing bacteria. The source of sugar also affects the damage it causes. Sugar in sticky foods, for example, clings to the teeth and encourages bacterial growth. Liberal use of sugar promotes the growth of plaque, the toxin-producing film that forms on teeth; plaque can lead to periodontal (gum) disease, the leading cause of tooth loss among U.S. adults. Research has recently linked periodontal disease with an increased risk of heart disease.[6]

Complex Carbohydrates

Complex carbohydrates, or starches, are a good source of minerals, vitamins, and fiber. These substances are found in breads, cereals, legumes, rice, pastas, and "starchy" vegetables such as beans and potatoes. Digestion breaks down complex carbohydrates into simple sugars. Complex carbohydrates take longer to digest than simple carbohydrates

■ Complex carbohydrates are a good source of minerals, vitamins, and fiber.

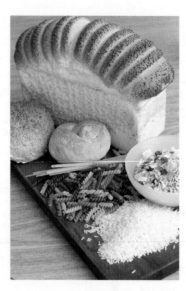

and, therefore, are a good long-term source of energy. According to USDA dietary guidelines, complex carbohydrates should provide the major supply of calories in diets, approximately 55% to 60% of total calories consumed.

Fiber is not a single substance, but rather a group of substances with varied physical properties. It is derived from the parts of plants that cannot be digested by enzymes in the human digestive tract. Although not considered a nutrient because it cannot be digested, it is essential because it aids in digestion. Fiber is found in foods composed of carbohydrates.

There are two kinds of fiber: soluble and insoluble. Both kinds benefit the body. Soluble fiber, once called crude fiber, absorbs water in the digestive tract and is easily fermented by bacteria in the large intestine. Oats, for example, are rich in soluble fiber, which helps lower blood cholesterol and manage blood sugar levels. In contrast, most insoluble fiber remains essentially unchanged during digestion. Wheat bran, whole-grain breads and cereals, broccoli, carrots, and pears are all rich in insoluble fiber, which tends to increase stool bulk. Studies now show an increased risk for heart disease, high blood pressure, and diabetes when diets low in fiber are consumed.[7]

The recommended daily intake for total fiber for women 50 and younger is 25 grams per day; for women older than 50, it is 21 grams per day. A woman should increase dietary fiber by slowly adding fiber to her diet over time. When choosing sources of fiber, opt for less-processed food, such as an apple rather than applesauce. Eating the skin of fruits and vegetables also increases fiber consumption (see **It's Your Health**).

Glycemic Index

Partly as a result of the recent popularity of high-protein, low-carbohydrate diets, much attention has been given to the glycemic index of foods. The **glycemic index** measures how fast glucose enters the bloodstream after a carbohydrate is eaten and thus how quickly the carbohydrate increases a person's blood sugar. In general, foods that are mostly simple sugars are highly processed, or contain refined sugars have a high glycemic index. This group includes refined breakfast cereals, white bread, white rice, white spaghetti, soft drinks, and sugar. Some complex carbohydrates, such as potatoes, behave just as simple carbohydrates do, elevating blood sugar to an excessive level. These complex carbohydrates have a high glycemic index, whereas complex carbohydrates that are high in fiber tend to have a lower glycemic index. Fiber aids in slowing digestion, so sugars tend to be absorbed into the bloodstream more slowly. Interestingly, ice cream has a fairly low glycemic index because the fat in ice cream tends to slow blood sugar absorption.

The rationale for avoiding high-glycemic-index foods relates to the resulting production of insulin. Avoiding high-glycemic-index foods and eating only low-glycemic-index foods may facilitate fat loss by reducing excess insulin. The weakness of this theory, however, is that obese and severely overweight individuals are already producing excess insulin; thus consuming a low-glycemic-index diet will not help them to achieve meaningful weight loss. A food's glycemic index is only part of the larger picture. Many fruits, for example, have very high glycemic indexes but are high in desirable fiber and vitamins.[8]

It's Your Health

Ways to Eat More Fiber

1. Eat whole fresh fruit instead of just drinking juice.
2. Eat the skins of fruits and vegetables, such as apples and potatoes.
3. Eat fruits with edible seeds, such as berries and kiwis.
4. Eat whole-grain foods.
5. Eat more of the stems when having broccoli or asparagus.
6. Peel citrus fruits and eat the sections with their membranes.
7. Eat more beans and peas.

Proteins

Protein provides the framework for muscles, bones, blood, hair, and fingernails. It is the main supply of amino acids—the building blocks that construct, repair, and maintain body tissues. The nine "essential" amino acids are the ones that the body cannot manufacture itself and must receive from dietary sources. Complete sources of protein contain all of the essential amino acids in their required amounts; incomplete sources of protein lack one or more of the essential amino acids. Complete proteins include meat, fish, poultry, and dairy products. Incomplete sources include beans, peas, peanuts, grains, and potatoes. Complementary proteins are protein sources that, when eaten together, supply the necessary amounts of all the essential amino acids. An example of complementary proteins is cooked dried or canned beans eaten with rice. One difficulty for vegetarians, vegans, or even people eating a diet low in animal proteins is that the body cannot store amino acids. To benefit the body, a person must consume all the essential amino acids at the same meal. Interestingly, vegetarian foods that complement each other in essential amino acids also often complement each other in taste. A peanut butter sandwich (containing wheat and peanuts), red (or black) beans and rice, or a bean burrito (beans wrapped in a corn or wheat tortilla) are all complete sources of protein.

The National Academy of Science recommends that women consume 0.8 gram of protein per kilogram of body weight (0.36 gram per pound of body weight)—a woman weighing 120 pounds, or 52 kg, should eat about 43 grams of protein a day.[9] Extra protein, like other excess calories, is stored as fat.

Many of the more recently publicized high-protein diets propose obtaining a significant percentage of daily calories from protein. A major problem with these diets is that they encourage consumption of proteins high in saturated fat, such as red meat and cheese, while discouraging consumption of healthy carbohydrates such as fruit, vegetables, and fiber. Diets high in saturated fat increase a person's risk for heart disease and certain types of cancer. High-protein diets also may increase a woman's risk for osteoporosis. Excess dietary protein increases calcium loss in the urine.

Soy is a type of protein that is being studied to determine its health benefits. Soy-based foods may lower cholesterol, ease hot flashes during menopause, prevent osteoporosis, and reduce the risk of breast and prostate cancer, all while helping a person lose weight. However, the evidence for some of these claims is still uncertain. Although several studies have found that soy-based products can provide significant health benefits, others have found little to no difference between groups eating soy products and control groups. However, soy-based products can still be a low-fat source of calcium, protein, and other nutrients. The FDA has limited use of the soy-related health claim to foods containing intact soy protein—the claim does not extend to isolated substances from soy protein such as isoflavones, a product found in soy that can act like estrogen in the human body, so manufacturers of such products cannot include this claim on their food labels. Women are advised to use caution in consumption of soy isoflavones. When consumed in moderation, soy-based products are probably not a major health risk.[8]

■ Complete proteins contain all the essential amino acids in their required amounts.

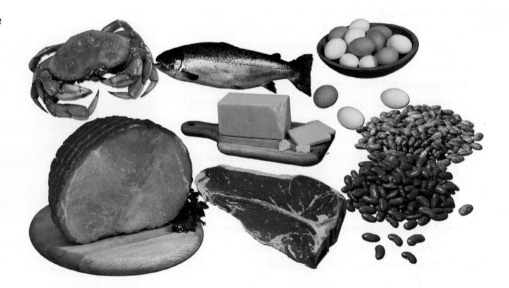

Fats

Fats perform many essential bodily functions. They store energy, maintain healthy hair and skin, carry **fat-soluble vitamins**, supply essential fatty acids, affect levels of blood cholesterol, and create a feeling of "fullness." **Cholesterol** is a type of fat produced by the liver. It is a vital constituent of cell membranes and nerve fibers and serves as a building block for estrogen, testosterone, vitamin D, and bile. Cholesterol is transported in the bloodstream in protein packages called lipoproteins, which are assembled in the intestinal tract and liver. **Low-density lipoproteins (LDLs)** —called the "bad" cholesterol—carry the cholesterol through the blood, dropping it off where it is needed for cell building and leaving any excess in arterial walls and other tissues. The excess accumulates in the arterial walls, causing blockage. **High-density lipoproteins (HDLs)**—known as the "good" cholesterol—pick up cholesterol deposits and bring them to the liver for reprocessing or excretion. Increased levels of LDLs are associated with an increased risk of heart disease, whereas increased levels of HDLs seem to have a protective effect against heart disease. The body normally produces all of the cholesterol that it needs, so dietary cholesterol (found in foods from animal sources such as eggs, meats, and dairy products) is actually unnecessary.

There are three types of fats:

1. **Saturated fats** come primarily from animal sources such as meat, poultry, milk, cheese, and butter. Some vegetable oils, such as coconut, palm kernel, and palm oil, also are saturated fats. At the molecular level, saturated fats are "saturated" with hydrogen atoms; each molecule holds as many as it can possibly carry. Saturated fats are generally solid at room temperature. They raise both LDL and HDL cholesterol, thereby increasing the risk of heart disease.

2. **Unsaturated fats** come from plants and include most vegetable oils. Carbon atoms in unsaturated fats have multiple bonds with each other. This prevents them from carrying the maximum number of hydrogen atoms they can carry (hence the name "unsaturated"). In turn, this configuration gives the molecules "kinks" that prevent unsaturated fat molecules from solidifying. They include two types:

   - **Monounsaturated fats**, such as those in olive, peanut, grapeseed, and canola oil
   - **Polyunsaturated fats**, such as those in safflower, sunflower, corn, and flaxseed oil

Unsaturated fats lower LDL cholesterol and raise HDL cholesterol, which has a positive effect on overall blood cholesterol levels and can therefore lower the risk of heart disease.

3. **Trans fats** form when vegetable oils are processed into margarine or shortening. They are found in snack foods such as potato chips, commercial baked goods with "partially hydrogenated vegetable oil" or "vegetable shortening," many types of fast foods (french fries and onion rings), stick margarine, and some dairy products. Trans fats are solid or semi-solid at room temperature. These types of fats are worse for cholesterol levels than saturated fats because they not only raise LDL cholesterol, but also lower HDL cholesterol. A report from the Institute of Medicine concluded that there is no safe level of trans fats in the diet. The FDA now requires that trans fats be listed on the Nutrition Facts food label used in the United States. The FDA estimated that the labeling requirement, which began in 2006, will have prevented 600 to 1,200 coronary heart attacks and saved 200 to 500 deaths per year by 2009.[9]

Lowering one's intake of saturated fat, trans fat, and dietary cholesterol is one of the major modifiable risk factors for coronary heart disease. Although it was once believed that dietary cholesterol alone was the culprit in heart disease, studies have since shown that lowering intake of dietary cholesterol has less effect on blood cholesterol levels than lowering intake of saturated fat.[10,11] In a study involving more than 80,000 female nurses, Harvard researchers found that increasing cholesterol intake by 200 mg for

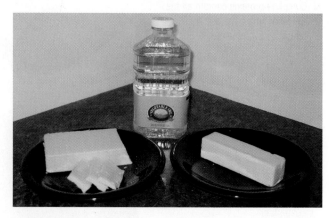

■ Fats are classified into three categories: saturated fats, which come primarily from animal sources; unsaturated fats, which come from plants; and trans fats, which form when vegetable oils are processed into margarine or shortening.

every 1,000 calories in the diet (about one egg per day) did not appreciably increase the risk for heart disease.[12]

It is recommended that 30% or less of daily calories come from fat, with 10% or less coming from saturated fat (**Table 9.1**). No daily limit has been set for trans fat, but any amount is harmful (**Table 9.2**). Additionally, diets should contain less than 300 mg of cholesterol per day.[10] These guidelines, which parallel the dietary guidelines endorsed by the USDA and the U.S. Department of Health and Human Services, emphasize the importance to women of following careful eating patterns from early childhood to old age. Currently, few American women are meeting these standards. **Self-Assessment 9.1** reviews the method for calculating daily fat intake.

Self-Assessment 9.1

Calculating Daily Fat Limits

To determine the maximum number of daily grams of fat:

1. Calculate approximately how many calories are consumed on a daily basis: _____

2. Divide the answer above by 33: _____

Women who find that they are eating more grams of fat than the calculated number should work on achieving this desired amount. Women with an intake of greater than 30% of calories from fat are at greater risk for many chronic diseases as well as obesity.

Table 9.1 Differences in Saturated Fat and Calorie Content of Commonly Consumed Foods

This table shows a few practical examples of the differences in the saturated fat content of different forms of commonly consumed foods. Comparisons are made between foods in the same food group (e.g., regular cheddar cheese and low-fat cheddar cheese), illustrating that lower saturated fat choices can be made within the same food group.

Food Category	Portion	Saturated Fat Content (grams)	Calories
Cheese			
■ Regular cheddar cheese	1 oz	6.0	114
■ Low-fat cheddar cheese	1 oz	1.2	49
Ground beef			
■ Regular ground beef (25% fat)	3 oz (cooked)	6.1	236
■ Extra lean ground beef (5% fat)	3 oz (cooked)	2.6	148
Milk			
■ Whole milk (3.24%)	1 cup	4.6	146
■ Low-fat (1%) milk	1 cup	1.5	102
Breads			
■ Croissant	1 medium	6.6	231
■ Bagel, oat bran	1 medium (4 inch)	0.2	227
Frozen desserts			
■ Regular ice cream	½ cup	4.9	145
■ Frozen yogurt, low-fat	½ cup	2.0	110
Table spreads			
■ Butter	1 tsp	2.4	34
■ Soft margarine with zero trans fat	1 tsp	0.7	25
Chicken			
■ Fried chicken (leg with skin)	3 oz (cooked)	3.3	212
■ Roasted chicken (breast, no skin)	3 oz (cooked)	0.9	140
Fish			
■ Fried fish	3 oz	2.8	195
■ Baked fish	3 oz	1.5	129

Source: U.S. Department of Agriculture. (2005). *Dietary Guidelines for Americans.*

Table 9.2   Trans Fatty Acid Content of Selected Foods

Food	Trans Fat as a Percentage of Total Fat
Bread, white	9.3%
Cake with chocolate frosting	18.3%
Cheesecake	12.0%
Cookies, chocolate chip	24.3%
Cookies, chocolate, cream filled	36.3%
Crackers, snack type	39.7%
Pastry, Danish	39.5%
French fries	23.9%
Granola bar	17.9%
Margarine, hard stick	29.4%
Shortening	22.2%
Popcorn, microwave	31.7%
Unprocessed vegetables, fruits, grains, nuts, vegetable oils, legumes, soy milk	0%

To find out whether a food contains trans fatty acids, look at the ingredient list. If the words "partially hydrogenated oils" are listed, it contains trans fats.

Source: U.S. Department of Agriculture.

Vitamins

Vitamins are organic substances that perform a variety of functions and are needed by the body in very small amounts. Vitamin supplements are one tool women can use to get their daily requirements for vitamins, but supplements should not be used to replace a balanced diet. Vitamin supplements cannot replace food or turn a junk-food meal into a healthy one. Vitamins are essential for life, promoting good vision, forming normal blood cells, creating strong bones and teeth, and ensuring proper functioning of the heart and nervous system. Although vitamins do not supply any energy, they do aid in the efficient conversion of foods into energy. There is no scientific information indicating that massive intake of vitamins far beyond the RDAs provides any benefit; in fact, overdosing on large amounts of vitamins can be harmful to people's health.

There are 13 essential vitamins: A, C, D, E, K, and the eight vitamins of the B complex. Fat-soluble vitamins (A, D, E, and K) are stored in the liver for relatively long periods of time; **water-soluble vitamins** (B-complex vitamins and C) are stored for very short periods of time. Each vitamin carries out specific functions. The body generally cannot manufacture vitamins; instead, they must be derived from food sources. A particular disease usually results if a certain vitamin is lacking or is improperly used by the body. **Table 9.3** summarizes facts known for each of the essential vitamins.

Folic Acid

Folate is a B vitamin found in foods such as chickpeas, spinach, strawberries, kidney beans, and citrus fruits and juices. Folic acid, a form of folate, is used to fortify grain-based foods, such as bread, flour, rice, pasta, and cereal. It is vital for cell growth and function and for the development of healthy neural tubes in fetuses. Neural tube defects, including spina bifida, are birth defects affecting the brain and spinal cord. Since fortification of cereal grains with folic acid began in the United States in 1998, the incidence of neural tube disorders has decreased by 20–30%. All women of childbearing age should include 400–600 micrograms (0.4–0.6 mg) of folic acid in their daily diet. Surveys have shown that as a group, women of childbearing age consume an average of 200 micrograms per day, only half of the recommended amount.[13] Folic acid also is important for maintaining levels of homocysteine, an amino acid found in the blood that builds and maintains tissues, but it can increase the risk of cardiovascular disease if it is consumed at excessive levels. Folic acid fortification is a public health intervention that, like immunization, actually saves money; one economic analysis concluded that folic acid fortification in the United States results in a cost savings of $88 million to $145 million annually and is associated with an overall economic benefit of $312 million to $425 million per year.[14]

Antioxidants and Phytochemicals

Antioxidants, which include vitamin E and vitamin C, are substances that can neutralize oxidants, harmful molecules that can build up in the body. Antioxidants and **phytochemicals** (substances such as carotenoids and flavonoids that appear to act as antioxidants) have been widely studied for their roles in disease prevention and health promotion. Evidence has shown that diets rich in fruits, vegetables, and grains—all of which are rich sources of antioxidants—are associated with a decreased risk of cardiovascular disease and cancer. Damage to cells from oxidation is associated with an increased risk of various diseases. Antioxidants are thought to block some of the oxygen-induced cell damage by stabilizing and neutralizing the effects of free radicals (toxic particles) in the body.

Table 9.3 Facts About Vitamins

Vitamin	Women's RDA*	Sources	What It Does
Vitamin A	700 μg	Liver, eggs, dairy products, carrots, bell peppers, green leafy vegetables, squash	Promotes good vision; helps form and maintain healthy skin and mucous membranes; helps fight infections
Vitamin B₁ (thiamin)	1.1 mg	Whole grains, dried beans, lean red meats, fish, sunflower seeds	Helps release energy from carbohydrates; necessary for healthy brain and nerve cells and for functioning of heart
Vitamin B₂ (riboflavin)	1.1 mg	Dairy products, liver, whole grains, spinach, broccoli	Aids in the release of energy from food; helps form antibodies and red blood cells
Vitamin B₃ (niacin)	14 mg	Nuts, dairy products, liver, enriched grains, poultry	Aids in the release of energy from food; involved in the synthesis of DNA; maintains normal function of skin, nerves, and digestive system
Vitamin B₅ (pantothenic acid)	5 mg	Whole grains, dried beans, eggs, nuts	Aids in the release of energy from food; essential for synthesis of numerous body materials
Vitamin B₆ (pyridoxine)	1.3 mg	Fortified breakfast cereals, meat, nuts, beans	Important in chemical reactions of proteins and amino acids; involved in normal functioning of brain and formation of red blood cells
Vitamin B₁₂ (cobalamin)	2.4 μg	Liver, beef, eggs, milk, shellfish	Necessary for development of red blood cells; maintains normal functioning of nervous system
Biotin	30 μg	Yeast, liver, eggs, milk	Important in the formation of fatty acids; helps metabolize amino acids and carbohydrates
Vitamin C† (ascorbic acid)	75 mg	Citrus fruits and juices, bell peppers, tomatoes, spinach, broccoli	Promotes healthy gums, capillaries, and teeth; aids iron absorption; maintains normal connective tissue; aids in healing wounds
Choline	425 mg	Whole grains, egg yolks, legumes, liver, soybeans, green leafy vegetables	Manages cholesterol in body; important for brain function; involved in production of hormones; necessary for functioning of folic acid
Vitamin D (calciferol)	5 μg	Dairy products, mackerel, sardines, salmon and other cold-water fish	Promotes strong bones and teeth; necessary for absorption of calcium
Vitamin E (tocopherol)	15 mg	Nuts, vegetable oils, whole grains, margarine, dark green vegetables	Protects tissue against oxidation; important in formation of red blood cells; helps body use vitamin K
Folate (folic acid/folacin)	400 μg	Liver, fortified breakfast cereals, lentils, chickpeas, spinach, beans	Important in the synthesis of DNA; acts together with vitamin B₁₂ in the production of hemoglobin; vital to healthy fetal development
Vitamin K	90 μg	Leafy green vegetables, soybeans, broccoli, cauliflower	Aids in the clotting of blood

*Pregnant or breastfeeding women need additional levels of these vitamins.
†Smokers should consume an additional 35 mg daily of vitamin C.
Sources: Willet, W. C. (2002). *Eat, Drink and Be Healthy: The Harvard Medical School Guide to Healthy Eating*. New York: Simon and Schuster. Editors of the *University of California at Berkeley Wellness Letter*. (1995). *The New Wellness Encyclopedia*. Boston: Houghton Mifflin.

Some studies show that vitamin E protects against damage in the artery lining, thereby decreasing the risk of coronary artery disease. Many studies indicate that eating fruits and vegetables rich in vitamin C and beta-carotene (the carotenoid that is the precursor of vitamin A) is linked to a reduced risk of many cancers. Carotenoids and flavonoids, which are found in foods such as onions, broccoli, red wine, green tea, and black tea, appear to have a positive effect on heart disease; however, the association between phytochemicals and heart disease is still uncertain.

It is obvious that a healthy diet helps prevent disease. However, evidence for more specific claims, such as those that mention individual foods preventing specific diseases, is uncertain at best. For now, experts recommend that people meet the RDAs by eating foods high in carotenoids, such as red, orange, and deep yellow fruits and vegetables (e.g., tomatoes, carrots, sweet potatoes) and dark green leafy vegetables (e.g., spinach, broccoli); foods high in vitamin E (e.g., vegetable oils, salad dressings, margarine, whole grains, peanut butter); and foods rich in vitamin C (e.g., citrus fruits, strawberries, broccoli). Eating a variety of fruits and vegetables promotes health by supplying the body not only with vitamins and fiber, but also with antioxidants that may reduce the risk of heart disease and some kinds of cancer.[8]

Minerals

Minerals are inorganic substances essential to bone formation (calcium), enzyme synthesis (iron), blood pressure maintenance (sodium), and normal functioning of the digestive process (potassium). Minerals make up the earth's surface. Carried into the soil, groundwater, and sea by erosion, they are taken up by plants and subsequently consumed by animals and humans. As components of the body, minerals are present in small amounts. Six minerals (calcium, chloride, magnesium, phosphorus, potassium, and sodium) are generally designated as macrominerals, or major minerals. Calcium and iron are especially important for women's health.

Because of the complex interactions between minerals and the dangers of overdosing, self-administration of mineral supplements in doses greater than the RDAs should be avoided. Megadoses of certain minerals may do serious harm. The best way to ensure an adequate, but not excessive, supply of minerals is to eat a varied, balanced diet. **Table 9.4** summarizes facts about each of the essential minerals.

Calcium

Calcium is a mineral of special concern to women. Calcium is an integral component of bones and teeth, and calcium deficiency is a major contributor to osteoporosis. When calcium levels in the blood fall too low, the body draws the mineral from the supply in the bones to meet its needs elsewhere. This process accelerates the gradual bone loss that occurs most dramatically in postmenopausal women. Calcium helps regulate heartbeat, blood clotting, muscle contraction, and nerve conduction. Evidence suggests that this mineral also helps prevent high blood pres-

sure, is essential in the development of the fetus during pregnancy, and may reduce the risk for colon cancer.

The RDA's recommendation that women receive 1,000 mg of calcium per day is deceptive. Adolescents, young women (ages 11 to 24), and postmenopausal women are advised to consume 1,200 mg daily. However, many health experts believe that lower dosages may be adequate. Three to five cups of milk or servings of other calcium-rich foods such as collard greens, cheese, tofu, cornbread, or sardines can supply the 1,000 mg recommendation. (See **It's Your Health**.) Daily supplements can also be a viable calcium source.[8]

The 2005 food pyramid continues to emphasize dairy products as an important part of a healthy diet. However, some nutrition experts believe that the U.S. dietary guidelines exaggerate the benefits and underestimate the dangers of a diet high in dairy foods. Dairy foods are an excellent source of calcium as well as protein, vitamin D, and other nutrients; however, they often contain large amounts of saturated fat and calories, and they are not an option for lactose-intolerant individuals. Women do not have to rely on dairy products for their calcium. A cup of collard greens, for example, has virtually the same amount of calcium as a cup of skim milk (see **It's Your Health**). In many Asian countries that have lower osteoporosis rates than the United

It's Your Health

Calcium Sources

Food	Amount	mg Calcium	Percentage of RDA 1,000 mg/day	1,200 mg/day
Plain yogurt	1 cup	415	41%	35%
Sardines with bones	3 oz	372	37%	31%
Skim milk	1 cup	302	30%	25%
Collard greens	1 cup	290	29%	24%
Swiss cheese	1 oz	262	26%	22%
Cheddar cheese	1 oz	213	21%	18%
Canned salmon, with bones	3 oz	167	17%	14%
Low-fat cottage cheese	1 cup	154	15%	12%
Blackstrap molasses	1 tbsp	137	14%	12%
Cooked broccoli	1 cup	136	14%	12%
Dried and cooked beans	1 cup	90	9%	7%
Orange	1 (medium)	54	5%	4%

Table 9.4 Facts About Minerals

Mineral	Adult RDA*	Sources	What It Does
Calcium	1,000–2,500 mg*	Milk and milk products, sardines and salmon eaten with bones, dark green leafy vegetables, certain types of tofu and soy milk, fortified orange juice	Builds bones and teeth and maintains bone density and strength; helps prevent osteoporosis; plays a role in regulating heartbeat, blood clotting, muscle contraction, and nerve conduction; helps prevent hypertension
Chloride	700 mg	Table salt, fish, pickled and smoked foods	Maintains normal fluid shifts; balances pH of the blood; forms hydrochloric acid to aid digestion
Magnesium	310–320 mg*	Whole grains, raw leafy green vegetables, nuts (especially almonds and cashews), soybeans, tofu, hard water	Aids in bone growth; assists function of nerves and muscles, including regulation of normal heart rhythm; important in energy metabolism
Phosphorus	700 mg*	Meats, poultry, fish, egg yolks, dried peas and beans, milk and milk products, nuts; present in almost all foods	Aids bone growth and strengthening of teeth; important in energy metabolism
Potassium	4,700 mg†	Oranges and orange juice, melons, bananas, dried fruits, dried peas and beans, potatoes	Promotes regular heartbeat; active in muscle contraction; regulates transfer of nutrients to cells; controls water balance in body tissues and cells; contributes to regulation of blood pressure
Sodium	500 mg (estimated safe amount for dietary intake)	All from salt and foods containing salt	Helps regulate water balance in body; plays a role in maintaining blood pressure
Chromium	50–200 µg†	Meat, cheese, mushrooms, oysters, peanuts, brewer's yeast, potatoes	Important for glucose metabolism; may be a cofactor for insulin; regulates cholesterol production in liver; aids in digestion of protein
Copper	900–10,000 µg†	Wheat, peanuts, shellfish (especially oysters), nuts, beef and pork liver, dried beans	Formation of red blood cells; cofactor in absorbing iron into blood cells; assists in production of several enzymes involved in respiration; interacts with zinc
Fluorine (Fluoride)	3.1 mg†	Fluoridated water, foods cooked with or grown in fluoridated water, fish, tea, gelatin	Contributes to solid bone and tooth formation; prevents dental cavities; may help prevent osteoporosis
Iodine	0.15 mg*	Primarily from iodized salt, but also seafood, seaweed food products, vegetables grown in iodine-rich areas, eggs, certain cheeses, whole milk	Necessary for normal function of the thyroid gland; essential for normal cell function; keeps skin, hair, and nails healthy; prevents goiter
Iron	18–45 mg*	Liver (especially pork liver), kidneys, red meats, egg yolks, peas, beans, nuts, dried fruits, green leafy vegetables, enriched grain products, blackstrap molasses	Essential to formation of hemoglobin, the oxygen-carrying factor in the blood; part of several enzymes and proteins in the blood
Manganese	320–350 mg†	Nuts, whole grains, vegetables, fruits, instant coffee, tea, cocoa powder, beets, egg yolks	Required for normal bone growth; helps maintain healthy skin; important for metabolism of glucose and fatty acids
Molybdenum	75–250 µg†	Peas, beans, cereal grains, organ meats, some dark green vegetables	Important for normal cell function
Selenium	50–55 µg	Fish, shellfish, red meat, egg yolks, chicken, legumes, whole grains	Protects cells against effects of free radicals that can damage cells; essential for normal functioning of the immune system and thyroid gland
Zinc	8–40 mg	Meat, liver, eggs, oysters, legumes, whole grain cereals, nuts	Essential for growth and skeletal development; important for immune system; assists in production of DNA and RNA

*These figures are not applicable to pregnant or breastfeeding women, who need additional minerals.

†Although there is no RDA for these minerals, the Food and Nutrition Board recommends this value as an average healthy intake.

Sources: Willet, W. C. (2002). *Eat, Drink and Be Healthy: The Harvard Medical School Guide to Healthy Eating*. New York: Simon and Schuster. Editors of the *University of California at Berkeley Wellness Letter*. (1995). *The New Wellness Encyclopedia*. Boston: Houghton Mifflin Co.

States, dairy products are marginal to nonexistent in traditional diets; leafy green vegetables are the main sources of calcium in these regions.

People who cannot meet the daily calcium intake recommendations through consumption of calcium-rich foods may use calcium-fortified foods and calcium supplements. Women who are susceptible to kidney stones should avoid such supplements to prevent an increased risk of stone formation. Because large amounts of calcium may lead to constipation, kidney stones, and poor kidney function, as well as interfere with the absorption of other minerals, women should not consume calcium levels significantly beyond their RDA.

Iron

Iron is found in the human body primarily in **hemoglobin**, a key component of red blood cells and the oxygen-carrying protein that gives blood its red color. When hemoglobin is not produced, the body becomes fatigued and weak. Reduced levels of hemoglobin result in anemia, a serious risk for women whose diets are chronically deficient in iron. Symptoms of iron-deficiency anemia include headaches, fatigue, general weakness, and pallor. In severe cases, anemia can lead to an irregular or increased heart rate. Iron-deficiency anemia is relatively common in the United States today, with 12% of women ages 12 to 49 experiencing some form of iron deficiency.[15] In addition to being found in hemoglobin, iron is stored in the liver, spleen, bone marrow, and other tissues.

Iron absorption is a complex process that varies with the types and combination of foods consumed and the body's needs. Women can use several strategies to increase their dietary intake of iron. Eating lean red meats is one method. Liver is one of the best sources of iron, but it should not be eaten more than once a week owing to its high cholesterol content. Chicken and fish typically contain one-third to one-half the iron of red meat. Vegetarian sources of iron include chickpeas, soybeans, kidney beans, and lentils. Choosing breads, cereals, and pasta labeled "enriched" or "fortified" and unrefined whole grains, such as whole-wheat bread, supplies a fair amount of iron. In addition, eating foods high in vitamin C facilitates the body's absorption of iron. For vegetarians and vegans, consuming vitamin C with meals is a must. Cooking in cast-iron cookware also helps to increase the iron content of foods. The more acidic the food (such as spaghetti sauce) and the longer it cooks, the more iron will be absorbed. Other compounds, such as coffee, tea, and dietary fiber, block the body's ability to absorb iron.

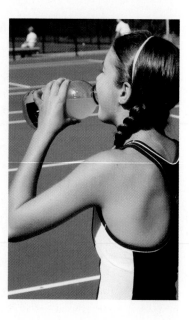

■ Sports and energy drinks may claim to "replenish" body fluids, but water alone is usually a more healthful (and cheaper) option.

Water

The human body is approximately 50% to 70% water. Water is manufactured only in small amounts by the body and must be consumed in the form of liquids and solids to meet daily needs. Every system in the body depends on water to function: Water regulates body temperature and chemical actions, disposes of waste, lubricates joints, cushions the fetus during pregnancy, transports nutrients, prevents bowel problems, and helps enzymes function properly.

The average female requires eight to nine cups of fluid per day; pregnant women have a slightly higher requirement due to the needs of the fetus. Some of this fluid comes from the food a woman eats; the rest must come from what she drinks. Drinking water is one healthful option. Another is drinking milk, skim milk, or fruit juice, which can also supply the body with minerals, protein, and vitamins. Sweetened sodas and sports drinks are less healthy options because they are typically loaded with sugar and calories and provide no additional nutritonal benefit.

Water is so essential that the human body can survive only three days without it, even though the body can be denied food for a few weeks and still recover. As little as 2% to 5% loss of body weight from water loss results in symptoms of dehydration, including headache, fatigue, flushed skin, and excessive thirst. Greater need for fluids occurs during exercise and conditions of high temperature, high altitude, and low humidity, and when it is necessary to counter the effects of high intakes of caffeine and alcohol, which promote fluid loss. Many studies are examining the effects of water consumption on the risk of various conditions, including kidney stones, certain cancers, obesity, and oral health.

Exercise and Fitness

Being physically active provides benefits to health at all stages of life. (This book uses the term physical activity to describe activity that brings health benefits—generally, any movement of a moderate intensity that lasts a few minutes or more. Many day-to-day activities, such as climbing a flight of stairs, count as physical activity. **Exercise** refers to a deliberate session of physical activity for the purpose of improving health.) Regular physical activity makes the body healthier and stronger; it also reduces the risk for disease and other negative health outcomes. This physical activity can come in the form of intense exercise sessions or from more moderate-intensity activities, such as walking, dancing, or yoga.

However, physical inactivity remains a serious national problem. More than half of U.S. adults do not get enough physical activity to provide significant health benefits. Men are more likely to be physically active than women, but this gap is shrinking. From 2001 to 2005, the percentage of women who were regularly physically active increased slightly, from 43% to 46.7%. Physical activity decreases with age and is less common among those with lower incomes, less education, and non-white ethnicity/race (see **Table 9.5**); however, these disparities also appear to be shrinking.[16]

Physical Fitness

"Physical fitness" means different things to different people. A dancer and a long-distance swimmer may both think of themselves as "fit" but they probably have different strengths, stretch different muscles, and have different workout goals. Fitness is also relative—a woman may be "more fit" this year than she was last year, and there is no clear endpoint at which fitness occurs. One definition of fitness is the ability to meet routine physical demands while maintaining a reserve to meet sudden challenges. Fitness provides short-term and long-term benefits. Women who exercise just an hour per week or more are 33% less likely to die from cancer, 50% less likely to die from cardiovascular disease, and 66% less likely to die early than women who do not excercise.[17]

Benefits of Exercise

Regular exercise offers many physical and psychological benefits that improve quality and quantity of life (**Table 9.6**). Adults and children of all age groups and body types, including people with disabilities, benefit greatly from

Table 9.5	Percentage of U.S. Women Regularly Engaging in Physical Activity, 2005
Age Groups	
18-24	52.7%
25-34	50.5%
35-44	49.7%
45-64	45.5%
65 or older	36.3%
Race/Ethnicity	
White, non-Hispanic	49.6%
Black, non-Hispanic	36.1%
Hispanic	40.5%
Other race	46.6%
Education Level	
Less than high-school graduate	37.1%
High-school graduate	43.2%
Some college	47.9%
College graduate	53.3%
Total	**46.7%**

Source: Centers for Disease Control and Prevention. (2007). *Prevalence of regular physical activity among adults—United States, 2001 and 2005.*

Table 9.6	Benefits of Regular Physical Activity

- Reduces the risk of early death
- Reduces the risk of developing coronary heart disease, stroke, and breast, lung, and colon cancer
- Reduces the risk of developing type 2 diabetes, osteoporosis, and depression
- Lowers high blood pressure and cholesterol
- Improves aerobic capacity, muscle strength, and muscle endurance
- Can reduce symptoms of depression and increase cognitive functioning
- For older adults, improves ability to complete day-to-day tasks, reduces the risk of falls, and improves mental cognition
- Helps maintain healthy muscles, joints, and bones
- Helps control weight, build muscle, and reduce body fat
- Can reduce symptoms and severity of diabetes and arthritis

Source: Department of Health and Human Services. (2008). *2008 Physical Activity Guidelines for Americans.*

I've made a real effort to incorporate exercise into my daily routine this semester. On Mondays, Wednesdays, and Fridays I go straight to the gym after class, and I go running Tuesdays, Thursdays, and Saturdays, taking Sunday off. It's funny, because I never really thought about exercise much until this year, but now it's a normal part of my life.

20-year-old student

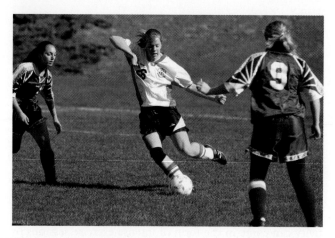

■ Organized sports are one form of exercise.

regular physical activity. Substantial health benefits occur if a person gets at least 150 minutes (2.5 hours) of moderate-intensity activity a week, and 75 minutes (1 hour and 15 minutes) of high-intensity exercise a week. Alternatively, a combination of both high- and moderate-intensity exercise can also be used to reach the total of 150 minutes, with every minute of high-intensity exercise counting for two minutes of moderate-intensity exercise. Greater health benefits occur if a person gets twice that amount or more (300 minutes a week of moderate-intensity activity, 150 minutes of high-intensity activity, or a combination of both).[18] However, even small amounts of physical activity are better than none at all. Regular exercise reduces death and injury from heart disease, the leading cause of death in the United States. Physical activity not only improves overall cardiovascular status, but also affects other risk factors for heart disease. For example, regular physical activity lowers blood pressure, reduces body fat, builds lean body weight, improves blood cholesterol levels, and reduces stress. Exercise reduces the risk of developing colon cancer, type 2 diabetes, osteoporosis, obesity, and other diseases. This association also may be a consequence of exercise's ability to reduce the risk factors for various chronic diseases, such as high body fat and smoking behaviors.

Physical activity is extremely important for maintaining the health of muscles, bones, and joints; ensuring normal skeletal development; increasing bone mass and density; and slowing the rate of bone loss as women age—hence its role in reducing the risk of osteoporosis. Regular physical activity also improves balance and coordination, which reduce a woman's risk of fall-related fractures in later life.

The basic fact that exercise burns calories and increases lean body weight is important not only for the prevention of obesity (a major risk factor for many chronic diseases), but also for a woman's overall sense of well-being. Although most individuals who exercise regularly report that they "feel better" when they exercise, until recently the scientific community has not been able to measure this phenomenon objectively. Many studies have confirmed the potential value of aerobic exercise, along with medication if necessary, as a complementary therapy for depression.[18–20] People who exercise regularly report feeling happier, feeling better about themselves, and in general experience a better quality of life than people who do not.[20] Regular exercise may also reduce the anxiety and depression that can appear during pregnancy.[21] Other studies found various psychological benefits from exercise, including decreased stress, increased sense of well-being, and improvements in cognitive function and mood.[18] Proper exercise during pregnancy also has many benefits, including improved psychological well-being, shorter labor, and speedier recovery after childbirth (see Chapter 6).

Components of Physical Fitness

Exercise physiologists usually define fitness in four major areas:

- Cardiovascular endurance
- Muscular strength
- Muscular endurance
- Flexibility

Modern lifestyles do not require much physical movement, and few U.S. women are naturally fit as a result of day-to-day activities. Most women who wish to become fit in today's society will need to make a commitment of time and energy to exercise.

Cardiovascular endurance, the ability to carry on vigorous physical activity for an extended period of time, is the most vital element of fitness. It is a measure of the ability of the heart to pump blood efficiently through the body. The development of cardiovascular endurance enhances the ability of the heart, blood vessels, and blood to deliver oxygen to the body's cells and then remove waste products. Although muscles are able to draw on quick sources of energy for short-term exertion, when exercise lasts more than a minute or two, the muscles require oxygen from the blood. Such physical activity is called aerobic exercise. With repeated regular exercise, the heart becomes able to pump more blood and deliver more oxygen with greater efficiency. The muscles' capacity to use this oxygen also improves. The coupled events are referred to as the "training effect." The heart rate, both at rest and exertion, decreases as a result of this regular exercise, and the heart acquires the ability to recover from the stress of exercise more quickly.

Muscular strength is the total force that muscle groups produce in one effort, such as a lift, jump, or heave. Working out with weights, either free weights or weight machines, is the best way to increase muscle strength. Strength gains come most quickly from heavy resistance and few repetitions.

Muscular endurance is the ability to perform repeated muscular contractions over a period of time without tiring. Although muscle endurance requires strength, it is not a single, all-out effort. The keys to increasing endurance are repetition, working at a moderate level, and building up to a specified goal. Sit-ups, push-ups, and pull-ups can be used to build endurance.

Flexibility is the ability of the joints to move through their full range of motion. It is best improved through static stretching exercises that apply steady pressure at the extreme range of motion without undue bouncing. Flexibility varies from person to person and from joint to joint. Women tend to be more flexible than men because of differences in their skeletons, muscle mass, and body composition. Good flexibility protects the muscles against pulls and tears because short, tight muscles may be more likely to be overstretched. Exercises intended to increase flexibility must be selected carefully, however, because some movements may actually cause injury to the lower back and knees. Some women find that stretching certain muscle groups helps relieve or prevent pain. Stretching hamstring and lower back muscles may alleviate lower back pain, and calf stretches may help prevent leg cramps.

Body composition refers to the ratio of lean body weight (muscle and bone) to fat weight. Exercise affects body composition in two major ways: by reducing excess body weight through energy expenditure and by increasing the body's overall metabolism rate. The body burns calories not only during the period of physical exercise, but also for several hours after exercise ends (known as afterburn). The longer and more intense the exercise, the longer the **basal metabolic rate (BMR)** remains elevated. Regular exercise improves overall muscle tone, contributing to a trimmer

appearance. Exercise can also improve balance, coordination (the ability to skillfully use different body parts and the senses together), and agility (the ability to coordinate multiple movements and to react quickly and safely).

Total Fitness

Activities to improve fitness are often referred to as conditioning programs or training regimens. Fitness programs tend to fall into two categories: aerobic training and strength training. Aerobic training increases the body's ability to use oxygen and improves endurance. Strength training enhances the size and strength of specific muscles and body regions. The best fitness programs combine aerobic exercise with strength training. Both types of exercise provide unique benefits. Strength training builds muscle and bone, and aerobic exercise improves cardiovascular fitness. Together, aerobic and strength training provide better benefits than either form of exercise alone. Coupled with a healthy diet, the combination program also may be the most efficient way to lose weight. In addition to burning calories while working out, the resultant muscle mass from strength training boosts the basal metabolic rate further because muscle consumes more energy than does fat.

Warm-Up

A warm-up is essential before any aerobic or strength training session. Warming up prepares the body for exercise by gradually increasing the heart rate and blood flow, raising the temperature of the muscles, and improving muscle function. It may also decrease the chance of sports-related injury. Stretching is not a wise way to begin a workout, because stretching cold muscles increases the risk of injury. Sudden exercise without a gradual warm-up can lead to an abnormal heart rate and blood flow and changes in blood pressure, which can be dangerous, especially for older exercisers.

Activities such as jogging in place or stationary cycling are full body warm-ups that can be performed for 5 to 10 minutes to raise body temperature.

Strength Training

Strength training, like aerobic exercise, helps prevent or delay many of the declines associated with aging or inactivity. Three components determine the amount of muscle that a strength-training program provides: intensity (the amount of weight lifted or pulled), repetitions (the number of times the weight is lifted or pulled), and frequency (the number of sessions in a given period). Experts generally

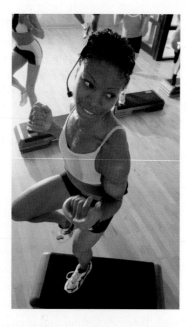

■ Strength training can help prevent or delay many of the declines associated with aging or inactivity.

Women tend to have less muscle mass than men, especially in the upper body. This discrepancy has been attributed to gender differences in size, hormones, and normal activity levels. Women who work out, however, gain strength at the same rate as men. Many women have avoided strength training out of fear of becoming "muscle bound." A moderate program will not create obvious muscle bulk in men or women but will result in a firmer, trimmer physique.

Aerobic Exercise

Aerobic exercise significantly raises the heart rate and provides different benefits than strength training. Aerobic exercise seems to lower body cholesterol levels and blood pressure more than strength training. It also improves cardiovascular fitness, the ability of the heart and lungs to supply the muscles with oxygen; strength training generally does not provide such a benefit. Examples of aerobic exercise include running, bicycling, and rollerblading.

Components of Aerobic Exercise.   When exercising, there are three important variables to consider: intensity, duration, and frequency. Intensity, duration, and frequency all affect the amount of health benefits any exercise program provides; no one of these variables is more important than the others.

Exercise intensity is the work per unit of time. It can be monitored by measuring the target heart rate—the exercise heart rate needed to produce a training effect—for 20 to 30 minutes during each workout. See **Table 9.7** for examples of moderate- and high-intensity activities.

Exercise duration is the length of one exercise session. To benefit the heart, aerobic exercise must be intense enough

agree that a person should use enough weight so that she can just barely do 8–12 repetitions in a row, and that a good frequency is two to three sessions per week.

Strength training does not have to mean lifting massive weights to build bulging muscles. Instead, it often calls for working out against moderate resistance to tone muscles and build muscle endurance. Free weights, dumbbells, barbells, or weight machines can provide this resistance. Body weight can also be used as resistance, as in push-ups or pull-ups.

Strength training offers many benefits:

- Well-toned muscles help maintain good posture and may help prevent injuries.

- Muscle strength produces benefits in daily living, from lifting items to engaging in physical activity, by increasing stamina and self-confidence.

- Strength training increases bone density, thereby helping to delay or minimize osteoporosis and vulnerability to fractures.

- Injury prevention is another important benefit of strength training, especially for musculoskeletal injuries induced by exercise, such as runner's knee or shin splints. These injuries are due in part to muscle weakness and imbalances as well as joint instability. Such conditions are often corrected with strength training.

- Maintaining a strong back through strength training protects it from injury. Lower back pain often results from weakness of back and abdominal muscles, both of which help support the back.

- Strength training helps improve posture, a source of many back problems.

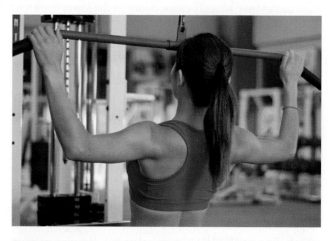

■ Maintaining a strong back through strength training protects it from injury.

Table 9.7 — Examples of Moderate- and High-Intensity Activities

Moderate-Intensity Activities

Walking briskly (3 mph or more)

Ballroom dancing

Playing tennis, doubles

Bicycling 5 to 9 mph, level terrain

Weight-lifting

High-Intensity Activities

Swimming laps

Hiking with a heavy backpack or on hilly terrain

Aerobic dancing

Playing tennis, singles

Jumping rope

Source: Department of Health and Human Services. (2008).
2008 Physical Activity Guidelines for Americans.

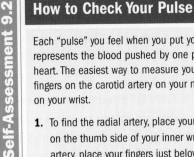

Self-Assessment 9.2 — How to Check Your Pulse

Each "pulse" you feel when you put your fingers on an artery represents the blood pushed by one pump of a person's heart. The easiest way to measure your pulse is to place your fingers on the carotid artery on your neck or the radial artery on your wrist.

1. To find the radial artery, place your first two or three fingers on the thumb side of your inner wrist. To find the carotid artery, place your fingers just below the edge of the jaw bone. Apply gentle pressure. Do not use your thumb.

2. Using a stopwatch or clock with a second hand, count the number of pulses in 30 seconds. Multiply by 2 to get the number of beats per minute.

to increase the heart rate and must continue for a minimum amount of time depending on the intensity of the workout. Many experts agree that aerobic activity should last for 30 minutes or more to provide the most benefit, but the evidence for this statement is not conclusive.[18]

Exercise frequency measures the number of exercise sessions over the long term. Engaging in regular periods of exercise is essential for any exercise program. Exercising in three to five half-hour periods per week builds muscle and improves fitness faster and more safely than exercising for the same length of time in one long weekly workout.

Maximum and Target Range Heart Rates. No aerobic exercise program will be beneficial unless it forces the heart to pump beyond its normal output. To determine this ideal pace, check whether the heart is beating within the target heart range—fast enough to ensure that the activity pushes the heart muscle to the point of improving fitness, but not so fast that it will become exhausted within too short a time or cause physical harm. (See **Figure 9.3** to determine maximum and target heart rates.) Checking the pulse during or immediately after exercise is useful for determining if the exercise is at the appropriate intensity (see **Self-Assessment 9.2**). An exercise program that keeps the heart rate within the desirable range provides a training effect in as safe a manner as possible. If the heart does not reach the lower limit of the target heart range during an exercise

Figure 9.3

Maximum and targeted heart rates.

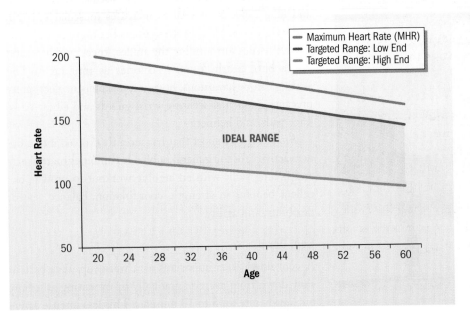

activity, increase the intensity by exercising more vigorously. If the heart rate exceeds the upper limit of the target heart range, particularly in the early phases of an exercise program, reduce the intensity to stay within the range.

Many Options of Aerobic Exercise.   Regular exercise is important. The form it takes is of secondary importance. Many women find that they are able to maintain their interest in exercise by changing their physical activity on a regular basis to avoid boredom. Seasonal variations and access to recreational facilities also influence exercise decision making. The following examples describe currently popular forms of aerobic exercise that are enjoyed by many women.

Moderate- to brisk-paced walking is an easy, safe, simple, and enjoyable way to stay healthy; walking for 30 to 45 minutes per day lowers the risk of heart disease, lowers blood pressure, helps control adult-onset diabetes, guards against osteoporosis, helps keep weight under control, and helps reduce stress. Most problems with walking can be avoided by simply wearing good walking shoes, warming up beforehand, practicing good walking technique, and working up slowly to the desired pace.

Jogging is aerobic exercise somewhere between a fast walk and a run, usually defined as moving at a pace slower than a 9-minute mile. Jogging is the classic aerobic exercise because it strengthens the heart and lungs, boosts stamina, improves bone strength, and improves circulation. Runners and joggers should be careful not to put too much stress on their knees, ankles, and other joints. Ways to reduce joint stress while running or jogging include using good running shoes; running on grass, dirt, or asphalt rather than con-

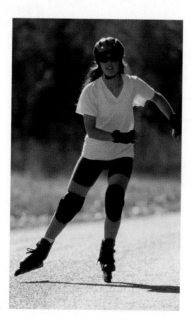

■ Aerobic exercise can take many forms. It is not limited to running or exercise classes.

crete; and alternating between running or jogging, and other forms of aerobic exercise.

Bicycling, whether on a stationary bike or outdoors, can be an excellent cardiovascular conditioner as well as an effective way to control weight. Stationary biking in aerobic settings, often referred to as "spinning," offers a variety of speed resistances to simulate biking a hilly course or race.

Stair climbing, either in buildings or on stair machines, is another excellent form of aerobic exercise. A major advantage of stair climbing, particularly with machines, is that it involves less impact on the joints and feet than many other forms of aerobic exercise. Step aerobics is another form of this exercise.

Swimming is an excellent way to strengthen and tone muscles as well as promote aerobic fitness. It does not, however, appear to be as effective an exercise modality for losing weight as other forms of exercise. A major benefit of swimming is that it places no excess stress on the joints, as do many other forms of aerobic exercise.

Aerobic dance is exercise combining music with kicking, stretching, bending, and jumping, to deliver the same benefits as running, cycling, or swimming. Aerobics can be especially good for cardiovascular fitness but presents risks to the joints and feet. Low-impact aerobics evolved in response to the many injuries incurred during traditional aerobic activities. This form of aerobics replaces jogging and jumping with steps that minimize the risk of injury or joint trauma. The third generation of aerobics, called "nonimpact aerobics," combines techniques of modern dance and martial arts with a focus on cardiovascular fitness.

In-line skating, also known as *rollerblading*, is a low-impact sport that improves cardiovascular development and lung capacity, as well as increases muscular strength and weight loss. Skating strengthens the muscles and connective tissues surrounding the ankles, knees, and hips, and it can burn nearly as many calories as running. In-line skating can be hazardous, however, if skaters neglect safety precautions such as wearing wrist guards and elbow pads, knee pads, and helmets.

Kickboxing is a sport that has recently evolved into a fitness activity for the general public. It combines martial arts and boxing skills with an aerobic workout to provide excellent benefits in strength, coordination, balance, speed, flexibility, and agility.

Cool-Down

A cool-down is as important as a warm-up. It is best to slow down from exercise gradually by exercising at a slow but steady rate for 5 to 10 minutes. This less intense activ-

> *Tennis was a big part of my life when I was in high school. Our school's women's tennis team was one of the best in the state, but we were always a second priority to the men's team, which was pretty mediocre. The female players weren't even allowed to wear our letters on our school jackets. My younger daughter plays soccer, and I love seeing her play. It's nice to see the women's teams getting some recognition!*
>
> **55-year-old doctor**

ity helps to prevent muscle stiffness and potentially dangerous sudden drops in blood pressure that occur when vigorous activities stop abruptly. Stretching after exercise is essential to protect against injury.

Physical Fitness and Women

Psychological, social, historical, and cultural factors all affect how women think about fitness and exercise. Historically, women were labeled "the weaker sex" and were not encouraged to become as fit as their male counterparts. Sociocultural prejudices have traditionally limited women's access to and full participation in sports. Self-esteem and self-confidence with physical activity are developmental tasks of childhood. Because young girls were traditionally not encouraged to excel or compete in the physical arena, they often lacked the self-esteem and confidence necessary to participate in sports as they grew older. It was not until 1978 that legislation known as **Title IX** mandated that public schools provide equal funding for girls' sports. Even since its passage, opportunities, resources, and, perhaps most importantly, encouragement for physical fitness have not been equally distributed to children, regardless of gender. Groups like the Women's National Basketball Association and a new generation of popular women's sports stars are revising the societal rule that says only male athletes can be admired.

Traditionally, men have excelled in physical competition against women. In general, men are able to run longer and faster, jump higher and farther, lift more and longer, and so forth. The traditional assumption has been that men are inherently physically gifted whereas women are not. In recent years, however, women have become more competitive in all athletic arenas. Several questions naturally flow from these advances that seek to better define gender similarities and differences in sports and exercise. Nevertheless, resolving these issues is difficult, because young girls and boys have not been raised with equivalent levels of emphasis, encouragement, and training in physical fitness.

Biologically, men and women are different. The influence of these differences on athletic performance is not fully understood. No apparent differences exist between the muscles of men and women. Rather, the fact that men are stronger than women reflects the larger absolute quantity of their muscle mass. The individual muscle fibers do not appear to be different. Women appear to be about half as strong as men in the upper body areas of the shoulders, arms, and backs and two-thirds as strong in the legs and lower body, primarily because men have larger muscle fiber areas and greater lean body weight (total weight minus body fat). Women's naturally higher percentage of body fat, essential for reproduction and general health, may have more of an effect on their physical performance than any other factor. Typically about 25% of a woman's body weight is fat, compared with 15% for men. Women's extra body fat may be a hindrance in sports such as running, but an advantage in sports such as swimming. In general, women also have a lower blood volume, about 5% less hemoglobin, smaller hearts, and less lung capacity than men.

In recent years, women's performances in endurance sports have dramatically improved. Women are increasingly being recognized as proficient athletes, whether in competition with each other or in mixed sports. The gender gap in such sports as biking is gradually shrinking. Female professional athletes may or may not reach the same levels of absolute performance as their male counterparts. In any case, it is important that women do not let prejudice or feelings of inferiority prevent them from reaching their own optimal fitness levels. Women's bodies respond to training as quickly as do men's. Reaching the level of fitness that best fits a person's individual preference and goals is the responsibility of an adult of either gender.

Exercise Myths and Facts

Fear and misinformation about fitness, workouts, or muscles cause many women to avoid exercise or to exercise inappropriately. Current medical knowledge shows that these fears are usually unfounded and that their resultant behaviors are often harmful.

Myth: Exercise increases the appetite.

Fact: Increased appetite is not necessarily a consequence of exercise. Some evidence suggests that exercise may even suppress the appetite for a short while. Those who do eat more when they exercise usually add fewer calories than they burn in their workouts. Exercise raises the basal metabolic rate, which remains elevated not only for the exercise period, but also for an extended time

after the physical activity ends. Calories are thus consumed at a higher rate for an extended period of time.

Myth: I am too out of shape or old to exercise.

Fact: People of all ages and body types benefit from physical activity. Exercise programs can begin by adding a few minutes of activity per day, such as walking or climbing a flight of stairs, and gradually increasing the amount of activity. Even small amounts of physical activity offer health benefits.

Myth: Exercising special spots will reduce local fat.

Fact: There is no such thing as effective "spot reduction." Although gadgets and gimmicks such as weighted belts, body wraps, rubberized workout suits, and other specialized devices are widely advertised, none of them will fulfill the promise of delivering a "flat stomach" or "slender thighs" in return for just minutes of exercise a day (and, of course, a few dollars). Fat tissue cannot be converted into muscle. When a woman exercises, she uses energy produced by burning fat in all parts of the body—not just around the muscles that are doing the most work. Sit-ups will not take fat off the abdomen any faster than any other body area. Sit-ups can, however, strengthen the abdominal muscles, which may help hold the abdomen in more.

Myth: No pain, no gain.

Fact: Exercise does not have to hurt to provide benefits. During the initial phase or the beginning of an exercise program or when intensifying an exercise program, some muscle discomfort is probable. Once a regular routine has been established, however, there is no requirement to keep pushing beyond that level for benefit. It is best to avoid pain during and after exercise by intensifying workouts slowly and by beginning each session with a warm-up and ending it with a cool-down.

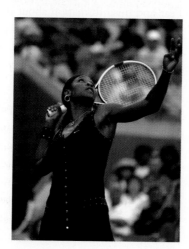

■ Women are increasingly being recognized as proficient athletes, whether in competition with one another or in mixed sports.

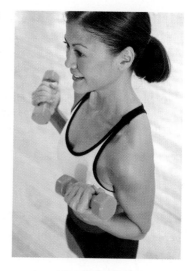

■ It is a myth that a woman will develop bulging muscles if she lifts weights.

Myth: Lifting weights gives women a bulky masculine physique.

Fact: Because most women have relatively low levels of the hormone testosterone, it is difficult for them to build large muscles. Both men and women can build firmer rather than bulkier muscles by lifting lighter weights more times rather than heavier weights fewer times.

Myth: The more sweat produced, the more fat lost.

Fact: Exercising in extreme heat or while wearing a plastic suit will, indeed, cause a person to sweat and lose weight. But sweat reflects the loss of water, not fat. Normal consumption of food and water will soon cause the weight to return. An individual who sweats too much during exercise without replenishing essential liquids runs the risk of developing heat exhaustion or dehydration. The amount of sweat produced is not a measure of energy expended. Sweating depends more on temperature, humidity, lack of conditioning, body weight, and individual variability.

Myth: Exercise is not good for trimming down because weight is gained in muscle.

Fact: Aerobic exercises, such as bicycling, jogging, and swimming, burn more fat than they add muscle. With exercises such as weight-lifting, muscle gain may indeed weigh more than burned-off fat. Usually, however, this tradeoff results in increased trimness because the added muscle is less dense and bulky than the lost fat. One added benefit is that the few extra pounds of muscle do not carry the health risks of excess fat. Another is that the body burns 15 to 20 times the calories to maintain a pound of muscle than it burns to maintain the same amount of fat.

Myth: Women cannot perform well athletically while menstruating.

Fact: Most women can perform physical activities consistently throughout their menstrual cycles. Researchers have found no significant differences in physical capabilities, such as oxygen intake, throughout the menstrual cycle. In fact, exercising during menstruation helps relieve pain and discomfort associated with the menstrual cycle.

Exercise and Aging

Exercise becomes more important with age. Many problems commonly associated with aging, such as increased body fat, decreased lean body weight (muscle mass), decreased muscle strength and flexibility, loss of bone mass, lower metabolism, and slower reaction times, are often signs of inactivity that can be minimized or even prevented by exercise. Reduced muscle strength is a major cause of physical disability in the elderly. Maintaining muscle strength and flexibility are critical components of maintaining the ability to walk and remain independent. For people 65 years and older, falls account for 80% of injuries requiring a hospital visit. When paired with calcium and vitamin D supplements, exercise can dramatically improve balance, coordination, and bone strength, greatly reducing the likelihood and severity of a fall.[22] In addition to improving physical fitness, exercise reduces the risk of developing type 2 diabetes and osteoporosis, and can reduce symptoms for people with osteoporosis and diabetes (see Chapter 11). The combination of weight-lifting and aerobic exercise seems to be the best method for preventing these chronic debilitating conditions. Exercise also promotes a sense of well-being and reduces symptoms of depression, a common problem among aging women.

Exercise Abuse

Pressure to be svelte and physically attractive bombards women from many directions. Being healthy and fit are desirable and noble goals, but occasionally individuals become so zealous in the pursuit of fitness or the desire to be attractive that injury results. Exercise abuse occurs when exercise or fitness supplants family, friends, work, and education in importance, or when athletic injuries are ignored. In an overuse syndrome, a body part or the entire body is exercised beyond its biological limit to the point of injury. Common overuse injuries affect the muscles, tendons, ligaments, joints, and skin. Overuse injuries are most commonly caused by excessive exercise, faulty technique, and poor equipment. "Going for the burn" is dangerous because the pain of overexertion is the body's message indicating that something is wrong; such a problem should be addressed, not ignored.

Some women may exercise so much that they stop menstruating. This condition, known as athletic amenorrhea, usually is the direct result of excessive exercise and an abnormally low ratio of body fat to body weight. The long-term consequences of prolonged athletic amenorrhea include the early onset of osteoporosis and its resultant risk for injury and debilitation. Athletic amenorrhea often affects adolescent female athletes who are involved in sports that emphasize slenderness, such as long-distance running, gymnastics, figure skating, and ballet, or women who are endurance athletes, such as distance swimmers and runners.[23] The **female athlete triad** is the relationship among disordered eating, amenorrhea, and osteoporosis. This problem usually begins with disordered eating. The combination of poor nutrition and intense athletic training causes weight loss and a decrease in or shutdown of estrogen production. Consequently, amenorrhea occurs. The final condition in the triad, osteoporosis, may follow if estrogen levels remain low and the woman's diet continues to lack calcium and vitamin D.

Anabolic steroid use is another form of exercise abuse. Anabolic steroids are synthetic derivatives of the male hormone testosterone. Although steroid use is particularly popular among teenage males, many women use these drugs as well. Men and women who take steroids with heavy resistance training increase their muscle and lean body mass, but also experience severe physical and psychological side effects. Documented adverse physical effects of steroid use in women include enlargement of the clitoris, growth of facial hair, changes in or cessation of the

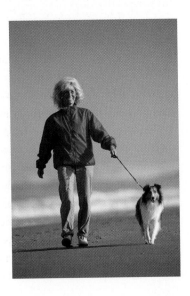

■ Exercise throughout the life span can help minimize or prevent many of the health problems associated with aging.

menstrual cycle, deepened voice, and breast diminution. Other potential side effects include increased risk of heart disease and stroke, increased aggression, liver tumors and jaundice, aching joints, bad breath, and acne.

In adolescents, steroid use can halt growth prematurely. The AIDS epidemic has introduced another liability from steroid use: increased risk of human immunodeficiency virus (HIV) transmission from sharing needles. The psychological effects of long-term, high-dose anabolic steroid use may lead to a preoccupation (addiction) with drug use, difficulty stopping, drug cravings, and withdrawal symptoms when use of the drugs is stopped.[24] Hepatitis B and C, two diseases that can seriously damage the liver, are also easily spread by needle sharing. Clearly, anabolic steroids should be totally avoided.

Maintaining a Healthy Weight

To maintain a healthy weight, a woman should balance the number of calories she consumes as part of a healthy diet with the number of calories she burns through daily physical activities. Weight loss should occur at the level of no more than 0.5 to 1 pound per week. Adults can evaluate their weight-for-height ratio, or **body mass index (BMI)**. (See **It's Your Health** and Self-Assessment 9.3.) Studies show that BMI is closely correlated with total body fat content for most people; however, a person who has a lot of muscle, a large body frame, and little fat may have a BMI above the healthy range but may still be healthy. Women who have a lot of fat and little muscle may have a BMI in the healthy range, but may not be at their most healthy weight. A BMI of between 25 and 29.9 is used to identify overweight and a BMI of 30 is used to identify

obesity in adults. Another way to define overweight is to measure the proportion of fat in the body, though it is a difficult measurement to perform accurately, even with professional training.

In addition to total weight, weight distribution is an important consideration. Women whose body-fat distribution favors the upper body ("apples") rather than the hips and thighs ("pears") are at higher risk of developing type 2 diabetes, coronary artery disease, hypertension, gallbladder disease, and polycystic ovarian syndrome.[25] Consequently, waist measurement has been used as a loose measure of one's chance of developing heart disease, cancer, or other chronic diseases. A waist larger than 35 inches for a woman and 40 inches for a man is considered to be a risk factor for the aforementioned diseases.

What Causes Weight Gain

Genetic, metabolic, behavioral, environmental, cultural, and socioeconomic factors all influence body weight. Some people may have a genetic predisposition to gain weight or a genetic need to eat more than they need for energy. For the vast majority of individuals, however, overweight and obesity result from excess calorie consumption and/or inadequate physical activity: When a woman takes in more calories than she burns, she will gain weight. Burning calories through physical activity helps to offset the amount of calories consumed and can help a person maintain or lose weight.

In the United States, weight gain is typically viewed from an individual perspective. People who are overweight or obese are often assigned responsibility for overindulging or overeating, while people who lose weight or stay at a healthy weight are praised for their discipline. Although this perspective does have elements of truth, taking a population-based perspective can also yield insights into the problems of obesity, overweight, and difficulty maintaining weight. It is not only discipline and a desire to be fit that influence whether a person chooses to exercise—it is also how much free time a woman has; whether she lives in a neighborhood with safe and satisfying places to walk, run, or play sports; and whether her work schedule allows her to visit a health club while it is open.

Similarly, if a woman lives in an area where healthful foods are unavailable, inconvenient, or considerably more expensive than processed foods high in fats and sugars, she is less likely to eat a healthful diet than if she lives in an area where healthful foods are easily accessible. The processed food industry uses a variety of tactics to sell its products, many of which are unhealthy. One of these tac-

---

It's Your Health

Evaluate Your Weight (Adults)

1. Weigh yourself and have your height measured. Find your BMI category in Self-Assessment 9.3. The higher your BMI category, the greater your risk for health problems.

2. Measure around your waist while standing, just above your hip bones. If it is greater than 35 inches for women or 40 inches for men, you probably have excess abdominal fat. This excess fat may place you at greater risk of health problems, even if your BMI is about right.

The higher your BMI and waist measurement, the more you are likely to benefit from weight loss.

Self-Assessment 9.3

Are You at a Healthy Weight?

Body Mass Index Table

Height (inches)	Normal						Overweight					Obese										Extreme Obesity														
BMI	19	20	21	22	23	24	25	26	27	28	29	30	31	32	33	34	35	36	37	38	39	40	41	42	43	44	45	46	47	48	49	50	51	52	53	54
												Body Weight (pounds)																								
58	91	96	100	105	110	115	119	124	129	134	138	143	148	153	158	162	167	172	177	181	186	191	196	201	205	210	215	220	224	229	234	239	244	248	253	258
59	94	99	104	109	114	119	124	128	133	138	143	148	153	158	163	168	173	178	183	188	193	198	203	208	212	217	222	227	232	237	242	247	252	257	262	267
60	97	102	107	112	118	123	128	133	138	143	148	153	158	163	168	174	179	184	189	194	199	204	209	215	220	225	230	235	240	245	250	255	261	266	271	276
61	100	106	111	116	122	127	132	137	143	148	153	158	164	169	174	180	185	190	195	201	206	211	217	222	227	232	238	243	248	254	259	264	269	275	280	285
62	104	109	115	120	126	131	136	142	147	153	158	164	169	175	180	186	191	196	202	207	213	218	224	229	235	240	246	251	256	262	267	273	278	284	289	295
63	107	113	118	124	130	135	141	146	152	158	163	169	175	180	186	191	197	203	208	214	220	225	231	237	242	248	254	259	265	270	278	282	287	293	299	304
64	110	116	122	128	134	140	145	151	157	163	169	174	180	186	192	197	204	209	215	221	227	232	238	244	250	256	262	267	273	279	285	291	296	302	308	314
65	114	120	126	132	138	144	150	156	162	168	174	180	186	192	198	204	210	216	222	228	234	240	246	252	258	264	270	276	282	288	294	300	306	312	318	324
66	118	124	130	136	142	148	155	161	167	173	179	186	192	198	204	210	216	223	229	235	241	247	253	260	266	272	278	284	291	297	303	309	315	322	328	334
67	121	127	134	140	146	153	159	166	172	178	185	191	198	204	211	217	223	230	236	242	249	255	261	268	274	280	287	293	299	306	312	319	325	331	338	344
68	125	131	138	144	151	158	164	171	177	184	190	197	203	210	216	223	230	236	243	249	256	262	269	276	282	289	295	302	308	315	322	328	335	341	348	354
69	128	135	142	149	155	162	169	176	182	189	196	203	209	216	223	230	236	243	250	257	263	270	277	284	291	297	304	311	318	324	331	338	345	351	358	365
70	132	139	146	153	160	167	174	181	188	195	202	209	216	222	229	236	243	250	257	264	271	278	285	292	299	306	313	320	327	334	341	348	355	362	369	376
71	136	143	150	157	165	172	179	186	193	200	208	215	222	229	236	243	250	257	265	272	279	286	293	301	308	315	322	329	338	343	351	358	365	372	379	386
72	140	147	154	162	169	177	184	191	199	206	213	221	228	235	242	250	258	265	272	279	287	294	302	309	316	324	331	338	346	353	361	368	375	383	390	397
73	144	151	159	166	174	182	189	197	204	212	219	227	235	242	250	257	265	272	280	288	295	302	310	318	325	333	340	348	355	363	371	378	386	393	401	408
74	148	155	163	171	179	186	194	202	210	218	225	233	241	249	256	264	272	280	287	295	303	311	319	326	334	342	350	358	365	373	381	389	396	404	412	420
75	152	160	168	176	184	192	200	208	216	224	232	240	248	256	264	272	279	287	295	303	311	319	327	335	343	351	359	367	375	383	391	399	407	415	423	431
76	156	164	172	180	189	197	205	213	221	230	238	246	254	263	271	279	287	295	304	312	320	328	336	344	353	361	369	377	385	394	402	410	418	426	435	443

BMI measures weight in relation to height. The BMI ranges shown above are for adults. They are not exact ranges of healthy and unhealthy weights, but rather show that health risk increases at higher levels of overweight and obesity. Even within the healthy BMI range, weight gains can carry health risks for adults.

Directions: Find your weight on the bottom of the graph. Go straight up from that point until you come to the line that matches your height. Then look to find your weight group.

Healthy Weight: BMI from 18.5 to 24.   **Overweight:** BMI from 25 to 29.   **Obese:** BMI 30 or higher.

Source: Adapted from *Clinical Guidelines on the Identification, Evaluation, and Treatment of Overweight and Obesity in Adults: The Evidence Report.* Available at http://www.nhlbisupport.com/bmi/bmicalc.htm.

tics has been to increase portion sizes to market the idea of customers getting a "better deal." These tactics have earned hundreds of millions of dollars for the fast-food and carbonated-beverage industries in particular. Unfortunately, these same tactics have also resulted in millions of people eating extra, unneeded calories without adding nutrients to their diet. **Table 9.8** provides examples of changes in portion size over the past 20 years.

Table 9.8   Portion Distortion

Food Item	Size and Calories		Ways to Burn the Extra Calories
	20 Years Ago	Today	
Bagel	3-inch diameter/ 140 calories	6-inch diameter/ 350 calories	Rake leaves for 50 minutes to burn extra 210 calories
French fries	2.4 ounces/ 210 calories	6.9 ounces/ 610 calories	Walk 2 hours, 20 minutes to burn extra 400 calories
Soda	6.5 ounces/ 85 calories	20 ounces/ 250 calories	Garden for 35 minutes to burn extra 165 calories
Turkey sandwich	320 calories	820 calories	Bike for 1 hour, 25 minutes to burn extra 500 calories

Source: National Heart, Lung and Blood Institute. *Stay Young at Heart.*

Overweight and Obesity

Overweight is defined as a BMI of 25 to 29.9, with obesity beginning at a BMI of 30. **Obesity** is a medical term meaning the excessive storage of energy in the form of fat. Obesity is a complex, multifactorial chronic disease. Overweight and obesity are increasing in both genders and among all population groups. Today there are more than twice as many overweight children and three times as many overweight adolescents as there were in 1980.[26] Overweight children and adolescents are more likely to become overweight or obese adults. Surveillance data reveal that more than two-thirds of adults in the United States are overweight or obese, and more than 1 out of 20 are extremely obese (see **Figure 9.4**). Approximately one out of five U.S. children are overweight, and one-third of those who are at a healthy weight are at risk of soon becoming overweight.[27] The prevalence of obesity is higher among African American women and Mexican American women than among women in any other ethnic groups. This condition is also more common among people with low incomes and low education.[26]

It has been suggested that the major factor behind this increase in rates of obesity is the jump in average calorie intake over the past 30 years. In 2003, the average daily calorie consumption was roughly 300 calories more than the average consumption in 1980. Refined grains, added fats, and added sugars accounted for most of this increase.[28]

Being overweight or obese can lead to many health problems, including adult-onset diabetes, hypertension, coronary heart disease, cancers, gout, gallbladder disease, and arthritic conditions. Women suffer from additional obesity-related problems, including irregular menstrual cycles, amenorrhea, infertility, and polycystic ovarian syndrome. Studies show that the risk of death rises with increasing weight. Moderate weight excess (10 to 20 pounds for a person of average height), even for women who exercise, increases the risk of death, particularly among adults age 30 to 64 years. Obese women may be at a slightly higher risk of developing breast cancer, but researchers are investigating whether the effects of obesity on breast cancer depend on weight gained as an adult or as a child. The risk for endometrial cancer also goes up with increasing fat tissue. According to the American Cancer Society, being 30 pounds overweight can increase a woman's risk of endometrial cancer threefold and being 50 pounds overweight can increase her risk tenfold.[29] People who are obese also are subject to discrimination and social stigmatization, and consequently they may suffer from low self-esteem and depression.

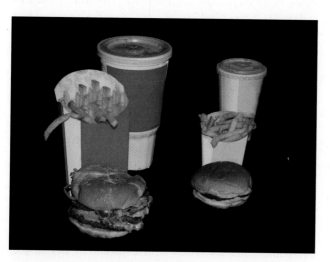

■ Food portions have become noticeably larger in the past 20 years, often providing enough food for at least 2 people.

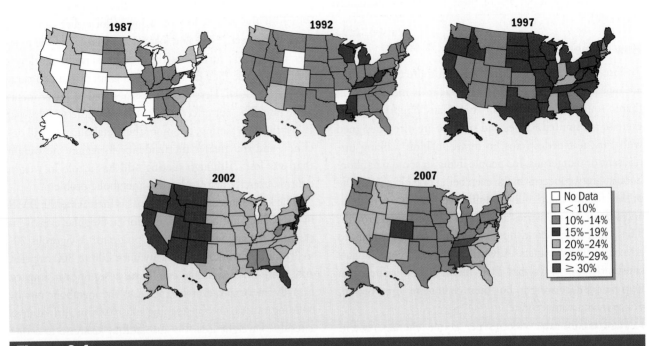

Figure 9.4

Obesity trends* among U.S. adults.

*BMI ≥ 30, or about 30 pounds overweight for a 5'4"person

Source: Centers for Disease Control and Prevention. (2008). *Behavioral Risk Factor Surveillance System.*

It has been estimated that current obesity in the United States could account for 14% of all deaths from cancer in men and 20% of those in women.[29] Left unabated, overweight and obesity may soon cause as much preventable disease and death as cigarette smoking. The recognition of obesity as the second leading cause of preventable death in the United States was somewhat slow to develop. In the 1970s, controversy arose over the significance of obesity as an effect on general health. Not until 1985 at the NIH Consensus Development Conference was it acknowledged that obesity leads to increased morbidity and mortality. Since then, the prevalence of people who are obese or overweight has continued to grow.

The root causes of obesity lie in genetics, environment, economics, and culture. Although its development is complex, the benefits of treatment are certain. Obesity treatments often begin with weight loss, employing low-calorie diets in conjunction with physical activity, behavior therapy, and pharmacotherapy and weight-loss surgery for people who are severely obese (BMIs equal to or greater than 40). Recent developments in weight-loss medications are allowing the estimated more than 100 million adults in the United States who are obese to have a much better chance for decreased morbidity and mortality.

Economic Dimensions of Obesity and Overweight

One recent study estimated that the annual cost of obesity and overweight in the United States is $117 billion.[30] This figure includes the direct medical costs to treat diseases associated with obesity such as diabetes, joint problems, and heart disease, and the indirect costs of morbidities associated with the condition. These indirect costs are measured in terms of lost productivity, premature disability, and early death. Health-care costs and the likelihood of complications from surgery for obese and overweight people are higher than those for people of healthy weight. Additional costs may be felt at the individual or household level, when overweight or obese people need to purchase specially designed chairs and beds to support them, specialty clothes, and higher-than-average numbers of medications. Together these items can create a significant cost burden to families.

Americans spend billions of dollars every year, most of it unsuccessfully, addressing weight concerns. In 2007, Americans spent $60 billion trying to lose weight. This money includes health-club memberships, home gym equipment, diet books, and participation in weight-loss programs. About 70 million people—almost one out of four people in the United States, attempt to lose weight

every year. Only about 5% of these people are ultimately successful.[32]

How Women Can Lose Weight

To lose weight, it is necessary to burn more calories than are ingested. However, this simple claim is more difficult than it sounds. For millions of Americans, opportunities to exercise are limited. Cities and suburbs are often designed with cars, not pedestrians, in mind, making walking unpleasant or dangerous; for people living in some neighborhoods, safety concerns make even being outside a risk. The profits of the multi-billion-dollar weight-loss, fast-food, and soft-drink industries all depend on continued growth: These industries spend hundreds of millions of dollars to advertise their products. Advertisements and commercials constantly tout ways that their methods or products can help people lose weight, but their claims are often biased, exaggerated, or inaccurate.

Fat contains nine calories per gram, whereas protein and carbohydrates have four calories per gram. The most important way that the body burns calories is through one's resting metabolism, or basal metabolic rate (BMR), the process that maintains body heat and controls automatic activities such as breathing and heartbeat. Nearly 75% of calorie use is devoted to these functions. When a woman attempts to lose weight by cutting calories, her body responds as it would to starvation, by burning fewer calories. Shifting from an intake of about 2,000 calories per day to a 1,200-calorie diet reduces resting metabolism by 5% to 10%, and a more stringent 800-calorie diet lowers it by 10% to 20%. Even after resuming a more normal calorie

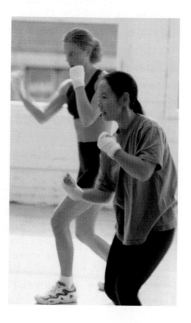

■ Regular exercise is an essential component of any weight-control program.

consumption, other changes keep the metabolic rate low. Much of the weight lost on a low-calorie diet can come from lost muscle tissue and lost water weight, and the muscles may shrink further as the woman stays at the lower weight because they do not have to work as hard to carry the body around. Less muscle tissue means a lower metabolic rate. The net effect is simple: The more weight that is lost through dieting, the more the metabolic rate will decline—and the greater the tendency to regain the weight that was lost. Although dieting still has a role in weight control, exercise helps solve this metabolic problem.

The key to successful weight loss is increasing the BMR by exercising, not by counting calories. Regular exercise is essential for any weight-control program. A vigorous 20- to 30-minute workout can easily burn 200 to 300 calories, and even brisk walking can have a significant impact. Equally important, exercise increases the metabolic rate by building muscle and by keeping muscle from shrinking as a result of weight loss. Because adding exercise to a diet program helps steady the metabolic rate, it makes it easier to keep the weight off.

Exercise alone does directly burn calories. Another advantage of exercise is that the metabolism remains higher for several hours afterward, so calories are burned at a higher rate, even during inactivity. Aerobic exercise burns calories faster than weight training, but weight training builds muscle, which is of critical importance in weight loss. A pound of muscle needs 30 to 50 calories per day just for maintenance, whereas fat needs only two maintenance calories per day. Substituting muscle for fat will therefore result in an increased daily caloric expenditure. Rather than simply promoting weight loss, exercise appears to affect the body in a more complex, integrated way, bringing appetite and energy expenditure into balance. In addition, exercise trims a physical profile even without weight loss. Muscle is denser than fat, so it is possible to appear thinner while the weight holds steady if a larger amount of fat is replaced with a smaller amount of muscle. Bathroom scales do not measure these changes. Regardless of its direct effects on weight and body fat, exercise serves to improve overall health by lowering blood pressure, improving cholesterol levels, strengthening the cardiovascular system, helping prevent type 2 diabetes, and reducing stress.

Keeping a food diary may help some women by allowing them to better identify their eating and exercising patterns. Meals, snacks, and drinks should all be recorded in the diary. After a review of a few days of diary notes, a woman can objectively examine her own eating habits and set realistic goals that rely on a diet based on healthy foods.

Women can monitor their progress through the food diary and weekly (not daily) checks with the scale. Once the reasonable desired weight loss is achieved, the focus should be on maintenance, again through sensible eating and exercise.

Ways Not to Lose Weight

U.S. women (and increasingly, U.S. men) spend countless hours worrying, thinking, and obsessing over weight loss. Diet books, programs, and plans make enormous profits by preying on women's insecurities about their weight, and then offering their new product as an easy solution to this "problem." When women do not lose weight, or lose weight but gain it back, they often blame themselves, even if the diets themselves are flawed, ineffective, or unrealistic.

Starvation or hunger is not the solution to any weight-loss effort. Food substitution, in which a woman consumes twice as many calories from carbohydrates as she does from fat, is far better than food restriction. Foods such as pasta and whole-grain bread are nutritious, filling, and low in calories when they are not smothered in high-fat products, such as butter, mayonnaise, and margarine. Alcohol should also be considered contraindicated in a weight-loss effort. Alcohol provides empty calories that contribute to weight gain without providing any nutritional benefit. Furthermore, alcohol affects the BMR because the body burns fat more slowly in the presence of alcohol; thus alcohol promotes the storage of body fat.

Dieting without exercise is the least effective way to lose weight. **Yo-yo dieting** is a term used to characterize the repeated, chronic pattern of dieting that describes most dieters' behavior. In addition to being frustrating, yo-yo dieting may be hazardous to health. Yo-yo dieting may be associated with a greater risk of coronary heart disease, although separating the direct physiological effects of the behavior and the resulting stress that comes with trying and failing to lose weight is difficult.[33] Yo-yo dieting may also weaken the immune system, making dieters more likely to become and stay sick.[34] Yo-yo dieters may even store more and more fat in the abdominal area with each failed diet; abdominal fat has been shown to be more harmful to one's health than fat in other places.

Diet supplements are another unhealthy way to lose weight. Weight-loss supplements often contain stimulants, which in high amounts may lead to an increased heart rate, heart attacks, nervousness, insomnia, headaches, seizures, or death. Many women have begun to use supplements such as Ephedra, which has been linked to adverse health outcomes and even possible mortality. Because the products

It's Your Health

Helpful and Unhelpful Weight-Loss Strategies

Helpful

Allow occasional treats or servings of favorite foods.

Develop realistic, long-term goals that can be maintained.

Concentrate on reducing, but not eliminating, fat from the diet. Monounsaturated fats like olive oil are best.

Stick with the program even if there are lapses.

Plan meals and snacks to include more complex carbohydrates, fruits, and vegetables.

Limit intake of fatty foods, oils, and dressings.

Avoid packaged snack foods.

Develop new interests that do not involve food.

Eat foods slowly.

Exercise regularly.

Drink water rather than carbonated beverages or sports drinks.

Reduce sugar intake—look for levels of simple carbohydrates.

Join a support group or share the process with a friend.

Clean the pantry—give away foods that are not part of the new healthy eating plan.

Try a new low-fat recipe each week.

Eat small meals throughout the day to keep from getting too hungry.

Unhelpful

Setting unrealistically high expectations.

Focusing solely on short-term goals.

Choosing a program that makes eating unpleasant.

Unconventional theories to explain how food combinations add or decrease body weight.

Following a diet that omits any one food group, or focuses on one particular food, such as grapefruit or yogurt.

Daily caloric intake less than 1,200 calories unless under medical supervision.

Any diet that promotes megadoses of vitamins to make up for nutritional deficits.

Fasting or starvation diets.

Any pill or potion that "melts fat."

Appetite-suppressant drugs.

Giving up all sweets or breads.

Using muscle stimulators or body wraps.

I have tried every diet in the book. I have had times where I have eaten only grapefruit, only rice, or only salads. I have also tried all the gimmicks—pills, liquids, body wraps. You name it, I've tried it. But nothing has really worked. I quickly gain the weight back, sometimes more, within a short time after I lose it. I always swear I won't try another stupid method, but as soon as I read an ad or see a new product, I feel that I have to give it a try.

22-year-old woman

Chapter Nine ■ Nutrition, Exercise, and Weight Management

are not subjected to the same testing standards as substances regulated by the FDA, supplements may have a higher rate of contamination or contraindications not stated on warning labels. Other weight-loss products, although not necessarily harmful, simply may be ineffective.

Other Weight-Loss Strategies

Many popular diets encourage different eating regimens to attain maximum weight loss. In the 1990s, diets typically focused on high-carbohydrate/very-low-fat daily regimens. Later, the high-protein, high-fat, low-carbohydrate (Atkins) diet reemerged as a popular weight-loss strategy. Many people were not able to lose weight on these diets because they mistakenly believed that they could eat unlimited amounts of certain foods. In reality, excessive calories from any food source cause weight gain. Low-fat foods are often packed with sugar to make up for the loss of flavor when fat is removed. In contrast, several high-profile diets, including the Atkins diet and the Zone diet, identify high-protein/low-carbohydrate meals as being optimal. These diets have become financial empires unto themselves, with books, snacks, prepared meals, and energy drinks all being sold to the millions of people who are subscribing to them. A *Consumer Reports* analysis found that people in Atkins and the Zone weight-loss programs were at least as likely as people in other top-rated weight-loss programs to lose weight in the short term but were more likely to drop out in less than a year. They were also more likely to eat too much saturated fat and not enough fruits and vegetables.[35]

Weight-loss surgery has gained attention as a tool for people who are severely overweight or obese. Gastrointestinal surgery for obesity, also called **bariatric surgery**, alters the digestive process. The operation promotes weight loss by closing off parts of the stomach to make it smaller. Operations that only reduce stomach size are known as "restrictive operations" because they restrict the amount of food the stomach can hold. Other operations, known as malabsorptive operations, combine stomach restriction with a partial bypass of the small intestine. These procedures create a direct connection from the stomach to the lower segment of the small intestine, literally bypassing portions of the digestive tract that absorb calories and nutrients. These operations often make eating and swallowing food extremely painful, literally making an ordeal out of every meal. All of these procedures are appropriate only for severely obese individuals who have not been able to control their weight with diet, exercise, and appropriate pharmaceutical interventions.

Body Image and Shape

Body image is a result of a complex interrelationship among self-perception, family attitudes toward bodies and food, social norms, and individual experiences. Standards for beauty and desirability are not absolute; they vary over time and from culture to culture. The ideal promoted by Madison Avenue and Hollywood has ranged from images of emaciation to women whose images have been altered

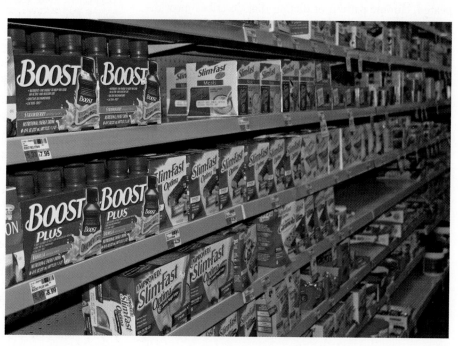

■ Weight-loss products should be used only when prescribed by a health-care provider; in these selected patients, the products should be used in combination with lifestyle changes to increase the success of long-term weight loss.

by computer design software. In Greek and Roman representations of Aphrodite and Venus as well as in paintings by Titian, Rubens, and Rembrandt, "ideal" women often had ample thighs, hips, waists, and abdomens. The Venus de Milo, one of the most beautiful of the classical female torsos, is muscular and rounded. Contemporary society is weight conscious, fashion conscious, exercise conscious, diet conscious, and not very tolerant of perceived physical imperfection.

Women have been socialized to believe that their physical attractiveness determines their social value. The media have further distorted this message by airbrushing images to produce flawless complexions, whitening and brightening of teeth and eyes, digital enhancement to increase breast size and decrease fat, and celebration of models and movie stars who are not representative of the average woman. These images, which appear on commercials, Internet advertisements, magazines, movies, and other locations, have unconscious but serious psychological effects. A study examining physical measurements of Miss America contestants, models, and Playboy Playmates over the course of the twentieth century found that women in all three groups were likely to be underweight and were often thin enough to meet the World Health Organization's definition of anorexic. The weight and BMI of all three groups of women have also fallen even as the weight of the

average American woman has increased over the past 50 years.[36] The gulf between what women see in the media and what they see in the mirror results in excessive dieting, eating disorders, a perceived need for plastic or cosmetic surgery, and feelings of self-loathing and inadequacy in many women, as seen in the following statistics:

- A 2003 poll found that 24% of the people who said they would try any diet to lose weight were obese women, whereas only 9% were obese men. Obese women were also much more likely than men to feel guilty about eating.[37]

- Females account for 90% of the estimated 8 million sufferers of eating disorders.[38]

- Nearly 12 million cosmetic surgical and nonsurgical procedures were performed in the United States in 2007, according to the American Society for Aesthetic Plastic Surgery (ASAPS). This represents an increase of more than 450% compared to the number of procedures performed in 1997. Although the number of surgical procedures, such as liposuction, breast augmentation, and eyelid surgery, also grew, the biggest increase has been in procedures that do not require actual surgery, such as Botox injections and laser hair removals.[39]

In the early 1990s, studies found that compared with women in other countries, girls and women in the United States dieted more and were less satisfied and more self-conscious about their bodies.[40] But a 1997 international study of body language showed increased discontent with bodies, appearance, and weight by women across Western nations, suggesting a more global problem.[41] This phenomenon begins early, with inappropriate eating habits and high anxiety about being overweight prevalent among adolescent girls. A large U.S. school-based study found that more than one-third of adolescent girls believed they were overweight, and more than 60% of female adolescents were trying to lose weight.[42] High school girls use methods such as starvation, fad diets, and purging methods, which can result in disordered eating behaviors to lose weight. This finding is especially disturbing given the importance of high calcium intake for building healthy bones and developing critical bone mass, as well as the need for dietary fat to ensure healthy breast development in adolescents. Another concern is that a girl's preoccupation with body image and discontent with body shape during adolescence may persist for life.

Excessive dieting and bodily preoccupation among young women are believed to be causal factors in the

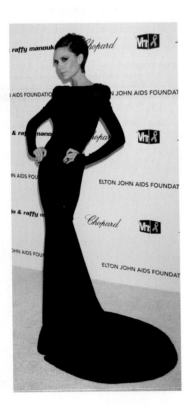

■ Women have been socialized to believe that an ultra-thin body shape is desirable.

I guess when I look in the mirror I see only the things that I feel are wrong. I wish I was thinner and taller, with a flatter stomach and a bigger chest. When I think about it, I realize that there are many things I actually like about myself but I can't seem to focus on them. When I look at other women, I notice their attributes. I wonder why I can't do that with myself.

25-year-old woman

It's taken me most of my life, but I've finally gotten comfortable with my body. I'm not skinny. But you know what? I'm not overweight or out of shape, either. I exercise, I eat a good diet, and I don't smoke. And guess what? I can stay out dancing at a club hours after most of the skinny girls are wiped out.

25-year-old librarian

millions of women who suffer from eating disorders. New research findings and growing numbers of activists are seeking to influence the women and girls who are alienated from their bodies and obsessed with dieting (**Table 9.9**).

Sociocultural Perspectives on Body Image

Women who grew up in largely African American communities often have a very different perspective on body ideals than women who grow up in white-dominated communities. Similarly, girls who grow up in families where their mothers had their own disordered eating habits or poor body images are more likely to internalize those signals and adopt similar attitudes. Religion also can influence a girl's or woman's concept of her body, through either doctrines of self-restraint, hard work, or negative viewpoints on sloth. Even when these attitudes are not specifically directed toward body size, these messages can translate into feelings of blame for girls and women who struggle to control their weight. Cultural norms can significantly influence weight management. A woman who wishes to change her eating habits may have to rebel against the traditions of her family or community.

Eating Disorders

When health-care professionals speak of eating disorders, they generally mean **anorexia nervosa**, **bulimia nervosa**, or **binge eating disorder (BED)**. Although eating disorders may seem to be modern afflictions, medical history indicates otherwise. A disease similar to anorexia was described as early as 1694, and the term "anorexia," meaning loss of appetite or desire, was first used in 1874.[43] Since that time, many other researchers have documented what is now referred to as anorexia nervosa. Bulimia, meaning "appetite like an ox," also has been described in historical writings. Ancient Egyptians believed that purging was a way to prevent disease, and women of the Middle Ages often purged for religious reasons.[44]

Today eating disorders are most common among young, educated white and Hispanic females from middle to upper social classes, with incidence rates peaking at age 18. Eating disorders can have roots in social, emotional, and even biological factors in women's lives; pressure to "fit in" with popular cliques or peers, a desire to avoid consumption as a way of dealing with strong emotions or maintaining control over one's life, and even feelings of euphoria

■ Women's perceptions about their bodies often are inaccurate.

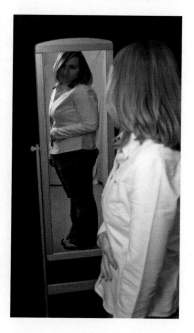

Table 9.9	Comparison of the Average Woman with Unrealistic Models		
	Average Woman	Barbie	Store Mannequin
Height	5′ 4″	6′ 0″	6′ 0″
Weight	145 lb	101 lb	Not available
Dress size	11–14	4	6
Bust	36–37″	39″	34″
Waist	29–31″	19″	23″
Hips	40–42″	33″	34″

Sources: *Health* magazine, September 1997; NEDIC, a Canadian eating disorders advocacy group; Anorexia Nervosa and Related Eating Disorders, Inc., 2003.

EXTREME DIETING

Many women who try restrictive or long-term diets experience trouble-some changes in the way they think, feel, and act. These women may feel cold, listless, and tired; have recurring, obsessive thoughts about food; grow anxious or afraid; and feel a reduced sex drive. Society has often designated these feelings as somehow feminine in nature. But the results of a landmark study conducted more than 50 years ago found that these symptoms are not unique to either gender, but instead reflect the body's reaction to starvation. This same study also found that diets that severely restrict calorie intake are ultimately unproductive in producing lasting weight loss.

In 1944, researcher Ancel Keys enrolled 36 male volunteers in what would be known as the Minnesota starvation experiment. This experiment was designed to examine the effects of a "semi-starvation diet" that many Europeans had been forced to adopt during World War II, with the goal of learning how to best help such people. The study results of the experiment, first published in 1950, are still cited by scientists studying the thought and behavioral patterns of people with eating disorders.

All of the participating men were young, healthy, tested to be emotionally stable, and of normal weight. The requirements of the semi-starvation diet were actually less restrictive than the diets many women put themselves through today. Participants received a low-fat, low-protein diet of 1,800 calories a day over a six-month period, with the goal of losing about 25% of their body weight. The men also were required to walk about three miles a day.

Physical symptoms appeared soon after the men started the diet and increased as time progressed. They became gaunt, lost hair, and broke out in rashes. The men reported feeling dizzy, tired, slow, clumsy, and cold. Participants slept under layers of blankets during the warm summer weather, and their sex drive plummeted.

But the researchers were even more surprised by the psychological changes that occurred. The men became withdrawn and irritable. Several men who were taking classes at the university had to withdraw because they couldn't concentrate. The men also became increasingly obsessed with food: They developed rituals, such as chewing food slowly, watering down meals, or drinking cup after cup of tea, that today are associated with eating disorders.

Even after the six-month period of food restriction was over, the men's metabolism continued to be affected by the diet restrictions. Symptoms continued for weeks after the restrictions were lifted. Many men did not feel full, no matter how much they ate; several men gorged themselves in attempts to do so. Most of the weight they gained back returned as fat, not muscle. Although the men eventually made full recoveries, the process was painful, difficult, and slow. The study found that vitamins and minerals weren't enough—participants also needed to consume a diet containing 4,000 calories a day for weeks to fully recover.

Interviewed more than 50 years later, the surviving study participants said they would do the experiment again because of the beneficial research it produced. Nevertheless, they all cited the study as the most difficult part of their lives.

Now that the risks of severely limiting calorie intake are known, the Minnesota starvation experiment would never be allowed today. The participants of the study enrolled because they believed their results could help victims of war. Women (or men) who are considering a similar diet plan today may want to ask themselves if their sacrifice is worth the effort.

Source: Kalm, L., & Semba, R. (2005). They starved so that others might be better fed: remembering Ancel Keys and the Minnesota experiment. *Journal of Nutrition* 135: 1347-1352.

that can occur when a person skips meals can all encourage a woman (or man) to adopt or continue an eating disorder. At the same time, these behaviors undermine one's health, self-esteem, and sense of competency. (For more on eating disorders, see Chapter 12.)

Global Perspectives on Hunger

Millions of people die each year from chronic hunger and malnutrition. **Hunger** is the painful or uneasy feeling caused by the continuous, unwanted lack of food. Chronic hunger results when a person's daily calorie intake is not enough for the individual to lead an active, healthy life. **Malnutrition** refers to an imbalance between the body's nutritional needs and the intake or digestion of nutrients. Malnutrition may result in disease or death, and can be caused by an unbalanced diet, or from problems in digesting or absorbing food. Although most people think of mal-nutrition as **undernutrition**, this term also includes **overnutrition**, which results from overeating, insufficient exercise, and excessive intake of vitamins and minerals. Overnutrition can lead to overweight and obesity, epidemics that are growing around the world.

Hunger is everywhere. Almost 1 billion people around the world regularly do not get enough food to eat.[45] Most of these people live in the developing world. For people living in hunger, securing food typically takes more time, resources, and effort than for people who do not live in hunger. In 2007, the number of people living in hunger increased by 75 million people. Many factors contributed to this increase: artificially low food prices that make it hard for local farmers to compete with large farms in the developed world, global warming, increased demand for energy, and the recent global financial crisis.[45] Today, one out of five people in the world lives on less than $1 a day; twice that population lives on less than $2 a day. One out every

five people around the world has no regular access to clean water, and two out of every five people lack access to sanitation.[46] Providing these simple services could save millions of lives per year and prevent much pain and suffering.

In 2006, 11% of households (12.6 million) in the United States were **food insecure**, meaning they did not have consistent access to a varied diet throughout the year. Considerable variety existed within food-insecure households. About one-third of these households (about 4 million households) had very low food security; people in these homes not only went hungry from time to time, but had to make serious changes to their eating habits at some point during the year. People living in the remaining food-insecure households were typically able to use strategies such as reducing the variety in their diets, obtaining food from emergency kitchens, or participating in federal food programs.[47] People at greatest risk of food insecurity live in households with the following characteristics:

- Having children and headed by a single woman
- Hispanic or black
- Located in the South
- Located in large cities or rural areas[47]

Populations at risk of malnutrition include infants and children, women who are pregnant or breastfeeding, the elderly, vegetarians, fad dieters, alcoholics or substance abusers, and people with certain chronic diseases. Malnourishment magnifies the effects of every disease, causing malnourished children to be ill nearly 160 days each year, almost half of their daily lives. The most destructive form of malnutrition, which mainly affects infants and young children, is **protein-energy malnutrition (PEM)**. Children have high energy and protein needs, and therefore they suffer most when protein is lacking in their diets. PEM affects more than one-fourth of the world's children. More than 70% of PEM-afflicted children live in Asia, 26% in Africa, and 4% in Latin America and the Caribbean.[48]

Other nutrients that are extremely important for health include the following:

- *Vitamin A.* Vitamin A deficiency (VAD) is the leading cause of preventable blindness, reduces the body's resistance to disease and infection, and can cause growth retardation in children. An estimated 250,000 to 500,000 children lose their sight every year due to VAD, and half of these children die within 12 months after becoming blind. This deficiency also poses a risk to pregnant women and their fetuses, causing night blindness, increased risk of maternal mortality, premature birth, low birthweight, and infection. Breastfeed-

ing is the best way to protect babies from VAD, because breast milk is a natural source of vitamin A.

- *Iron.* Iron deficiency is the principal cause of anemia, which affects more than 30% of the world's population. Iron deficiency and anemia impose a heavy economic burden on society, because affected individuals are less able to work and be productive members of a community. In many developing countries, malaria and worm infections consume iron from the body, making problems caused by iron deficiency even worse. Health consequences for pregnant women and their fetuses include premature birth, low birthweight, and increased risk of maternal death. Twenty percent of all maternal deaths have been attributed to anemia.

- *Iodine.* Iodine deficiency is primarily known for causing goiters (enlarged thyroid glands), a condition that can be dramatically disfiguring. Iodine deficiency disorders (IDDs) threaten the mental health of children, representing the world's most prevalent cause of brain damage. Iodine deficiency during pregnancy may result in stillbirth, miscarriage, congenital abnormalities, and mental impairment in the baby. More than 13% of the world's population (740 million people) is affected by this problem. Salt iodization has improved iodine status in many countries.[48]

■ ■ ■ ■

Informed Decision Making

Nutrition

Healthful eating is essential to health promotion and disease prevention. To develop sensible eating habits, women should eat balanced meals containing carbohydrates, fats, and proteins, as well as the essential vitamins and minerals. Understanding the Nutrition Facts label will help women choose foods based on their nutrient content. Women should also be aware of the dangers of nutrient deficiencies as well as nutritional excesses.

Maintaining a Personal Exercise Program

Exercise provides enormous benefits to health and disease prevention. Exercise should be not just a means to an end, such as "losing another five pounds," but a permanent part of a person's life. The most health benefits come from at least 150 minutes (2.5 hours) of exercise per week of moderate-intensity physical activity. High-intensity physical activity (activity that, when you are performing it, works you hard enough that conversation is difficult) can be included in this total, with every one minute of high-

intensity activity counting for two minutes of moderate-intensity activity. The ideal exercise program should include both aerobic and muscle-building activity. Additional exercise beyond 150 minutes per week provides additional benefits, and any amount of exercise is better than none at all.

Common perceived barriers to exercise for women include lack of time to exercise, lack of encouragement from family and friends, not wanting to exercise alone, the desire to avoid exertion or soreness, and a fear of looking silly.[49] Staying committed to exercise can also be a challenge. About 50% of people who start structured exercise programs drop out in 6 to 12 months. Habits that can make sticking with an exercise program easier include:

- Keeping an exercise log
- Recording total calories burned in a workout, distance traveled, or improvements in performance
- Exercising with a friend or in a class
- Choosing activities that are personally enjoyable
- Switching to new programs or rotating between programs to maintain interest
- Giving oneself periodic rewards for continuing to exercise

Imagining exercise as a normal part of one's routine maintenance (like brushing one's teeth) can also help a woman stay on a program: A woman who misses an exercise session or who forgets to brush her teeth before going to bed one night should not give up on either activity, but should continue both habits the next day as if nothing unusual had happened.[49]

Body Image and Weight Management

A woman who decides to lose weight should begin by examining her diet and activity level, as well as her motives for doing so. Some women want to lose weight to improve their health; others to improve their physical appearance. Many women feel a combination of both desires. However, women who feel an especially powerful desire to lose weight may want to reflect on their own body image. Society places an enormous pressure on women to be thin and to conform to artificial body types that may be unhealthy or impossible to achieve. Developing a healthy body image, with the help of a medical professional if necessary, may benefit some women more than an Olympian-level fitness program.

Extra weight neither accumulates nor disappears overnight. Weight-loss programs that focus on slow but steady weight loss are healthier and more likely to keep weight off

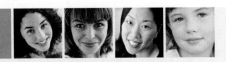

Profiles of Remarkable Women

Billie Jean King (1943–)

Billie Jean Moffit started out playing softball, but knowing there was no significant future for women in the sport at the time, she concentrated her efforts on tennis. At the age of 18, King upset Margaret Smith Court, the world's leading women's tennis player, at Wimbledon. In 1967, after becoming the first woman player since 1939 to win the triple crown of singles, doubles, and mixed doubles in both the British and U.S. championships, she was selected as "Outstanding Female Athlete of the World." By 1968, King had won three Wimbledon championships as well as the U.S. title and was the world's top-ranked women's amateur.

In 1972, King was named *Sports Illustrated*'s "Sportsperson of the Year," the first woman to win the award. In 1973, in front of a still-standing record crowd for the most people ever to attend a single tennis match, the 29-year-old King beat 55-year-old tennis professional Bobby Riggs in three straight sets. The "Battle of the Sexes" match was arranged after Riggs claimed that a woman player would never be able to beat a man. King continued winning competitions, and throughout her professional tennis career she was ranked number one in the world five times and number one in the United States seven times. She holds 20 Wimbledon titles and was ranked in the top 10 in the world for 17 years.

King also became the first woman athlete to earn $100,000 in a single season. Even while displaying her outstanding athletic ability, she stayed committed to women's issues by speaking out and lobbying for women and their right to earn comparable money in tennis and other sports. She was founder and president of the Women's Tennis Association, a labor union for players; a founder of two leagues for professional women athletes, including the Women's Professional Softball League; and publisher, with her husband Larry King, of *WomenSport*, a magazine depicting women's progress as athletes. King established tennis camps, shops, and clinics across the country and created World Team Tennis, a league for professionals. As a coach for World Team Tennis, she became the first woman to coach male professional athletes. King has been inducted into the Women's Sports Foundation Hall of Fame and into the International Tennis Hall of Fame.

than programs that focus on dramatic short-term results. An average weekly loss of one pound is a realistic, safe goal for weight loss. Joining a group or making a serious arrangement for support with a friend can help sustain a long-term commitment.

A woman who adopts a healthy diet or starts an exercise program should not stop either activity once she reaches her initial weight-loss goal. A balanced diet and exercise continue to provide benefits only for as long as they are practiced. Reverting to unhealthy habits not only harms the body, but also is likely to result in the return of lost weight.

Summary

The human body needs six nutrients to function and stay healthy:

- Carbohydrates, which can be simple (sugars) or complex (starches), provide fuel for the body.
- Proteins supply amino acids, which construct, repair, and maintain body tissues.
- Fats store energy and perform many other functions. Many Americans consume too much fat; however, no diet should eliminate this vital nutrient.
- Vitamins, which the body uses for nearly all aspects of function, are needed in small but regular amounts.
- Minerals are inorganic substances that help with bone formation, enzyme synthesis, maintaining blood pressure, and digestive function. Calcium and iron are especially important minerals for young women.
- Water is something the body needs for all its actions. Women should consume eight to nine cups of water per day.

U.S. women spend most of their waking hours in sedentary activity. By incorporating regular exercise into their daily routine, women can become more fit, improve their quality of life, and reduce their risk of chronic disease and premature death. These dramatic benefits to activity can also be pleasurable.

Topics for Discussion

1. How can an older sister best advise a younger sister about weight management? What are the important issues to be taken into consideration when talking to a girl about her weight?

2. What should a woman do if she has a friend whom she suspects to have an eating disorder but the friend denies it?

3. Women who are physically active are healthier and therefore at lower risk of chronic disease and early mortality than those who are inactive. Should they have to pay the same insurance rates as those women whose lifestyles place them at greater risk for illness? If so, how should insurance policies be implemented to be fair and accurate?

4. Some believe that the physical fitness craze has been detrimental to the women's movement because it has added another layer of pressure to conform to an "ideal" body shape or size. Is that argument valid?

5. What can be done to improve women's attitudes toward exercise and physical fitness?

6. What are the biggest challenges to regular exercise and a healthy diet that you face? How are these challenges going to change over the next five years? How do they differ from the challenges your female friends have in these areas?

Web Sites

American Council on Exercise: http://www.acefitness.org

American Dietetic Association: http://www.eatright.org

American Society of Bariatric Physicians: http://www.asbp.org

Center for Nutrition Policy and Promotion: http://www.usda.gov/cnpp

Dietary Guidelines for Americans: http://www.health.gov/dietaryguidelines

International Food Information Council Foundation: http://www.ific.org

National Eating Disorders Association: http://www.nationaleatingdisorders.org

National Institute of Mental Health Center on Eating Disorders: http://www.nimh.nih.gov/publicat/eatingdisorders.cfm

Nutrition.gov: http://www.nutrition.gov

The Obesity Society: http://www.obesity.org

The President's Council on Physical Fitness and Sports: http://www.fitness.gov

U.S. Department of Agriculture: http://www.usda.gov

U.S. Food and Drug Administration: http://www.fda.gov

USDA: Center for Food Safety and Applied Nutrition: http://www.cfsan.fda.gov

References

1. Mokdad, A. H., Marks, J. S., Stroup, D. F., & Gerberding, J. (2004). Actual causes of death in the United States, 2000. *Journal of the American Medical Association* 291: 1238–1245.

2. U.S. Department of Health and Human Services & U.S. Department of Agriculture. (2005). *A Healthier You—Dietary Guidelines for Americans*. Washington, DC: U.S. Government Printing Office.

3. Putnam, J., Allshouse, J., & Kantor, L. S. (2003). U.S. per capita food supply trends: more calories, refined carbohydrates, and fats. *FoodReview: Weighing in on Obesity* 25(3): 33–37.

4. Lowry, R., Galuska, D. A., Fulton, J. E., Wechsler, H., & Kann, L. (2002). Weight management goals and practices among U.S. high school students: associations with physical activity, diet, and smoking. *Journal of Adolescent Health* 31(2): 133–144.

5. Centers for Disease Control and Prevention. (2007). Fruit and vegetable consumption among adults—United States, 2005. *Morbidity and Mortality Weekly Report* 56(10): 213–217.

6. Rufail, M. L., Schenkein, H. A., Barbour, S. E., Tew, J. G., & van Antwerpen, R. (2005). Altered lipoprotein subclass distribution and PAF-AH activity in subjects with generalized aggressive periodontitis. *Journal of Lipid Research* 46: 2752–2760.

7. James, S. L., Muir, J. G., Curtis, S. L., & Gibson, P. R. (2003). Dietary fibre: a roughage guide. *Internal Medicine Journal* 33(7): 291–296.

8. Willet, W. C. (2002). *Eat, Drink and Be Healthy: The Harvard Medical School Guide to Healthy Eating*. New York: Simon and Schuster.

9. U.S. Department of Health and Human Services & Food and Drug Administration. (July 9, 2003). *FDA Backgrounder—FDA Acts to Provide Better Information to Consumers on Trans Fats*. Available at: http://www.fda.gov/oc/initiatives/transfat/backgrounder.html.

10. Mensink, R. P., Zock, P. L., Kester, A. D., & Katan, M. B. (2003). Effects of dietary fatty acids and carbohydrates on the ratio of serum total to HDL cholesterol and on serum lipids and apolipoproteins: a meta-analysis of 60 controlled trials. *American Journal of Clinical Nutrition* 77(5): 1146–1155.

11. Caro, J., Huybrechts, K. F., Klittich, W. S., Jackson, J. D., & McGuire, A.; CORE Study Group. (2003). Allocating funds for cardiovascular disease prevention in light of the NCEP ATP III guidelines. *American Journal of Managed Care* 9(7): 477–489.

12. Hu, F. B., Stampfer, M. J., Rimm, E. B., et al. (1999). A prospective study of egg consumption and risk of cardiovascular disease in men and women. *Journal of the American Medical Association* 281: 1387–1394.

13. Egen, V., & Hasford, J. (2003). Prevention of neural tube defects: effect of an intervention aimed at implementing the official recommendations. *Soz Praventivmed* 48(1): 24–32.

14. Grosse, S. D., Waitzman, N. J., Romano, P. S., & Mulinare, J. (2005). Reevaluating the benefits of folic acid fortification in the United States: economic analysis, regulation, and public health. *American Journal of Public Health* 95: 1917–1922.

15. Iron deficiency—United States, 1999–2000. (2002). *Morbidity and Mortality Weekly Report* 51(40): 897–899.

16. Centers for Disease Control and Prevention. (2007). Prevalence of regular physical activity among adults—United States, 2001 and 2005. *Morbidity and Mortality Weekly Report* 56(46): 1209–1212.

17. Hu, F. B., Willet, W. C., Li, T., Stampfer, M. J., Colditz, G. A., & Manson, J. E. (2004). Adiposity as compared with physical activity in predicting mortality among women. *New England Journal of Medicine* 351(26): 2694–2703.

18. Department of Health and Human Services. (2008). *2008 Physical Activity Guidelines for Americans*. Available at: http://www.health.gov/PAGuidelines/.

19. Moore, K. A., & Blumenthal, J. A. (1998). Exercise training as an alternative treatment for depression among older adults. *Alternative Therapies in Health and Medicine* 4: 48–56.

20. Elavsky, S., McAuley, E., Motl, R. W., et al. (2005). Physical activity enhances long-term quality of life in older adults: efficacy, esteem, and affective influences. *Annals of Behavioral Medicine* 30(2): 138–145.

21. Da Costa, D., Rippen, N., Drista, M., & Ring, A. (2003). Self-reported leisure-time physical activity during pregnancy and relationship to psychological well-being. *Journal of Psychosomatic Obstetrics and Gynaecology* 24(2): 111–119.

22. Kannus, P., Sievanen, H., Palvenen, M., Jarvinen, T., & Parkkari, J. (2005). Prevention of falls and injuries in elderly people. *Lancet* 366(9500): 1885–1893.

23. Warren, M. P., & Goodman, L. R. (2003). Exercise-induced endocrine pathologies. *Journal of Endocrinological Investigation* 26(9): 873–878.

24. Hall, R. C., Hall, R. C. W., & Chapman, M. J. (2005). Psychiatric complications of anabolic steroid use. *Psychosomatics* 46(4): 285–290.

25. Savard, M. & Svec, C. (2005). *The Body Shape Solution to Weight Loss and Wellness*. New York: Atria Publishers.

26. Centers for Disease Control and Prevention. (2008). *Obesity and Overweight: U.S. Obesity Trends*. Available at: http://www.cdc.gov/nccdphp/dnpa/obesity/trend/maps/.

27. Hedley, A. A., Ogden, C. L., Johnson, C. L., Carroll, M. D., Curtin, L. R., & Flegal, K. M. (2004). Prevalence of overweight and obesity among U.S. children, adolescents, and adults, 1999–2002. *Journal of the American Medical Association* 291: 2847–2850.

28. Food and Agriculture Organization of the United Nations. (2006). *County Profile: United States, 2004*. Rome: FAO.

29. Calle, D., Rodriguez, C., Walker-Thurmond, K., & Thun, M. (2003). Overweight, obesity, and mortality from cancer in a prospectively studied cohort of U.S. adults. *New England Journal of Medicine* 348: 1625–1638.

30. U.S. Department of Health and Human Services, National Institutes of Health, & National Institute of Diabetes and Digestive and Kidney Diseases. (January 31, 2006). *Statistics Related to Overweight and Obesity*. Available at: http://win.niddk.nih.gov/statistics/#econ.

31. Wolf, A. M., Manson, J. E., & Colditz, G. A., (2002). The economic impact of overweight, obesity, and weight loss. In Eckel, R., ed. *Obesity: Mechanisms and Clinical Management*. New York: Lippincott, Williams and Wilkins.

32. Palmer, H. (May 30, 2007). *Our Loss, Diet Industry's Gain*. American Public Media radio broadcast. Available at: http://marketplace.publicradio.org/display/web/2007/05/30/our_loss_diet_industrys_gain/.

33. Ward, E. M. (1994). Researchers disagree on the dangers of yo-yo dieting. *Environmental Nutrition* 17(6): 2.

34. Shade, E. D., Ulrich, C. M., Wener, M. H., et al. (2004). Frequent intentional weight loss is associated with lower natural killer cell cytotoxity in postmenopausal women; possible long-term immune effects. *Journal of the American Dietetic Association* 104(6): 903–912.

35. Rating the diets from A to Z. (June 2005). *Consumer Reports* 70(6): 18–22.

36. Byrd-Bredbenner, C., Murray, J., & Schlussel, Y. (2005). Temporal changes in anthropometric measurements of idealized females and young women in general. *Women and Health* 41(2): 13–20.

37. Yin, S. (2004). Size and gender. *American Demographics* 26(2): 14.

38. Rome, E. S. (2003). Eating disorders. *Obstetrics and Gynecology Clinics of North America* 30(2): 353–377, vii.

39. American Society for Aesthetic Surgery. (2004). *Quick Facts*. Available at: http://www.surgery.org/press/index.php.

40. Rothblum, E. (1990). Women and weight: fad and fiction. *Journal of Psychology* 124: 5–24.

41. Garner, D. M. (January–February 1997). The 1997 body image survey results. *Psychology Today*. Available at: http://www.psychologytoday.com/articles/pto-19970201-000023.htm.

42. Centers for Disease Control and Prevention. (2008). *2007 Youth Behavior Risk Survey*. Atlanta: CDC.

43. Hsu, L. K. G. (1990). *Eating Disorders*. New York: Guilford Press.

44. Crowther, J. H., Tennenbaum, D. L., Hobfoil, S. E., & Paris-Stephens, M. A. (1992). *The Etiology of Bulimia Nervosa*. Washington, DC: Hemisphere.

45. Food and Agriculture Organization of the United Nations. (2008). *Clinton at UN: Food, Energy, Financial Woes Linked*. Available at: http://www.fao.org/newsroom/en/news/2008/1000945/index.html.

46. UNICEF. (2007). *State of the World's Children, 2008*. New York: United Nations.

47. Nord, M., Andrews, M., & Carlson, S. (2007). *Household Food Security in the United States, 2006*. Washington, DC: U.S. Department of Agriculture.

48. World Health Organization. (2003). *Nutrition*. Available at: http://www.who.int/nutrition/index.htm.

49. Harne, A. J., & Bixby, W. R. (2005). The benefits and barriers of strength training among college-age women. *Journal of Sport Behavior* 28(2): 151–166.

Chapter Ten

Understanding and Preventing Cardiovascular Disease and Cancer

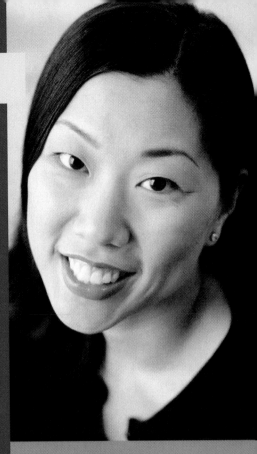

Chapter Objectives

On completion of this chapter, the student should be able to discuss:

1. The main components and functions of the circulatory system and blood.
2. The processes leading to atherosclerosis and myocardial infarction.
3. The conditions that contribute to congestive heart failure.
4. Types of congenital heart disease and its associated prevalence and mortality rates.
5. The cause and effects of rheumatic heart disease.
6. The significance of angina pectoris.
7. Conditions that lead to peripheral artery disease.
8. The major causes of cerebrovascular accidents.
9. The major modifiable risk factors for cardiovascular disease.
10. Gender and race differences that determine risk for cardiovascular disease.
11. The process of cancer development and metastasis.
12. Cancer from an epidemiological perspective and racial, ethnic, and socioeconomic dimensions.
13. Types of benign conditions of the breast, cervix, uterus, and ovaries.
14. Risk factors, screening methods, and treatment modalities for breast, cervical, uterine, and ovarian cancer.
15. The purpose of Pap smears and HPV tests and how they relate to benign cervical conditions as well as cervical cancer.
16. Risk factors, screening methods, and treatment modalities for lung cancer, colorectal cancer, and skin cancer.
17. Prevention of cardiovascular disease and cancer through lifestyle changes and health screening.

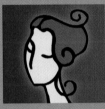

womenshealth.jbpub.com

Women's Health Online is a great source for supplementary women's health information for both students and instructors. Visit

http://womenshealth.jbpub.com

to find a variety of useful tools for learning, thinking, and teaching.

Introduction

Genetics and lifestyle are major contributors to chronic diseases. Genetics clearly plays a role in determining who is at highest risk for developing certain diseases and conditions. Lifestyle alone cannot totally counter a heavy genetic loading for certain conditions; however, among those who are genetically predisposed lifestyle changes can make a difference. This chapter provides an overview of cardiovascular disease and cancer, which are the major killers of women today. Each disease is discussed in terms of epidemiological considerations, risk factors, screening, treatment, and personal decision making to reduce the risk of disease.

Cardiovascular Disease

Cardiovascular disease (CVD) comprises a group of diseases that includes two major categories: diseases of the heart and cerebrovascular disease (primarily stroke). Nearly 460,000 women die annually in the United States of CVD, equaling a rate of about one death every 37 seconds. Stroke accounts for approximately 19% of these deaths.[1,2] According to the Centers for Disease Control and Prevention (CDC)/National Center for Health Statistics (NCHS), if all major forms of CVD were eliminated, life expectancy would increase by almost seven years. More lives are claimed by CVD than by the next five leading causes of death combined. Cardiovascular deaths usually occur in later years when women are beset with a variety of co-morbid conditions, such as high blood pressure, high blood cholesterol, osteoporosis, and diabetes. **Figures 10.1** and **10.2** illustrate the death rates from CVD among women of different races as they age.[2]

Cardiovascular disease is also among the leading causes of disability in women. Heart disease can be severely disabling, creating lifestyle limitations. Stroke can lead to paralysis, incontinence, language impairments, and loss of memory. Although it was once believed that heart conditions and stroke were an inevitable consequence of aging, it is now realized that these diseases are greatly influenced by negative lifestyle behaviors, such as cigarette smoking, poor nutrition, and lack of exercise.

Perspectives on Cardiovascular Disease

Epidemiology

Cardiovascular disease is the leading cause of death for women, regardless of racial or ethnic group. Of the various forms of CVD, coronary heart disease (CHD) is the leading cause of death. In 2004, 217,800 women (48%), compared to 233,500 men (52%) died of CHD. Among these women, 64% died suddenly with no warning symptoms. Stroke, the third leading cause of death among women, after heart disease and cancer, killed 91,300 women (61%) compared with 58,800 men (39%).[4]

Although some cardiovascular diseases occur among children and adolescents, the majority are diseases of individuals who are middle-aged (50 years) or older. The incidence of CHD begins to rise for women between the ages

Figure 10.1

Death rates for diseases of the heart for women 45 or older.

Source: Centers for Disease Control and Prevention, National Center for Health Statistics. (2008). *Health United States,* Table 36.

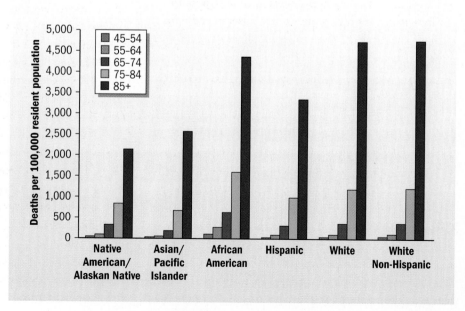

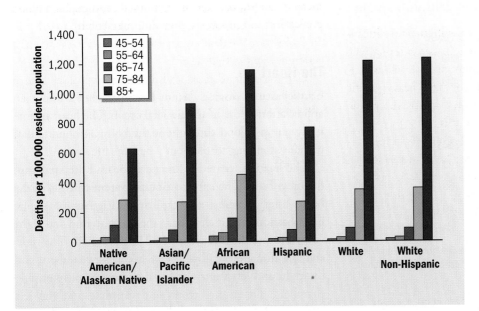

Figure 10.2

Death rates for cerebrovascular disease for women 45 or older.

Source: Centers for Disease Control and Prevention, National Center for Health Statistics. (2008). *Health United States,* Table 37.

of 55 and 60, about 10 years later than for men. The incidence of stroke begins to sharply rise in both women and men between the ages of 55 and 64.[1,2]

Economic Dimensions

Cardiovascular disease imposes a heavy burden on the medical care system in the United States, particularly on emergency medical departments and hospitals. Clinical care of CVD patients is costly and often prolonged. The estimated cost of cardiovascular disease and stroke in the United States in 2008 was $448.5 billion. This figure includes both direct and indirect costs.

- Direct costs: health expenditures including those for physicians and other professionals, hospital and nursing home services, medications, home health care, and other medical durables

- Indirect costs: lost productivity resulting from morbidity and mortality

An estimated $296.4 billion was spent for the care of persons with cardiovascular diseases and stroke in 2008. The estimated indirect costs (those costs related to lost work days and lost future earnings) from these diseases include $37.6 billion for lost productivity due to morbidity and $114.5 billion for lost productivity due to mortality.[1] Cardiovascular disease often affects individuals during their peak productive years at work, causing significant disruption to families who depend on the person's income.[1] The high rate of CVD also carries a burden for the countries that lose productive workers to disease. The emotional cost to women and their families and friends from such disease is incalculable.

Global Dimensions

During the past century, CVD has been increasingly recognized as a leading cause of disability and death worldwide. With an ever-increasing life expectancy, countries that once were overwhelmed with infectious and communicable diseases, maternal and infant deaths, and malnutrition are now besieged with CVD. CVD ranks as a leading cause of death among women worldwide.[3] The ability to acquire fast foods (which are often loaded with saturated fats and high in calories), a decrease in physical exercise, and high rates of cigarette smoking have further contributed to the problem. Of particular concern is the increasing number of children in developing countries who engage in these dangerous health habits.[4] According to the World Health Organization (WHO), more than 20% of women are obese in Eastern Europe, the Middle East, the Pacific Islands, the United Kingdom, the United States, and some South American countries.[4] Cardiovascular disease death rates vary widely among women across the continents (see **Table 10.1**). The Russian Federation leads in death rates whereas rates in Japan and France are much lower.

Smoking rates among women are beginning to plateau or decline, in part because of strong and widespread public health education and intervention. Nevertheless, some women still smoke and compromise their health.[6] **Table 10.2** presents examples of smoking trends among women in selected countries.

Table 10.1 CVD Deaths per 100,000 Women

Country	CVD Deaths
Russian Federation	659
Hungary	303
Argentina	174
United States	150
Republic of Korea	133
Canada	92
Israel	83
Japan	69
France	66

Source: World Health Organization, http://www.who.int/whosis/mort/download/en/index.html; National Center for Health Statistics; National Heart, Lung and Blood Institute.

Table 10.2 Smoking Trends Among Women in Selected Countries

Country	1980	1990	2003–2005
France	17	20	21 (2003)
Israel	30	16	18 (2005)
Poland	N/A	29	26 (2005)
Russian Federation	N/A	12	15 (2004)
Sweden	28	25	18 (2005)
United Kingdom	34	28	23 (2004)

Source: World Health Organization. (2007). *European Health for All Statistical Database*. http://www.euro.who.int/hfadb.

Cultural attitudes affect lifestyle habits. Women in many countries have moved from rural areas to urban areas—from physically active lifestyles such as farming to more sedentary work in offices and industry. Another concern is the "migration" effect that often occurs among women who migrate from developing to developed countries. As with migration from farm to city, women who migrate to more developed countries are exposed to different cultures and styles of living. Unhealthy foods may be convenient and present in greater quantities, while healthy foods and opportunities for physical activity may be more rare. These lifestyle changes put immigrant women at particularly high risk for obesity, high blood pressure, high blood cholesterol, and diabetes—all risk factors for CVD. Unfortunately, in many countries and for many women immigrants, disease prevention and health care remain fragmented.[7]

The Heart

Cardiovascular disease cannot be understood without an appreciation of the heart as a vital organ. The heart relentlessly pumps blood throughout the body 24 hours a day, without stopping, throughout a person's life.

The heart is located in the chest behind the **sternum**, the breastbone. The **cardiovascular system** consists of the heart, arteries, veins, and capillaries (**Figure 10.3**). The heart has four major chambers: the **right atrium** and **right ventricle** and the **left atrium** and **left ventricle**. The right and left atria are the upper blood-receiving chambers, and the right and left ventricles are the lower blood-pumping chambers. The right atrium and ventricle and the left atrium and ventricle are each separated by a valve. The right atrium and ventricle are separated by the **tricuspid valve**; the left atrium and ventricle are separated by the **bicuspid** or **mitral valve**. Blood flows from the atrium through the valve to the ventricle below. A thick muscular wall known as the **septum** separates the right and left sides of the heart.

Oxygen-poor blood from throughout the body travels to the heart so that it can be pumped to the lungs for oxygenation. The oxygen-poor blood enters the right atrium of the heart from the **inferior** and **superior vena cava** (major veins). From the right atrium, blood flows through the tricuspid valve into the right ventricle, where it is pumped to the lungs via the **pulmonary arteries**. In the lungs, carbon dioxide and waste products are removed from the blood and exchanged for fresh oxygen. The newly oxygen-rich blood leaves the lungs via the **pulmonary veins** and flows into the left atrium. From the left atrium, it passes through the mitral valve into the left ventricle. The left ventricle contracts and forces the oxygen-rich blood through the **aortic valve** into the **aorta** (the main artery) and from there throughout the major **arteries**, flowing gradually into smaller and smaller arteries, **arterioles**, and finally **capillaries** throughout the body. The capillaries—microscopic vessels with thin walls—are the sites where the nutrients and oxygen in the blood are exchanged for waste and carbon dioxide at the cellular level. From the capillaries, the oxygen-poor but carbon dioxide–rich blood flows into the **venules** and veins as it makes its way back to the heart. The cycle then begins again.

For this system to function properly, the pump—the heart—must remain strong and forceful. It must contract

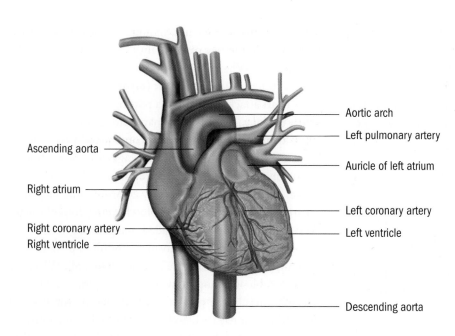

Figure 10.3

Cardiovascular system.

Aortic arch

Left pulmonary artery

Auricle of left atrium

Left coronary artery

Left ventricle

Ascending aorta

Right atrium

Right coronary artery

Right ventricle

Descending aorta

forcefully and quickly when a woman runs a marathon, yet it must slow for rest during sleep. The heart is activated to perform its pumping function by electrical stimuli pulsed from specialized tissues called nodes buried in the cardiac muscle. This electrical stimulation can be detected by a special device known as an **electrocardiograph (ECG)**, sometimes known as an EKG. An ECG can detect a normal heart rhythm or abnormalities such as a heart attack or a congenitally damaged tricuspid valve.

Similar to the heart, the arteries have muscles and must expand and contract vigorously to meet the demands placed on the body, yet remain supple and open. Veins, although they must also remain supple and open, do not have muscles and must therefore rely on surrounding mus-

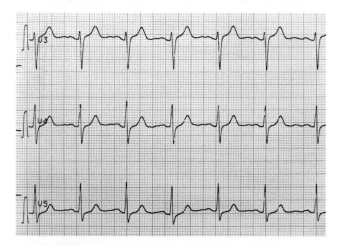

■ An electrocardiograph (ECG) can detect a normal heart rhythm or abnormalities such as a heart attack or a congenitally damaged tricuspid valve.

cles to move the blood along through the venous system to its destination.

Blood is the vehicle for transporting the food and waste throughout the body. An average woman circulates about six quarts of blood per day. Blood consists of many critical components, which are all suspended in plasma. The primary components are as follows:

- The **red blood cells (erythrocytes)** carry oxygen and carbon dioxide. Hemoglobin is an important protein in the red blood cells that carries oxygen from the lungs throughout the body; it also gives blood its red color.

- The **white blood cells (leukocytes)** act as scavengers to rid the blood and body of bacteria and waste. Several types of white blood cells exist, each of which has its own role in fighting bacterial, viral, fungal, and parasitic infections.

- The **platelets (thrombocytes)** cause the blood to clot.

If the heart's electrical signal loses its regular pattern, the heart can begin to beat irregularly and less effectively, a condition called **arrhythmia**. Arrhythmias are very common and can occur in an otherwise healthy heart; in some cases, however, they may indicate a serious problem and can lead to heart disease. When the atria emit uncoordinated electrical signals, the condition is called **atrial fibrillation** (AF); when disordered electrical activity causes rapid, uncoordinated contractions of the ventricle, the condition is called **ventricular fibrillation** (VF). AF is not usually life threatening in itself, but it can lead to other, more serious conditions. For example, when the atrium doesn't pump blood evenly, some blood may remain in the atrium and form a clot. If this clot enters the bloodstream, it can travel to the brain and cause a stroke. In VF, little or no blood may be pumped from the heart, which can result in collapse and sudden death. Physicians can detect heart abnormalities and will first determine the origination of the arrhythmia and its severity before considering treatment.

Pathophysiology of the Heart

Cardiovascular disease encompasses both heart disease (coronary heart disease, congestive heart failure, rheumatic heart disease, angina pectoris, peripheral artery disease, hypertension) and cerebrovascular disease (stroke). Many of these diseases can be prevented or controlled with lifestyle modifications or medications (see "Risk Factors for Cardiovascular Disease").

Heart conditions, in general, can be diagnosed by a variety of tests. Which test is used often depends on a woman's risk factors, her history of heart problems, and her current symptoms. Types of tests include noninvasive tests such as electrocardiograms and magnetic resonance imaging (MRI), nuclear imaging tests that require a needle puncture, and possibly invasive imaging tests such as cardiac catheterization. (For more information on diagnostic tests, visit the Web sites listed at the end of this chapter.)

Treatment also varies greatly for each patient depending on the severity of the condition. This chapter describes the many medications, surgical interventions, and lifestyle changes that can be used to prevent and treat heart disease.

Coronary Heart Disease

Coronary heart disease (CHD) is a result of narrowed or clogged arteries. **Arteriosclerosis** is a generic term that describes any disease of the arteries that leads to thickening and hardening of the artery walls. **Atherosclerosis**, a form of arteriosclerosis, is the major culprit in CHD. It causes the heart vessels to become clogged, thereby impairing a woman's ability to function. This can happen in a variety of ways:

- The arteries can become clogged with waste, usually fat deposits (**plaques**). These waste deposits build up over years on the inner portion of the arteries, impeding the flow of blood.

- The arteries can become stiff with age or disease, rendering them less able to respond to the demands placed on them. If the blood flow is compromised, the area being fed by that particular artery or arteries does not receive proper nutrients and can become damaged or die.

Because the arteries surrounding the heart are so twisted and tortuous, they are particularly prone to developing atherosclerosis. When that occurs, a woman is at increased risk of suffering a **heart attack (myocardial infarction)**.

A heart attack, or death of a portion of the heart, occurs when one or more of the coronary arteries in the heart become damaged or clogged and, consequently, the arteries close off (**Table 10.3**). Such blockages can occur from a circulating blood clot called an **embolus**. As an embolus moves through the bloodstream, it can become lodged in an artery, blocking any further blood from getting through. The resulting blockage is called a **thrombus** (stationary blood clot). A clot can also form as a result of plaque (cholesterol) build-up within the arterial inner wall. Whatever the cause, blood cannot flow downstream from the blockage. As a result, the part of the body fed by the blocked artery does not receive blood carrying oxygen and nutrients and becomes severely impaired or dies. Blockages within different coronary arteries create different problems. For example, if the blockage occurs within the major artery feeding the left ventricle (the main pump of the heart), the entire ventricle can cease to pump. This stops blood flow to the rest of the body. If this situation is not reversed immediately, a woman can die or suffer irreversible brain damage within a matter of minutes from lack of oxygen to the brain. The heart also can become damaged from other diseases or conditions, such as rheumatic heart disease, or from injury, such as a heart attack, which can lead to congestive heart failure, a condition in which the heart is impaired and cannot pump effectively.

Atherosclerosis cannot be cured, but its progression can be slowed. Treatment often depends on which organs are involved. For heart conditions, cholesterol-lowering med-

---

Table 10.3 Warning Signs of a Heart Attack

- Chest discomfort: tightness, pressure, squeezing, fullness, or pain lasting a few minutes. The discomfort can go away and come back.

- Shortness of breath with or without chest discomfort

- Other signs: cold sweat, nausea, lightheadedness

Less Common Symptoms in Women

- Atypical abdominal pain

- Palpitations, paleness, dizziness

- Fatigue

Source: American Heart Association. *Heart Attack, Stroke and Cardiac Arrest Warning Signs.* Available at: http://www.americanheart.org/presenter.jhtml?identifier=3053.

ications can be used to control high cholesterol levels and are a critical factor in treatment. **Balloon angioplasty** is a procedure used to open narrowed or blocked coronary arteries. A small, hollow tube called a catheter is inserted into an artery near the blockage, and then a balloon near the end of the catheter is inflated. This action helps to widen the vessel and allow blood to flow more freely. A wire mesh **stent** is usually placed at the site of the original narrowing to keep the artery open. In contrast, **coronary artery bypass graft (CABG) surgery** creates a new passage around the blocked part of the coronary artery to restore blood flow to the heart muscle. When the brain is affected, antiplatelet medications, including aspirin, and anticoagulant medications, such as warfarin and heparin, may be used to prevent strokes. When atherosclerosis narrows arteries that supply the bowel, balloon angioplasty may be used or a bypass arterial graft may be performed.

Some of these treatments also may be useful in treating a patient after a heart attack. The ultimate goal of such treatment is to minimize damage by restoring blood flow to the heart muscle.

Research has shown that people with heart disease are more likely to suffer from depression than otherwise healthy people. People with depression also are at greater risk for developing heart disease. Furthermore, depression and low perceived social support after a heart attack are associated with higher morbidity and mortality. Data show that treating depression in recent heart attack patients does not reduce the risk of death or second heart attack; however, it may help the symptoms of depression and improve quality of life for the patients.[7–9]

Acute Coronary Syndrome

Acute coronary syndrome (ACS) is a term that is used to describe individuals who present with specific cardiac symptoms: myocardial infarction (heart attack) or unstable angina (chest pain that is unexpected or unusual and may be more severe than usual). This important diagnostic category seeks to identify individuals when they are moving toward a heart attack (unstable angina) or are in the early stages of a heart attack. The goal is to intervene before serious damage occurs.

Congestive Heart Failure

Congestive heart failure (CHF) occurs when heart muscles are weak and cannot pump with proper vigor. In such a case, the heart loses its ability to contract properly or sufficiently to meet the demands placed on it. Even if the arteries remain open, without a strong pumping action from the heart, the ability of the nutrient-rich and oxygen-rich blood to reach cells is hampered, and the cells may suffer damage or die. Additionally, the heart muscle itself depends on a rich blood supply from the coronary arteries, which must remain open and supple if the heart is to function with vigor. As a result, circulation suffers and fluids begin to accumulate in veins, causing breathing problems, kidney problems, and swelling in the extremities, particularly the legs. CHF may have many causes, but it is often a disease of older women who have suffered heart damage from high blood pressure, atherosclerosis, arteriosclerosis, or heart attack. In some cases, CHF occurs because of a congenital defect or damage to the heart from a bacterial disease, such as rheumatic heart disease.

In many cases, congestive heart failure can be prevented or minimized by controlling high blood pressure, treating underlying bacterial infections, and following lifestyle modifications that prevent other forms of CVD. Medication, salt reduction, and possibly surgery to alleviate blockages in coronary arteries may help to improve heart function once CHF has been diagnosed. CHF is the single most frequent cause of hospitalization for people age 65 or older, with women accounting for more than half of all cases.[1]

Congenital Heart Disease

Congenital heart disease is an abnormality of the heart that is present at birth. It can include one or more of the following:

- A hole in the septum
- Imperfectly formed blood vessels
- Valvular damage
- Left ventricular imperfections

Patent ductus arteriosus is a congenital condition in which the ductus arteriosus (passageway between the pulmonary artery and aorta) does not close. It is a common condition in premature babies. Another congenital heart disease, called **pulmonary stenosis**, occurs when the valve between the ventricle and the pulmonary artery is defective and does not open properly. Atrial or ventricular septal defects occur when an opening appears between the two upper or lower chambers of the heart. The majority of these imperfections can be corrected with surgery.

Nearly 36,000 babies are born each year with congenital heart defects; these defects claim the lives of approximately 4,300 young people per year. Forty-three percent of the deaths occur in infants less than one year old.[1] Mortality associated with congenital heart defects has been declining, however, due to advances in diagnosis and surgical treatments. From 1994 to 2004, for example, death rates declined 31.6%. Congenital heart defects or imperfections often can be corrected with surgery.

Rheumatic Heart Disease

Rheumatic heart disease results from a bacterial infection (*Streptococcus*) that has been inadequately treated and causes damage to the heart valves. Rheumatic heart disease is a downward progression from an inadequately treated strep throat, which progresses to rheumatic fever and affects the entire body. The brain, heart, and joints can be permanently damaged. In the heart, rheumatic heart disease can damage the valves by closing them off either completely or partially. This condition may require surgery and valve replacement. The best treatment is prevention—for example, treatment of the initial strep throat, which precludes further damage. Modern antibiotic therapy has sharply reduced mortality from rheumatic heart disease. In 1950, approximately 15,000 Americans died of this disease; in 2007, there were 3,200 deaths. The highest death rates were in women.[1]

Angina Pectoris

Angina pectoris (or just *angina*) is chest pain resulting from an insufficient supply of blood, and thus oxygen, to the heart muscle. The symptoms can range in severity from a mild cramping ache to a crushing pain in the chest. The impairment of blood flow can result from atherosclerosis or a spasm of a normal artery. The estimated prevalence of angina is greater in women than in men—angina affects more than 3 million women in the United States.[1] Angina is also a symptom of CVD and may be a predictor of future myocardial infarction. Depending on the cause of the impairment, the pain can be relieved by medication, often nitroglycerin, which is a strong vasodilator (opening the closed blood vessel).

Peripheral Artery Disease

Peripheral artery disease (PAD) is a disease of the extremities (hands, arms, but mainly legs and feet) in which the blood supply is diminished and sufficient oxygen and nutrients do not reach these areas properly. Because waste is not removed from these areas sufficiently, a woman can experience symptoms that range from cramping and numbness to gangrene (tissue death), which may require amputation of the extremity. The cause of PAD is related to atherosclerosis and arteriosclerosis and is particularly associated with diabetes, smoking, and hypertension. Of all the known risk factors, smoking is the most strongly re-

lated to PAD. Treatment options include lifestyle modifications, such as smoking cessation, anticoagulant or antiplatelet medications, angioplasty, or bypass surgery.

Metabolic Syndrome

Metabolic syndrome is the name for a group of diseases that can occur together and create a greater risk for CVD. The National Heart, Lung and Blood Institute and the American Heart Association note that the presence of three or more of the following diseases predisposes a person to an increased risk for metabolic syndrome[10]:

- Elevated waist circumference
  - Men: Equal to or greater than 40 inches (102 cm)
  - Women: Equal to or greater than 35 inches (88 cm)
- Elevated triglycerides
  - Equal to or greater than 150 mg/dL
- Reduced HDL ("good") cholesterol
  - Men: Less than 40 mg/dL
  - Women: Less than 50 mg/dL
- Elevated blood pressure
  - Equal to or greater than 130/85 mm Hg
- Elevated fasting glucose
  - Equal to or greater than 100 mg/dL

The principal factors contributing to metabolic syndrome appear to be central obesity and insulin resistance—factors that are increasingly common among women. Both organizations recommend weight loss and control, healthy eating, and increased physical activity as ways to prevent metabolic syndrome.[10]

Cerebrovascular Accident (Stroke)

Cerebrovascular accident, commonly called **stroke**, is a condition in which blood vessels leading to and within the brain become damaged. The process of blood flow blockage that occurs in the coronary vessels of the heart is similar to that which occurs in the brain. The other major process involved in stroke is vessel rupture, often resulting from atherosclerotic vessels. When the blood vessel either is blocked or bursts, part of the brain cannot get blood and therefore oxygen, which it needs to survive. The most common type of stroke, **ischemic stroke**, is caused by blockage; the clot in such cases is called a cerebral thrombus or cerebral **embolism**. **Hemorrhagic strokes** are caused by ruptured blood vessels.

An **aneurysm** is one type of weakened blood vessel that can cause a stroke. It entails a ballooning of a weakened region of a blood vessel resulting from several factors including a congenital defect, chronic high blood pressure, or an injury to the brain. If left untreated, the aneurysm will continue to weaken until it ruptures and bleeds in the brain (**Figure 10.4**).

Warning signs (**Table 10.4**) may precede a stroke in the form of a **transient ischemic attack (TIA)**. In a TIA, the artery may close momentarily in a spasm, and the woman may have a brief memory lapse or garbled speech. Such an event often occurs very quickly, and the woman may have little memory of it.

A variety of tests can diagnose a stroke by examining the brain and outlining the injured brain area:

- Imaging tests, such as a CT (computed tomography) or CAT (computerized axial tomography) scan, produce a picture of the brain similar to X rays.

- Electrical tests, such as an EEG (electroencephalogram) or an evoked response test, record the electrical impulses of the brain.

- Blood flow tests, such as B-mode imaging, Doppler testing, duplex scanning, and angiography (arteriography or arteriogram), show any problem that may cause changes in blood flow to the brain.

Surgery, drugs, acute hospital care, and rehabilitation are all accepted stroke therapies. Treatment of an ischemic stroke focuses on removing the obstruction and restoring blood flow. The most promising medication for ischemic

Figure 10.4
Types of cerebrovascular accidents.

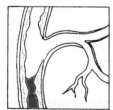
Thrombus

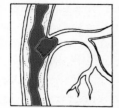
Embolism

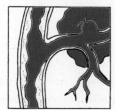
Aneurysm (ruptured)

Table 10.4 Warning Signs of Stroke

- Sudden numbness or weakness of the face, arm, or leg, especially on one side of the body
- Sudden confusion, or trouble speaking or understanding
- Sudden trouble seeing in one or both eyes
- Sudden trouble walking, dizziness, loss of balance or coordination
- Sudden, severe headache with no known cause

In the event of a stroke, immediate action is required. Call 911 or the local emergency system and get medical treatment immediately.

Source: American Heart Association. *Stroke Warning Signs.* Available at: http://www.americanheart.org/presenter.jhtml?identifier=4742.

stroke is the clot-busting drug tissue plasminogen activator (tPA). For maximum benefit, tPA therapy must be started within three hours of the onset of stroke symptoms. Generally, only 3% to 5% of people who suffer a stroke reach the hospital in time to be considered for this treatment. Although tPA carries a risk of bleeding in the brain, its benefits generally outweigh the risks when an experienced doctor uses it properly. A five-year study by the National Institute of Neurological Disorders and Stroke (NINDS) found that stroke patients who received tPA within three hours of the start of stroke symptoms were at least 30% more likely to recover with little or no disability after three months.[11]

Doctors sometimes use balloon angioplasty and the implantable steel screens called stents to remedy fatty build-up clogging a vessel. When the carotid artery (a neck artery) is partially blocked by a fatty build-up, surgery might be performed to remove the plaque—a technique called carotid endarterectomy. Antiplatelet agents, such as aspirin, and anticoagulants, such as warfarin, interfere with the blood's ability to clot and can play an important role in preventing ischemic stroke.

To treat a hemorrhagic stroke, an obstruction needs to be introduced to prevent rupture and bleeding of the affected blood vessel. Surgical treatment is often recommended to either place a metal clip at the base of the aneurysm or to remove the abnormal vessels. Endovascular procedures are less invasive and involve the introduction of a catheter through a major artery in the leg or arm; the catheter is then guided to the aneurysm, where it deposits a mechanical agent, such as a coil, to prevent rupture.

After a stroke, rehabilitation is often necessary to help survivors relearn skills that are lost when part of the brain is damaged and learn new ways of performing tasks to

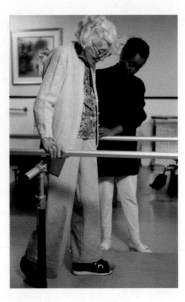

■ Recovery from a stroke can be very difficult.

compensate for any disabilities. Therapy begins in the acute-care hospital after the patient's medical condition has been stabilized, often within 24 to 48 hours after the stroke. Post-stroke rehabilitation requires the services of physicians; rehabilitation nurses; physical, occupational, recreational, speech-language, and vocational therapists; and mental health professionals.

The types and degrees of disability that follow a stroke depend on which area of the brain is damaged. Generally, stroke can cause five types of disabilities:

■ Paralysis is one of the most common disabilities resulting from stroke. It usually appears on the side of the body opposite the side of the brain damaged by stroke,

and may affect the face, an arm, a leg, or the entire side of the body.

■ Stroke patients may lose the ability to feel touch, pain, temperature, or position. Some experience pain, numbness, or odd sensations of tingling or prickling in paralyzed or weakened limbs. The loss of urinary continence and/or bowel control is fairly common immediately after a stroke and often results from a combination of sensory and motor deficits. Permanent incontinence after a stroke, however, is uncommon.

■ At least one-fourth of all stroke survivors experience language impairments, involving the ability to speak, write, and understand spoken and written language. Interestingly, sex-related differences have been noted depending on which portion of the brain is affected. Functional MRI scans have shown that males predominantly rely on areas of the left hemisphere of the brain, whereas females activate both the left and right regions for certain aspects of language. A stroke that occurs in the left hemisphere can therefore have disastrous results for men in terms of speech, whereas women can use the other, unaffected side to regain speech. This knowledge helps to explain why women seem to be more resilient to the effects of such injury and are more likely than males to recover language ability after suffering a left-hemisphere stroke.[12]

■ Stroke can damage parts of the brain that are responsible for memory, learning, and awareness. Stroke survivors may have dramatically shortened attention spans or may lose their ability to make plans, comprehend

■ Functional MRI scans show that male subjects predominantly rely on areas of the left hemisphere of the brain, while females activate both the left and right regions for certain aspects of language. (© Shaywitz, et al., 1995 NMR Research/Yale Medical School)

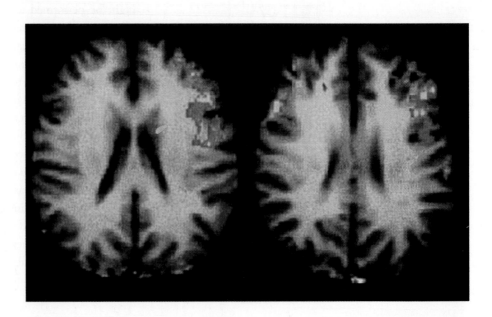

meaning, learn new tasks, or engage in other complex mental activities.

- Survivors of stroke often feel fear, anxiety, frustration, anger, sadness, and a sense of grief for their physical and mental losses. The physical effects of brain damage are responsible for some of these emotional disturbances and personality changes. Clinical depression appears to be the emotional disorder most commonly experienced by stroke survivors.

Whatever the cause of the stroke, the damage to the artery prevents oxygen and nutrients from reaching a particular area of the brain. As a result, that portion of the brain dies. Depending on where the stroke occurs in the brain, speech, memory, thought, and movement can be diminished or lost. Stroke is a leading cause of severe, long-term disability. Recovery is dependent on many factors, many of which stem from the individual's pre-stroke status: age, mental status, physical abilities, economic support, and cultural perceptions. Often women are older when they experience a stroke and frequently do less well compared to men in recovering physical and mental functioning. [8,9,13]

Although a stroke can happen at any time to anyone, it is generally a condition that occurs in older individuals. The incidence of a stroke doubles each decade for people older than 55. Of those women with an initial stroke, 25% die within a year, although this varies with age and race. Those who suffer a stroke at age 65 or older have an even greater chance of dying. Among women younger than 65, 53% of those who have a stroke will die within eight years.[1]

Risk Factors for Cardiovascular Disease

Cardiovascular diseases result from a complex interaction of genetics, lifestyle, and environmental factors that lead to different pathological conditions of the cardiovascular system. The major risk factors (those that make a significant contribution to the development of a disease) for CHD that can be modified or controlled include cigarette smoking, high blood pressure, high blood cholesterol, diabetes, obesity, and sedentary lifestyle (see **Self-Assessment 10.1**). The major risk factors for stroke that can be modified or controlled are high blood pressure, cigarette smoking, and diabetes. Risk factors that cannot be changed or controlled include increasing age, family history of CVD,

---

Self-Assessment 10.1

Personal Risk Factors for Cardiovascular Disease

Age
A woman's risk of cardiovascular disease increases as she gets older, most noticeably after menopause.

Genetics
A family history of cardiovascular disease increases a woman's risk.

Race
Until age 75, African American women are twice as likely to die of cardiovascular disease as white women; after age 75, white women are more likely to die of cardiovascular disease.

Obesity
Being 20% over recommended body weight is a risk factor for cardiovascular disease.

Smoking
For women, smoking is the most significant risk factor for cardiovascular disease.

Hypertension
Elevated blood pressure is a risk factor for cardiovascular disease. A woman's blood pressure is likely to rise after menopause.

Elevated cholesterol
Elevated cholesterol is a major risk factor for cardiovascular disease.

Sedentary lifestyle
Failure to achieve adequate levels of physical activity predisposes an individual to cardiovascular disease.

Diabetes
Diabetes is more prevalent in women and is a major risk factor for cardiovascular disease.

Menopause (natural or surgical)
A woman's risk of heart disease rises as she approaches menopause (loss of estrogen) and continues to rise thereafter.

Having one or more of these risk factors increases the risk of developing heart disease. The more risk factors a woman has, the greater her risk.

Source: American Heart Association.

and race. Although these factors can contribute to a person's risk of disease, they are not perfect predictors of disease. A woman with normal cholesterol levels, for example, may have heart disease. Conversely, a woman with high cholesterol may not have heart disease even though she does have one of the factors that put her at risk.

Cigarette Smoking

As discussed in detail in Chapter 13, cigarette smoking is the greatest preventable cause of death in the United States. Not only does it increase the risk of several kinds of cancers, but it also sharply increases the risk of heart attack (especially sudden death from heart attack), stroke, and PAD. Although smoking rates have declined sharply since 1960, too many women still smoke. Current estimates are about 18.1% of women.[14] Furthermore, smoking is highest among women with little education and lowest among women with a bachelor's degree or higher.[1,15]

Certain components in cigarette smoke act as **vasoconstrictors**, meaning they narrow the blood vessels. One such compound is carbon monoxide, a gas that reduces the amount of oxygen that red blood cells can carry. This poor oxygen-carrying ability decreases the amount of oxygen available to the heart, brain, muscles, and every organ in the body. Nicotine is another vasoconstrictor. By narrowing the blood vessels, it increases the likelihood of a blood clot forming. Over time in a chronic smoker, vasoconstriction contributes to the increased fragility and brittleness of arteries, which in turn contributes to atherosclerosis.

The good news is that when a woman stops smoking, her risk for heart disease begins to decline within months. According to the World Health Organization, one year after quitting, the risk of coronary heart disease decreases by 50%; within 15 years, the relative risk of an ex-smoker dying from CHD approaches that of a lifetime nonsmoker.[16]

Secondhand smoke, also known as **environmental tobacco smoke (ETS)**, comes from nearby tobacco products that are burning. The toxins contained in secondhand smoke include more than 60 cancer-causing agents, nicotine, and carbon monoxide.[17,18] Secondhand smoke is associated with a number of potentially lethal conditions: lung cancer, sinus cancer, lung conditions (such as asthma, or impaired lung function, especially in young children), heart

disease, low birthweight in babies (especially when mothers smoke during pregnancy), and others. Repeated exposure to secondhand smoke almost doubles the risk of heart disease.[18]

Hypertension

Blood pressure is the pressure exerted against the walls of the arteries when the heart pumps, specifically when the left ventricle contracts. This pressure is crucial in maintaining equilibrium throughout the vascular system as different forces affect this system. For example, when an athlete runs a race, the heart must pump faster and harder to meet the demands of the cells for oxygen. As part of this process, the arteries must constrict to keep the pressure constant to accomplish the task of running.

Blood pressure is measured with a **sphygmomanometer**. This cuff device is connected to a hose, which is in turn connected to a measuring device. The cuff is wrapped around the woman's upper arm (or in rare instances the leg) and inflated, thereby constricting the underlying artery and stopping the blood flow and with it the sound of the heartbeat. Gradually the pressure in the cuff is released, and the blood begins to flow back through the artery and the sound of the heartbeat returns. The first sound heard as the blood begins to flow back into the artery is called the **systolic**, and the last sound heard before it disappears again is called the **diastolic**. The measurement is shown as millimeters of mercury (mm Hg) and is expressed as a fraction, such as 115/75 mm Hg, or 115 mm Hg systolic and 75 mm Hg diastolic. The first number,

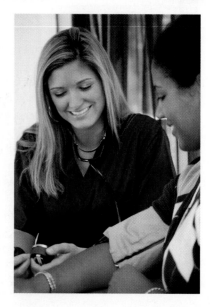

■ All women should know their personal risk for hypertension and regularly monitor their blood pressure.

Hey, smoking is cool, and it helps me stay thin. Sure I hear all the no-smoking ads, but I see people lighting up all the time. So why not! Besides, my friends and I know we can quit anytime.

15-year-old female student

which expresses the systolic pressure, represents the amount of force the blood exerts against the wall of the artery when the heart contracts. The second number, which expresses the diastolic pressure, represents the amount of pressure the blood exerts against the wall of the artery when the heart rests between beats.

Hypertension, also known as high blood pressure, is a blood pressure that remains elevated above what is considered a safe level. Hypertension is not the same as excessive stress or tension, as some individuals mistakenly imagine. Although numbers such as 120/80 mm Hg have been noted over the years as "normal" blood pressure, there is no true normal number because blood pressure varies throughout the day and during different activities. A young woman may have a blood pressure of 90/70 mm Hg during a visit to the doctor, whereas an older woman may have a blood pressure of 138/80 mm Hg during her doctor's visit. Both may be deemed appropriate. The numbers used by the National Heart, Lung and Blood Institute's National High Blood Pressure Education Program and by the American Heart Association to indicate high blood pressure are 140 mm Hg systolic and 90 mm Hg diastolic. Although blood pressure can reach heights such as 140/90 mm Hg or greater in a healthy adult during exercise, these levels return to a lower level after exercise. Continuing levels of blood pressure at 140/90 mm Hg or higher, however, are considered high blood pressure and, as such, increase an individual's risk for heart disease and stroke (see **Table 10.5**). One out of every three adults in the United States has high blood pressure.[1]

Over time, high blood pressure exerts a damaging effect on small arteries, known as arterioles. Arterioles become thicker and less elastic, resulting in arteriosclerosis. This condition, coupled with the effects from atherosclerosis, creates an explosive situation. When faced with the demands of heavy exertion (such as running or shoveling snow), arterioles, particularly in the brain, heart, or kidneys, can close off, rupture, or leak, causing a stroke, heart attack, or renal accident (in kidneys). About half of the people who have a first heart attack and two-thirds of people who have a first stroke have blood pressures greater than 160/95 mm Hg.[1]

The highest rates of high blood pressure occur among African American and Hispanic women; those who are older, overweight, or obese; and those who are poor or near poor.[1] The risk of high blood pressure increases with age. More than half of women older than age 55 have elevated or high blood pressure. With the rise in blood pressure comes a higher risk of heart disease and death. According to the American Heart Association, the estimated death rate associated with high blood pressure was 14.5 per 100,000 for white women and 40.8 per 100,000 among black women.[1]

Women who are obese tend to have higher levels of blood pressure than do women who are more slender. In many cases, high blood pressure can be brought under control by diet, weight loss, and weight control. In some women, especially African American women, salt sensitivity appears to be important in the development and control of high blood pressure. To counter this problem, women may have to reduce the amount of salt they consume. When necessary, medication can be used to lower elevated blood pressure. A woman with high blood pressure should be under the supervision of a health-care provider. Blood pressure should be checked periodically, especially as a woman ages.

High Blood Cholesterol

Cholesterol is a fatty substance found in all cells that is essential for the manufacture and maintenance of cells, sex hormones, and nerves throughout the body. In most individuals, the body manufactures an appropriate amount of cholesterol to serve its needs. In some individuals, however, blood cholesterol levels may be excessively high, due to obesity, poor diet, or genetic abnormalities. High blood levels of cholesterol (greater than 240 mg/dL) are associated with an increased risk of mortality and morbidity from CHD.

When an excessive amount of cholesterol is present, the body can become overwhelmed, and the unused cholesterol is deposited on the inner walls of the arteries. Over

Table 10.5	Classification of Blood Pressure for Adults		
BP Classification	**Systolic Blood Pressure (mm Hg)**	**Diastolic Blood Pressure (mm Hg)**
Normal	Less than 120	And less than 80
Prehypertension	120–139	Or 80–89
Stage 1 hypertension	140–159	Or 90–99
Stage 2 hypertension	Equal to or greater than 160	Or equal to or greater than 100

Source: U.S. Department of Health and Human Services, National Institutes of Health, National High Blood Pressure Education Program. (2003). *The Seventh Report of the Joint National Committee on Prevention, Detection, Evaluation, and Treatment of High Blood Pressure.*

time (usually decades), these deposits gradually accumulate, slowly narrowing the artery (**Figure 10.5**). The inner walls become clogged and brittle, and pieces of the artery tear, leaving jagged edges. These jagged edges stick up and catch material that flows by in the bloodstream, thereby adding more waste deposits to the wall. The artery is gradually closed off either by a fatty plaque or by a transient embolus, which may become lodged in the narrowed artery. Another type of smaller plaque, called an unstable plaque, also may cause blood to clot. If the plaque bursts within the artery wall, its contents are released into the bloodstream and can trigger a blockage. In any case, the blood does not reach a part of the body, and that part will die unless the artery is once again opened. If this blockage happens in a coronary artery, a heart attack occurs.

Cholesterol is made in the liver and small intestine, and it is transported throughout the body in a **lipoprotein**. Lipoproteins consist of fats and protein bound together in a chemical structure that enables them to be transported in the blood. They are made up of the following key elements: low-density lipoproteins (LDL), high-density lipoproteins (HDL), very-low-density lipoproteins (VLDL), and triglycerides. Everyone has each of these substances in varying amounts in each lipoprotein molecule.

- LDL cholesterol is often referred to as "bad" cholesterol because of its affinity for sticking to the wall of the artery and lodging there.

- HDL cholesterol is often referred to as "good" cholesterol because it functions somewhat like a trash collector, taking the LDL cholesterol out of the body.

- **VLDL** is associated with the transport of fats known as triglycerides.

- **Triglycerides** are a form of fat that comes from food and is also made in the body. High triglycerides are often a sign of high total cholesterol.

When speaking of cholesterol levels in the blood, healthcare professionals generally refer either to the total blood cholesterol level, or to the LDL cholesterol and HDL cholesterol levels. Cholesterol levels are measured from a small amount of blood (about one teaspoonful) drawn from a vein. To obtain a total blood cholesterol measurement, the person does not have to fast for 12 hours before the drawing. If the physician wishes to obtain an accurate measurement of the LDL cholesterol and the HDL cholesterol, however, the person must fast for 12 hours before the sample is drawn. The measurement is shown in milligrams per deciliter (mg/dL). As with blood pressure measurements, there is no one "normal" level for blood cholesterol. **Table 10.6** summarizes the cholesterol-related recommendations from the National Heart, Lung and Blood Institute's National Cholesterol Education Program.

A low level of HDL has been found to be a predictor of mortality from CHD in both young and older women, and is a stronger predictor in women than in men.[1] Women, particularly those who are fit and slender and who have not experienced menopause, tend to have slightly elevated HDL cholesterol levels compared with men or with postmenopausal women. Elevated HDL cholesterol levels are shown to be protective against heart disease. After menopause, a woman's hormone levels begin to drop and so do her HDL cholesterol levels—sometimes by as much as 10% to 20%. During this time, a woman's risk for heart

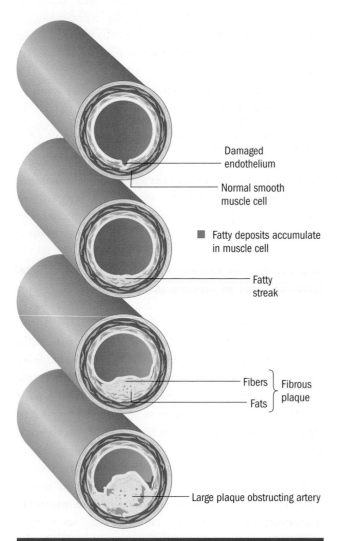

Damaged endothelium

Normal smooth muscle cell

■ Fatty deposits accumulate in muscle cell

Fatty streak

Fibers ⎫
Fats ⎬ Fibrous plaque

Large plaque obstructing artery

Figure 10.5

Narrowing arteries.

disease continues to rise.[19,20] Research has shown that elevated triglyceride levels sharply increase a person's risk of dying from a heart attack, even if a person's blood cholesterol is normal.[20,21]

As discussed in Chapter 9, cholesterol levels can often be controlled by diet. A diet low in cholesterol and saturated fat is crucial in maintaining a low overall total cholesterol level. Saturated fats eaten in food actually have a greater effect on blood cholesterol than cholesterol eaten in food. Eating saturated fats increases the total blood cholesterol, particularly the LDL cholesterol—the "bad" cholesterol. This means that a woman should watch the amount of cholesterol she consumes; she also should be careful to limit both the dietary cholesterol and the dietary saturated fat she eats. Daily consumption of essential nutrients remains crucial.

Despite cholesterol being a strong predictor of potential heart attack or stroke, almost half of people who have heart attacks have normal levels of cholesterol. Studies have shown that levels of **C-reactive protein** (CRP), a protein found in the blood when inflammation is present, may actually be a stronger predictor of potential cardiovascular disease than cholesterol levels. CRP levels can be measured by a simple blood test.[23] The American Heart Association and the Centers for Disease Control and Prevention issued guidelines for the use of such testing; the guidelines recommend that CRP screening should be reserved for people with moderate cardiovascular risk and that it should not replace assessment for major risk factors.[24] If CRP levels are high, treatment that is used to lower cholesterol—such as exercise, aspirin, and **statins**—can also be used to lower CRP. Although CRP can be useful as a predictor, high levels of this protein can indicate a number of other acute and chronic conditions, including arthritis, tuberculosis, cancer, pneumonia, or the common cold. Positive CRP also can occur during the last half of pregnancy or with the use of oral contraceptives.

Whether C-reactive protein should be used as a screening mechanism in women remains unclear. Even when controlling for other risk factors, C-reactive protein levels are generally higher in women of all racial and ethnic groups compared with men. More research is required.[25]

Another substance found in the blood is **homocysteine**, an essential amino acid. Increased levels harm the arterial lining and increase the risk for heart disease.[26,27] Folic acid and vitamins B_6 and B_{12} can lower homocysteine levels. Whether such efforts reduce the rates of heart disease is not yet clear. Until the studies are more clear, women at high risk for heart disease should make certain that their

Table 10.6 What Do Cholesterol Numbers Mean?

Level	Category
Total Cholesterol	
Less than 200 mg/dL	Desirable
200–239 mg/dL	Borderline high
240 mg/dL or greater	High
LDL Cholesterol	
Less than 100 mg/dL	Optimal
100–129 mg/dL	Near optimal/above optimal
130–159 mg/dL	Borderline high
160–189 mg/dL	High
190 mg/dL or greater	Very high
HDL Cholesterol	
Less than 40 mg/dL	Major risk factor
40–59 mg/dL	Borderline
60 mg/dL or greater	Protective factor
Triglyceride	
Less than 150 mg/dL	Desirable
150–199 mg/dL	Borderline high
200 mg/dL or greater	High

Note: Cholesterol levels are measured in milligrams (mg) of cholesterol per deciliter (dL) of blood.

Source: National Heart, Lung and Blood Institute, National Cholesterol Education Program. (2005). *High Blood Cholesterol: What You Need to Know.* NIH Publication No. 05-3290.

diet is rich in folic acid and vitamins B_6 and B_{12} (fruits and green leafy vegetables).

Lp(a), a lipoprotein, is one variation of LDL cholesterol. It is not yet clear whether this is a useful risk marker for CVD in women; however, a group of otherwise healthy women with very high levels of Lp(a) showed an increased risk of the disease. In addition, high levels of Lp(a) could also be modified by taking hormone replacement therapy. Yet the question remains as to whether measuring Lp(a) should be a routine clinical measure for health-care providers. More research is required.[28,29]

Diabetes

Diabetes is a disorder of the pancreas in which naturally occurring insulin (a hormone that is used to convert sugar, starches, and other types of food into energy, mainly glucose) is not properly manufactured or used. The most common form of diabetes is type 2 diabetes (see Chapter 11).

Diabetes causes many serious problems and can lead to life-threatening situations. Yet the number of women with diabetes is rising, most often in those who are overweight or obese. Women who develop diabetes during pregnancy (gestational diabetes) are at higher risk of developing the disease again later in life.[30]

The prevalence of diabetes among Hispanic, African American, American Indian, Alaskan Native, and Asian and Pacific Islander women is two to four times greater than among non-Hispanic white women. This translates into a substantially greater risk for heart disease and stroke. The reasons for this greater prevalence are not entirely clear, although higher rates of overweight and obesity certainly contribute to the risk. The role of genetic predisposition to the disease among certain racial and ethnic groups is being explored. The critical issue for anyone with diabetes is to understand the disease and its effects on their health and well-being, and to assure that they maintain proper nutrition, exercise habits, and medication.[1]

Overweight and Obesity

Overweight and obesity are major risk factors for a number of diseases, especially for heart disease. Overweight is defined as having a body mass index (BMI) of 25 or greater; obesity is defined as having a BMI of 30 or greater. More than 61% of U.S. women are considered overweight and 36% are considered obese.[1] The highest rates of both are among African American and Hispanic women. Perhaps one of the most troubling issues is the number of children who are overweight and obese: 16.3% of girls 6 to 19 years of age are overweight. This condition is considered a major risk factor for the development of CHD through the heightened risk of developing high blood pressure, high blood cholesterol, and diabetes. Overweight and obesity are also correlated with poor nutrition and sedentary lifestyle—other CHD risk factors. Eating a diet rich in saturated fats and cholesterol can lead to clogged arteries. This compromises blood flow, especially to the heart, and can lead to a heart attack or stroke.

The way that fat is distributed on a woman's body may also affect her risk for heart disease. Truncal distribution of fat (around the stomach and upper body), as opposed to

I am overweight and know that I need to lose weight, but how can I afford all those expensive weight-loss foods in the supermarket? My kids need the fat in their diet, and I can't afford to buy and fix two separate meals.

35-year-old mother

hip and thigh distribution, appears more risky. The truncal distribution pattern has been referred to as an "apple" shape, and the hip and thigh distribution a "pear" shape. More information on obesity can be found in Chapter 9.

Sedentary Lifestyle

Sedentary lifestyle is another important modifiable risk factor for cardiovascular disease. Sedentary lifestyle simply means that a woman is not getting enough regular aerobic exercise—any movement that raises the heart rate significantly for an extended period of time. More than 27% of women do not participate in the recommended amount of physical activity.[1] For all races, women are less physically active than men on average. Aerobic exercise is a critical factor in keeping the heart and other muscles strong and in good working condition. Regular exercise also aids in controlling weight, helping to raise HDL cholesterol levels, and both controlling and reducing the risk of developing diabetes. The Nurses' Health Study, a large ongoing study observing female nurses, showed similar protective effects against coronary heart disease for brisk walking and vigorous exercise.[31,32] See Chapter 9 for more information.

Other Factors Affecting CVD Risk

Menopause.   After menopause (the cessation of menses), the risk for heart disease and stroke increases significantly for women. Coronary heart disease rates in women after menopause are two to three times higher than those in women of the same age who have not yet reached menopause. One reason appears to be related to the loss of natural estrogen. Scientists believe that during and after menopause, women experience a decrease in HDL cholesterol and an increase in LDL cholesterol and triglycerides. Increased plaque is noted in the arteries, and heart attacks and strokes begin to occur. Research also has shown that the decrease in estrogen as a result of natural and surgical menopause is associated with these changes in serum lipid profiles (blood cholesterol levels).[33]

Estrogen loss during menopause and the use of hormone replacement therapy (HRT) have inspired tremendous debate in the last several years. Observational studies in both animals and humans, carried out largely in the 1970s and 1980s, showed that HRT could be beneficial in slowing the onset of heart disease. More recent clinical trials, carried out in the 1990s and early 2000s, however, showed that HRT had no effect or was even dangerous. Recent examination of some of those clinical trials has shown where some of the differences in findings may lie. The increased risk appears to be greatest for women who started HRT after they had been menopausal for several years or more, and those with established heart disease, especially for women on a particular regimen of HRT. Women who started HRT during or immediately after cessation of menstrual periods generally did not show an increased risk. (See Chapter 8 for more information.)[33,34] In addition, different types of medication, dosage, and routes of administration clearly affect how a woman responds.

Oral Contraceptives. Oral contraceptives (the "pill") were officially introduced in the 1960s.[35] With them came better birth control and some beneficial side effects: decreased risk of ovarian and endometrial cancers, pelvic inflammatory disease, and dysmenorrhea (painful periods). However, negative side effects also became evident: cardiovascular disease, especially in women who had risk factors for CVD, such as smoking and high blood pressure. Over time, scientists and drug manufacturers changed the formulation of oral contraceptives, significantly lowering dosages of estrogen and progestin, key hormonal agents. The question remained, however, as to whether the changed dosage would change the CVD risk. Recent studies examining the risks associated with oral contraceptives, especially the lower dosages, and CVD have shown that changing the dosage did reduce the risks for CVD, especially heart attack and stroke, but did not eliminate them. The risk of heart attack and stroke are uncommon in women of childbearing age. However, for women who are at risk for CVD, such as women who smoke and have high blood pressure, taking oral contraceptives can pose a risk.[36,37]

People who smoke may have an increase in blood pressure from oral contraceptives, especially women on higher dose pills. Older women and obese women have the highest risk of increased blood pressure from oral contraceptives.

Concerns also have been raised regarding thromboembolism, also known as deep-vein thrombosis (VTE), with oral contraceptive use. The estimated risk of VTE is low with all modern low-dose oral contraceptives.[28]

Several studies have found that oral contraceptive users with a history of migraine are two to four times more likely to have an ischemic stroke than women with a history of migraine who do not use this form of birth control. Studies suggest the risk is greater among women who have severe migraine headaches with "aura"—focal neurologic symptoms such as blurred vision, temporary loss of vision, seeing flashing lights or zigzag lines, or trouble speaking or moving. Experts now recommend that a woman who has migraine headaches with focal neurologic symptoms should not start combined oral contraceptives and a woman age 35 or older should choose another method if possible if she has migraine headaches even without focal neurologic symptoms. Mild or severe headaches that are not migrainous do not rule out use of birth control pills.[38,39]

Because the risk of cardiovascular disease increases in oral contraceptive users with other risk factors, women should have a complete medical checkup before choosing oral contraceptives as their method of birth control.

Alcohol and Illicit Drugs. Research has shown that consuming modest levels of wine or other alcohol has a beneficial effect on CVD risk—namely, a daily intake of no more than one drink per day can reduce the risk of coronary heart disease in women. Research is being conducted to find out whether these benefits are due to an increased intake of antioxidants, which can be found in red wine; the increase in HDL cholesterol that alcohol produces; or the prevention of platelets sticking together due to certain substances in alcoholic beverages. There is, however, an increase in risk of stroke and other causes of morbidity and mortality with moderate to heavy consumption of alcohol.[30] Therefore, nondrinkers should not take this as a recommendation to begin drinking, and those who are drinking more than the recommended amount should cut back. One "drink" equals

- 1 to ¹/₂ fluid ounce (fl oz) of 80–100 proof alcohol *or*
- 4 fl oz wine *or*
- 12 fl oz beer.

Illicit drugs, such as cocaine, LSD (acid), and heroin, may cause short-term cardiovascular effects as well as long-term cardiovascular complications. Cocaine and LSD both increase heart rate and blood pressure while constricting the blood vessels. Cocaine can lead to medical complications such as ventricular fibrillation (disturbances in heart rhythm) and heart attacks. Cocaine-related deaths are often a result of cardiac arrest.[40] Heroin slows down cardiac function during use. Its long-term effects include scarring and collapsing of the veins and bacterial infections of the blood vessels and heart valves, often leading to death. These drugs also are associated with many other short- and long-term negative effects. See Chapter 13 for more details.

Stress. Stress is a normal part of everyday life and, in fact, is essential to proper functioning of the body.

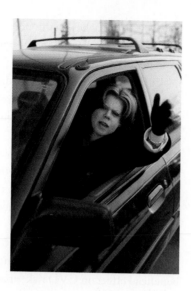

■ Continuous stress is associated with cardiovascular disease.

External stimulation can push a person to action—to study for a test, or to sprint the final lap in a race. A kiss from a loved one can also create stress, but most would not want to do without it. Distress can have negative side effects. The extent to which these negative side effects influence a person's sense of self and well-being differs greatly.[41] A number of studies have associated heart disease with job stress, defined as low job control and high job demands. Researchers are also investigating the link between anger in stressful conditions and increased risk of premature cardiovascular disease. Whether women manifest stress differently from men requires additional study.[42] What does seem clear is that women are affected by negative stress, which can make them more susceptible to heart disease and stroke.

Compounding Risk Factors

Cardiovascular risk factors play a crucial role in the development of CVD. The existence of multiple risk factors has a cumulative effect. For example, consumption of a diet high in cholesterol and saturated fats leads to high blood cholesterol and deposition of fatty plaques in the arteries. That same diet, which is often also high in calories, leads to overweight and obesity, which strain the heart and arteries and contribute to high blood pressure and diabetes. These factors place additional strain on arteries already carrying increasing amounts of plaques. The addition of cigarette smoking compounds the problem, making the arteries fragile and more constrictive. Arteries become clogged with waste, and the supreme pump—the heart—becomes sluggish and weak. In short, the combination of these risk factors produces a scenario for disaster: heart attack, stroke, CHF, and peripheral vascular disease.

Such disaster events are not always fatal. If a woman survives the heart attack or stroke, she may be severely limited by a damaged heart or the effects of the stroke, such as impaired vision, memory, speech, or movement. Thus, even though she may be alive, the quality of her life and that of her family may be seriously diminished. Although no one can predict what will happen, this scenario can usually be prevented or controlled by establishing and maintaining good health habits early in life.

Sex/Gender Differences in Cardiovascular Disease

Cardiovascular disease, particularly heart attack, is sometimes not considered a disease of women by women, their families, and even some health-care professionals. Part of the reason may be that women present with signs and symptoms of the disease some 10 to 15 years later than men. Between the ages of 20 and 39, CVD is more prevalent in men. By ages 40–59, however, the sexes are about equal. These differences in prevalence may in part stem from estrogen loss as women age. Estrogen has been shown to have a positive effect on the cardiovascular system. As women approach menopause, their rates of CVD begin to rise.[1,2]

Overall, more women than men die from CVD. In 2005, 329,250 women died of heart disease and 86,993 of stroke, whereas 322,841 men died of heart disease and 56,586 of stroke (see **Table 10.7**). Heart disease and stroke are the first and third leading causes of death for women, respectively; in contrast, heart disease is the leading cause for men, yet stroke is the fifth leading cause for men. That does not imply that men are in better cardiovascular health than women, it simply means that other diseases, conditions, and behaviors affect men and their health differently than they do women. For example, unintentional injuries (traffic and other accidents) rank higher in men, whereas Alzheimer's disease is higher in women.

The signs and symptoms of a myocardial infarction (heart attack) also underscore these differences. Both men and women may experience the following symptoms.

- Pain or discomfort in the chest region, *and/or*
- Pain or discomfort in the upper torso (trunk and arms)
- Shortness of breath, *and/or*
- Cold sweat, nausea, or dizziness.

However, women appear more prone to other symptoms, especially shortness of breath, nausea/vomiting, and back or jaw pain. Some women may not even be aware they are

Table 10.7 Leading Causes of Death by Gender

Cause of Death	Number of Females	Cause of Death	Number of Males
Diseases of the heart	329,250	Diseases of the heart	322,841
Malignant neoplasms (cancer)	268,890	Malignant neoplasms (cancer)	290,422
Cerebrovascular disease (stroke)	86,933	Unintentional injury	76,375
Chronic lower respiratory disease	68,498	Chronic lower respiratory disease	62,435
Alzheimer's disease	51,040	Cerebrovascular disease (stroke)	56,586
Unintentional injuries	41,434	Diabetes mellitus	36,538
Diabetes mellitus	38,581	Influenza and pneumonia	28,052
Influenza and pneumonia	34,949	Suicide	25,907
Nephritis, nephritic syndrome, nephrosis	22,633	Nephritis, nephritic syndrome, nephrosis	21,268
Septicemia	18,814	Alzheimer's disease	20,559

Source: National Center for Health Statistics. (2007). *Health United States*, Tables 36 and 37.

having a heart attack. These differences in symptoms present a challenge not only to the woman and her family/friends/co-workers, but also to health-care professionals. Rather than a heart attack, they may suspect gastrointestinal symptoms (gas, upset stomach) and thus not act quickly. Immediate action is essential at the first signs and symptoms of a heart attack. The sooner the person gets to treatment, preferably within the first three hours of symptom onset, the less heart damage may occur. Further complicating the issue is that women often experience a "silent" heart attack in which there are no signs or symptoms. This lack of symptoms puts them at great risk: Sixty-four percent of women who experienced sudden death from CHD had no symptoms. Within five years of a heart attack, 43% of women 40 or older will die; 6% will have a stroke. Rehabilitation, a key factor in post–heart attack recovery, was 55% less likely to be used by women compared to men.[1]

The reasons for these sex-related differences are not entirely clear. One key factor may be the age differential between women and men at the time of the event—women

are generally older and have more compromising risk factors. Scientists are exploring these differences, but such studies take time because it is important to follow groups of individuals over decades to determine what occurs and why. Such long-term studies, which have already provided important CVD data on women and men, include, but are not limited to, the Framingham Heart Study, the Nurses' Health Study, the Bogalusa Heart Study, the Rancho Bernardo Study, and many others.

Racial Differences in Cardiovascular Disease

The age-adjusted death rates for heart disease and stroke vary significantly among women in the five major U.S. designated racial and ethnic groups. Although the rates are highest among African American women, white and Hispanic women also have elevated rates. The lowest rates are among Asian American women.[1,2]

The reasons for these disparities are not fully understood. Examination of CVD risk factors demonstrates that Mexican American and African American women have the highest rates of obesity, high blood pressure, and diabetes. Note that comparable data are not available for all racial and ethnic groups.[1] These risk factors are interrelated. Obesity enhances high blood pressure and diabetes. Smoking increases blood pressure and enhances blood clotting.

- Among Mexican American women,
  - 73% are overweight or obese and 39.4% are obese
  - 22.6% are pre-diabetic

I started having chest pains, but I thought they were just due to stress. I didn't want to make a big deal of it. My doctor didn't suspect anything either—I guess I look pretty healthy. But when they did the tests, they found that I had had a "silent heart attack." I wish I had paid closer attention to the pain, and I wish that my doctor had been more sensitive about the possibility of my having a heart attack.

60-year-old woman

- 31.4% have high blood pressure
- 50% have a total cholesterol greater than 200 mg/dL
- 19.2% smoke

- Among African American women,
  - 79.6% are overweight or obese
  - 22.6% are pre-diabetic and 13.2% have physician-diagnosed diabetes
  - 46.6% have high blood pressure
  - 42.1% have a total cholesterol greater than 200 mg/dL
  - 17.3% smoke

- Among white women,
  - 57.6% are overweight or obese and 30.7% are obese
  - 21.6% are pre-diabetic and 5.6% have physician-diagnosed diabetes
  - 31.9% have high blood pressure
  - 49.7% have a total cholesterol greater than 200 mg/dL
  - 20% smoke

Of particular concern is the number of children and youth who are also at elevated risk for CVD earlier in life because of these risk factors[1]:

- Overweight is increasing among girls ages 6–11 years: whites 15.6%, African Americans 24.8%, and Mexican Americans 16.6%. For adolescent females: whites 14.5%, African Americans 23.8%, and Mexican Americans 17.1%.

- Yet many did not meet the recommended levels of physical activity: whites 30.2%, African Americans 21.3%, and Mexican Americans 26.5%.

- Current cigarette smoking among female high school students in grades 9–12 is: whites 27%, African Americans 11.9%, and Mexican Americans 19.2%.

These elevated risk factors, together and over time, lead to disease, disability, and death. Yet, these negative behaviors persist. The question is why? Despite extensive research, no clear explanation has emerged. Critical factors such as perception, socioeconomic status, neighborhood environment (rural vs. urban), culture, immigrant status, and education all play an important role individually and in combination.

Diabetes rates are rising along with obesity and high blood pressure rates. From 1994 to 2002, the prevalence of diabetes among adults in the United States rose 54%. One of the greatest increases was observed among Native Americans/Alaskan Natives.[37] The 2003 death rates from diabetes were 47 per 100,000 for African American women and 20 per 100,000 for white women. The risk of CVD among diabetic women is double that among nondiabetic women.

The presence of two or more CVD risk factors compounds this risk. For example, women who are obese and smoke lose about seven years of life expectancy compared with non-obese nonsmokers.[44] African American and American Indian/Alaskan Native women had the highest rates of multiple risk factors for CVD.[45]

Other, less obvious factors play a role in the development of CVD in women. When examining women of comparable socioeconomic status, one study showed that African American and Mexican American women still have higher rates of risk factors for CVD.[44] Yet another study showed that at younger ages, women of lower socioeconomic status had higher rates of CVD. By 60 years of age, however, those differences had disappeared.[45] Other factors that have not been fully studied but that appear to have an important impact are culture and neighborhood environments. The force of a community or culture can have an important effect on how a woman sees herself—fat, thin, just right—what she eats, and how she maintains her health.

Cancer

Cancer is a disease characterized by uncontrolled cellular growth and reproduction. It is not new to science. The term **carcinoma**, meaning a cancerous growth, was coined by Hippocrates in the fourth century B.C. There are more than 100 different diseases categorized as "cancer." **Table 10.8** provides a summary of the major types of cancer. Many distinctions may be made among these types of cancer, although they all follow similar basic processes.[46]

A **tumor**, also referred to as a neoplasm or "new growth," is any abnormal growth of cells. Some tumors are solid, whereas others known as cysts consist of a thin-walled sac filled with fluid. A **benign tumor** is one that remains localized and confined in its original growth site; that is, it does not invade the surrounding tissue or spread to distant body sites. Examples of benign tumors include skin warts or cysts. Because benign tumors are confined and localized, they often are left alone, drained, or surgically removed. Usually benign tumors are not life threatening unless they are located in a surgically inaccessible location.

In contrast to benign tumors, **malignant tumors**, also called malignant neoplasms, are capable of spreading to other tissues and organs and invading adjacent tissue, the definition of a cancerous growth. The process of cancer cell

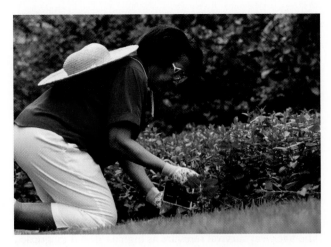

■ African American women bear a disproportionate burden of stroke disability and death.

invasion and spreading is known as **metastasis**. Cancer cells circulate through the blood or lymphatic system and can invade healthy cells in other parts of the body. These circulating cells often become trapped in the first network of capillaries that they encounter, usually the lungs. Blood leaving every organ other than the intestines travels to the lungs to get oxygenated, so the lungs are the most common site for metastasis. Blood leaving the intestines goes to the liver, the second most common site of metastasis. Some

Table 10.8 Types of Cancer

Main Groups of Cancer

Carcinoma: the most common of all tumors—accounting for approximately 90% of all cancers; affects cells that cover the body, line the organs, and form glands.

- Adenocarcinoma—cancer that originates in an organ or gland
- Squamous cell carcinoma—cancer that originates in the skin

Sarcoma: rare type of cancer that originates in the connective tissue, such as muscle and bone.

Leukemia: cancer that originates within the blood and blood-producing organs.

Lymphoma: cancer that originates from lymph tissue, which is part of the body's immune system.

Other Types of Cancer

Hepatoma: a cancer that originates from liver cells.

Melanoma: a cancer that originates within the melanocytes (skin cells that produce the pigment melanin).

Neuroblastoma: a cancer that originates from cells in the nervous system.

cancer cells have an affinity for other receptors and, therefore, may metastasize to certain types of tissues. Once metastasis has occurred, localized surgical treatment is usually impossible.

Two kinds of **carcinogens** (cancer-causing substances) appear to lead to cancer: carcinogens that damage genes that control cell reproduction and migration and carcinogens that enhance the growth of tumor cells. Many agents, including chemical substances, viral or bacterial carcinogens, physical agents, and natural substances in the blood can cause **carcinogenesis**. Smoking is one of the major causes of carcinogenesis. Smoking cigarettes is associated with increased risk for cancers of the lung, mouth, nasal cavities, pharynx, larynx, esophagus, stomach, pancreas, liver, cervix, kidney, and bladder. The frequency of smoking, tar content, and duration of the habit all play important roles in the initiation and promotion of cancer-cell growth.

Factors in the diet also affect the development of cancer. What a woman consumes as part of her diet is just as important as what she avoids. Saturated fat; non-nutrient food additives such as salt, nitrates, and nitrites; and alcohol all have been associated with increased risk of cancer. In contrast, vegetables and fruits containing phytochemicals (see Chapter 9) may act as protective factors against cancer.

Radiation, occupational carcinogens such as asbestos, and even certain drugs or medications can cause cancer. Viral carcinogens also have been recognized as contributors to cancer. For example, the human papillomavirus (HPV) and hepatitis B virus are responsible for a majority of cancers in the anal–genital region and the liver, respectively. Scientific evidence suggests that approximately one-third of the 565,650 cancer deaths in 2008 were related to nutrition, physical inactivity, obesity, and other lifestyle factors and could be prevented.[47]

Perspectives on Cancer
Epidemiological Overview

Cancer is the second leading cause of death for women in the United States, with an estimated 271,530 women dying from this disease in 2008.[48] When examined by racial and ethnic group, cancer is the second leading cause of death for black, white, Hispanic, and American Indian/Alaskan Native women. For Asian women, however, it is the leading cause.[2] Although anyone can develop cancer, most cases affect adults beginning in middle age. More than 77% of cancers are diagnosed in people age 55 or older.[48]

Although lung cancer is the leading cause of cancer deaths in women, breast cancer has the highest prevalence among new cancer cases among women in the United States (**Figure 10.6**). Breast cancer is estimated to have caused more than 40,000 deaths among women in 2008. The vast majority of new cases and deaths are in women age 40 or older. Death rates, however, appear to be declining since 1990 at about 3.3% per year, with the greatest decline among women younger than 50 years of age.[48] White and black women have higher rates of new cases and deaths than all other racial and ethnic groups.[44]

Cancer of the lung is the second most commonly diagnosed cancer among both men and women. Breast cancer is the most common cancer among women, but lung cancer is the most deadly. Less than one out of every five women who develop breast cancer will die from it, but lung cancer kills most of the women who have it (**Figure 10.6**). Until recently, women's death rates from lung cancer were steadily increasing. That trend appears to be leveling off, reflecting a decline in smoking rates. Nevertheless, women still lag behind men in smoking cessation. The reasons for these differences are not entirely clear, but one important contributor is that women's smoking rates were highest about 20 years later than they were in men. Regional variation is also interesting. For example, new cases of lung

cancer in women ranged from 20.9 cases per 100,000 population in Utah to 74.9 per 100,000 in Kentucky.[47] The five-year survival rate for lung cancer is low (15%), and early detection of the disease is difficult because symptoms often do not appear until the disease has reached an advanced stage.[48]

Colorectal cancer is the third leading cancer diagnosed in women, although the number of cases declined sharply in the 1990s. Nevertheless, an estimated 25,700 women died from colorectal cancer in 2008. The death rate also has declined over the past 20 years. When diagnosed at an early stage, the death rates from this type of cancer are low. The five-year survival rates are as high as 90% if diagnosed at a localized stage and as low as 9% if diagnosed at a distant stage.[49]

Endometrial cancer, or cancer of the uterine lining, is the fourth most common cancer in women. Cases of endometrial cancer for 2008 totaled more than 40,100 in the United States, with 7,470 deaths.[50] Ovarian cancer causes more deaths than any other cancer affecting the female reproductive system. Although there are fewer cases of ovarian cancer, more than twice as many deaths are attributable to this cause than to endometrial cancer. If diagnosed and treated early, there is a 95% survival rate for endometrial cancer. Only 19% of cases are diagnosed at an early stage,

Figure 10.6

Estimated cancer cases and deaths in women, 2005.

Source: *Surveillance Epidemiology and End Results 2006*, National Cancer Institute, U.S. National Institutes of Health.

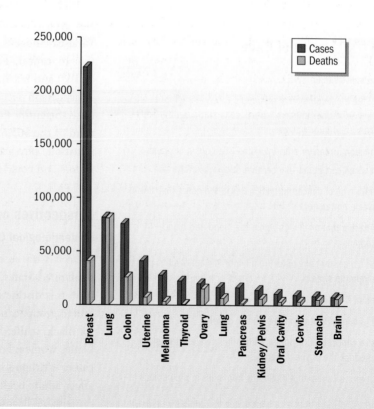

however.[51] Approximately 11,070 cases of cervical cancer were expected to be diagnosed in 2008, despite the fact that cervical cancer is nearly 100% preventable. The significant decline in the death rate from cervical cancer over the past 40 years is largely attributed to widespread cervical cancer screening programs using the Papanicolaou (Pap) test, but other techniques and prevention methods may reduce this number even further (see Chapter 7).[52]

Skin cancer is one of the 10 most common cancers in women. Approximately 1 million cases of basal cell and squamous cell carcinomas were expected to be diagnosed in 2008, along with 27,530 cases of melanoma in women. Since 1974, the rate of skin cancer has been increasing about 6% per year; however, the rate of increase has recently slowed to a little less than 3% per year. If detected at a localized stage, the five-year survival rate for skin cancer is 98%. Some 6,800 deaths in women from skin cancer occurred in 2008.[53]

Racial/Ethnic and Socioeconomic Dimensions

The morbidity and mortality of cancer and chronic diseases are not evenly distributed across women in the United States. The extent to which African American women experience higher cancer mortality than white women is striking. Although overall death rates from cancer have dropped for both white and African American women since 1973, African American women continue to experience greater overall cancer incidence rates, breast cancer death rates, colorectal and lung cancer incidence rates, and colorectal cancer death rates compared with women of any other racial and ethnic group (see **Table 10.9**). Although white women have higher rates of breast cancer, African American women have the highest mortality rate from breast cancer. These racial differences in breast cancer mortality rates may be due to a combination of factors, including the lower likelihood of African American women with breast cancer being diagnosed in the early disease stages and a lower survival rate in women whose disease has advanced.

Although incidence and mortality rates for cervical cancer have declined markedly during the last several decades, the numbers still remain too high. African American women have the highest mortality rates from cervical cancer, while Hispanic women have the highest incidence rates. The racial disparity is even more pronounced in the incidence and mortality rates among older (age 65-plus) women of color as compared to older white women.[54]

Because cancer risk is strongly associated with lifestyle and behavior, differences in ethnic and cultural groups—

| **Table 10.9** | Cancer Death Rates in Women by Educational Attainment and Race, 2001 |

Cancer	African American	Non-Hispanic White
All-sites		
≤ 12 yrs education	148.1	128.79
> 12 yrs education	103.3	73.02
Lung		
≤ 12 yrs education	30.8	37.0
> 12 yrs education	17.9	114.2
Colorectal		
≤ 12 yrs education	14.1	9.36
> 12 yrs education	10.8	5.44
Breast		
≤ 12 yrs education	36.0	25.2
> 12 yrs education	31.1	18.5

Rates are for individuals 25–64 years of age at death, per 100,000, and age adjusted to the 2000 U.S. population.

Source: Adapted from Albano, J. D., Ward, E., & Jemal, A. (2007). Cancer mortality in the United States by education level and race. *Journal of the National Cancer Institute* 99: 1384-1394.

such as dietary patterns, alcohol and tobacco use, and sexual and reproductive behaviors—can provide clues to factors involved in development of the disease. Cultural values and belief systems can also affect attitudes about seeking medical care or following screening guidelines. Screening programs are particularly important for early detection of cancer. Socioeconomic factors, such as lack of health insurance, transportation, or child care, can impede women's access to care and lead to late diagnosis and poor survival. Lack of participation in and reduced access to screening have been hypothesized as possible contributors to the disproportionate cancer burden in minority women. For example, mammography use has been found to be higher among nonminority women with a higher income and more education. To be effective, screening programs must be culturally sensitive and readily available. Language barriers, lack of health insurance, lack of availability and access to health care, and mistrust of the medical profession all have been identified as significant barriers to effective prevention programs in minority populations.

Economic Dimensions

The National Institutes of Health (NIH) estimated overall costs for cancer in 2007 at $219 billion, with $89 billion for direct medical costs and over $112 billion in lost productivity.[60] There is also a great economic burden placed on the individual cancer patient and family in terms of time, reduced employment opportunities, and payments for cancer treatments not covered by insurance. The emotional costs to the patients and their friends and families are incalculable.

Global Perspective

Cancer knows no boundaries. Women across the world are affected, but better prevention, early detection, and improved treatment have helped many nations lower cancer incidence and mortality rates. Yet, in many developing countries, cancer rates continue to rise, especially in those where Western lifestyles—cigarette smoking, high-fat diets, and less physical activity—have been adopted. Eastern Europe has some of the highest rates of cancer worldwide. Among women, North America has the highest cancer incidence rates, while Northern Europe has the highest cancer mortality rates. The highest rates for lung cancer incidence and mortality are among North American women, followed by Northern European and Chinese women. Breast cancer incidence is highest in North America, Western Europe, and Australia/New Zealand, with the lowest rates being found in Africa and China. Breast cancer mortality rates are highest in the United States, Canada, Europe, Argentina, and Brazil. The highest incidence and mortality rates for cervical cancer are among East African and Western South American women, and the lowest among Middle Eastern and Western Asian women.[55]

Breast Conditions

More than half of all women who menstruate regularly go through the frightening experience of finding a lump in a breast. In more than 90% of these cases, the lump is benign and needs no treatment. Being able to understand the issues and concerns about breast conditions is an important dimension of women's health.

Benign Breast Diseases

Most breast lumps are not cancer. **Fibrocystic breast disease**, also called **cystic mastitis**, is the most common breast disorder and the most frequent cause of a breast lump in women younger than age 25. This disease is most prevalent in women between the ages of 30 and 50. Typical symptoms of this condition include lumpy, tender breasts, particularly during the week before menses. Fibrocystic changes also may cause pain and swelling. Several modalities have been used to treat fibrocystic breast disease, including hormonal therapy and vitamin E, but none

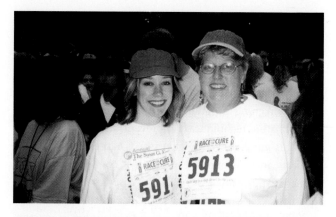

■ Breast cancer survivors and advocates have raised awareness and billions of dollars for research.

has emerged as the definitive treatment. Restricting dietary fat and eliminating caffeine intake can decrease symptoms. Although fibrocystic breast changes are not a medical problem, affected women may find it more difficult to detect lumps during breast self-exams. Only a small subgroup of women with fibrocystic breast disease is at increased risk for breast cancer. These women have an atypical cell condition known as **hyperplasia**, which can be diagnosed by a breast **biopsy**, a procedure in which a small sample of breast tissue is removed and examined under a microscope.

Another nonmalignant form of breast tumor is **fibroadenoma**, which is common in women in their twenties and thirties. This type of tumor produces a firm, movable, nontender lump. Fibroadenomas are usually removed both to confirm the diagnosis and to prevent further damage to breast tissue from continued localized tumor growth.

Breast Cancer

Breast cancer is a frightening condition for women. Before 1974, when U.S. First Lady Betty Ford underwent a mastectomy, breast cancer was not considered to be a public news item. Since then, news reports about breast cancer victims and breast cancer research have become more common. Women, however, still feel that information can be frightening, conflicting, and sometimes misleading. An understanding of breast cancer is important for all women, because this disease is one of the most treatable cancers if it is detected early.

The classification system for breast cancer consists of five levels:

■ In situ stage breast cancer can be diagnosed by mammogram, but the tumors are usually too small to be felt. The five-year survival rate for in situ tumors is nearly 100%.

- Stage I breast cancer remains localized to the breast, generally is smaller than 2 cm in size, and has not spread to the lymph nodes.

- Stage II breast cancer tumors generally are larger—2 to 5 cm in size—and have not spread to the lymph nodes. Stage II tumors also may be smaller than 2 to 5 cm but have spread to nearby lymph nodes.

- Stage III tumors are growths that are larger than 5 cm in size or that have grown into the chest wall, skin, or distant lymph nodes.

- Stage IV tumors are classified as growths that have spread to other parts of the body.

Five-year breast cancer survival rates decline with increasing size and invasiveness of the tumor.

Risk Factors

Genetics also plays a role in breast cancer risk. Women with mothers or sisters (first-degree relatives) who have had breast cancer are generally at double the risk of developing the disease. Approximately 5–10% of breast cancer cases are believed to be inherited. Most of the hereditary cases result from mutations in two breast cancer genes: BRCA1 and BRCA2. These genes reduce the risk for breast cancer by manufacturing a protein that prevents abnormal cell growth. However, if the gene is mutated, it increases a woman's risk for breast cancer and ovarian cancer. Mutated BRCA1 or BRCA2 account for up to 10% of all breast cancer cases. Although BRCA1 and BRCA2 are generally the most common gene defects leading to breast cancer in women, other mutations such as ATM, CHEK2, P53, and PTEN also exist.[56] Although any woman can have such mutated genes, they are most common in Ashkenazi Jewish women (generally of Eastern European origin). In fact, white women are more likely to develop breast cancer, but African American women are more likely to die of it. Two possible reasons for this are that African American women may have more aggressive tumors and many may not have the cancer identified or obtain treatment in the early stages of the disease.

Exposure to two hormones, estrogen and progesterone, plays an important role in a woman's development and her ability to become pregnant and bear children.[57] These hormones can also create some increased risk depending on a woman's lifetime exposure, the type of medication used, and how it is administered. Some examples follow:

- Women who have early onset of menstruation (less than 12 years of age) or later menopause (after 50 years of age) have a somewhat great risk. Part of the reason may be the longer exposure to the naturally occurring hormones estrogen and progesterone.

- Never having had a child or having a child later in life (after age 30) may present an increased risk. These hormones play a crucial role in pregnancy.

- Overweight and obesity: Estrogen is made largely in the ovaries; however, it is also manufactured in fat cells. After menopause, the estrogen in a woman's body comes largely from fat cells. The heavier the woman, the greater the exposure.

- Hormone replacement therapy: The use of estrogen alone or estrogen and progesterone in combination for menopausal women has been strongly debated for a number of years. Recent studies, however, now suggest that women who begin HRT immediately after the onset of menopause do not have a substantially great risk of developing breast cancer.[58]

- Oral contraceptives: Since the first release of oral contraceptives four decades ago, the hormonal type, dosage, and delivery (how and when they are taken) have been changed to enhance the positive effects and lower the negative effects. Recent analyses of scientific studies suggest that with the changes in oral contraceptives the risk of breast cancer is small for most women. However, some women are at greater risk and should not take oral contraceptives. They include women over 35 who smoke and/or have high blood pressure, women who have had or are at risk for heart disease or stroke, women who have migraines, women who have breast or estrogen-dependent cancers, and women who have liver disease.[59]

- Diethylstilbestrol (DES) exposure: Women who took this medication 40–60 years ago to prevent miscarriage have a slightly increased risk of developing breast cancer. Some evidence suggests that their daughters may also have an increased risk.

- Alcohol use: Women who drink more than two drinks of alcohol a day are at about $1\frac{1}{2}$ times the risk of women who do not drink alcohol.

- Exposure to chest radiation for other types of cancer puts some women at higher risk.

There is a family history of breast cancer. I am learning everything I can. I do monthly BSE, and I have regular clinical exams and mammograms. There is so much research going on today. I am trying to stay informed because I know that I need to know.

32-year-old woman

Screening and Diagnosis

Many of the identified risk factors for breast cancer cannot be modified by lifestyle behaviors. Early detection of breast cancer, however, can be lifesaving. Indeed, the prognosis for breast cancer strongly depends on the stage at which it is detected (**Table 10.10**). There are three basic methods for early detection of breast cancer, all of which are important prevention behaviors for women to reduce their risk of breast cancer:

■ **Breast self-examination** (BSE) consists of the systematic palpation of the breast tissue of each breast while lying on one's back. The most common sign of breast cancer is a new lump or mass in the breast, although other signs, such as swelling of the breast, skin dimpling, or nipple changes, may be present as well. The American Cancer Society recommends that women over the age of 20 years examine their breasts monthly after menses and at the same time each month. For women who have reached menopause, regular BSE should be done on a scheduled monthly basis. In addition to examining for lumps, women should check for breast discharge. **Figure 10.7** provides detailed guidance on the BSE procedure.

■ Clinical breast examinations (CBE) are conducted by a woman's health-care provider and should be performed every three years for women ages 20–39 and every year for women age 40 or older. The exam consists of observing the breasts for signs such as dimpling, feeling the breast and underarm for abnormal areas or swollen lymph nodes, and squeezing the nipples to check for discharge.

■ **Mammography**, a low-dose radiograph of the breast tissue, can detect smaller breast lesions that cannot be felt through BSE or CBE. This technology has the potential to detect breast cancer at its earliest stages of development. Mammography involves compressing the breast between two flat disks. Two radiographs are taken of each breast, and one is taken from above the breast. Although mammograms can detect some breast cancers before they can be felt, other tumors may be felt through BSE or CBE that could not be detected by a mammogram. For this reason, it is extremely important to perform regular BSEs and have regular CBEs. The use of mammography is recommended by several major medical and health organizations as part of an early detection program for breast cancer, in conjunction with regular physical examinations. The National Cancer Institute and the American Cancer Society recommend screening mammograms for women age 40 years or older every one to two years. Women with a family history of breast cancer should discuss when to begin mammograms with their health-care provider.

Although a breast tumor may be suspected with an examination or mammography, the ultimate diagnosis is made by biopsy. The biopsy removes a sample of tissue, which is then examined for abnormal cell growth.

Table 10.10   Breast Cancer Survival Rates

Stage*	Tumor Size	Five-Year Survival Rates
I	Less than 2 cm or about 1 inch—no metastasis	98%
IIA IIB	2–5 cm with no or lymph node involvement in the same side of the breast—no metastasis	81–92%
IIIA IIIB	More than 5 cm with lymph node involvement on same side of breast—no metastasis	54–67%
IV	Not applicable because of metastasis	20%

*The stages are expressed in Roman numerals: I = 1, II = 2, III = 3, and IV = 4.

Source: The 2002 American Joint Committee on Cancer TNM System. Revised 9/2/2005. http://www.cancer.org.

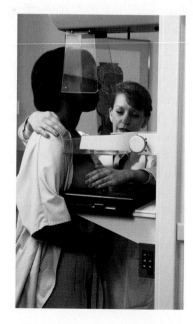

■ Mammography is an important screening method currently available for detecting nonpalpable tumors in the breast.

Breast Self-Examination

Breast self-examination should be done once a month so you become familiar with the usual appearance and feel of your breasts. Familiarity makes it easier to notice any changes in the breast from month to month. Early discovery of a change from what is "normal" is the main idea behind BSE. The outlook is much better if you detect cancer in an early stage.

If you menstruate, the best time to do BSE is 2 or 3 days after your period ends, when your breasts are least likely to be tender or swollen. If you no longer menstruate, pick a day such as the first day of the month, to remind yourself it is time to do BSE.

Here is one way to do BSE:

1. Stand before a mirror. Inspect both breasts for anything unusual, such as any discharge from the nipples or puckering, dimpling, or scaling of the skin.

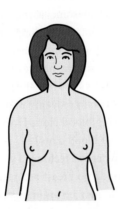

The next two steps are designed to emphasize any change in the shape or contour of your breasts. As you do them, you should be able to feel your chest muscles tighten.

2. Watching closely in the mirror, clasp your hands behind your head and press your hands forward.

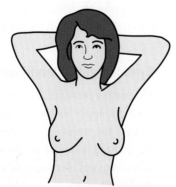

3. Next, press your hands firmly on your hips and bow slightly toward your mirror as you pull your shoulders and elbows forward.

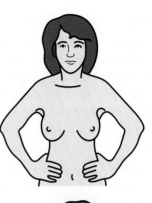

Some women do the next part of the exam in the shower because fingers glide over soapy skin, making it easy to concentrate on the texture underneath.

4. Raise your left arm. Use three or four fingers of your right hand to explore your left breast firmly, carefully, and thoroughly. Beginning at the outer edge, press the flat part of your fingers in small circles, moving the circles slowly around the breast. Gradually work toward the nipple. Be sure to cover the entire breast. Pay special attention to the area between the breast and the underarm, including the underarm itself. Feel for any unusual lump or mass under the skin.

5. Gently squeeze the nipple and look for discharge. (If you have any discharge during the month– whether or not it is during BSE–see your doctor.) Repeat steps 4 and 5 on your right breast.

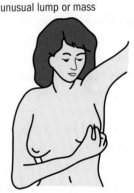

6. Steps 4 and 5 should be repeated lying down. Lie flat on your back with your left arm over your head and a pillow or folded towel under your left shoulder. This position flattens the breast and makes it easier to examine. Use the same circular motion described earlier. Repeat the exam on your right breast.

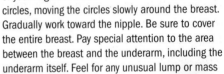

Figure 10.7

Breast self-exam.

Magnetic resonance imaging (MRI) is a procedure that has been in use for years, but until recently has not been used for breast cancer screening. The scans appear to be especially usefully in pre- and perimenopausal women, especially those who have dense breast tissue. For women who are at increased risk for breast cancer, MRI scans appear to be better at detecting tumors at an earlier stage. However, sometimes the test can show abnormalities when none exist. Therefore, this screening test is still being studied in a series of clinical trials.[62]

Treatment and Reconstruction

Surgery is the primary treatment for breast cancer, although it may be combined with radiation therapy or hormone therapy. Breast cancer surgery may be performed immediately following a positive biopsy, thereby avoiding the need for a second round of anesthesia and procedure. Most women, however, prefer a two-step procedure in which the biopsy and the necessary surgery are separate events. The two-step process enables the woman to review her options better and make her decision carefully.

Different types of breast removal surgical procedures are used to treat breast cancer.[63]

- A **lumpectomy** is often used for early-stage localized tumors when it is possible to remove only the tumor and some surrounding tissue. A separate incision may be made to remove the axillary lymph nodes (lymph nodes in the armpit area). In women with early cancer, a lumpectomy with subsequent radiation therapy has become the primary alternative to modified radical mastectomy. Lumpectomies are usually limited to those breast tumors that are well defined and less than one to two inches in total diameter.

- A **partial** or **segmental mastectomy** involves the removal of some breast tissue and some of the lymph nodes.

- A **simple mastectomy** involves the complete removal of the breast but not the lymph nodes under the arm or the chest wall muscles.

- A **radical mastectomy** is the removal of the entire affected breast, the underlying chest muscles, and the lymph nodes under the arm. Although once a very common surgery, this procedure is used less often today because of the disfigurement and the side effects it causes.

- A **modified radical mastectomy** has become the standard surgical procedure for most breast cancers that require removal of the entire breast. It involves removing

the breast, some of the lymph nodes, and the lining over the chest muscles. This procedure has survival rates comparable to those with the radical mastectomy, but it is more conducive to breast reconstruction and results in greater mobility and reduced swelling.

Adjuvant therapies—treatments that enhance surgical effectiveness—include **chemotherapy**, hormone therapy, and **radiation therapy**. Chemotherapy and hormone therapy may be used in the treatment of localized tumors, as well as for the control of metastatic conditions. Hormone therapy is used to block the effects of estrogen, which promotes the growth of some breast cancers. Tamoxifen is the most commonly used antiestrogen drug. It is also being studied as a chemopreventive agent to reduce the risk of breast cancer in high-risk women. Although studies from the Breast Cancer Prevention Trial have shown that tamoxifen is beneficial in reducing breast cancer incidence among high-risk women, serious side effects have been reported in some users, including endometrial cancer and blood clots in the lungs. Raloxifene, a drug used to reduce osteroporosis in women, has also been shown to be effective in treating breast cancer. Like tamoxifen, raloxifene reduced invasive breast cancer by about 50%, but it was more effective in reducing uterine cancer and had a lower risk of causing blood clots. However, both drugs still increase the risk of blood clots.[64]

After mastectomy, a woman faces the decision of whether to undergo breast reconstruction. Reconstruction of breast tissue may be an important part of breast cancer recovery for some women. The degree of difficulty associated with reconstruction varies with the extent of surgery.

In addition, emotional support and social support are important components of recovery. Local support groups may provide valuable information and assistance with physical and psychological breast cancer recovery issues.

Gynecological Conditions

The term *gynecological conditions* refers to any disease in a woman's upper or lower reproductive tract. This section reviews the major gynecological conditions of the cervix, uterus, and ovaries; it also discusses the risk factors, screening, and treatment of malignant and nonmalignant conditions.

Benign Cervical Changes

Polyps are small benign growths that develop in the endocervical canal, often after the onset of menstruation. Polyps usually produce mild symptoms such as abnormal vaginal bleeding or discharge. Although they are rarely cancerous, the growths should still be examined. Treatment of a cervical polyp consists of removing the polyp and examining the tissue to rule out malignancy.

Cervical dysplasia, which involves abnormal changes in the cells of the cervix, also is a benign condition. It is considered precancerous, however, because severe untreated **dysplasia** can result in invasive cervical cancer. Low-grade or mild dysplasia usually occurs in women from the ages of 25 to 35 years and usually can be detected with a Pap smear. High-grade or moderate to severe dysplasia refers to the presence of a large number of precancerous cells covering the surface of the cervix. Also referred to as **carcinoma-in-situ**, severe dysplasia is more likely to become cancerous but can be successfully cured if detected and treated rapidly. Treatment varies depending on the severity of the dysplasia.

Cervical Cancer*

Cervical cancer is a type of uterine cancer affecting the lower part of the uterus, which is referred to as the cervical canal. Most cancers of the cervix originate on the cells lining the surface of the cervix. Cervical cancer is classified into five stages, 0 through IV[65]:

- In its localized first stage, or stage 0, cervical cancer involves only the outer layer of skin.
- Stage I cancer has spread throughout the cervix.
- Stage II cancer has spread beyond the uterus but not to the pelvic wall.
- Stage III cancer has spread to the pelvic wall and the vagina, and may affect the kidney.
- Stage IV cancer affects the regional nodes and has spread past the pelvic wall. It also may be found on the bladder or rectum.

As with other forms of cancer, survival rates decline as the condition becomes more invasive.

Risk Factors. Cervical cancer is primarily caused by persistent infection with certain high-risk strains of the human papillomavirus (HPV). These high-risk types of HPV that are associated with cervical cancer are not the same types that produce genital warts, however. HPV infection is a sexually transmitted disease that most sexually active women contract during their twenties. In fact, nearly 80% of women will have HPV at some point in their lives. Most women who become infected with HPV will clear the virus on their own, through their body's natural immune response. A few women will not clear the virus, however, and instead develop a long-term persistent infection. These women are at higher risk for developing cervical cancer. Factors that may contribute to whether a woman develops a long-term persistent infection with high-risk HPV may include having HIV/AIDS (lower immune system suppression), taking immunosuppressant drugs, having multiple sexual partners, having other sexually transmitted diseases, smoking cigarettes, having a mother who took the drug diethylstilbestrol (DES),* and having a family history of cervical cancer.[66,67] Women age 30 or older can now be tested for HPV when they get their Pap smear.

Invasive cervical cancer rarely occurs in women who have regular gynecological examinations. When it does, however, symptoms may include bleeding between menstrual periods, spotting after intercourse, and increased vaginal discharge. By the time symptoms of cervical cancer appear, a tumor is usually quite large and may have already invaded nearby tissue.

Screening and Diagnosis. Cervical cancer is preventable through regular screening; it is one of the few cancers with a truly effective screening modality. The **Pap smear**, also referred to as a Pap test, provides a method of screening for the cellular changes before cancer develops and to detect cancer at its earliest stages. The Pap test has played a significant role in reducing cervical cancer rates and deaths in the United States. This screening test is usually performed during a routine gynecological examination (see Chapter 7). A sample of cells is obtained from the cervix and then sent to a laboratory for microscopic analysis. A Pap smear can be done in one of two ways: The collected cells can be smeared on a slide or they can be put in a liquid solution.

A newer screening method, the HPV test, looks for the DNA of cancer-causing types of HPV. The HPV test was first approved in the United States by the FDA for follow-up evaluation in women whose Pap results are uncertain—typically referred to as ASC-US (atypical squamous cells

---

*AUTHOR'S NOTE. The cervix is technically part of the uterus, but because the characteristics and risk factors for uterine and cervical cancer are distinctive, they are discussed separately.

---

*Diethylstilbestrol (DES)** was prescribed from 1938 to 1971 to prevent miscarriages or premature deliveries in pregnant women. In 1971, the FDA advised physicians to stop prescribing DES because it was linked to a rare vaginal cancer.

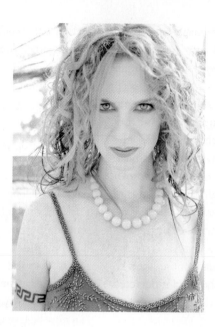
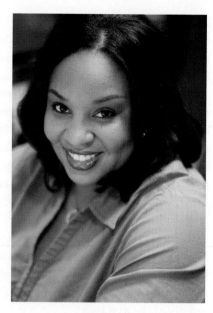

■ Cervical cancer survivors Christine Baze (*left*) and Tamika Felder (*right*) have created nonprofit organizations to educate women about HPV and cervical cancer. They spread the message that through screening with Pap tests and HPV tests, as well as immunizing with the new HPV vaccine, no woman should suffer or die from cervical cancer. Christine shares her message through her music via The Yellow Umbrella Tour (www.popsmear.org), while Tamika Felder conducts educational "House Parties" on HPV and cervical cancer (www.tamikaandfriends.org).

of undetermined significance). More recently, it has been approved for cervical cancer screening in women age 30 or older. The HPV test can be done at the same time as the Pap test using a similar method of collecting cervical cells. Once collected, the cell sample is sent to the laboratory for analysis and detection. Studies show that when used in conjunction with the Pap test, the HPV test's ability to identify a woman needing early intervention to stop the disease is nearly 100%.

The American College of Obstetricians and Gynecologists and the American Cancer Society have released new guidelines for cervical cancer screening.[52,53] Both guidelines recommend that women begin cervical cancer screening within three years of becoming sexually active or at age 21, whichever comes first. Women should be screened every year with a conventional Pap test and every two years with a liquid-based Pap test until age 30. Women age 30 or older can have a Pap test with an HPV test; if both are normal, she can safely wait to have a repeat test in three years. Having a positive HPV test does not mean that a woman will get cervical cancer; it just means that she should be followed more closely by her health-care provider. If a Pap smear is abnormal, regardless of the results of the HPV test, the clinician will want to perform a colposcopy and possibly a biopsy to view the cervical cells more closely. If Pap test results are inconclusive (also referred to as ASC-US), the HPV test can help the clinician clarify a woman's risk of cervical cancer. A negative HPV test means a woman is not at risk of developing cervical cancer in the next few years. Even when results are nega-

tive, all women should still continue to visit their health-care provider for an annual exam.

In 2006, a vaccine against select types of the HPV virus was approved by the Food and Drug Administration and recommended by the Centers for Disease Control and Prevention's Advisory Committee for Immunization Practices for use in females 11–12 and as a "catch-up" for females 13–26 who had not been previously vaccinated. The vaccine is effective against four types of HPV, types 16 and 18, and types 6 and 11, which cause genital warts. Although there have been suggestions that the vaccine be mandatory for young girls, such actions have not yet been put in place. However, the vaccine appears to be a powerful tool that could dramatically reduce—but not eliminate—cases of cervical cancer.[68,69] For more information on HPV, see Chapter 7.

Treatment. Treatment following an abnormal Pap smear depends on the results of the cervical biopsy. Inflammation of the cervix, known as **cervicitis**, may be associated with a vaginal infection or discharge that requires only local treatment with specific vaginal creams or suppositories. Treatment for dysplasia depends on its severity and usually consists of cryosurgery, cone biopsy, or laser cone biopsy.[70]

Cryosurgery is a procedure that destroys tissue by a freezing process. It is most often used to treat mild or moderate dysplasia. As a procedure, cryosurgery has the advantage of producing little or no discomfort. It also presents few risks for complications, such as bleeding, further infection, or infertility from scarring. A watery vaginal discharge is common for about two weeks after cryosurgery. It is generally recommended that women avoid intercourse, douching, or tampons during this recovery time.

A cone biopsy (or **conization**) is considered to be both a diagnostic and a therapeutic procedure because it provides tissue for an accurate diagnosis while removing the abnormal tissue. Cone biopsy procedures are less common today than they were a few years ago because of the widespread use of **colposcopy**. Colposcopy is performed in the physician's office using a **colposcope**, a special microscope that permits close examination of the cervix and vagina as well as biopsy.

Treatment of cervical cancer depends on the tumor's stage when diagnosed. Carcinoma-in-situ may be treated with cone biopsy in a woman who wishes to have more children. Surgery to remove abnormal tissue in or near the cervix will remove the tumor but leave the uterus and the ovaries intact. Definitive treatment of carcinoma-in-situ, however, may require a hysterectomy, surgical removal of the uterus, to ensure complete removal of the cancerous cells. Lymph nodes, as well as the fallopian tubes and ovaries, may also need to be removed. Depending on the stage of the cancer, radiation therapy or chemotherapy may be used as adjuvant therapy. Even after hysterectomy, a small percentage of women experience a recurrence of cancer in the vagina, so lifelong gynecological follow-up is important.

Benign Uterine Conditions

Fibroids are benign tumors composed of muscular and fibrous tissue in the uterus (see **Figure 10.8**). They often begin developing in women between the ages of 25 and 35. Fibroids are the primary cause of an abnormally enlarged uterus and one of the most common reasons for hysterectomy. Although single fibroid tumors occur, multiple tumors are more common. Symptoms depend on the size and location of the tumors and may include the following:

- Irregular vaginal bleeding
- Vaginal discharge
- Pain in the lower back
- Pain during sexual intercourse
- Frequent urination

Fibroids may increase in size under the influence of estrogen produced during pregnancy, from oral contraceptives, or from HRT. They often shrink and disappear with menopause. These tumors are usually detected during routine pelvic examinations because they create an enlarged and irregular uterus.

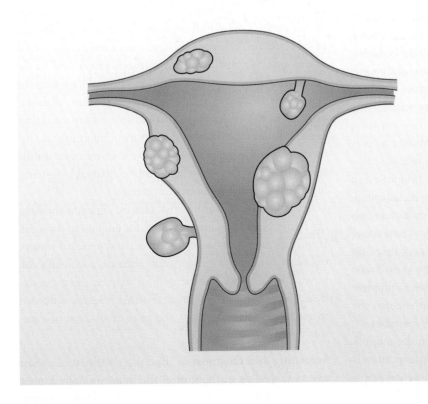

Figure 10.8

Uterine fibroids. Uterine fibroids are classified according to their location within the uterus. They may develop in the outer portion of the uterus, within the uterine wall, or under the lining of the uterine cavity; some fibroids grow on a stalk inside or outside of the uterus.

Hormone-based treatments are useful for temporarily reducing the size of the fibroid and relieving symptoms. A gonadotropin-releasing hormone (GnRH) agonist may be used to block the production of hormones, particularly estrogen, by the ovary. The most commonly used GnRH agonist in the United States is Lupron, which is given by an injection either once a month or every three months. Fibroids usually regrow, however, once treatment stops.

Surgery may be indicated for fibroids if they cause severe pain or bleeding. Surgery involves removing either the fibroid alone (**myomectomy**) or the entire uterus (hysterectomy). A hysteroscopic resection may be used for certain types of fibroids; in this procedure, a fiber-optic scope is inserted through the vagina while a dilation and curettage is used to remove the fibroid. Uterine artery embolization is a newer procedure in which small particles of plastic or gelatin sponge are injected through a catheter that is placed in the uterine artery. The particles block the blood supply to the fibroid, resulting in the death of the fibroid tissue. The fibroid shrinks and symptoms are usually relieved without the need for surgery.[71]

Endometriosis is another benign condition of the uterus. In this condition, tissue that looks and acts like endometrial tissue begins to grow outside the uterine lining. When it grows directly into the muscle wall of the uterus (**myometrium**), the condition is termed **adenomyosis**. This progressive condition is most common in women ages 30 to 40 years. Because endometrial tissue responds to hormonal influences during the menstrual cycle, women who have this disorder often feel pain just before or during menstruation. Endometriosis also may cause abdominal upset during menstruation and abnormal vaginal bleeding. Many women, however, have advanced lesions without any symptoms.

Treatment of endometriosis involves hormones to prevent ovulation. When hormonal drugs fail to relieve symptoms of pain or when the endometriosis has progressed to the point of forming large cysts, surgery may be indicated. Through operative **laparoscopy**, deposits of endometriosis as well as more extensive disease involving cysts and adhesions can be removed using either electrocautery (burning of tissue) or a laser. The most radical surgery as well as a more definitive cure for endometriosis involves a complete hysterectomy. If diseased tissue remains after surgery, the pain of endometriosis may continue to affect a woman.

Endometrial hyperplasia is an increase in the number of normal cells lining the uterus. Although the condition is not cancer, it may develop into cancer in some women if left untreated. Hyperplasia is caused by a constant production of estrogen and a lack of progesterone, which results in an abnormal thickening of the endometrium. Its most common symptoms are heavy menstrual periods and bleeding between periods. Treatment depends on the extent of the condition (mild, moderate, or severe) and on the age of the woman. Young women are usually treated with progesterone, and the endometrial tissue is checked often. Hyperplasia in women near or after menopause may be treated with hormones if the condition is not severe. Hysterectomy is the usual treatment for severe cases.

Malignant Uterine Tumors

Uterine cancer typically begins in the tissue lining of the uterus, the **endometrium**. Endometrial cancer is most common in women age 55 or older.

Carcinoma-in-situ is found only on the surface layer of the endometrium. As the cancer progresses to stage I, it spreads to the muscle wall of the uterus. Stage II cancer spreads to the cervix and, possibly, regional glands (tissue supporting the cervix). By stage III, cancer has spread to the vagina, pelvic lymph nodes, and other membranes or organs in the pelvic cavity. The final stage of cancer involves the bladder, rectum, and possibly the abdominal lymph nodes.[73]

Risk Factors.   Endometrial cancer accounts for most uterine cancers. The greatest risk factor for endometrial cancer is being older than 55 years of age. Risk factors of uterine cancer in general are believed to involve excess stimulation of endometrial cell proliferation by estrogen in the absence of progesterone. Obesity is believed to increase endometrial cancer risk, perhaps owing to estrogen production in fat cells. Other risk factors that may be a result of high levels of estrogen in the body include high blood pressure, diabetes, early menarche (before age 12), and late menopause (after age 55). Failure to ovulate and a history of infertility also increase risk and may be associated with an estrogen imbalance. Other risk factors include postmenopausal long-term, high-dose estrogen replacement therapy.

In addition to hormonal risk factors, cigarette smoking has been linked to an increased risk for endometrial cancer. Family history of endometrial cancer and personal history of breast, ovarian, or colon cancer increase a woman's risk as well. Finally, risk is increased for women using tamoxifen treatment for breast cancer. Further research is needed to ascertain the mechanisms and roles of all these risk factors for endometrial cancer.[73]

Screening and Diagnosis.   Because endometrial cancer affects the inside of the uterus, the tumor initially cannot be seen or felt during a pelvic examination. Unfortunately, a pelvic exam and Pap smear are only partially effective in the diagnosis of endometrial cancer and the disease is not usually detected until symptoms appear. The most common symptom of endometrial cancer after menopause is vaginal bleeding. Other symptoms may include pain in the pelvic area, difficult or painful urination, pain during intercourse, and change in bowel patterns.

The American Cancer Society recommends that women at increased risk for endometrial cancer (i.e., those with a history of infertility or obesity) have an endometrial biopsy at menopause. Women on unopposed estrogen replacement therapy should have such biopsies repeated on a regular basis. A **transvaginal ultrasound** also has proven useful as a screening tool for endometrial cancer.

Diagnosis of endometrial cancer is by biopsy, ultrasound, dilation and curettage (D&C), or **hysteroscopy**. These procedures permit the evaluation of the tissue and cells lining the uterine cavity.

Treatment.   Treatment of endometrial cancer depends on several factors, including the stage of the disease. Because uterine cancer may spread rapidly, treatment of early-stage disease involves removal of the uterus as well as the fallopian tubes and ovaries. A combination of surgery and radiotherapy is effective in the treatment of localized disease. Regional spread of the cancer outside of the uterus is treatable by radiation. Advanced, metastatic endometrial cancer is generally treated by the administration of progesterone, which results in prolonged survival but not cure. Treatment for later-stage disease includes removal of not only the uterus, fallopian tubes, and ovaries, but also the cervix, part of the vagina, and lymph nodes.

Benign Ovarian Growths

Cysts are fluid-filled growths that are extremely common. Ovarian cysts are usually benign and rarely cause discomfort or pain. If symptoms do occur, they often include pain or pressure in the pelvic cavity, irregular periods, and pain during intercourse.

A number of different types of cysts exist, which are differentiated by the tissue that makes up the cyst. The most common type results from the follicle that surrounds a mature egg. If the follicle does not rupture to release the egg during ovulation, it becomes a cyst. Many of these cysts go away without treatment within a few months. Other types of cysts include the following:

- Hemorrhagic cysts formed by blood
- Epithelial cysts formed by epithelial cells from the ovary
- Dermoid cysts formed from skin precursor cells

Epithelial cysts and dermoid cysts must be removed surgically to avoid continued growth. Birth control pills are often used as a form of treatment for women who have recurrent cysts.

Polycystic ovarian syndrome, a condition that affects women of reproductive age, causes the formation of numerous cysts in the ovaries. The disorder results from increased levels of hormones, including estrogen and testosterone. Women with polycystic ovarian syndrome are often obese (an effect of excess estrogen) and have excess body or facial hair (an effect of testosterone).

Ovarian Cancer

Ovarian cancer, the fourth most common cancer in women, causes more deaths than any other cancer of the female reproductive system. This cancer usually affects women around the time of menopause or later (ages 50 to 70). Stage I ovarian cancer is limited to the ovaries. Spreading to areas elsewhere in the pelvis is representative of stage II cancer. Stage III cancer spreads to the lymph nodes or other areas inside the abdominal cavity. Once the cancer has spread to distant sites, stage IV has been reached.

Risk Factors.   The risk factors for ovarian cancer are difficult to define; those that appear to be related do not necessarily mean that a woman will get the disease. However, several risk factors appear to be associated with the disease:

- A family or personal history of cancer, especially breast, uterine, colon, or rectal
- Older than 55
- Never been pregnant
- Use of fertility drugs for more than a year
- Possibly the use of hormone replacement therapy, especially estrogen
- Possibly obesity[74]

Screening and Diagnosis.   Ovarian cancer, often called the "silent cancer," usually remains asymptomatic until it is relatively advanced. It is not detected by Pap smears. Early detection is best accomplished through regular pelvic examinations, transvaginal ultrasound, and a laboratory test for an ovarian tumor marker in the blood, called CA-125. Elevated levels of CA-125 are associated with ovarian cancer, but also may indicate other conditions.

Early symptoms of ovarian cancer may include pelvic pressure, abdominal swelling, gas pains, indigestion, and vague abdominal discomfort. Rarely, however, are any of these symptoms attributed to ovarian cancer because they are all symptoms of other common benign conditions.

Diagnosis of ovarian cancer is confirmed through ultrasound or biopsy.

Treatment. Definitive treatment for ovarian cancer consists of surgery, radiation, and chemotherapy. Surgical treatment involves removal of the uterus, fallopian tubes, and ovaries. If a woman desires to have children and has a slow-growing tumor, her doctor may remove only the affected ovary. Chemotherapy and radiation therapies are used after surgery to kill remaining cancer cells and improve survival.

Other Cancers of Special Concern to Women

Women are susceptible to cancer anywhere in their bodies. Lung cancer, colorectal cancer, and skin cancer, however, all deserve special consideration. The following section discusses the risk factors, screening guidelines, and treatment for each of these cancers.

Lung Cancer

For the past 20 years, more women have died from lung cancer than from breast cancer. Lung cancer remains the leading cause of cancer deaths among women. Lung cancer is deadlier than breast cancer, which is almost twice as common in women (100,000 new cases of lung cancer compared to 180,000 new cases of breast cancer in 2008). About one in four (26%) of women with lung cancer die from the disease compared to 15% of women with breast cancer. Although overall death rates from lung cancer declined during the 1990s, they have only remained relatively stable for women after increasing for several decades. New lung cancer cases and deaths in women vary considerably by state. Some of the lowest rates of new cases in women are in the West while some of the highest are in the Northeast and Midwest. Death rates also vary, with the highest female death rates in Kentucky, West Virginia, and Nevada.[76]

Most cases of lung cancer start in the lining of the bronchi, but the disease can originate anywhere. Lung cancer is believed to develop over many years, and it often spreads before it can be detected radiographically. Causes of lung cancer vary, but most cases share a common factor—a persistent exposure to lung irritants, particularly those that are inhaled such as cigarette smoke.

Risk Factors. Although exposure to radon, asbestos, radioactive materials, and some industrial compounds has been associated with lung cancer, cigarette smoking is clearly the most significant risk factor. This risk factor is responsible for more than 80% of lung cancer cases and al-

My mom died of lung cancer at the age of 50. She never smoked a day in her life. But my dad smoked, my uncle who lived with us smoked, all her friends smoked, and many of her co-workers smoked in her office before her workplace became smoke free. It makes me so angry when I see people smoking. Don't they realize that they're not just killing themselves but they're also killing their family and friends?

32-year-old woman

most 90% of lung cancer deaths. A diagnosis of cancer usually reflects the cumulative effect of many years of smoking. Lung cancer mortality rates are about 22 times higher for current male smokers and 12 times higher for current female smokers compared with lifelong nonsmokers.[76]

Secondhand smoke is also a risk factor. A nonsmoker married to a smoker has a 30% greater risk of developing lung cancer than the spouse of a nonsmoker. Each year, over 3,000 nonsmoking adults die of lung cancer as a result of breathing secondhand smoke. A family history of lung cancer may increase a person's risk, although this increase may be associated with exposure to secondhand tobacco smoke from smoking family members as opposed to being a hereditary factor.[77]

Asbestos exposure is a less common, but still powerful, risk factor. It increases a person's risk of developing lung cancer sevenfold. Asbestos workers who smoke have a 50–90 times greater risk than people in general. Other cancer-causing environmental agents exist, such as radon, radioactive ores, mineral exposures, and, potentially, air pollution.[78]

Diagnosis. Early detection of lung cancer is difficult because symptoms do not appear until the disease has reached an advanced stage. A persistent cough may then present as a predominant symptom. Along with cough, common symptoms of lung cancer include weight loss, bloody **sputum**, recurring bronchitis or pneumonia, and chest pain. There are no specific screening techniques or guidelines for the early detection of lung cancer. Newer tests, such as low-dose helical CT scans and molecular markers in sputum, have the potential to detect early lung cancer. A person with symptoms may have a chest radiograph, sputum tests, and fiber-optic examination of the bronchial passages for a more definitive diagnosis.

Treatment. Because most lung cancers are not diagnosed until they are in advanced stages, treatment options are usually limited. Treatment typically includes surgical removal of the affected regions, followed by radiation and chemotherapy. A **lobectomy** removes a lobe of the lung; a

pneumonectomy removes an entire lung; and a **segmentectomy** removes a section of a lobe of a lung.

Colorectal Cancer

Colorectal cancer is the third most common cancer in men and women. This type of disease develops in a gradual, progressive manner and may present anywhere in the colon and rectal areas. Cancer affecting different areas of this anatomical region often presents with different symptoms. By far the most common colon cancer is **adenocarcinoma**, which begins in the glandular structure lining the colon. This is a slow-growing cancer, and it may not manifest symptoms for years. Carcinoma-in-situ, or stage 0 cancer, is found in the lining of the colon or rectum. Stage I cancer spreads to other layers of the lining, whereas stage II disease spreads to nearby tissue. Lymph node involvement indicates stage III cancer, and spreading to other parts of the body indicates stage IV cancer. Colon cancer is about twice as common as rectal cancer.[78]

Risk Factors.   Increasing age is the primary risk factor for colorectal cancer. Ninety percent of people with colorectal cancer are older than 50 years of age. The risk of developing colon and rectal cancers is about twice as high for individuals with an immediate family member who has had colorectal cancer or certain conditions such as **familial adenomatous polyposis (FAP)**. FAP is characterized by the presence of hundreds of polyps in the colon and rectum (see **Figure 10.9**). Likewise, a history of inflammatory bowel disease is associated with a high risk of developing colon cancer. An individual who has developed a polyp or carcinoma in the past is also at increased risk of developing a second carcinoma.

Dietary factors are important determinants of colon and rectal cancer risk. An increased incidence of these cancers is associated with diets that are high in fat and low in fiber or other components of fruits and vegetables. In particular, the most definitive dietary risk for colorectal cancer is a high-fat diet.[79]

Screening and Diagnosis.   In its early stages, colorectal cancer usually causes no symptoms. Warning signs for advanced colorectal cancer include rectal bleeding, blood in the stool, a change in bowel habits, and cramping in the lower abdomen.

Similar to other forms of cancer, early detection of colorectal cancer greatly improves the likelihood of complete recovery. Approaches to the detection of colorectal cancer include **digital rectal examination**, **sigmoidoscopy**, **fecal occult blood testing**, and **colonoscopy**. In contrast to

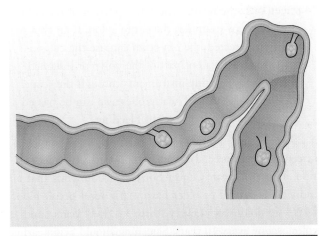

Figure 10.9

Colon polyps. An individual who has a history of polyps in the colon is at increased risk of developing colorectal cancer.

breast cancer and cervical cancer studies, there are fewer and more limited studies demonstrating the efficacy of these measures in terms of reducing mortality, although studies do support the efficacy of screening in terms of earlier cancer detection.

Each test for colorectal cancer screening has inherent advantages and disadvantages:

- Digital rectal examination is a simple part of a routine physical examination; however, it is relatively insensitive as a screening test because very few colorectal lesions develop within the range of the examining finger.

- Sigmoidoscopy entails examination of the rectum and lower part of the colon with a thin, lighted tube. Although more tumors can be detected with this procedure, a significant disadvantage is discomfort for the patient.

- Screening for tumors by fecal occult blood testing has the potential advantage over the other two methods to detect a tumor in any part of the colon. This type of test employs a simple procedure of smearing a small sample of stool on a slide containing a chemical that changes color in the presence of hemoglobin. Developing tumors cause minor bleeding, which results in the presence of occult blood (small amounts of blood in the stool). Unfortunately, the testing process is plagued by a significant number of false-positive and false-negative findings.

- Colonoscopies are often used when a sigmoidoscopy detects a polyp or abnormality, or the person is at high risk for colorectal cancer. While sigmoidoscopies screen only the rectum and lower portion of the colon, a colonoscopy examines the entire colon. If an abnormality is detected, the physician can use the colonoscope to remove all or part of the polyp or inflamed tissue by passing tiny instruments through the scope. Medicines, lasers, and heat probes also can be passed through the scope to stop any bleeding.

Despite the limitations of each of these methods, screening for colorectal cancer is important for early detection. The American Cancer Society recommends that all individuals age 50 or older have yearly fecal occult blood tests, sigmoidoscopy every three to five years, and a colonoscopy every 10 years. Screening should begin earlier if there is a strong family or personal history of polyps, colorectal cancer, or chronic inflammatory bowel disease.

Treatment.   Treatment depends largely on the stage of the tumor and can include surgery, chemotherapy, biological therapy, radiation therapy, or a combination of these treatments. Surgery to remove the tumor can be done through a colonoscopy, laparoscopy (use of a thin tube inserted into a small incision in the abdomen), or open surgery where the abdomen is opened. Chemotherapy employs anticancer medications that destroy the tumor. Biological therapy employs monoclonal antibodies that attach to the cancer cells and prevent cancer cell growth. Radiation therapy uses powerful "high energy" rays to destroy the cells. The death rates in colorectal cancer have decreased in the past 20 years, suggesting better detection and treatment.[79]

Skin Cancer

Cancer of the skin—the most common of all cancers—can be classified as either nonmelanomas or melanomas. The nonmelanoma skin cancers are the most common skin cancers and include two types[53]:

- **Basal cell carcinomas**. Approximately 75% of all skin cancers are basal cell carcinomas, with more than 1 million cases occurring annually. Basal cell carcinomas

usually develop in areas exposed to the sun, such as the head and neck. The growth rarely spreads, but, if left untreated, it can invade other tissues. Many people with basal cell carcinomas will have recurring growths in the same or other places on their body.

- **Squamous cell carcinomas**. Squamous cell carcinomas also appear on areas of the body commonly exposed to sun. These growths are more likely to spread and invade other tissues than the basal cell carcinomas, although very few affect other areas of the body if treated promptly.

Melanoma is a cancer arising from pigment-producing cells in the skin, called **melanocytes**. Although not nearly as common as basal and squamous cell carcinomas, it is a much more serious condition. Melanoma often appears as brown or black growths on the legs of fair-skinned women, although the growths can form on people with darker skin. This form of skin cancer is curable in its early stages, but if left untreated, it will metastasize to other areas of the body and can be deadly.

Risk Factors.   The major risk factor for melanoma is ultraviolet radiation from sunlight. The rates of melanoma are significantly greater in whites than in African Americans.[80] It is believed that the greater pigmentation of dark skin affords more protection against radiation. The presence of moles is also an indicator of increased risk of melanoma. Although they are benign, certain types of moles, such as **dysplastic nevi**, can increase a person's risk. Dysplastic nevi is the term for irregular moles (*nevi* is the medical term for multiple moles), and this condition often runs in families. Moles are considered irregular when they have an uneven border or color. A family history of melanoma is another important risk factor; individuals with a

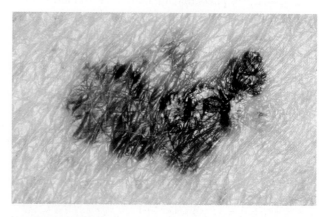

■ The American Cancer Society emphasizes four warnings of melanoma: Asymmetry; Border irregularities; Color irregularities; and Diameter.

first-degree relative who has had melanoma are eight times more likely to develop melanoma themselves.

Similar to melanomas, nonmelanoma skin cancers are caused by solar ultraviolet radiation. Fair skin and male gender also increase the risk of nonmelanoma skin conditions. All forms of sun tanning and sun exposure are potentially hazardous to the skin. Exposure to ultraviolet radiation from the sun is the greatest single cause of cancer in the United States. Basal cell carcinoma and squamous cell carcinoma are associated with frequent exposure to the sun over many years. In contrast, melanoma has been associated with a single, blistering sunburn early in life. Occupational exposure to coal tar, pitch, creosote, arsenic compounds, or radium is also a risk factor.

Preventive measures for skin cancer include limiting or avoiding sun exposure during midday hours (10 A.M. to 4 P.M.), using sun lotion with a sun protective factor (SPF) of 15 or greater, and avoiding tanning beds and sun lamps. According to the American Cancer Society, if everyone used sun protection, 1 million cases of skin cancer could be prevented each year.

Screening and Diagnosis.   Early detection of all skin cancers is critical and is essential to the outcome of melanoma. Recognition of changes in skin growths or the appearance of new growths is the best way to find early skin cancer.

Screening is best accomplished by skin examination. Basal cell carcinomas often appear as flat, scaly red areas or small, raised, translucent areas. Squamous cell carcinomas are growing lumps or flat, reddish patches. Melanomas may develop within a mole or as a new mole-like growth. They are characterized by increasing size and changes in color. The American Cancer Society emphasizes four warnings of melanoma (the ABCD system):

- Asymmetry—the shape of one-half of a lesion or mole is different from the other.

- Border irregularities—the edge may be uneven, ragged, or blotched.

- Color irregularities—different colors may be present in the mole or lesion.

I had so many sunburns as a child. My mom has had basal cells removed from her face and my grandfather had melanoma, so I know I'm at high risk for skin cancer. I get checked regularly by a dermatologist, but so far, the moles that she has removed from my back have been normal. I finally understand how important it is to protect myself from the sun.

30-year-old fair-skinned woman

- Diameter—the mole or lesion is usually greater than 6 mm (about 1/4 inch) in diameter.

If a skin growth looks suspicious, diagnosis will be performed through a skin biopsy (sample of the growth). A woman should check her own body on a monthly basis for new skin growths or changes. A cancer check by a dermatologist is recommended every three years for women ages 20 to 40 years, and every year for those older than age 40.

Treatment.   There are five primary treatments for nonmelanoma skin cancer. Surgery is used in 90% of the cases.[53] Radiation therapy, electrodesiccation, cryosurgery, and laser therapy are also employed for early forms of nonmelanoma skin cancer. Treatment for melanoma usually consists of surgical removal of the mole or lesion and possibly regional lymph nodes. Advanced cases of disease are treated with chemotherapy, radiation therapy, or immunotherapy. Survival rates are high for localized lesions, but metastatic disease is not responsive to therapy. Because melanomas are able to metastasize quickly, early detection is the major determinant of survival.

Informed Decision Making

There are several things that a woman can do to try to reduce her risk of CVD and cancer. For most women, prevention is the most important step, and taking good care of one's long-term health. The old adage, "An ounce of prevention is worth a pound of cure," is still correct. It is much smarter to do everything you can to reduce your risk of suffering a life-threatening or disabling heart attack at 55 by never smoking, eating a prudent diet, and exercising—all behaviors that should begin in childhood. Although it's better to begin these behaviors earlier in life rather than later, it is never too late to change.

Prevention Through Lifestyle

Lifestyle is a critical part of maintaining a woman's health and preventing disease. Such efforts also help to minimize problems when a woman is affected by a disease. Prevention and health enhancement include quitting smoking (or never starting), limiting alcohol intake, avoiding illegal and dangerous substances, practicing safe sex, being physically active, using sunblock while in the sun, maintaining an appropriate weight, and eating a proper diet. Enjoying life and maintaining a positive mental outlook are other important factors. These activities should be put in place as children and maintained throughout life. Another important part of maintaining health and preventing disease is for each woman to work in partnership with her physician or other health-care provider. This is a partnership for health.

Prevention Through Health Screening

Cardiovascular disease prevention involves getting screened and knowing one's family history of heart disease and stroke. When a woman visits the doctor, she should discuss her smoking, alcohol, and dietary status. Her blood pressure, blood cholesterol and triglycerides, and fasting blood glucose should be measured. In addition, her waist circumference should be measured to check for signs of excess fat around her waist.[81]

Mammography is the best way to detect breast cancer in its earliest, most treatable stage—an average of 1.7 years before a woman can feel the lump. Clinical breast exams and monthly breast self-exams are recommended for women younger than age 40 and should supplement mammograms for women older than age 40. Any breast lumps; skin changes, such as flaking or crusting, or weeping eruptions around the nipple; discharge from the nipple; or dimpling or retraction of the skin should be evaluated by a physician.

Pap smears and HPV testing are screening methods that can greatly reduce invasive cervical cancer morbidity and mortality rates. Because cervical cancer is a slow-growing disease, screening programs started at age 21 dramatically decrease the risk of developing advanced disease.

I had a lump in my breast, and it had been there for some time. It didn't hurt. I guess that I was hoping it was nothing and would go away. I waited too long. This has been a rough year, but I am trying to tell other women not to make the same mistake. If you feel a lump, regardless of the size, have it checked right away.
42-year-old woman

In fact, when cervical cancer is detected at its earliest stage, the five-year survival rate is more than 90%. Pelvic exams are also essential for women to detect any abnormal changes of the reproductive system.

Self-examination of one's skin enables a woman to detect early forms of skin cancer. Women should become familiar with their bodies to be able to recognize any of the warning signs of cancer.

Table 10.11 summarizes the current cancer screening recommendations.

Summary

Cardiovascular disease and cancer together represent the greatest risks to women's health. The underpinnings of disease causality and progression have been shown to be a complex interrelationship among an individual's family history, environment, lifestyle, and comorbid conditions. Though family history is not the only risk factor, it has been shown that women with genetic predispositions to

Table 10.11 Screening Tests

These findings are from HINTS, a nationally representative survey carried out in 2002-2003 and 2005. The purpose of this survey was to determine how people obtain information about cancer and what can be done to reach people most effectively.[82]

Most people know about screening tests—mammograms, Pap smears, colonoscopies—but most do not know when the tests should be started.

Women
- Only 32% of women knew that they need to begin mammogram screenings at age 40.
- 74% did, however, get mammogram screenings as recommended.
- 87% of women respondents stated that they had an annual Pap test, but the majority of women respondents did not realize that they did not have to have one every year.
- Only 47% of women knew that HPV causes cervical cancer

The knowledge base among women also varies substantially across the country.

Lung Cancer
- Only 27.9% of respondents knew lung cancer was the leading cancer death in the United States, but 84% knew that smoking causes lung cancer. The lowest knowledge base was in the Midwest and South.

Colorectal Cancer Screening
- Many respondents could not name even one screening method for colorectal cancer.
- 67% did not know that individuals over 50 should be screened.

Race/Ethnicity
- Lack of knowledge about when to begin colorectal cancer screening:
  - 79% Hispanic
  - 75% African American
  - 70% American Indian/Alaskan Native
  - 38% white

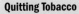

It's Your Health

Quitting Tobacco

The positive effects of quitting begin very soon after you stop using tobacco and continue long after you've quit.

Short-Term Benefits

- Your blood pressure, pulse, and body temperature, which were abnormally elevated by nicotine, return to normal. Persons taking blood pressure medication should continue doing so until told otherwise by their physician.

- Your body starts to heal itself. Carbon monoxide and oxygen levels in your blood return to normal.

- Your chance of having a heart attack goes down.

- Nerve endings start to regrow. Your ability to taste and smell improves.

- Your breathing passages (bronchial tubes) relax, lung capacity goes up, and your breathing becomes easier.

- Your circulation improves.

- Your lungs become stronger, making it easier to walk.

- In your lungs, the cilia (hairlike structures on the lining) begin to regrow, increasing the ability of your lungs to handle mucus, to clean themselves, and to reduce infection.

- Coughing, sinus congestion, fatigue, and shortness of breath decrease. Your overall energy level increases.

Long-Term Benefits

- As a former smoker, your chance of dying from lung cancer is less than it would be if you continued to smoke. Your chance of getting cancer of the throat, bladder, kidney, or pancreas also decreases.

Source: National Cancer Institute, U.S. National Institutes of Health. Available at http://www.cancer.gov/cancertopics/factsheet/Tobacco/quitting-benefits.

---

cardiovascular disease and certain types of cancers are at increased risk for developing disease. Recognizing that these diseases affect women of all ages should be an incentive for women to begin making lifestyle changes in diet, physical activity, tobacco use, and health screening as early as possible.

Adopting healthy lifestyle choices can greatly reduce a woman's risk. Women must challenge themselves to become familiar with the risk factors for cardiovascular disease and cancer, and their changing risk status as they age. Women should be vigilant about following prevention recommendations and screening guidelines for disease. By

Gender Dimensions

SEX/GENDER DIFFERENCES IN BREAST CANCER

Breast cancer is well known and feared among women. Unfortunately, because it is far less common, breast cancer is not usually thought of as a threat to men's health, often with disastrous consequences. In 2008, an estimated 1,990 breast cancer cases were diagnosed in men—about 100 times less than among women—and about 450 men died from the disease.[83]

Men and women both have breast tissue. Both sexes also have "male" and "female" hormones, such as testosterone and estrogen, just in different amounts. The major difference in females and males is the amount of breast tissue and the hormonal influence on it. Females have more breast tissue than men and make far more female hormones than men do. These female hormones cause the breasts to develop and grow. In men, male hormones, made largely in the testicles, inhibit breast growth spurred by female hormones. Yet breast tissue, in both males and females, can become cancerous.

Several risk factors are associated with breast cancer in men:

- Radiation exposure in the chest area, as in radiation treatment for a disease

- Diseases that produce high levels of estrogen (female hormone) in the body, such as cirrhosis of the liver or Kleinfelter's syndrome (a genetic disorder in which men have more than one X chromosome, e.g., XXY)

- Female relatives who have alternations of the BRCA1 or BRCA2 genes

- Obesity: fat cells produce estrogen

Known mutations in breast-cancer susceptibility genes—BRCA1, BRCA2, and CHEK2—pose a heightened breast cancer risk in women. BRCA1 and BRCA2 are also associated with breast cancer in men, and CHEK2 may also prove a risk. BRCA2 is the genetic mutation that appears most commonly in men and accounts for an estimated 5–10% risk. BRCA1 is less common and seems to appear more often in men of Jewish heritage.[84,85]

A study on the incidence of male and female breast cancer in a Veteran's Affairs population showed that men appeared to develop the disease later than women, and the median overall survival was 7 years for men and 9.8 years for women. The following were some of the important differences noted between the sexes in the study:

- Men presented with a greater disease stage.

- Men had greater lymph node involvement.

- Hormone treatment was less successful in men.

- Men were less likely to receive chemotherapy.[86]

This is a disease that deserves attention in both sexes. Yet, for many reasons men are more reluctant to acknowledge or be tested for the disease. Fortunately, men are becoming more aware and making efforts to educate both men and women about the disease in men. Web sites are more prevalent and men are becoming more comfortable discussing it. However, much work remains to be done to promote public awareness of breast cancer in men.

Profiles of Remarkable Women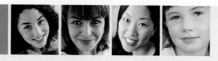

Elizabeth Barrett-Connor, M.D. (1935–)

Dr. Elizabeth Barrett-Connor is a world-renowned epidemiologist who has greatly increased the knowledge base regarding cardiovascular disease, diabetes, cancer, and osteoporosis, and the relationships of these diseases to lifestyle and behavior. Among her many accomplishments, she is widely recognized for conducting the Rancho Bernardo study, a long-term observational study of a group of largely middle-class women and their lifestyles and behaviors. This study has provided substantial knowledge about women as they age, particularly in the area of menopause.

She has been honored many times and has been the recipient of grants from organizations for her research in areas ranging from heart disease to diabetes to aging. Barrett-Connor is a member of numerous professional societies, a reviewer of 14 journals, and has been on the editorial boards of more than 10 journals.

Long an advocate for studies that bring exacting science to women's health issues, Barrett-Connor is noted for her work in chronic diseases that are common in older women. Her studies and her advocacy have advanced women's health knowledge substantially. For example, her studies on the role of hormone replacement therapy in the possible prevention of heart disease are internationally recognized. Barrett-Connor entered medicine at a time when few women had followed this path. She persevered and became a leader in the field. Over the years, Barrett-Connor has established herself as a role model through her leadership in medicine and her dedication to mentoring other women physicians and health-care professionals.

Profiles of Remarkable Women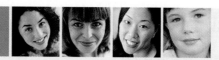

Nanette K. Wenger, M.D. (1930–)

Dr. Nanette Wenger is a Professor of Medicine (Cardiology) at Emory University School of Medicine. She is now also the Director of Cardiac Clinics, Chief of Cardiology, and Director of the Ambulatory Electrocardiography Laboratory at Grady Memorial Hospital in Atlanta, and a consultant at the Emory Heart Center.

Wenger has been honored and recognized numerous times, including being the recipient of the Atlanta Woman of the Year in Medicine award, the American College of Sports Medicine 1994 citation, the Best Doctor in America award for 1994–1998, and the Physician of the Year award from the American Heart Association in 1998. She has also been cited in *Time* magazine's "Women of the Year" issue for her accomplishments in cardiac rehabilitation and international medical teaching.

Wenger has been appointed as a member and chair on numerous boards and committees. At present, some of her appointments include member of the review board for the National Heart, Lung and Blood Institute's Cardiovascular Health Study, a member of the Expert Advisory Panel in Cardiovascular Disease for the World Health Organization, Editor-in-Chief of the *American Journal of Geriatric Cardiology*, and consultant, editor, or reviewer for numerous journals.

Much of Wenger's work has highlighted gender and age differences in clinical outcomes. She has been involved in cardiac rehabilitation and education of heart disease in women for many years.

Profiles of Remarkable Women

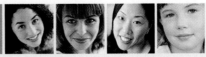

Mary-Claire King (1946–)

Mary-Claire King is an American Cancer Society Professor in the Departments of Medicine and Genetics at the University of Washington in Seattle. King has received many honors, including election to the American Epidemiological Society, fellow in the American Association for the Advancement of Science, and election to the American Academy of Arts and Sciences. She has participated in numerous public advisory committees, including the Breast Cancer Program Review Group with the National Cancer Institute, the Board of Scientific Consultants at Memorial Sloan Kettering Cancer Center, the National Institutes of Health Office of Women's Health Scientific Advisory Committee, and the United Nations War Crimes Tribunal. King has been politically active since the Vietnam War, working with Ralph Nader's consumer-interest group, and consulting on a project to reunite kidnapped children from the Argentinean civil war with their grandparents.

King was the first person to suggest the idea that familial breast cancer could be traced to a particular gene. In 1990, she proved the existence of the gene for hereditary breast cancer, now known as BRCA1. She later found that the same gene could stop and in some cases reverse breast and ovarian cancers. King is also working on genetic research focused on AIDS and inherited deafness.

working cooperatively with health-care providers, women can diminish their risk of developing disease, and most effectively deal with treatment should the need arise. Knowledge, personal preventive measures, and lifestyle modifications are the best ways for a woman to reduce her chances of morbidity and mortality associated with these diseases.

Topics for Discussion

1. What factors can influence women of different ages to adopt healthier lifestyles and engage in preventive action to reduce their risks of cardiovascular disease and cancer? Discuss factors for different age groups beginning with the teen years.

2. What can women do to increase their general awareness of cardiovascular and cancer threats? Discuss for different age groups beginning with the teen years.

3. What can public health agencies and community organizations do to increase the general awareness of women regarding cardiovascular and cancer risk factors?

4. Substantial differences exist in the incidence and prevalence of cancer and cardiovascular diseases across racial and ethnic groups. Discuss which factors influence these differences and why.

5. How can academic institutions take a more active role in disease prevention for young women?

Web Sites

American Cancer Society: http://www.cancer.org

American Heart Association: http://www.heart.org

Breast Cancer Network of Strength:
      http://www.networkofstrength.org

CDC: Cancer Prevention and Control:
      http://www.cdc.gov/cancer/

Gynecological Cancer Foundation: http://www.thegcf.org

LungCancer.org: http://www.lungcancer.org

Lung Cancer Online: http://www.lungcanceronline.org

National Cancer Institute: http://www.cancer.gov

National Cervical Cancer Coalition:
      http://www.nccc-online.org

National Heart, Lung and Blood Institute:
      http://www.nhlbi.nih.gov

National Ovarian Cancer Coalition:
      http://www.ovarian.org

Ovarian Cancer National Alliance:
      http://www.ovariancancer.com

Skin Cancer Foundation: http://www.skincancer.org

Susan G. Komen for the Cure: http://www.komen.org

Women's Cancer Network: http://www.wcn.org

References

1. Rosamund, W., et al. (2008). Heart disease and stroke statistics—2008 update: a report from the American Heart Association Statistics Committee and Stroke Statistics Subcommittee. *Circulation* 117: e25–e146.
2. National Center for Health Statistics. (2007). Available at: http://www.cdc.gov/nchs/data/hus/hus07.pdf.
3. World Health Organization. (2008). *The Top 10 Causes of Death*. Available at: http://www.who.int/mediacentre/factsheets/fs310/en/index.html.
4. World Health Organization. (2008). *World Health Statistics 2008*. Geneva, Switzerland. Available at: http://www.who.int/whosis/whostat/2008/en/index.html.
5. World Health Organization. (2008). *WHO Database*. Available at: http://www.who.int/whosis/databases/en.
6. World Health Organization. (2007). *European Health for All Database*. Available at: http://www.euro.who.int/hfadb.
7. Writing Committee for the ENRICHD Investigators. (2003). Effects of treating depression and low perceived social support on clinical events after myocardial infarction: the Enhanced Recovery in Coronary Heart Disease Patients (ENRICHD) randomized trial. *Journal of the American Medical Association* 289: 3106–3116.
8. Lai, S. M., et al. (2005). Sex differences in stroke recovery. *Preventing Chronic Disease* 38(8): A13.
9. Ostwald, S. K., et al. (2008). Predictors of functional independence and stress level of stroke survivors at discharge from inpatient rehabilitation. *Journal of Cardiovascular Nursing* 23(4): 371–377.
10. American Heart Association. (2008). *Metabolic Syndrome*. Available at: http://www.americanheart.org/presenter.jhtml?identifier=4756.
11. National Institute for Neurological Disorders and Stroke. (August 24, 2004). *Review of the t-PA Review Committee*. Available at: http://www.ninds.nih.gov/funding/review_committees/t-pa_review_committee/t-pa_committee_report.pdf.
12. Shaywitz, B. A., et al. (1995). Sex differences in the functional organization of the brain for language. *Nature* 373: 607–609.
13. Chiou-Tan, F. Y., Keng, M. J. Jr., Graves, D. E., Chan, K. T., & Rintala, D. H. (2006). Racial/ethnic differences in FIM scores and length of stay for underinsured patients undergoing stroke inpatient rehabilita-tion. *American Journal of Physical Medicine and Rehabilitation* 85(5): 415–423.
14. American Lung Association. (2007). *Women and Smoking Fact Sheet*. Available at: http://www.lungusa.org/site/c.dvLUK9O0E/b.33572/k.985F/Women_and_Smoking_Fact_Sheet.htm.
15. Centers for Disease Control and Prevention. (2001). *Surgeon General's Report—Women and Smoking*. Chapter 5. Available at: http://www.cdc.gov/tobacco/data_statistics/sgr/sgr_2001/index.htm#full.
16. World Health Organization. (2005). Female smoking. *Smoking Trends: 1960–2000*. Geneva, Switzerland: World Health Organization. Available at: http://www.who.int/entity/tobacco/en/atlas6.pdf.
17. U.S. Department of Health and Human Services. (2005). *Report on Carcinogens* (11th ed.). Research Triangle Park, NC. Available at: http://ntp.niehs.nih.gov/ntp/roc/toc11.html.
18. National Cancer Institute. (2007). *Cancer Progress Report*. Available at: http://progressreport.cancer.gov/.
19. LaRosa, J. C. (1997). Triglycerides and coronary risk in women and the elderly. *Archives of Internal Medicine* 157: 961–968.
20. McBride, P. (2008). Triglycerides and risk for coronary artery disease. *Current Atherosclerosis Reports* 10(5): 386–390.
21. Austin, M. A., et al. (2000). Cardiovascular mortality in familial forms of hypertriglyceridemia: a 20-year prospective study. *Circulation* 101: 2777.
22. Ridker, P. M., et al. (2002). Comparison of C-reactive protein and low density lipoprotein cholesterol levels in the prediction of first cardiovascular events. *New England Journal of Medicine* 347(20): 1557–1565.
23. Yeh, E. T. (2005). High-sensitivity C-reactive protein as a risk assessment tool for cardiovascular disease. *Clinical Cardiology* 28(9): 408–412.
24. Pearson, T. A., et al. (2003). Markers of inflammation and cardiovascular disease: application to clinical and public health practice: a statement for healthcare professionals from the Centers for Disease Control and Prevention and the American Heart Association. *Circulation* 107: 499–511.
25. Lakoski, S. G., et al. (2006). Gender and C-reactive protein: data from the Multiethnic Study of Atherosclerosis (MESA) cohort. *American Heart Journal* 152(3): 593–598.
26. American Heart Association. (2005). *Homocysteine, Folic Acid and Cardiovascular Diseases*. Available at: http://www.americanheart.org/presenter.jhtml?identifier=4677.

27. Wald, D. S., et al. (2002). Homocysteine and cardiovascular disease: evidence on causality from a meta-analysis. *British Medical Journal* 325: 1202.

28. Suk, D. J., et al. (2006). Lipoprotein(a), measured with an assay independent of apolipoprotein(a) isoform size, and risk of future cardiovascular events among initially healthy women. *Journal of the American Medical Association* 296(11): 1363–1370.

29. Suk, D. J., et al. (2008). Lipoprotein(a), hormone replacement therapy, and risk of future cardiovascular events. *Journal of the American College of Cardiology* 52(2): 124–131.

30. National Diabetes Education Program. (2006). *Type 2 Diabetes Risk After Gestational Diabetes.* Available at: http://www.ndep.nih.gov/diabetes/pubs/FS_Post-GDM.pdf.

31. Hu, F. B., et al. (2004). Adiposity as compared with physical activity in predicting mortality among women. *New England Journal of Medicine* 351(26): 2694–2703.

32. Irwin, M. L., et al. (2008). Effect of exercise on total and intra-abdominal body fat in postmenopausal women. *Journal of the American Medical Association* 289(3): 323–330.

33. Koledova, V. V., et al. (2007). Sex hormone replacement therapy and modulation of vascular function in cardiovascular disease. *Expert Review of Cardiovascular Therapy* 5(4): 777–789.

34. Qiao, X., et al. (2008). Sex steroids and vascular responses in hypertension and aging. *Gender Medicine* 5(Suppl A): S46–S64.

35. OrthoTri-Cyclen. *Oral Contraceptives: From Historical Evolution to Modern Revolution.* Available at: http://www.orthotricyclen.com/cyberdoctor.com/page9=html.

36. Baillargeon, J. P., et al. (2005). Association between the current use of low-dose oral contraceptives and cardiovascular arterial disease: a meta-analysis. *Journal of Clinical Endocrinology and Metabolism* 90(7): 3863–3870.

37. Gillum, L. A., Mamidipudi, S. K., & Johnston, S. C. (2000). Ischemic stroke risk with oral contraceptives: a meta-analysis. *Journal of the American Medical Association* 284(1): 72–78.

38. MacClellan, L. R., et al. (2007). Probable migraine with visual aura and risk of ischemic stroke: the stroke prevention in young women study. *Stroke* 38(9): 2438–2445.

39. Lampl, C., et al. (2006). Migraine and stroke—why do we talk about it? *European Journal of Neurology* 13(3): 215–219.

40. American Heart Association. (2008). *Cocaine, Marijuana and Other Drugs.* Available at: http://www.americanheart.org/presenter.jhtml?identifier=4552.

41. Ellins, E., et al. (2008). Arterial stiffness and inflammatory response to psychophysiological stress. *Brain, Behavior, and Immunity* 22(6): 941–948.

42. Stansfield, S. A., et al. (2002). Psychological distress as a risk factor for coronary heart disease in the Whitehall II Study. *International Journal of Epidemiology* 31: 248–255.

43. Centers for Disease Control and Prevention. (2005). Racial/ethnic and socioeconomic disparities in multiple risk factors for heart disease and stroke—United States, 2003. *Morbidity and Mortality Weekly Report* 54(5): 113–117.

44. Lee, J. R., et al. (2005). The association between educational levels and risk of cardiovascular disease fatality among women with cardiovascular disease. *Women's Health Issues* 15(2): 80–88.

45. Finkelstein, E. S., et al. (2004). Racial/ethnic disparities in coronary heart disease risk factors among WISEWOMAN enrollees. *Journal of Women's Health* 13(5): 503–518.

46. National Cancer Institute. (2008). *Common Cancers.* Available at: http://www.cancer.gov/cancertopics/commoncancers/.

47. American Lung Association. (2008). *Lung Cancer.* Available at: http://www.lungusa.org/site/pp.asp?c=dvLUK9O0E&b=4104583#lungcancer2.

48. American Cancer Society. (2008). *Cancer Facts & Figures 2008.* Atlanta: American Cancer Society.

49. Jemal, A., Siegel, R., Ward, E., et al. (2008). Cancer Statistics, 2008. *CA: A Cancer Journal for Clinicians* 58: 71–96. Available at: http://caonline.amcancersoc.org/cgi/content/full/58/2/71.

50. National Cancer Institute. *Endometrial Cancer.* Available at: http://www.cancer.gov/cancertopics/types/endometrial.

51. National Cancer Institute. *Ovarian Cancer.* Available at: http://www.cancer.gov/cancertopics/types/ovarian.

52. International Agency for Research on Cancer. *Globocan. Cervix Uteri.* Available at: http://www-dep.iarc.fr/GLOBOCAN/map.asp?cancer=142&rate=1&sex=2&type=1&submit=Execute&size=2&colour=1&output=1&scale=1.

53. National Cancer Institute. *Skin Cancer.* Available at: http://www.cancer.gov/cancertopics/types/skin.

54. American Cancer Society. (2008). *What Is Cervical Cancer?* Available at: http://www.cancer.org/docroot/

CRI/content/CRI_2_4_1X_What_is_cervical_cancer_8.asp.

55. World Health Organization. (2003). *Global Cancer Rates Could Increase by 50% to 15 Million by 2020.* Available at: http://www.who.int/mediacentre/news/releases/2003/pr27/en/.

56. U.S. National Library of Medicine. (2007). *Breast Cancer.* Genetics Home Reference. Available at: http://ghr.nlm.nih.gov/condition=breastcancer.

57. ESHRE Capri Workshop Group. (2004). Hormones and breast cancer. *Human Reproduction Update* 10(4): 281–283.

58. Prentice, R. L., et al. (2008). Conjugated equine estrogens and breast cancer risk in the Women's Health Initiative Clinical Trial and Observational Study. *American Journal of Epidemiology* 167(12): 1407–1415.

59. Casey, P. M., Cehran, J. R., & Pruthi, S. (2008). Oral contraceptive use and risk of breast cancer. *Mayo Clinic Proceedings* 83(1): 86–91.

60. American Cancer Society. (2008). Cancer Facts and Figures 2008.

61. National Cancer Institute. (2008). *Breast Cancer Screening.* Available at: http://www.cancer.gov/cancertopics/pdq/screening/breast/Patient/page3.

62. Pisano, E. D., Hendrick, R. E., Yaffe, M. J., et al. (2008). Diagnostic accuracy of digital versus film mammography: exploratory analysis of selected population subgroups in DMIST. *Radiology* 246(2): 376–383.

63. American Cancer Society. *How Is Breast Cancer Treated?* Available at: http://www.cancer.org/docroot/CRI/content/CRI_2_2_4X_How_Is_Breast_Cancer_Treated_5.asp.

64. National Cancer Institute. (2006). *Results of the Study of Tamoxifen and Raloxifene (STAR) Released: Osteoporosis Drug Raloxifene Shown to Be as Effective as Tamoxifen in Preventing Invasive Breast Cancer.* Available at: http://www.cancer.gov/newscenter/pressreleases/STARresultsApr172006.

65. National Cancer Institute. (2008). *Stages of Cervical Cancer.* Available at: http://www.cancer.gov/cancertopics/pdq/treatment/cervical/Patient/page2.

66. American Cancer Society, *What Are the Risk Factors for Cervical Cancer?* Available at: http://www.cancer.org/docroot/CRI/content/CRI_2_4_2X_What_are_the_risk_factors_for_cervical_cancer_8.asp.

67. National Cancer Institute. (2007). *General Information About Cervical Cancer.* Available at: http://www.cancer.gov/cancertopics/pdq/screening/cervical/Patient/page2.

68. Vetter, K. M., & Geller, S. E. (2007). Moving forward: human papillomavirus vaccination and the prevention of cervical cancer. *Journal of Women's Health* 16(9): 1258–1268.

69. Markowitz, L. E., et al. (2007). Quadrivalent human papillomavirus vaccine: recommendations of the Advisory Committee on Immunization Practices (ACIP). *Morbidity and Mortality Weekly Report* 56(RR02): 1–24. Available at: http://www.cdc.gov/mmwr/preview/mmwrhtml/rr5602a1.htm?s_cid=rr5602a1_e.

70. National Cancer Institute. (2008). *General Information About Cervical Cancer.* Available at: http://www.cancer.gov/cancertopics/pdq/treatment/cervical/Patient.

71. Medica. (2005). *Management of Benign Uterine Conditions.* Medica Guideline VI-GYN.01. Available at: http://provider.medica.com/C15/PolicyIndex/Document%20Library/VIGYN01.pdf.

72. Fiorelli, J. L., Herzog, T. J., & Wright, J. D. (2008). Current treatment strategies for endometrial cancer. *Expert Review of Anticancer Therapy* 8(7): 1149–1157.

73. National Cancer Institute. (2008). *Stages of Endometrial Cancer.* Available at: http://www.cancer.gov/cancertopics/pdq/treatment/endometrial/Patient/page2.

74. National Cancer Institute. (2006). *What You Need to Know About Ovarian Cancer, Risk Factors.* Available at: http://www.cancer.gov/cancertopics/wyntk/ovary/page4.

75. Johns Hopkins Pathology. *Ovarian Cancer Treatment.* Available at: http://ovariancancer.jhmi.edu/treatment.cfm.

76. American Cancer Society. (2008). *Cancer Facts and Figures 2008.* Atlanta, GA: American Cancer Society.

77. American Lung Association. *Secondhand Smoke Fact Sheet.* Available at: http://www.lungusa.org/site/pp.asp?c=dvLUK9O0E&b=35422.

78. Health Alliance Cancer Services. *Risk Factors for Lung Cancer.* Available at: http://www.health-alliance.com/Cancer/lung/risk_factors.html.

79. National Cancer Institute. (2006). *What You Need to Know About Cancer of the Colon and Rectum.* Available at: http://www.cancer.gov/cancertopics/wyntk/colon-and-rectal/page1.

80. Byrd-Miles, K., Toombs, E. L., & Peck, G. L. (2007). Skin cancer in individuals of African, Asian, Latin-American, and American-Indian descent: differences in incidence, clinical presentation, and survival compared to Caucasians. *Journal of Drugs in Dermatology* 6(1): 10–46.

81. Pearson, T. A., Blair, S. N., Daniels, S. R., et al. (2002). AHA guidelines for primary prevention of cardiovas-

cular disease and stroke: 2002 update. *Circulation* 106: 388.

82. Rutten, L. F., Moser, R. P., Bekjord, E. D., et al. (2007). *Cancer Communication: Health Information National Trends Survey*. Washington, DC, National Cancer Institute. NIH publication No. 07-6214.

83. National Cancer Institute. (2008). *General Information About Male Breast Cancer*. Available at: http://www.cancer.gov/cancertopics/pdq/treatment/malebreast/patient#Keypoint2.

84. American Cancer Society. *What Are the Risk Factors for Breast Cancer in Men?* Available at: http://www.cancer.org/docroot/CRI/content/CRI_2_4_2X_What_are_the_risk_factors_for_male_breast_cancer_28.asp?rnav=cri.

85. American Cancer Society. *Do We Know What Causes Breast Cancer in Men?* Available at: http://www.cancer.org/docroot/CRI/content/CRI_2_4_2X_Do_we_know_what_causes_male_breast_cancer_28.asp.

86. Nahleh, Z. A., Srikantiah, R., Safa, M., Jazieh, A. R., Muhleman, A., & Komrokji, R. (2007). Male breast cancer in the Veterans Affairs population: a comparative analysis. *Cancer* 109(8): 1471–1477.

Chapter Eleven

Other Chronic Diseases and Conditions

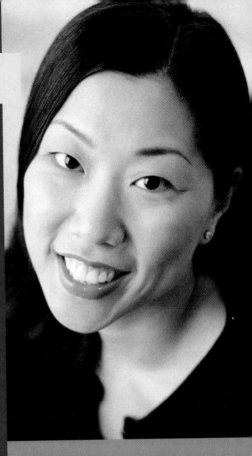

Chapter Objectives

On completion of this chapter, the student should be able to discuss:

1. Prevalence and incidence of various chronic diseases and their effects on women.

2. Differences between racial and ethnic groups in the incidence rates of chronic diseases.

3. The individual and societal costs of various chronic diseases.

4. Risk factors, screening tests, and preventive and treatment measures for osteoporosis.

5. The process of bone resorption, bone formation, and osteoporosis development.

6. The two major forms of arthritis that disproportionately afflict women.

7. Risk factors and symptoms of arthritis and methods for pain management.

8. The differences between the two major types of diabetes.

9. The special risks that pregnancy presents to the diabetic mother.

10. Diabetes management and responding in emergency situations.

11. Autoimmune diseases that most commonly affect women.

12. Types of lupus and the clinical manifestations of the disease.

13. The basics of Hashimoto's disease and Graves' disease.

14. The development of Alzheimer's disease and the resulting symptoms.

15. Methods for diagnosing Alzheimer's disease and ways to treat symptoms of the disease.

16. Ways that a woman can recognize symptoms of a disease so as to seek treatment and prevent future disease-related complications.

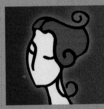

womenshealth.jbpub.com

Women's Health Online is a great source for supplementary women's health information for both students and instructors. Visit

http://womenshealth.jbpub.com

to find a variety of useful tools for learning, thinking, and teaching.

Introduction

Chronic diseases are diseases or conditions that persist or progress over a long time. Chronic diseases develop slowly, do not resolve spontaneously, and are rarely cured completely. Chronic diseases are often caused by malfunctions within the body, environmental factors, or a combination of the two, though bacteria or viruses can sometimes be responsible for these diseases. Many of these diseases manifest themselves in young women, creating health issues that these individuals must learn to live with for the rest of their lives.

Living with a chronic disease can become an encompassing process, especially when the disease causes frequent illness and necessitates many visits to physicians. Some women begin to consider the management of their illness to be a full-time job. Others try to live as they did before diagnosis, not wanting their condition to become central to their lives. Women's responses to chronic disease are as individual as the women themselves. In all cases, however, active support networks via family, friends, health-care providers, disease support groups, or therapy can help ease the burden of disease management. Support can help the woman cope with the physical and emotional ramifications of having a chronic disease.

Lifestyle factors greatly influence some chronic diseases. Chronic diseases of lifestyle share similar risk factors as a result of exposure, over many decades, to unhealthy diets, smoking, lack of exercise, continued stress, and other risks. These lifestyle risk factors contribute to high blood pressure, high cholesterol levels, diabetes, and obesity, which in turn lead to conditions such as stroke, heart attack, tobacco- and nutrition-induced cancer, chronic bronchitis, and emphysema, culminating in high mortality and morbidity rates.

Chronic diseases are the leading cause of death in the United States and around the world. The World Health Organization (WHO) estimates that chronic diseases cause about 35 million, or 60%, of the 60 million deaths every year.[1] Cardiovascular disease and cancer (see Chapter 10) are by far the biggest killers in this category, but other chronic diseases, like the ones discussed in this chapter, still kill 10 million people every year—more than twice the number of annual deaths from AIDS and tuberculosis combined.[1]

This chapter reviews osteoporosis, arthritis, diabetes mellitus, certain autoimmune diseases, and Alzheimer's disease—chronic diseases that have dramatic effects on the health of women in the world today. Discussions of some other chronic diseases, such as herpes and AIDS (Chapter 7) and cancer (Chapter 10), appear in other chapters.

Dimensions of Chronic Diseases

Epidemiological Overview

Understanding, preventing, and managing chronic conditions are important steps for maintaining satisfactory health. The prevalence of chronic conditions is difficult to ascertain because of differences and inconsistencies in diagnostic criteria and the lack of national reporting systems. Many chronic diseases affect women more often than they do men.

- Of the 10 million Americans estimated to have osteoporosis, 8 million are women and 2 million are men.[2]

- Osteoarthritis and rheumatoid arthritis, two of the most common health problems in the United States, are far more prevalent in women than in men.

- Diabetes affects 24 million people in the United States. Women make up almost half of this total; an estimated 10.2% of adult U.S. women have diabetes.[24]

- About 75% of autoimmune diseases occur in women and most often present during women's childbearing years. **Table 11.1** shows the disproportionate female-to-male ratios in autoimmune diseases. Reproductive hormones likely affect when (and how often) these diseases appear: Many autoimmune diseases improve during pregnancy and then reappear after delivery, appear after menopause, or get worse during pregnancy.[3]

Table 11.1 Female–Male Ratios in Autoimmune Diseases

Sjögren's syndrome	18:1
Hashimoto's disease/hypothyroiditis	9:1
Lupus	10:1
Scleroderma	4:1
Rheumatoid arthritis	2:1
Multiple sclerosis	2:1
Type 1 diabetes	1:1.1

Source: Adapted from Fairweather, D., & Rose, N. (2004). Women and autoimmune diseases. *Emerging Infectious Diseases* 10(11): 2005-2011.

- Women may be at greater risk for developing Alzheimer's disease (AD). Women's longer life spans make them more likely to develop AD, which is more likely to appear as a person ages. Even when they are not affected by the disease, women are affected by AD because they are most likely to be the primary care providers for their parents, spouses, and other family members.

Racial/Ethnic and Socioeconomic Dimensions

Rates and severity of chronic diseases vary among racial and ethnic groups. White and Asian American women have osteoporosis more often than African American women, owing to African Americans' higher bone mineral density. As they age, however, African American women's risk of osteoporosis changes to resemble that of white women, and their risk for hip fracture doubles approximately every seven years. African American women are more likely than white women to die following a hip fracture. Although it is not clear why this discrepancy exists, studies show that a woman's age, her health status, and the time frame in which she receives medical attention for the fracture are important predictors for a positive outcome following a hip fracture. Women who are older, have pre-existing medical conditions, and have a delay in surgery for a fracture are much more likely to die.

Racial differences are also evident with arthritis. U.S. survey data indicate that although blacks are about as likely as whites to have arthritis, they are more likely (10.1% ver-

sus 7.9%) to have more serious symptoms that limit their daily activities. Overall, blacks with doctor-diagnosed arthritis have a higher prevalence of severe pain attributable to arthritis, compared with whites (34.0% versus 22.6%).[4]

Diabetes is also more prevalent among non-white populations. As seen in **Figure 11.1**, non-Hispanic blacks have the highest prevalence rates of diabetes in the United States, followed by Hispanics and Asian Americans.[5]

Economic Dimensions

Chronic diseases dramatically affect both the national economy and individual lives. According to the CDC, more than 90 million Americans live with chronic diseases, and chronic diseases (including cardiovascular disease and cancer) account for 70% of all deaths in the United States. Overall, the medical care costs for chronic diseases account for more than 75% of America's $2 trillion in medical care costs. Chronic diseases decrease life expectancy and account for one-third of the years of potential life lost before age 65.[6]

Costs associated with specific chronic diseases are also staggering. Diabetes costs an estimated $132 billion per year. In 2003, the costs of arthritis and related conditions were $128 billion.[7] Bone fractures caused by osteoporosis cost Americans $12 to $18 billion per year.[8] National direct and indirect annual costs of caring for individuals with Alzheimer's disease are at least $100 billion.[9]

Individuals with chronic diseases sometimes struggle with paying for appropriate care, often having to turn to

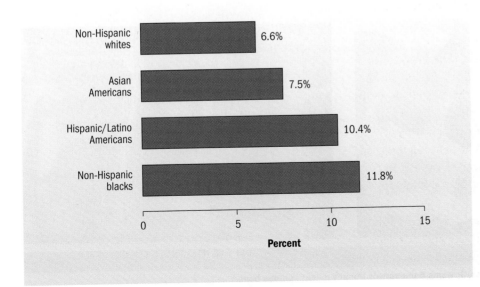

Figure 11.1

Age-adjusted total prevalence of diabetes in people aged 20 years or older, by race/ethnicity—United States, 2006.

Source: Centers for Disease Control and Prevention. (2007). *National Diabetes Fact Sheet.*

public insurance programs such as Medicaid or Medicare for coverage. Keeping a full-time job may become increasingly difficult for those with a chronic disease, so these people who desperately need health insurance may not be able to receive it from their employers. Others experience costs in their personal relationships as the strain of dealing with chronic disease damages marriages or other interpersonal relationships.

Women are also disproportionately affected by caregiving associated with chronic disease. Whether they or someone in their family is suffering, women carry the majority of the burden of care and support for patients.

Osteoporosis

Osteoporosis is an age-related, debilitating disorder characterized by a general decrease in bone mass and structural deterioration of bone tissue. Bone is living, growing tissue that changes throughout life. **Bone remodeling** is the process that removes older bone (resorption) and replaces it with new bone (formation) so as to maintain a healthy skeleton. Until a woman's mid-twenties, new bone forms faster than resorption occurs until peak bone mass is reached. After age 30, bone resorption begins to exceed bone formation. The first few years after menopause are the most significant for bone loss. As bone is lost, the skeletal structure weakens, leading to an increased risk of fracture. Osteoporosis develops when bone resorption occurs too quickly or bone replacement occurs too slowly (**Figure 11.2**).

Osteoporosis is a major cause of bone fractures in postmenopausal women and a leading cause of frailty. It affects approximately 8 million women, with millions more at increased risk of developing osteoporosis due to low bone mass. This translates to one in two women older than age 50 having an osteoporosis-related fracture in her lifetime. Osteoporosis is responsible for more than 1.5 million fractures per year, including 300,000 hip fractures, 700,000 vertebral fractures, 250,000 wrist fractures, and more than 300,000 fractures at other sites.[2]

Hip fractures are especially serious. Women have two to three times as many hip fractures as men, and white, postmenopausal women have a one in seven chance of hip fracture during their lifetime. The rate of hip fracture increases at age 50, doubling every five to six years. Nearly one-half of all women who reach age 90 have suffered a hip fracture.[10] Hip fractures present long-term problems when they occur. Only 25% of hip fracture patients will make a full recovery; 40% will require nursing home care, 50% will need a cane or walker, and 24% of those over age 50 will die within 12 months.[10]

Osteoporosis is often classified into three categories: primary, secondary, and fractures. Primary osteoporosis, the most common form, is diagnosed when other disorders known to cause osteoporosis are not present. Primary osteoporosis is also classified according to the age group of the patient:

- Juvenile osteoporosis affects prepubescent boys and girls.
- Idiopathic osteoporosis describes the condition in young adults when the cause is not related to another disease.
- Postmenopausal osteoporosis occurs in women within 15 to 20 years after menopause.

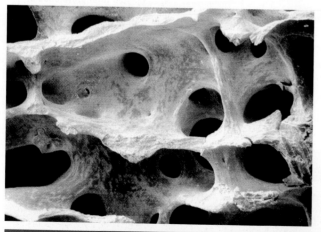 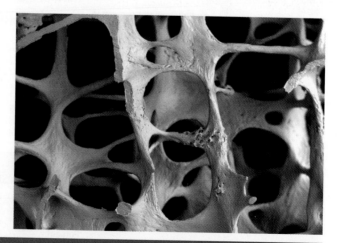

Figure 11.2

Left to right, healthy bone versus osteoporotic bone. Osteoporosis literally means "porous bone."

Table 11.2 Risk Factors for Osteoporosis

Risk Factors That Are Not Modifiable
- Being female
- Increased age/postmenopausal
- Small frame and thin-boned
- White or Asian race
- Family history of osteoporosis or fractures

Risk Factors That Are Modifiable
- Diet low in calcium and vitamin D
- Sedentary lifestyle
- Cigarette smoking
- Estrogen deficiency
- Low weight and body mass index
- Certain medications, such as glucocorticoids, some anticonvulsants, and thyroid hormones
- Abnormal absence of menstrual periods (amenorrhea)
- Anorexia nervosa or bulimia

Having one or more of these risk factors increases the risk of developing osteoporosis. The more risk factors a woman has, the greater her risk.

Postmenopausal osteoporosis, the most common form of primary osteoporosis, is characterized by low bone mass. **Table 11.2** outlines factors contributing to low bone mass. The use of alcohol and caffeine-containing beverages is inconsistently associated with decreased bone mass. Late menarche, early menopause, and low endogenous estrogen levels are also associated with low bone density.[11]

Secondary osteoporosis is diagnosed when the condition is related to another illness or to the use of medications or drugs. A variety of factors contribute to secondary osteoporosis, including congenital conditions, diet, drugs, endocrine disorders, and other systemic disorders.

Diet or nutritional disorders contributing to secondary osteoporosis include vitamin C deficiency, calcium or vitamin D deficiency, high-protein diet, high phosphate intake, and iron overload.

Risk Factors

Smoking is especially detrimental to bone health. Smoking is known to cause early menopause and can increase the rate of bone loss. The effects of smoking on bone health have been difficult to analyze in more detail because possible confounding factors, such as lifestyle differences between smokers and nonsmokers, may play a role. Smokers are often thinner, have higher alcohol intake, are more likely to lead sedentary lifestyles, and tend to have earlier menopause than nonsmokers do—all of which are risk factors for poor bone health. Additionally, inadequate calcium intake and a lack of regular weight-bearing exercise also increase the risk for developing osteoporosis.

Some medications may also cause bone loss. Many of these medications are used to treat other chronic conditions. For example, long-term use of glucocorticoids (medicines prescribed for a wide range of diseases including arthritis, asthma, Crohn's disease, and lupus) can lead to a loss of bone density and fractures. Antiseizure drugs, gonadotropin-releasing hormone (GnRH) analogs, excessive use of aluminum-containing antacids, certain cancer treatments, and excessive thyroid hormone also may cause bone loss. This possibility of bone loss is not a reason for women to stop taking these medications, however. Women using these medications should discuss their options for osteoporosis prevention with their health-care providers.

Certain medical conditions may lead to bone loss, including diseases of the thyroid gland such as hyperthyroidism and hypothyroidism. Amenorrhea (lack of menstrual periods) or diseases that lead to amenorrhea, such as anorexia nervosa, cause estrogen deficiencies, which in turn lead to accelerated bone loss (Table 11.2).

Signs and Symptoms

Osteoporosis is often called a "silent disease" because neither pain nor specific symptoms are associated with this condition. Only one out of four women who has osteoporosis is aware of the condition.[12] Some women notice a loss of height as the vertebrae weaken, collapse, and consequently fracture. When the bones in the spine fracture, a woman loses a small amount of height. The spine also begins to curve as multiple fractures occur.

Screening and Diagnosis

One "red flag" that signals a woman might have osteoporosis is a bone fracture that results from minimal trauma. To test for osteoporosis, a bone mass measurement (also referred to as a bone mineral density test) must be taken. Methods for measuring bone mineral density are painless,

My mother just found out that she has osteoporosis. I have watched my grandmother shrink with it. The doctor says that my mother can do some things to prevent further bone loss. The message for me is to prevent it from happening. I am now much more interested in diet and exercise.

26-year-old woman

Table 11.3   Bone Mineral Density Tests

- DXA (dual energy X-ray absorptiometry) measures the spine, hip, or total body.
- pDXA (peripheral dual energy X-ray absorptiometry) measures the wrist, heel, or finger.
- SXA (single energy X-ray absorptiometry) measures the wrist or heel.
- QUS (quantitative ultrasound) uses sound waves to measure density at the heel, shin bone, and kneecap.
- QCT (quantitative computed tomography) is most commonly used to measure the spine, but can be used at other sites.
- pQCT (peripheral quantitative computed tomography) measures the wrist.
- RA (radiographic absorptiometry) uses an X ray of the hand and a small metal wedge to calculate bone density.
- DPA (dual photon absorptiometry) measures the spine, hip, or total body (used infrequently).
- SPA (single photon absorptiometry) measures the wrist (used infrequently).

Source: National Osteoporosis Foundation. (2006). http://www.nof.org/osteoporosis/bonemass.htm.

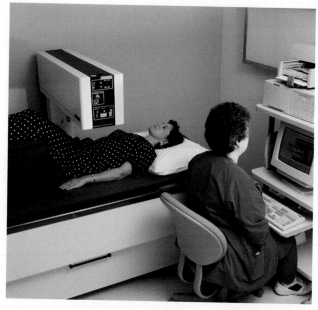

■ Bone mineral density tests are painless, noninvasive, and safe. Bone density may be measured in the spine, hip, wrist, finger, kneecap, shin bone, or heel, depending on the machine.

noninvasive, and safe. Traditional tests measure bone density in the areas most susceptible to fractures caused by osteoporosis: the spine, the hip, and the wrist. Newer machines measure density in the finger, the kneecap, the shin bone, and the heel (**Table 11.3**).

Women who should be tested include:

- All postmenopausal women younger than age 65 who have one or more additional risk factors for osteoporosis besides menopause.
- All women age 65 or older.
- Postmenopausal women with fractures.
- Women who are considering therapy for osteoporosis or who want to monitor the effectiveness of certain osteoporosis treatments.

Prevention and Treatment

In the absence of a cure for osteoporosis, prevention is the best strategy available. Lifestyle and personal behaviors are the key osteoporosis prevention strategies. A woman should not start smoking and she should quit if she already smokes.

An inadequate supply of calcium over a woman's lifetime is a major risk factor for developing osteoporosis. Calcium plays an important role in achieving peak bone mass, maintaining bone mass before menopause, and preventing bone loss in the postmenopausal years. Vitamin D is necessary for intestinal absorption of calcium. Studies show that supplemental calcium and vitamin D reduce the risk of fracture of the spine, hip, and other sites. Dietary calcium is preferable; however, supplements should be used if a woman cannot meet a daily intake of 1,000–1,200 milligrams per day (see Chapter 9). The typical diet of U.S. women contains less than 600 milligrams of calcium per day. Vitamin D is synthesized in the skin through exposure to sunlight and also can be provided through diet via vitamin D–fortified milk, cereal, egg yolks, saltwater fish, and liver. Those people who cannot obtain enough vitamin D naturally should include 200–600 IU (International Units) in their diets per day.

Participating in weight-bearing and muscle-strengthening exercises on a regular basis is important for osteoporosis prevention and overall health. These exercises improve agility, strength, and balance, thus reducing a woman's risk of falls, decreasing her risk of fractures. Weight-bearing exercises (exercises in which bones and muscles work against gravity) include walking, hiking, jogging, stairclimbing, dancing, and tennis. Muscle-strengthening exercise, such as weight-lifting, improves muscle mass and bone strength.

Bone loss accelerates after menopause, and long-term estrogen replacement therapy may help prevent osteoporo-

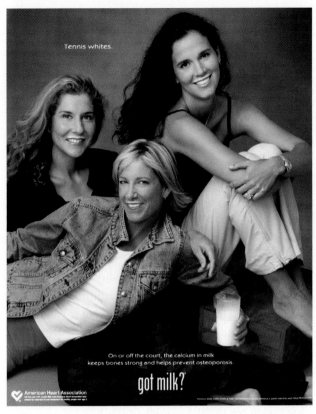

On or off the court, the calcium in milk keeps bones strong and helps prevent osteoporosis.

got milk?

American Heart Association

■ Fortified milk is one source of calcium and vitamin D, but foods such as leafy green vegetables can also supply this vital nutrient.

Table 11.4	Tips for Fall Prevention

Outdoors

- Use a cane or walker for added stability.
- Wear rubber-soled shoes for traction.
- Walk on grass when sidewalks are slippery.
- In winter, carry salt to sprinkle on slippery sidewalks.

Indoors

- Keep rooms free of clutter, especially on the floors.
- Be careful on highly polished floors that become slick and dangerous when wet.
- Avoid walking in socks, stockings, or slippers without rubber soles.
- Be sure carpets and area rugs have skid-proof backing or are tacked to the floor.
- Keep stairwells well lit.
- Attach handrails on both sides of all stairwells.
- Install grab bars on bathroom walls near tub, shower, and toilet.
- Use a rubber bath mat in shower or tub.
- Keep a flashlight with fresh batteries beside the bed.

sis and fractures in women by reducing bone resorption and slowing postmenopausal bone loss.[13]

Treating osteoporosis involves management of osteoporosis-associated fractures, universal prevention measures, and medical treatment of the underlying disease. Current osteoporosis recommendations indicate that all persons who have had osteoporotic vertebral or hip fractures and those with a bone mineral density diagnostic of osteoporosis should receive treatment. In women with a bone mineral density above the osteoporosis range, treatment may be indicated depending on the number and severity of other risk factors.[14]

Preventing fall-related fractures is also a special concern for women with osteoporosis. Many factors can cause falls, including impaired vision or balance, certain chronic diseases, and certain medications. A woman at risk should be aware of any factors that may affect her balance or gait, and she should discuss these changes with her health-care provider. Additionally, environmental factors can lead to falls; however, some of these factors can be easily prevented, as shown in **Table 11.4**.

Arthritis

Arthritis, defined as any inflammation of the joints, encompasses more than 100 diseases and conditions that affect joints, the surrounding tissues, and other connective tissues. Scientists do not fully understand the causes of arthritis. The most common forms of arthritis are osteoarthritis, rheumatoid arthritis, and gout. Regardless of the form, similar processes occur as the disease develops. All joints are encased in a capsule that contains lubricating fluid; if swelling and inflammation occur within the joint capsule, stiffness, rigidity, and pain during movement may result. Eventually a scar between the bones may develop, resulting in joint deformity. Recurrent joint pain in women is usually caused by arthritis.

Arthritis and other rheumatic conditions (conditions affecting the joints and muscles) are among the most common chronic conditions and the leading causes of disability in the United States. Arthritis affects at least 46 million Americans—more than one out of five adults.[14] The prevalence of arthritis is higher among women than among men. As the number of older Americans grows, so will the prevalence of arthritis, due to the high frequency of the disease among older adults. Although aging is a risk factor, nearly three of every five people with arthritis are younger than 65 years of age. Arthritis significantly affects quality of life, preventing more than 8.2 million people in the

United States from normally participating in their usual daily activities. By 2030, 65 million Americans 18 or older will have doctor-diagnosed arthritis.[15]

Osteoarthritis

Osteoarthritis, also called degenerative joint disease, is the most common form of arthritis, affecting more than 27 million people. A milder form of arthritis than rheumatoid arthritis, it is seen in all age groups but is most common among older adults. After age 50, osteoarthritis is more common in women than in men.[16]

In osteoarthritis, the surface layer of cartilage erodes, causing bones under the cartilage to rub together. This friction results in joint pain, swelling, and loss of movement of the joints. This disease most often affects the hips, knees, hands, neck, and lower back, but it may affect other joints as well. Joint stiffness and pain occur at the end of the day with osteoarthritis, and other body parts are usually not affected. Hip and knee osteoarthritis are the leading causes of arthritis disability and the primary reasons for joint replacement surgery.

Rheumatoid Arthritis

Rheumatoid arthritis is a chronic inflammatory disease with increasing prevalence among older adults. It currently affects 1.3 million people in the United States, and is twice as common in women as in men.[17]

Rheumatoid arthritis is an autoimmune disease, meaning that the person's immune system attacks the body's own cells. In this condition, the cells inside the joint capsule are attacked, causing inflammation and affecting the cells of the synovial (thin membrane inside the joint capsule). The abnormal synovial cells eventually invade and destroy cartilage and bone within the joint (**Figure 11.3**), which can lead to severe disability.

With this disease, inflammation occurs in the joint lining but may extend to other tissues and cause bone and cartilage erosion, joint deformities, movement problems, and activity limitations. Connective tissue and blood vessels also may be affected by inflammation; if inflammation affects other organs, such as the lung and the heart, a per-

I am twenty-three, and I have arthritis. Sometimes I am frightened that I will end up with gnarled hands like my grandmother. I hope that new treatments will prevent my disease progression.
23-year-old student

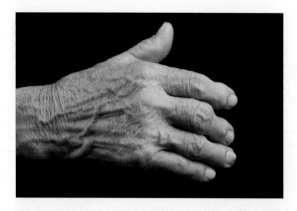
■ Arthritis can be phyically debilitating, as well as painful.

son may be at increased risk of mortality from respiratory and infectious diseases. Rheumatoid arthritis generally occurs in a symmetrical pattern, meaning that it will involve both the left and right hands, not just one of them. The disease varies significantly between individuals: Some people have flare-ups followed by periods of remission, whereas others have severe disease that is continuously active. Rheumatoid arthritis can also go away and not return.

Gout

Gout is a painful and potentially disabling form of arthritis that was first described more than 2,000 years ago by the Greek physician Hippocrates. Treatments can now control most cases of gout, but diagnosing gout can be difficult, and treatment plans often must be individualized. Gout is caused by an excess of uric acid in the body. This excess can result from an increased production of uric acid due to a metabolic disorder or the inability of the kidneys to adequately clear uric acid. Consumption of certain foods (such as shellfish) and an excess of alcoholic beverages may increase uric acid levels and precipitate gout attacks, but studies are not conclusive on these associations. Some medications and transplant drugs can also increase uric acid levels. With time, elevated levels of uric acid in the blood may be deposited around joints, especially in the feet and toes. Eventually, the uric acid may form needle-like crystals in joints, leading to acute painful gout attacks. Uric acid may also collect under the skin, where it is known as tophus, or in the urinary tract as kidney stones.

In the United States, gout afflicts an estimated 3.1 million people.[18] While gout and its complications occur more commonly in men, the disease also presents in women after menopause and in people with kidney disease. Gout is

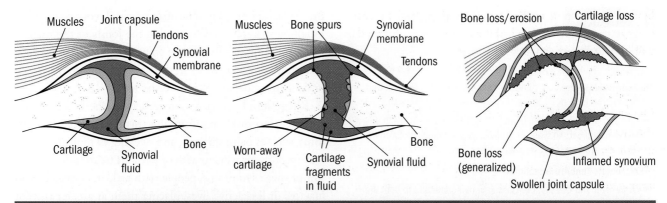

Figure 11.3

Left to right, healthy joint, joint affected by osteoarthritis, and joint affected by rheumatoid arthritis.

strongly associated with obesity, hypertension, hyperlipidemia, and diabetes. Some families have a genetic predisposition to gout. African Americans and people with poor kidney function are more likely to have gout attacks.

Diagnosis of gout can be tricky because several other kinds of arthritis can mimic a gout attack. Given that its treatment is specific to gout, proper diagnosis is essential. The definitive diagnosis of gout is dependent on finding uric acid crystals in the joint fluid during an acute attack. However, uric acid levels in the blood alone are often misleading and may be transiently normal or even low. Additionally, uric acid levels are often elevated in individuals without gout.

Since the 1800s, colchicine has been a standard treatment for acute gout. Although colchicine is very effective, its side effects may include nausea, vomiting, diarrhea, and other adverse events. Because of these side effects, nonsteroidal anti-inflammatory drugs (NSAIDs) have become the treatment of choice for most acute attacks of gout. NSAIDs may also have significant toxicity, but if used over a short term, they are generally well tolerated. However, some people are unable to take NSAIDs because of other medical factors such as ulcer disease, poor kidney function, or use of blood thinners. Elderly patients often cannot tolerate NSAIDs because of their multiple side effects. High doses of aspirin and aspirin-containing products should be avoided during acute attacks, but low-dose aspirin can be continued. Corticosteroid-type medications are also used to treat gout attacks and can be given as pills or by injection. Decisions about which treatment is appropriate must be tailored to the individual and depend on his or her kidney function and other medical factors. With correct treatment, gout should be well controlled in almost all cases.

Risk Factors

Arthritis is the leading chronic condition among women and a major cause of activity limitation.[19] Two to three times more women than men are affected by rheumatoid arthritis.[20] Risk also increases with age, with nearly half of the elderly population being affected by some form of arthritis. Some people are genetically predisposed to arthritis, placing them at higher risk for developing the disease. Other risk factors are modifiable, although altering these factors does not guarantee prevention. Obesity is one such factor. In 1971, obese people were approximately 20% more likely to develop arthritis than those who were not overweight. By 2002, that number jumped to 60%. These findings suggest that obesity has contributed to more cases of arthritis in recent years than in previous decades.[19] Joint injuries from sports, infectious diseases such as **Lyme disease**, and occupations that require repetitive joint use and knee bending are other factors that increase a person's risk of arthritis. **Table 11.5** summarizes the major risk factors associated with arthritis.

Because women are more likely than men to have rheumatoid arthritis, researchers have been studying the role of hormones in the development of the disease. The investigations conducted to date have produced contradictory results.

Arthritis is not uniformly distributed across the United States. The reasons for the inequitable distribution are unclear but are the subject of ongoing research. As

Table 11.5 Risk Factors for Arthritis

Risk Factors That Are Not Modifiable

■ Age: The risk of developing most types of arthritis increases with age.

■ Gender: Most types of arthritis are more common in women, who account for 60% of all cases. Gout is more common in men.

■ Genetic: Genes have been identified that are associated with a higher risk of certain types of arthritis, such as rheumatoid arthritis (RA) and systemic lupus erythematosus (SLE).

Risk Factors That Are Modifiable

■ Overweight and Obesity: Excess weight can contribute to both the onset and the progression of knee osteoarthritis.

■ Joint Injuries: Damage to a joint can contribute to the development of osteoarthritis of that joint.

■ Infection: Many microbial agents can infect joints and potentially cause the development of various forms of arthritis.

■ Occupation: Certain occupations involving repetitive knee bending are associated with osteoarthritis of the knee.

Source: Centers for Disease Control and Prevention. (2005). http://www .cdc.gov/arthritis/arthritis/risk_factors.htm.

Figure 11.4 shows, arthritis cases are most common in the middle eastern states and less prevalent in most other states.

Symptoms

Symptoms of arthritis depend on the specific disease affecting the joints. Osteoarthritis evolves slowly. Early in the disease, joints may ache after physical work or exercise. Small bony knobs may appear on the joints of the fingers, causing the fingers to become enlarged, gnarled, achy, stiff, and numb. Osteoarthritis in the knees or hips may make it difficult for a person to walk or bend.

Rheumatoid arthritis is regarded as the most painful and the most disabling form of arthritis in women. Symptoms, such as pain, stiffness, and swelling of multiple joints, may improve or worsen with or without treatment. As a result of these symptoms, people with arthritis typically lead inactive or less active lives, placing them at greater risk for other diseases, including heart disease, hypertension, diabetes, colon cancer, obesity, depression, and anxiety.

Diagnosis

No single test can diagnose arthritis. Instead, a medical and family history and a physical exam to check the joints, reflexes, and muscle strength are the first steps in diagnosis. Radiographs can determine the amount of damage done to a joint by showing cartilage loss, bone damage, and bone spurs. In the early stages of arthritis, before damage is evident, radiographs are not useful; however, they are helpful for monitoring the progression of the disease. Blood tests to determine the cause of the symptoms, a test for rheumatoid factor (an antibody present in most rheumatoid arthritis patients), and a joint aspiration (drawing fluid from the joint for examination) may also be used for diagnosing arthritis.

Figure 11.4

Percentage of adults with arthritis,* 2003.

Source: Centers for Disease Control and Prevention. (2005). *At a Glance— Targeting Arthritis: Reducing Disability for 43 Million Americans.* Atlanta, GA.

*People 18 or older with self-reported doctor-diagnosed arthritis.

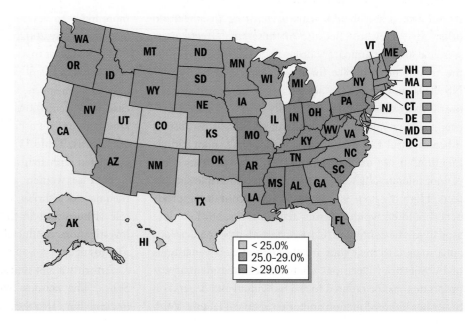

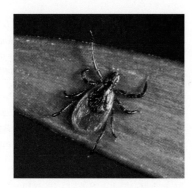

■ Infected deer ticks can transmit bacteria by biting humans, causing Lyme disease, which has many possible adverse outcomes, including arthritis.

Prevention and Treatment

Maintaining an appropriate weight is an important preventive measure. For people who are overweight, losing weight through healthful eating and regular exercise also can help reduce the effects of osteoarthritis. Precautions during, before, or after exercise can also reduce the chance of joint injury. Women should participate in warm-ups, strengthening exercises, and cool-downs when performing any type of exercise or sports-related activities. Other methods for preventing joint injury and damage to ligaments and cartilage, which in turn can prevent osteoarthritis, include avoiding contact sports and repetitive joint motion; wearing braces, pads, and proper shoes; and exercising on appropriate surfaces. Regular exercise decreases impairment by increasing muscle and joint function. Research has shown that weakness in a woman's quadricep muscles is a risk factor for osteoarthritis of the knee, and that exercise can significantly benefit knee osteoarthritis pathology.[21]

Another cause of arthritis is Lyme disease, a disease caused by the bacterium *Borrelia burgdorferi*. These bacteria are transmitted to humans by the bite of infected deer ticks and cause 24,000 infections in the United States each year.[22] After several months of being infected, more than half of people who are not treated with antibiotics experience recurrent attacks of painful and swollen joints. About 10% to 20% of these people develop chronic arthritis.[23] Strategies to prevent Lyme disease include using insect repellants, wearing long-sleeved shirts and pants when walking in wooded areas, and checking one's body for ticks immediately upon return.

The goals of treating arthritis are to decrease pain, improve joint care by slowing down or stopping joint damage, and improve a person's sense of well-being and ability to function. Exercise is one of the best treatments for arthritis. Such physical activity maintains healthy and strong muscles, preserves joint mobility, and maintains flexibility. It is important to exercise when pain is least severe and to recognize when rest is necessary. Resting the body reduces active joint inflammation and pain and prevents pain from over-exercising. Canes, splints, or braces may be used to temporarily take pressure off joints or to provide extra support. Controlling body weight through a healthful diet is also an important way to reduce stress on weight-bearing joints and limit further injury.

Many people with osteoarthritis or rheumatoid arthritis use medications to reduce pain and inflammation, as well as prevent joint damage:

- NSAIDs, either in prescription or over-the-counter form, can reduce pain, swelling, and inflammation.

- Topical pain-relieving creams, rubs, and sprays, such as those containing capsaicin, are applied directly to the skin to relieve pain.

- Corticosteroids (anti-inflammatory hormones) may be used for short-term pain relief, stiffness, and swelling and to reduce the risk of joint swelling.

- Hyaluronic acid, a medication for joint injection, is useful for relieving pain associated with osteoarthritis of the knee.

- For rheumatoid arthritis, disease-modifying anti-rheumatic drugs (DMARDs) may produce significant improvement. DMARDs are used to alter the course of rheumatoid arthritis and to prevent joint and cartilage destruction. Serious side effects can occur, however, so the medications are not appropriate for everyone.

- Biologic response modifiers (BRMs) inhibit proteins called cytokines that contribute to inflammation and joint damage in rheumatoid arthritis. BRMs must be injected under the skin or given as an infusion into a vein.

- Immunosuppressants appear to be very effective in restraining the active immune system, the key to the disease process. These medications can cause side effects, however, and their effectiveness appears to diminish over time.

Another option for treatment is surgery. Surgery may be performed to resurface and reposition bones, replace joints, remove loose pieces of bone or cartilage, reconstruct tendons, or remove inflamed synovial tissue. Some people may find relief through alternative treatments, such as acupuncture, nutritional supplements, relaxation techniques, and biofeedback. Although most of these approaches are not harmful, studies have not been conducted to prove that they offer a definite benefit.

Diabetes

Diabetes is a disease characterized by abnormal glucose production or metabolism. A person with diabetes has either a deficiency of insulin (the hormone produced by the pancreas and needed to convert glucose to energy), or a decreased ability to use insulin. As a result, glucose builds up in the bloodstream, and, without treatment, will damage organs and contribute to heart disease.

There are three major kinds of diabetes: type 1, type 2, and gestational diabetes. Type 1 diabetes is often classified as an autoimmune disease, though genetic and environmental factors can also influence its development. In this type of diabetes, the body's immune system attacks the cells that produce insulin, the hormone that regulates blood glucose. Type 1 diabetes often first appears in childhood or adolescence, and it accounts for about 5% of total cases of diabetes. About 90% to 95% of people with diabetes have type 2 diabetes. In this form of diabetes, cells are unable to use insulin properly. **Gestational diabetes** occurs when women become intolerant to glucose during pregnancy. After pregnancy, gestational diabetes usually but not always goes away. Women who have had gestational diabetes are at high risk of developing type 2 diabetes within the next 5 to 10 years.

Most people with type 1 diabetes develop the disease early in life, while type 2 diabetes generally occurs later in life; however, the rise in childhood obesity is leading to a dramatic surge in the incidence of type 2 diabetes among children and adolescents.

Diabetes is becoming more common in the United States (**Figure 11.5**). In 2007, 23.6 million people, or 7.8% of the U.S. population, had diabetes.[24] According to the CDC's most recent analysis:

- Almost half of the people with diabetes are female. About 10.2% of women age 20 or older have diabetes.

- Minority racial and ethnic groups are the hardest hit by type 2 and gestational diabetes; the prevalence is at least two to four times higher among black, Hispanic, American Indian, and Asian/Pacific Islander women than among white women.

- The risk of diabetic ketoacidosis (DKA), often called diabetic coma, is 50% higher among women than men.

- Heart disease is the leading cause of diabetes-related

> *Dramatic new evidence signals the unfolding of a diabetes epidemic in the United States. With obesity on the rise, we can expect the sharp increase in diabetes rates to continue. Unless these dangerous trends are halted, the impact on our nation's health and medical care costs will be overwhelming.*
>
> **Jeffrey P. Koplan, MD, MPH**
> **Director, Centers for Disease Control**
> **and Prevention, 1998–2002**

deaths. Adults with diabetes have heart disease rates and risk for stroke rates about two to four times higher than adults without diabetes.

Researchers have also identified pre-diabetes, a condition in which a person has abnormally high blood-glucose levels, but does not have diabetes. An estimated 57 million people in the United States—about one out of six Americans—had pre-diabetes in 2007.[24] Pre-diabetes often progresses to type 2 diabetes, but weight loss and regular exercise can prevent or delay this progression.

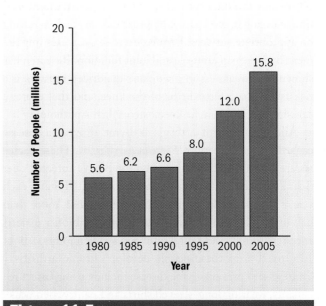

Figure 11.5

Number of persons with diagnosed diabetes, United States.

Source: Centers for Disease Control and Prevention, National Center for Health Statistics. (2007). National Diabetes Data and Trends. http://www.cdc.gov/diabetes/statistics/prev/national/figpersons.htm.

The number of cases of diabetes in the United States has nearly tripled over the last 25 years.

My grandmother had diabetes, but she was not always good about taking care of herself. She always loved taking us out for ice cream when I was a girl, and I worry that these habits may have contributed to her stroke. I also worry about myself and my father—a strong sweet tooth runs in our family, but I don't want either of us to suffer like my grandmother did.

24-year-old woman

Risk Factors

Risk factors for diabetes include having a first-degree relative (mother, father, or sibling) with diabetes, being overweight, and having hypertension or abnormal high-density lipoprotein (HDL) or triglyceride levels. African Americans, Hispanics, and American Indians/Alaska Natives are at increased risk for developing type 2 diabetes. American Indians have the highest rate of diabetes in the United States—for example, 14.9% of American Indians and Alaska Natives age 20 years or older and receiving care from the Indian Health Services have diabetes.[5] **It's Your Health** provides a checklist of factors to ascertain personal risk of diabetes.

Symptoms and Complications

Symptoms of type 1 diabetes usually develop over a short period of time. They may include increased thirst and urination, constant hunger, weight loss, blurred vision, and extreme tiredness. If not treated with insulin, a person can lapse into a coma and eventually die. Symptoms of type 2 diabetes develop gradually. Although they are not as noticeable as symptoms of type 1 disease, type 2 symptoms are similar and include frequent urination, unusual thirst, weight loss, blurred vision, feelings of fatigue or illness, frequent infections, and slow healing of sores.

The most alarming part of diabetes is the severity of the complications associated with the disease (**Table 11.6**). Diabetes is the leading cause of new cases of blindness in adults 20 to 74 years of age. Each year, an estimated 12,000 to 24,000 people become blind because of diabetic eye disease. Early detection and treatment can prevent 90% of these cases of blindness.[24] Diabetes is also the leading cause of end-stage renal disease (ESRD) or kidney failure, accounting for about 44% of new cases.[26] At least half of the new cases of diabetes-related kidney failure could be prevented each year.

Because unregulated diabetes causes thickening of blood, circulation issues are common. As a result, many

It's Your Health

Am I at Risk for Diabetes?

- I am 45 or older.
- I am overweight.
- I have a parent, brother, or sister with diabetes.
- My family background is Alaska Native, American Indian, African American, Hispanic/Latino American, Asian American, or Pacific Islander.
- I have had gestational diabetes, or I gave birth to at least one baby weighing more than 9 pounds.
- My blood pressure is 140/90 mm Hg or higher, or I have been told that I have high blood pressure.
- My cholesterol levels are not normal. My HDL cholesterol ("good" cholesterol) is below 35 mg/dL or my triglyceride level is above 250 mg/dL.
- I am fairly inactive. I exercise fewer than three times per week.
- I have polycystic ovary syndrome (PCOS) (women only).
- On previous testing, I had impaired glucose tolerance (IGT) or impaired fasting glucose (IFG).
- I have other clinical conditions associated with insulin resistance (acanthosis nigricans).
- I have a history of cardiovascular disease.

The more items you checked, the higher your risk.

Anyone 45 years old or older should consider getting tested for diabetes. If you are 45 or older and overweight, getting tested is strongly recommended. If you are younger than 45, are overweight, and have one or more of the risk factors above, you should consider testing. Ask your doctor for a fasting blood glucose test or an oral glucose tolerance test. Your doctor will tell you if you have normal blood glucose, pre-diabetes, or diabetes.

Source: NIH, NDIC. (2006). Am I at Risk for Getting Diabetes? Available at http://diabetes.niddk.nih.gov/dm/pubs/riskfortype2/.

Table 11.6 Complications of Diabetes

- Heart disease, including peripheral vascular disease, coronary heart disease, and cardiac failure
- Stroke
- High blood pressure
- Retinopathy (broken blood vessels in retina)/blindness
- End-stage renal disease (kidney failure)
- Damage of the nervous system
- Lower-extremity amputations
- Periodontal disease
- Congenital malformations/spontaneous abortions
- Neonatal mortality
- Macrosomia (large-birthweight babies)
- Diabetic ketoacidosis (coma)
- Susceptibility to infections and illness, such as pneumonia

people have trouble healing from injuries, especially in their extremities. About 60% to 70% of people with diabetes suffer mild to severe forms of damage to their nervous system, including impaired sensation or pain in the feet. If severe, the nerve damage can require lower-limb amputation. More than 60% of nontraumatic lower-limb amputations occur among people with diabetes.[24] Amputations are also caused by infection related to nonhealing diabetic foot ulcers. New treatments for nonhealing diabetic foot ulcers include genetically engineered replacement dermis, growth hormone products, and better wound management programs.

Adults with diabetes are two to four times as likely to develop heart disease or stroke as those without diabetes. In fact, heart disease is the leading cause of diabetes-related deaths. Women with poorly controlled diabetes also are at risk of diabetic ketoacidosis, a serious condition in which acid levels increase in the blood. Diabetes is known to affect brain function and increase the risk for cognitive decline, dementia, depression, and stroke. These complications frequently occur together, leading to poor quality of life with considerable social and economic implications. Although the results of different studies may be contradictory, the overall conclusion is that diabetes, often associated with high blood pressure, contributes to cognitive decline in elderly diabetics as well as to increased frequency and severity of cerebral vascular events.[25,26]

Pregnancy presents special risks to diabetic women. Women are more likely to have healthy pregnancies if their diabetes is well controlled before they become pregnant and throughout the pregnancy. The risk of serious congenital malformations and macrosomia (large birthweight) in babies born to mothers with diabetes is greater than in the general population. Due to the increased incidence of babies with large birthweights, women with diabetes are three to four times more likely to have a cesarean delivery than are women without diabetes. In addition, 3% to 5% of pregnancies among women with diabetes result in death of the newborn, compared with 1.5% for women who do not have diabetes.[24]

I was diagnosed with diabetes at the age of five. I still remember being in the hospital and how scared I was. My father died young from diabetes complications. I am determined to learn as much as I can to take care of myself.

32-year-old woman

Diagnosis

The routine test for diagnosing diabetes is a fasting plasma glucose test. A doctor may choose to perform an oral glucose tolerance test, which involves a fasting blood sample followed by numerous blood samples after glucose syrup is ingested. The "gold standard" for diagnosing diabetes is an elevated blood sugar level after an overnight fast (not eating anything after midnight). A value above 126 mg/dL on at least two occasions typically means a person has diabetes. People without diabetes have fasting sugar levels that generally run between 70 and 110 mg/dL. A fasting glucose level of 100 to 125 mg/dL indicates a form of prediabetes called impaired fasting glucose (IFG), meaning that the person is more likely to develop type 2 diabetes but does not have it yet.[27]

Prevention and Treatment

Type 1 diabetes can be managed through a strict regimen of multiple daily insulin injections, a carefully calculated diet, planned physical activity, and home blood glucose testing several times a day. Treatment of type 2 diabetes is also based on diet control, exercise, and blood glucose testing, and for some people may entail oral medications or insulin. Daily management is important to control blood sugar levels from going too high or too low. **Hypoglycemia** (low blood sugar levels) can cause a person to become nervous, shaky, and confused and can result in the person passing out. Consumption of food or drink with sugar in it can counteract low blood sugar. If levels rise too high, as in **hyperglycemia**, a person may become very ill. Early signs of hyperglycemia include high blood sugar, high levels of sugar in the urine, frequent urination, and increased thirst. Hyperglycemia should be treated as an emergency situation and emergency services (such as 911) should be called immediately.

Autoimmune Diseases

Autoimmune diseases, in which the immune system attacks normal components of the body, are more common among women than among men. More than 80 serious, chronic illnesses are collectively referred to as autoimmune diseases, and these diseases involve the nervous, gastrointestinal, and endocrine systems, as well as skin and other connective tissue, eyes, blood, and blood vessels. Approximately 75% of autoimmune diseases occur in women, most frequently first manifesting during the childbearing years.[28] These diseases include multiple sclerosis, type 1 diabetes, scleroderma, rheumatoid arthritis, thyroid disorders, Sjögren's syndrome, and systemic lupus erythematosus (SLE). Rheumatoid arthritis, diabetes, SLE, and thyroid disease are the most common autoimmune diseases. Together, autoimmune diseases represent the fourth largest cause of disability among women in the United States.[28]

Lupus

Lupus is a disease that is still not fully understood. In patients with lupus, the immune system forms antibodies that target healthy tissues and organs. Lupus can be a mild, moderate, or severe disease. Although lupus may affect men and women of any age, it is primarily a disease of young women of childbearing age. This condition affects women 10 to 15 times more often than it does men, and it affects African American women two to three times more often than it does white women.[29]

Lupus presents in three forms. Discoid lupus, also known as cutaneous lupus, only affects the skin and causes a rash that usually appears on the face and upper body. Only about 10% of people with discoid lupus will progress to the systemic form of lupus, which can involve any organ or system of the body. Systemic lupus erythematosus (SLE) is the most common and more severe form of the disease; it is characterized by unpredictable periods of disease activity and periods of symptom-free remission. SLE can affect many parts of the body, including joints, skin, kidneys, lungs, heart, blood vessels, nervous system, blood, and brain. Drug-induced lupus is a reaction to some prescription medicines. The symptoms of this type of lupus are similar to SLE, but do not affect the kidneys or central nervous system. Drug-induced lupus usually disappears when the medication is discontinued.[30]

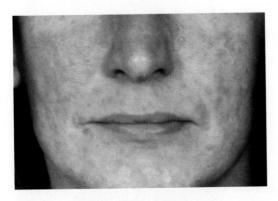

■ A rash is a common symptom of lupus.

Risk Factors

The cause of lupus is unknown, although genetic, hormonal, and environmental factors appear to play a role. Lupus is known to occur within families, although no specific gene for it has been found. Environmental factors, including infections, exposure to sunlight, stress, and certain medications, play a role in triggering flare-ups of the disease. Because the cause of lupus is unknown, it has been difficult to determine its risk factors.

Symptoms

Lupus has been called "the great imitator" because of its varied symptoms, which often mimic other, less serious illnesses. Lupus is characterized by periods of remission when no symptoms are present. The two most common symptoms are painful, swollen joints and a skin rash. In addition to being nonspecific, symptoms of lupus vary from person to person because lupus can affect any organ or organ system. Although lupus can affect any part of the body, most people experience symptoms in only a few organs. **Table 11.7** summarizes the symptoms of lupus.

Table 11.7 Lupus Symptoms

Symptom	Percentage of Cases
Achy joints (arthralgia)	95%
Frequent fevers of more than 100°F	90%
Arthritis (swollen joints)	90%
Prolonged or extreme fatigue	81%
Skin rashes	74%
Anemia	71%
Kidney involvement	50%
Pain in the chest on deep breathing (pleurisy)	45%
Butterfly-shaped rash across the cheek and nose	42%
Sun or light sensitivity (photosensitivity)	30%
Hair loss	27%
Abnormal blood clotting problems	20%
Raynaud's phenomenon (fingers turning white and/or blue in the cold)	17%
Seizures	15%
Mouth or nose ulcers	12%

Source: Courtesy of Robert G. Lahita, MD, PhD, from the LFA brochure, "What Is Lupus?" Reprinted with permission from the Lupus Foundation of America, Inc. All rights reserved.

The origins of lupus remain a mystery and are the subject of considerable speculation and research. Cigarette smoking is one of many environmental exposures, including infectious agents, silica exposure, and hormonal and dietary factors, such as vitamin D, hypothesized to be linked to the development of SLE.[31,32] However, the root causes of lupus likely involve more than these factors.

Diagnosis

The clinical diagnosis of systemic lupus involves taking note of symptoms of lupus, such as skin rash, joint pain, chest pain, seizures, and photosensitivity, and reviewing a person's history of medications. A complete blood count and urinalysis may provide evidence of the involvement of the kidneys and blood vessels. The antinuclear antibody test (ANA) may be used to rule out a diagnosis of lupus. It is positive in virtually all people with lupus and is the best diagnostic tool available for lupus. ANA is not a definitive test, however, because a positive ANA result can be found in people with certain other illnesses and conditions, people using certain medications, or even people in the general population without any illnesses.

Treatment and Prevention

Lupus is characterized by periods of symptoms called "flare-ups." The symptoms are unpredictable and inconsistent when they present.

Women with lupus can take preventive measures to help prevent flare-ups. People who are photosensitive should avoid sun exposure and regularly use sunscreen to prevent rashes. Exercise is important to prevent muscle weakness and fatigue, while stress reduction can be achieved through support groups and counseling. Treatment usually involves nonsteroidal anti-inflammatory drugs (NSAIDs) to ease muscle and joint pain. Corticosteroids are used on a short-term basis to treat skin rashes. Some people find antimalarial agents, such as Plaquenil or Aralen, helpful for skin and joint symptoms, as well as oral ulcers. Immunosuppressant drugs may be used in serious cases of lupus, when major organs are losing their ability to function. These drugs suppress, or turn down, the immune system to limit the damage done to the organ(s) and reduce inflammation. Serious side effects may occur with their use, including nausea, vomiting, hair loss, bladder problems, decreased fertility, and increased risk of cancer and infection.

Thyroid Disease

The thyroid is a small gland, shaped like a butterfly, located in the middle of the lower neck. Its primary function is to control the body's metabolism—the rate at which cells perform duties essential to living. To control body metabolism, the thyroid produces two hormones, T_4 and T_3, that regulate cell energy.

Figure 11.6

Thyroiditis.

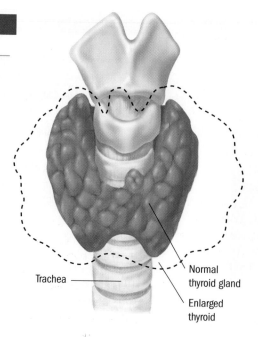
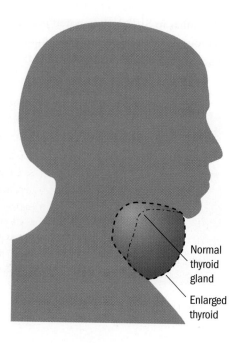

Trachea

Normal thyroid gland

Enlarged thyroid

Normal thyroid gland

Enlarged thyroid

A properly functioning thyroid will maintain the right amount of hormones needed to keep the body's metabolism functioning at a steady state. The quantity of thyroid hormones in the bloodstream is monitored and controlled by the pituitary gland, which is located in the center of the skull below the brain. When the pituitary gland senses either a lack of thyroid hormones or a high level of thyroid hormones, it will adjust its own thyroid-stimulating hormone (TSH) and send messages to the thyroid to regulate hormone production.

Thyroiditis is an inflammation of the thyroid gland (**Figure 11.6**). When the thyroid produces too much hormone, the body uses energy faster than it should; this condition is called hyperthyroidism. When the thyroid doesn't produce enough hormone, the body uses energy slower than it should; this condition is called hypothyroidism. The American Association of Clinical Endocrinologists estimates that more than 27 million Americans have overactive or underactive thyroid glands, but more than half are undiagnosed.[33]

Hypothyroidism results from an underactive thyroid. Hypothyroidism can be caused by a lack of iodine in the diet. Another common cause is a condition known as Hashimoto's thyroiditis, or Hashimoto's disease. This autoimmune condition is caused when the immune system reacts against the thyroid gland. About 8 million Americans have this condition, and most of them are women.[34] Because people with hypothyroidism lack enough thyroid hormones to properly run their metabolisms, they often

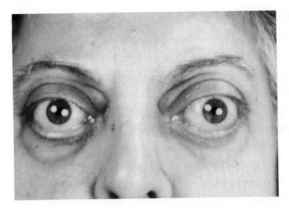

■ There are many symptoms of Graves' disease, including increased appetite, weight loss, nervousness, insomnia, and bulging appearance of the eyes.

have symptoms associated with having low energy. (See **Table 11.8** for a full list of symptoms.)

Hyperthyroidism occurs when the body produces too much thyroid hormone. Because the excess of thyroid hormone increases the body's metabolism by as much as 60% to 100%, people with hyperthyroidism often feel symptoms associated with being overstimulated. (See Table 11.8 for a full list of symptoms.)[35] Graves' disease, an autoimmune disorder in which the immune system stimulates the thyroid, causes about 80% of hyperthyroid cases. Hyperthyroidism is 8 to 10 times more common in women than in men.[36] In some cases, people with hyperthyroidism may have moderate to severe eye problems, which may cause bulging of the eyes, blurring of vision, or damage to the eyes.

Table 11.8 Symptoms of Hypothyroidism and Hyperthyroidism

Many people may have no symptoms.

Hypothyroidism		Hyperthyroidism	
■ Feeling tired and listless	■ Hoarse voice	■ Weight loss	■ Diarrhea
■ Fatigue	■ Slow heart rate	■ Heat tolerance	■ Vision problems, eye irritation
■ Difficulty concentrating	■ Leg cramps	■ Shakes and tremors of hands	■ For women, lighter periods, as well as difficulties in becoming pregnant or in carrying the child to term
■ Sensitivity to cold	■ Difficulty swallowing	■ Feeling nervous and irritable	
■ Dry skin	■ Sore muscles	■ Increased energy expenditure	
■ Dry, coarse hair and hair loss	■ Depression	■ Diarrhea	■ For men, loss of interest in sex, erectile dysfunction
■ Constipation	■ For men, loss of interest in sex, erectile dysfunction	■ Sweating more than normal	
■ Heavy and irregular menses		■ Fingernails growing faster	■ Sleep disturbances
■ Slow-growing and brittle fingernails	■ Weight gain due to fluid retention, but usually no more than 3–4 pounds	■ Muscle weakness, especially thighs and upper arms	■ Eyes that appear larger than normal
■ Feeling of fullness in throat	■ Goiter	■ Faster heart rate, sometimes irregular rhythms and an erratic pulse	

Risk Factors

Both Hashimoto's disease and Graves' disease are inherited conditions. Risk factors include being a woman over 20 years old, although the disorder may occur at any age and may affect men. Risk factors for thyroid disorders do not seem to be a direct cause of the disease, but seem to be associated with it in some way. Having a risk factor for thyroid disorders makes the chances of developing a condition higher but does not inevitably lead to a thyroid disorder. Likewise, people without known risk factors can still develop thyroid disorders.

Risk factors for thyroid conditions include the following:

- Family history of thyroid disease
- Previous thyroid concerns, nodules, enlargement, or goiter
- Previous transient thyroid condition during a pregnancy

Symptoms

Table 11.8 summarizes clinical manifestations of Hashimoto's disease and Graves' disease. However, many people have no symptoms, and symptoms rarely occur all at once.

Screening and Diagnosis

Thyroid disease can be difficult to diagnose because its symptoms are easily confused with other conditions. A comprehensive history and physical examination are integral to a diagnosis of thyroiditis. Such an examination would include weight and blood pressure, pulse rate and cardiac rhythm, and examination of the thyroid, neuromuscular system, eyes, skin, and the cardiovascular and lymphatic systems.[37]

Laboratory testing is also important. The thyroid-stimulating hormone (TSH) test is generally used as a screening test because it can often identify thyroid disorders before the onset of symptoms. Blood tests measuring levels of thyroxine (T_4) are also used to confirm the presence of thyroid disease.

When thyroid disease is caught early, treatment can control the disorder even before symptoms become evident.

Treatment

Treatment for Hashimoto's disease is based on determining the correct amount of thyroid hormone (thyroxine) needed to stimulate the thyroid gland. Gradually increasing doses of thyroxine are given until a person's blood levels become normal. Annual checkups are necessary to confirm that the prescribed dose is still appropriate. During pregnancy, doses of thyroxine usually increase; as a person

ages, doses usually decrease. Overtreatment of hypothyroidism with thyroid hormone can result in bone loss. Graves' disease is treated with antithyroid drugs to prevent the thyroid gland from manufacturing thyroid hormone.

Alzheimer's Disease

Alzheimer's disease is an irreversible, progressive brain disorder that evolves gradually and results in memory loss, behavior and personality changes, and a decline in cognitive abilities. It is one of a group of disorders that cause **dementia** (cognitive decline). The changes result from the death of brain cells and the breakdown of the connections between them. The progression of Alzheimer's disease and the resulting cognitive decline vary from person to person. People with this disease usually live anywhere from 3 to 20 years after first showing symptoms.[38] Alzheimer's disease is the most common cause of dementia among people age 65 or older, with approximately 5 million people currently suffering from it. This number will increase as the population ages.[39] The risk of developing Alzheimer's disease increases with age; however, the disease and symptoms of dementia are not a part of normal aging.

The main characteristics of the brain in a person with Alzheimer's disease include amyloid plaques and neurofibrillary tangles. Plaques are dense deposits of protein and cellular material that form outside and around the brain's neurons. Researchers are not certain whether the plaques cause the disease or are simply a by-product of the disease process. Tangles are insoluble twisted fibers that build up inside neurons. A form of a protein called tau is the main

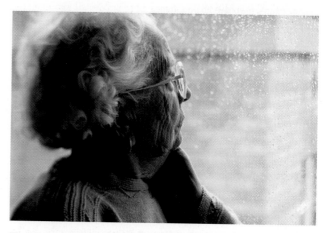

■ Alzheimer's disease is a devastating disease that results in memory loss, behavior and personality changes, and a decline in cognitive abilities.

component of the tangles. In healthy neurons, tau proteins help stabilize a cell's structure. In brains affected by Alzheimer's disease, the tau protein is chemically altered and cannot hold the structure together. The resulting collapse is responsible for malfunctions in communication.

Risk Factors

It is not fully understood what causes Alzheimer's disease, but it is clear that its onset can be triggered by age, genetic background, and possibly lifestyle. These factors can interact differently from person to person. Some studies have implicated female gender, severe or repeated head injuries, lower education levels, and environmental agents as risk factors; however, more studies are needed to determine the exact relationship among these risk factors and the development of Alzheimer's.

Familial Alzheimer's disease (FAD) follows a pattern of inheritance. It often has an early onset, meaning that it occurs most often in people younger than 65. FAD often progresses faster than the more common form of Alzheimer's disease, which typically occurs in people age 65 or older. As many as 50% of FAD cases are caused by defects in three genes located on three different chromosomes. Even if only one of these mutations is inherited from a parent, a person will inevitably develop a form of early-onset Alzheimer's. Genetics play a role in late-onset disease as well; however, a person can inherit the gene associated with late-onset Alzheimer's and not get the disease. Similarly, people with late-onset Alzheimer's may not have any genetic factor.

The risk of developing Alzheimer's increases with age. One out of every 10 persons 65 years or older is a victim of Alzheimer's disease, although early-onset victims may be in their forties or fifties. Approximately 20% of Americans between the ages of 75 and 84, or almost half of those 85 years or older, suffer from Alzheimer's disease.[40]

Symptoms

Alzheimer's disease disrupts three key processes in the brain: nerve cell communication, metabolism, and repair. This disruption causes many nerve cells to stop functioning, lose connections with other nerve cells, and die. The disease advances by stages, from early, mild forgetfulness to severe loss of mental function (i.e., dementia). Symptoms usually first appear after age 65.

The disease first destroys neurons in parts of the brain that control memory; as a result, a person's ability to do easy and familiar tasks begins to decline. People in the ini-tial stages of disease often think less clearly and forget the names of familiar people and common objects. Later in the disease, they may forget how to do simple tasks, such as brushing their teeth. The cerebral cortex, particularly the area responsible for language and reasoning, is affected next, disrupting a person's language skills and ability to make judgments. Personality changes also may occur. Emotional outbursts and disturbing behavior, such as wandering and agitation, become more frequent as the disease runs its course. Eventually, many other areas of the brain are involved. All of these brain regions atrophy, and the person becomes bedridden, incontinent, totally helpless, unresponsive to the outside world, and susceptible to a variety of illnesses and infections. People with Alzheimer's disease often die from pneumonia.

Diagnosis

At this time, there is no definitive diagnosis for Alzheimer's disease. The only way to conclusively diagnose it is through autopsy, by examining the characteristic plaques and tangles in the brain.

Currently, several tools are used to diagnose possible Alzheimer's disease in a person who is having difficulties with memory or other mental functions. A health-care provider will examine a person's history, do a complete physical exam, run various laboratory tests and brain scans, and perform tests that measure memory, language skills, and other abilities related to brain functioning. Using these special tests, clinicians can now diagnose Alzheimer's with up to 90% accuracy.[41] It is important to rule out other illnesses or medications that can cause dementia; severe depression in the elderly is often accompanied by memory loss and therefore is often confused with Alzheimer's. Depression and Alzheimer's disease do coexist in many patients.

Researchers are currently studying brain imaging techniques to improve their ability to detect biological changes or signs of dysfunction in the brain. The earlier an accurate diagnosis of disease can be made, the better the chance of managing symptoms and helping patients and their families plan for future care while the patient is still able to take part in the decision-making process.

My grandfather has Alzheimer's disease. My mother tries to take care of him but it is very difficult. Sometimes my sisters and I feel angry that she does not have time for us even when we understand that he needs her attention.

20-year-old woman

Treatment and Research

There is no cure for Alzheimer's disease, but the FDA has approved several medications for its treatment. These drugs may delay memory decline for some individuals, but they do not stop the underlying degeneration of brain cells. Research is producing new insights into many Alzheimer's concerns. Studies are showing how drug and nondrug approaches to treatment can improve daily functioning, treat specific symptoms, and maximize quality of life. Although drug therapy is important and beneficial, especially in early stages of the disease, the management of Alzheimer's has evolved to include nonpharmacological therapies as integral aspects of care. These therapies include the management of problematic behaviors, home or "environmental" modifications, and the use of appropriate communication techniques. Support and education for caregivers and family members are also crucial to the best care of people with Alzheimer's.

The care of a person who has Alzheimer's disease is challenging on many fronts. More than 70% of people with Alzheimer's live at home, where family and friends provide their care.[38] Care can be emotionally devastating, physically demanding, and a financial burden. Caregivers are subject to high levels of chronic stress, and caregiver burnout is a major factor in the inability to continue caring for a person with Alzheimer's at home.

Physical activity, good nutrition, and social interaction are important for keeping Alzheimer's patients as functional as possible. Maintaining a calm, safe, structured environment also helps patients feel better and remain independent longer. Drugs can help soothe agitation, anxiety, depression, and sleeplessness, and may help boost participation in daily activities. Newer medications can also improve or preserve thinking skills, at least temporarily.

Genetic research is an important area of Alzheimer's disease study. Scientists have found genetic links to the two forms of Alzheimer's disease. Early-onset Alzheimer's is a very rare form of the disease that can occur in people between the ages of 30 and 60. In the 1980s, researchers found that mutations (or changes) in certain genes on three chromosomes cause early-onset disease. A person has a 50% chance of developing early-onset disease if one parent has any of these genetic mutations.

Late-onset Alzheimer's disease, the more common form, develops after age 65. Certain forms of the apolipoprotein E (APOE) gene can influence this Alzheimer's disease risk. Scientists are now intensively searching for other genes that may be linked to Alzheimer's. Discovering these genes is essential for understanding the disease's etiology and identifying targets for new drug development and other prevention or treatment strategies.

In 2003, a major expansion of Alzheimer's genetics research efforts began. The Alzheimer's Disease Genetics Study, which will end in 2010, is collecting genetic material and cell lines from individuals in families with more than two living siblings who have late-onset Alzheimer's disease. This program helps geneticists find additional genes that may be risk factors for Alzheimer's.

■■■■
Informed Decision Making

Lifestyle changes are often the first step toward chronic disease prevention. A healthy diet, regular exercise, and avoidance of harmful substances are standard methods for health promotion. Other important approaches toward disease prevention include being knowledgeable about chronic diseases and their symptoms and visiting one's health-care provider regularly. A woman who knows her body can recognize changes or problems readily and prevent or slow progression of disease before symptoms begin or complications arise.

For osteoporosis prevention purposes, a woman usually only needs to have a bone mineral density test two or three times during her lifetime. If her bone density is decreasing, preventive measures such as medication may be an appropriate option.

A significant aspect of arthritis treatment involves learning ways to ease pain and perform daily activities. A diagnosis of arthritis should encourage women to become more active in their own health care and learn better ways to manage their diseases.

Some diseases can cause significant damage if left undiagnosed and therefore untreated. Uncontrolled diabetes, for example, can lead to serious illness and possibly death. With appropriate treatment, however, women with diabetes can live complete and satisfying lives.

A disease such as Alzheimer's presents different issues. Early diagnosis appears to have little effect on treatment or management of the disease. It does, however, afford both the patient and family members time to arrange for who will make future health-care, financial, long-term care, and any other decisions necessary for the patient. Many issues need to be considered with Alzheimer's disease because as the disease progresses, a person will no longer be able to make rational decisions or care for himself or herself. A woman who is considering becoming a caregiver for a person with this disease needs to understand the time and commitment involved before making such a decision. Early diagnosis assists people in this preparation.

Today, the Internet is playing an important role for patients and their families in dealing with the issues that arise from managing a chronic disease. It provides individuals with access to large networks of patients who may share their condition or situation. Sharing tales of common experiences is often very comforting, as is having a large, informal network for information dissemination. In addition, the Internet has provided a massive educational venue for chronic disease, acting as a resource on disease symptoms, diagnostic options, treatments, and support tools. As with all information sources, there are risks related to information received on the Internet, including claims for supposed "miracle cures" for certain disorders, and information that is misleading or inaccurate. As with all other topics, women should make every effort to go to trusted sources to get information about chronic diseases. (See the Web sites listed at the end of this chapter.)

■■■■
Summary

Knowledge, personal preventive practices, and lifestyle modifications are the best measures by which a woman can reduce her chances of developing chronic conditions and be proactive in seeking early diagnosis, treatment, and care. In the cases of chronic diseases that are genetically triggered, women can better understand their risks by learning about their family history. Health screenings can alert a woman to an increased risk of disease, allowing her to make decisions on lifestyle changes and treatment options. Although prevention is the first step, chronic diseases can affect a woman who has followed a healthy lifestyle and has adhered to screening guidelines for various conditions. The next step is understanding how to control or treat a condition, through both lifestyle modifications and treatment options.

Profiles of Remarkable Women

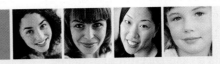

Mary Tyler Moore (1936–)

Mary Tyler Moore began her career as a dancer and actress in TV commercials. After a series of unsuccessful TV series and specials, she landed a role on *The Dick Van Dyke Show* in the early 1960s. From that point, Moore's career took off. *The Mary Tyler Moore Show* ran from 1970 to 1977 and was followed by *Mary* (1978), *The Mary Tyler Moore Hour* (1979), and *Mary* (1985–1986). Moore won five Emmy awards for her roles on *The Dick Van Dyke Show* and *The Mary Tyler Moore Show*. Her career has continued with roles in movies and on Broadway.

Moore has overcome many obstacles in her personal life. Her son committed suicide at the age of 24; soon thereafter, she divorced her husband. She later checked herself into the Betty Ford Clinic with alcohol abuse problems.

Since early adulthood, Moore has also had diabetes. Over the course of her disease, she has experienced several flare-ups of diabetic retinopathy that have been kept under control with laser surgery. As the International Chairwoman of the Juvenile Diabetes Foundation (JDF), Moore has advocated for diabetes education, awareness, and increased funding for diabetes research. She has been featured in a series of public service announcements for the JDF. In June 1999, Moore led 100 child delegates in the first Juvenile Diabetes Foundation Children's Congress before the Senate Committee on Appropriations, Subcommittee in Labor, Health and Human Services, and Education. She and the children, as well as other advocates, called on lawmakers to increase funding for diabetes research to help speed up the discovery of a cure. Moore has continued to lead the Children's Congress to Capitol Hill every other year, making the event one of the largest media and grassroots efforts held in support of finding a cure for juvenile diabetes, raising national awareness, and representing personal advocacy. Moore continues her fight against the disease that affects her life and the lives of the more than 16 million people with diabetes.

■■■■

Topics for Discussion

1. What type of ethical issues may arise with testing for genetic predisposition to various chronic diseases?

2. How can lifestyle changes affect chronic disease management?

3. How can chronic disease affect a woman's day-to-day life?

4. What differences exist between chronic diseases that occur early in life versus those that manifest later in life?

5. In what ways does early diagnosis help a woman and her family to cope with her disease?

■■■■

Web Sites

Alzheimer's Association: http://www.alz.org

Alzheimer's Disease Education and Referral Center (ADEAR): http://www.alzheimers.org

American Diabetes Association: http://www.diabetes.org

Arthritis Foundation: http://www.arthritis.org

Lupus Foundation of America: http://www.lupus.org

National Institute of Arthritis and Musculoskeletal and Skin Diseases: http://www.niams.nih.gov

National Institute of Diabetes and Digestive and Kidney Diseases: http://www.niddk.nih.gov

National Institutes of Health, Osteoporosis and Related Bone Diseases National Resource Center: http://www.niams.nih.gov/bone

National Multiple Sclerosis Society: http://www.nmss.org

National Osteoporosis Foundation: http://www.nof.org

■■■■

References

1. World Health Organization. (2005). *Preventing Chronic Diseases: A Vital Investment.* Department of Chronic Diseases and Health Promotion. WHO Library. Geneva, Switzerland: WHO Press.

2. National Osteoporosis Foundation. (2006). *Osteoporosis Fast Facts.* Available at: http://www.nof.org/osteoporosis/diseasefacts.htm.

3. National Institutes of Health. (2005). *Progress in Autoimmune Disease Research: Report to Congress.* Available at: http://www.niaid.nih.gov/dait/pdf/ADCC_Final.pdf.

4. Centers for Disease Control and Prevention. (2005). Racial/ethnic differences in the prevalence and impact of doctor-diagnosed arthritis—United States, 2002. *Morbidity and Mortality Weekly Report* 54(5): 119–123.

5. Centers for Disease Control and Prevention. (2005). *National Diabetes Fact Sheet.* National Center for Chronic Disease Prevention and Health. Available at: http://www.cdc.gov/diabetes/pubs/estimates.htm#prev4.

6. Centers for Disease Control and Prevention. (2005). *Chronic Disease Overview.* Available at: http://www.cdc.gov/nccdphp/overview.htm.

7. Centers for Disease Control and Prevention. (2007). National and state medical expenditures and lost earnings attributable to arthritis and other rheumatic conditions. *Morbidity and Mortality Weekly Report* 56(1): 4–7.

8. Centers for Disease Control and Prevention. (2004). *Improving the Clinical Use of Biochemical Bone Marker in Metabolic Bone Diseases.* Available at: http://www.cdc.gov/nceh/dls/osteoporosis.htm.

9. Alzheimer's Association. (2006). *Alzheimer's Facts and Figures.* Available at: http://www.alz.org/AboutAD/statistics.asp.

10. American Academy of Orthopaedic Surgeons. (2001). *Falls and Hip Fractures.* Available at: http://orthoinfo.aaos.org/fact/thr_report.cfm?Thread_ID=77&topcategory=Hip.

11. National Institutes of Health. (2000). *Osteoporosis Prevention, Diagnosis, and Therapy. Consensus Development Conference Statement. March 27–29, 2000.* Available at: http://consensus.nih.gov/2000/2000Osteoporosis111html.htm.

12. Delaney, M. F. (2006). Strategies for the prevention and treatment of osteoporosis during early menopause. *American Journal of Obstetrics and Gynecology* 194(2 suppl): S12–S23.

13. Cosman, F. (2005). The prevention and treatment of osteoporosis: a review. *Medscape General Medicine* 7(2): 73.

14. Centers for Disease Control and Prevention. (2006). Prevalence of doctor-diagnosed arthritis and arthritis attributable to activity limitations, 2003–2005. *Morbidity and Mortality Weekly Report* 55(40): 1089–1092.

15. Centers for Disease Control and Prevention. (2005). *Arthritis Related Statistics.* Available at: http://www.cdc.gov/arthritis/data_statistics/arthritis_related_statistics.htm#1.

16. Arthritis Foundation. (2005). *Osteoarthritis Fact Sheet.* Available at: http://www.arthritis.org/conditions/fact_sheets/OA_Fact_Sheet.asp.

17. Helmick C. G., et al. (2008). Estimates of the prevalence of arthritis and other rheumatic conditions in the United States: part I. *Arthritis and Rheumatism* 58(1): 15–25.

18. Lawrence R. C., et al. (2008). Estimates of the prevalence of arthritis and other rheumatic conditions in the United States: part II. *Arthritis and Rheumatism* 58(1): 26–35.

19. Leveille, S. G., Wee, C. C., & Iezzoni, L. I. (2005). Trends in obesity and arthritis among baby boomers and their predecessors, 1971–2002. *American Journal of Public Health* 95(9): 1607–1613.

20. Messier, S. P., Loeser, R. F., Miller, G. D., et al. (2004). Exercise and dietary weight loss in overweight and obese older adults with knee osteoarthritis: the Arthritis, Diet, and Activity Promotion Trial. *Arthritis and Rheumatology* 50(5): 1501–1510.

21. Miyaguchi, M., Kobayashi, A., Kadoya, Y., Ohashi, H., Yamano, Y., & Takaoka, K. (2003). Biochemical change in joint fluid after isometric quadriceps exercise for patients with osteoarthritis of the knee. *Osteoarthritis and Cartilage* 11: 252–259.

22. Centers for Disease Control and Prevention. (2004). Lyme disease—United States, 2001–2002. *Morbidity and Mortality Weekly Report* 53(5): 365–369.

23. National Institutes of Health. (2005). *Lyme Disease: The Facts, the Challenge.* National Institute of Allergies and Infectious Diseases and National Institute of Arthritis and Musculoskeletal and Skin Diseases. NIH Publication #05-7045.

24. Centers for Disease Control and Prevention. (2005). *National Diabetes Fact Sheet: General Information and National Estimates on Diabetes in the United States, 2005.* Atlanta, GA: U.S. Department of Health and Human Services, CDC.

25. Bauduceau, B., Bourdel-Marchasson, I., Brocker, P., & Taillia, H. (2005). The brain of the elderly diabetic patient. *Diabetes Metabolism* 2: 92–97.

26. Kumari, M., & Marmot, M. (2005). Diabetes and cognitive function in a middle-aged cohort: findings from the Whitehall II study. *Neurology* 65(10): 1597–1603.

27. National Institutes of Health. (2005). *Diagnosis of Diabetes.* National Diabetes Information Clearing House. Available at: http://diabetes.niddk.nih.gov/dm/pubs/diagnosis/.

28. American Autoimmune Related Diseases Association. *Autoimmune Disease in Women—the Facts.* Available at: http://www.aarda.org/women.html.

29. Lupus Foundation of America. (2001). *Lupus Fact Sheet.* Available at: http://www.lupus.org/education/factsheet.html#4.

30. U.S. Department of Health and Human Services. (2003). *Frequently Asked Questions: Lupus.* Available at: http://www.4woman.gov/faq/lupus.htm.

31. Kamen, D. L., Cooper, G. S., Bouali, H., Shaftman, S. R., Hollis, B. W., & Gilkeson, G. S. (2006). Vitamin D deficiency in systemic lupus erythematosus. *Autoimmune Review* 5(2): 114–117.

32. Costenbader, K. H., & Karlson, E. W. (2005). Cigarette smoking and systemic lupus erythematosus: a smoking gun? *Autoimmunity* 38(7): 541–547.

33. American Association of Clinical Endocrinologists. (2006). *Thyroid Awareness Month—March 2006.* Available at: http://www.aace.com/public/awareness/tam/2006/.

34. Thyroid Foundation of America. (2004). *Thyroid Disorders and Treatments.* Available at: http://www.tsh.org/disorders/index.html.

35. MayoClinic.Com. (2005). *Hyperthyroidism.* Available at: http://www.mayoclinic.com/health/hyperthyroidism/DS00344.

36. Thyroid Foundation of America. (2004). *Racing the Engine—Hyperthyroidism.* Available at: http://www.tsh.org/disorders/hyperthyroidism/hyperthyroidism.html.

37. AACE Thyroid Task Force. (2002). American Association of Clinical Endocrinologists medical guidelines for clinical practice for the evaluation and treatment of hyperthyroidism and hypothyroidism. *Endocrinology Practice* 6: 457–469.

38. Alzheimer's Association. (2005). *Fact Sheet—Alzheimer's Disease.* Available at: http://www.alz.org/Resources/FactSheets/FSADFacts.pdf.

39. Answers 4 Families. (2004). *Alzheimer's Disease and Other Dementias: Statistics on Alzheimer's Disease (AD).* Available at: http://nncf.unl.edu/alz/info/alz.stats.html.

40. American Health Assistance Foundation. (2005). *Alzheimer's: Risk Factors and Prevention.* Available at: http://www.ahaf.org/alzdis/about/adrisk.htm.

41. Alzheimer's Disease Education and Referral Center (2005). *Alzheimer's Information—Diagnosis.* Available at: http://www.alzheimers.org/diagnosis.htm.

Chapter Twelve

Mental Health

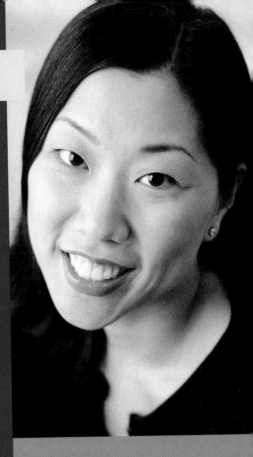

Chapter Objectives

On completion of this chapter, the student should be able to discuss:

1. The importance of maintaining good mental health, as well as reasons why objectively defining "mental health" is difficult.

2. How biological, social, and environmental factors contribute to and affect mental health.

3. Epidemiological, economic, legal, and political dimensions of mental health.

4. Basic categories of mental disorders, including mood, anxiety, and eating disorders, as well as their symptoms, treatment, and effects on women.

5. Risk factors for suicide among adults, adolescents, and children.

6. Major factors that contribute to a woman's overall mental health.

7. Strategies for coping with life's daily stresses and improving mental health in general.

8. Factors to consider before seeking treatment for a mental disorder.

9. Different methods of treating mental disorders, including pharmaceutical treatments and counseling.

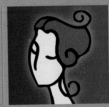

womenshealth.jbpub.com

Women's Health Online is a great source for supplementary women's health information for both students and instructors. Visit **http://womenshealth.jbpub.com** to find a variety of useful tools for learning, thinking, and teaching.

Introduction

Mental health is at least as important as physical health for a person to live a happy, meaningful life. Poor mental health can interfere with maintaining relationships, having a sense of satisfaction in one's self and one's work, and functioning in day-to-day life. Mental illnesses can dull or block even our basic interests in food, sleep, and sexual contact.

So how should a topic as important, yet as nebulous, as "mental health" be defined? One definition of mental health is "how we think, feel, and act as we cope with life."[1] By this definition, good mental health could be considered a state of well-being that allows a person to be productive, have fulfilling relationships with other people, adapt to changes, and cope with difficult circumstances. Mental disorders can be defined as health conditions marked by changes or abnormalities in mood, thinking, or behavior (or a combination of the three) that produce distress or impair functioning.[2]

Making more specific definitions without going into extensive detail is difficult. The *Diagnostic and Statistical Manual of Mental Disorders*, fourth edition (DSM-IV-TR), the manual the American Psychological Association uses to classify mental disorders, uses more than 140 words to define "mental disorder," and 943 pages (17 major diagnostic classes along five axes) to define every recognized mental disorder.

One reason contributing to the difficulty of defining "mental health," "mental disorders," and "mental illness" is the fact that the distinction between mental and physical health is largely artificial. The brain governs our ability to think, feel, and respond—everything we think of as "mental health." The brain, like any other organ, requires nutrients and oxygen, and can be damaged or otherwise affected by nutritional deficiencies, thyroid problems, tumors, or physical trauma. Mental health also influences physical health: Depression, for example, makes people less likely to exercise, more likely to engage in substance abuse, and less able to take good care of themselves, greatly increasing their risk for heart disease and other conditions. The environment also affects a person's mental health. If you restrict a person's vitamin C intake, that person will be very likely to develop scurvy, even if that person is otherwise "healthy." Similarly, if you prevent a person from getting enough oxygen, he or she will have a panic attack, even if that person is otherwise a brave, disciplined person in good mental health.

Social context also influences how cultures conceptualize mental health. The DSM once, but no longer, classified

homosexuality as a mental illness. Today, suicide is considered the ultimate symptom of mental illness, but in feudal Japan, this act was expected of an honorable person under some circumstances. Freud said the mark of a mentally healthy individual was the ability to love and to work, but even this definition carries certain social judgments about what is important for a good life.

Finally, mental health is difficult to define because it is a matter of degree. People who may be considered "mentally healthy" may engage in behaviors that, if taken further, are associated with mental illness. A woman may be considered mentally healthy, and even sensible, for washing her hands several times a day during cold or flu season, but if that same woman begins washing her hands 30 or 40 times a day and her hand washing begins interfering with her ability to work, she could be diagnosed with obsessive-compulsive disorder (OCD). Drawing a line between the mentally healthy and people with mental disorders requires a judgment call that may vary from person to person. (Similarly, different people have different definitions about at what point water turns from "hot" to "cold," even if everyone agrees that boiling water is hot and ice is cold.)

Mental illness is extremely common. Just as a person's physical health varies throughout his or her lifetime, so, too, does his or her mental health. Most people with mental disorders are otherwise normal people who love and are loved, and who contribute to society. People with mental illnesses can be politicians, artists, writers, accountants, doctors, or any other profession. They may seek treatment and recover fully, or they may cope with their disorder as best they can by themselves. In some cases, the perspectives these people gain from dealing with a mental disorder may be of great value to society; some historians have argued that Abraham Lincoln and Winston Churchill were better leaders because of their depressive tendencies.

Half of all Americans experience mental illness in their lifetimes, but most of these people will not seek professional treatment.[2] Many factors contribute to this lack of care. Sometimes good mental health care is not available or affordable, or people do not know where they can find it. The stigma associated with mental illness—many people are afraid to seek help because they are afraid of being thought of as "crazy"—also prevents many people from seeking needed care. Even as science continues to make enormous strides in mapping the brain and understanding cognitive function, the basic problem of improving access to mental health care will remain one of the major health challenges of the twenty-first century.

Factors Affecting Mental Health

Biological, psychosocial, and environmental factors, and even the food a person eats all influence mental health. Genetics, for example, clearly predispose some people to some forms of mental illness. Studies following separated identical twins find that if one twin has bipolar disorder, the other twin has about a 59% chance of also developing the disease—clearly greater than the proportion of bipolar disorder in the general population.[2] Yet genes are clearly not the only factor: Since identical twins share the same genetic code, some other factor in their environment is responsible for the other 41%. Psychosocial and cultural factors influence how a woman views herself, responds to stress, interacts, and is treated by other people. Factors such as low self-esteem and experiences such as abuse or trauma, all of which women are more likely than men to experience, can make a person more vulnerable to mental illness.

Biological Factors

Biological factors vary among mental illnesses, but often include genetic predisposition to a disease, abnormal brain structure or function, irregular levels or activity of neurotransmitters or hormones, head or brain injuries, or prenatal exposure to illegal drugs or alcohol.

Many studies have examined patterns in twins and families to determine genetic factors that create vulnerability to certain types of mental illness. Most people with mental disorders have a history of mental illness in their family, providing evidence of a genetic link. Other studies have found that if one identical twin has a mental illness, the other one often has the same illness.

The influence of hormones during reproductive-related events is another important biological factor in women's mental health. Although studies have produced conflicting findings, it appears that changes in hormone levels have some effect on mental well-being and may be a factor in depression during premenstrual syndrome, postpartum depression, and postpartum psychosis. Brain structure and function, as well as neurotransmitter levels, also have been studied to identify gender-related differences and differences between people with and without mental illness.

Social and Psychosocial Factors

Social and psychosocial factors change throughout a woman's lifetime and influence the way a woman views herself and interacts with others. Women with low incomes, low levels of education, and who work in difficult, stressful, and low-status jobs have higher rates of mental illness than do women who have a higher socioeconomic status, higher education level, and higher-status job. These higher rates likely result from a combination of the undervalued or nonvalued roles that these women fill and the financial difficulties that accompany such roles. Women in roles that society does not highly value, such as full-time homemakers, often suffer from low self-esteem. Women who are trying to fill multiple roles as career women, mothers, and caretakers often feel overwhelmed, which may lead to low self-esteem and, in some cases, depression.

Gender roles are created by the way parents view their male and female children and the expectations and values that society has for each gender. Societal constraints often present a black-and-white picture of gender—for example, seeing men as aggressive and women as passive, men as independent and women as dependent, men as stoic and women as emotional, men as strong and women as weak. Consequently, many parents interact with girls and boys differently, encouraging girls to be delicate, nurturing, nonaggressive, and sensitive to the feelings of others, and teaching boys to be assertive, aggressive, and dominant. For many women, aggression can turn inward, resulting in aggression directed at themselves rather than at others, and manifested as depression or another mental illness.

As children reach puberty, gender differences become even more apparent. A girl's success is often based on popularity and attractiveness, whereas a boy's success is often based on athleticism and academic achievement. Factors such as these lead many girls to base their self-esteem on their physical appearance and body weight. These pressures are especially difficult given that the physical and

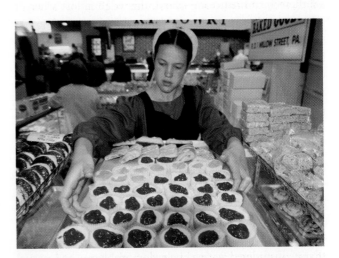

In modern American society, rates of depression are much greater in women than in men. In Amish society, rates of depression are equal by gender. Social and cultural factors are the likely cause for the difference.

Gender Dimensions

GENDER DIFFERENCES IN MENTAL ILLNESS

Strong gender differences exist not only in the prevalence of specific mental disorders, but also in the way the diseases manifest themselves. Some of these differences are:

- Women have twice the rate of clinical depression as men.
- Women have four times the incidence of seasonal affective disorder as men.
- Women experience more of the depressed phase of bipolar disorder and have more rapid cycling between mania and depression.
- Women are nine times more likely to suffer from anorexia nervosa and bulimia nervosa.
- Twice as many women suffer from panic disorder.
- Women are more likely to have phobias and experience more intense symptoms.
- Borderline personality disorder and histrionic personality disorder are diagnosed in more women.
- Men are more than three times as likely to be diagnosed with antisocial personality disorders than women.
- More women attempt suicide, although more men die from their attempts.

hormonal changes of puberty and other stressors already make adolescence difficult.

Research shows that at all grade levels, girls continue to receive less attention than boys in academic settings. Girls generally make better grades than boys do, but despite this academic success, girls experience more internal costs—worry, anxiety, and depression. As the authors of one study note, "although girls may have the edge over boys in terms of their performance in school, this edge is lost when it comes to the experience of internal distress."[3] Another study showed that women tend to attribute their successes to luck and their failures to lack of ability, whereas men tend to attribute their successes to ability and their failures to bad luck.[4]

During and after adolescence, girls must create an identity for themselves, deal with their sexuality, make education and possibly career choices, and become independent. For adolescents, risk factors for mental disorders include lack of parental support, sexual abuse, low self-esteem, and weak relationships with friends or family. Some teens may not exhibit obvious signs of emotional distress and may express their lack of mental wellness through substance abuse, disordered eating, behavior problems, and sexual promiscuity. Teenage girls are more likely than teenage boys to experience depression. Studies show that female high school students have significantly higher rates of anx-

- Young girls often lag behind boys in self-esteem and they are more likely to experience depression.

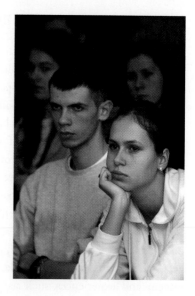

iety disorders, eating disorders, and adjustment disorder than their male counterparts, who have higher rates of disruptive behavior disorders, attention deficit disorder, autism, and learning disabilities.

Early adulthood brings many decisions, including those concerning career choices, relationships such as marriage or intimate partnerships, and childbearing. Reproductive events at this time in a woman's life, such as pregnancy, postpregnancy, infertility, or the decision not to have children, may create personal stress and relationship tension. Many women also experience increased independence at this time in their lives, as well as increased financial obligations and responsibilities at work and at home. All of these factors can affect a woman's mental health.

Many women begin to experiment with recreational drug use during adolescence and early adulthood. Among women with mental health disorders, substance abuse is a common occurrence. This problem may result from these women attempting to self-medicate and cope, or from the fact that their mental disorders inhibit their reasoning skills. The prolonged use of illicit drugs can put people at higher risk for developing mental disorders and can make existing disorders worse, causing people to self-medicate with drugs with more intensity or more frequency. This pattern creates a vicious cycle in the relationship between drug use and mental disorders.

Studies have shown that between 30% and 60% of drug abusers have mental health disorders; depression and attempted suicide are especially common among female substance abusers. For many of these abusers, their depressive symptoms predated their use of alcohol and other drugs. Rates of drug abuse or dependence among anorexics range from 5% to 19%; among bulimics, these rates are signifi-

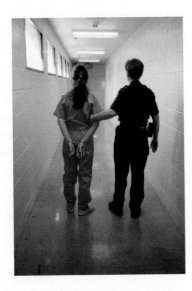

■ Data reveal that about 16% of all inmates are mentally ill.

cantly higher, ranging from 8% to 36%.[5] These women may abuse cocaine, heroin, or methamphetamines to lose weight because these substances act as appetite suppressants. Estimates of the number of patients with bipolar disorder who also have a substance abuse problem range from 30% to 60%. In fact, substance abuse is more likely to be present with bipolar illness than with any other disorder. Individuals with bipolar disorder who abuse drugs or alcohol may have an earlier onset and worse course of illness than those who do not.

As women reach midlife, many continue to deal with career issues and financial burdens and struggle to balance their many roles of mother, wife, daughter, friend, sibling, employer, employee, and self. Women also may be dealing with stress from growing children and aging parents. The support and joy that good relationships offer a woman are often important counterbalances to the stress of managing her everyday life. As she nears late adulthood, a woman may be fortunate enough to feel satisfied with her accomplishments and be financially secure. Women who struggle with retirement issues, physical health, unaccomplished areas of their lives, ill parents, or adult children with difficulties, however, may feel overwhelmed by stressors not fully within their control.

Depression and **dementia** resulting from Alzheimer's disease (Chapter 11) are serious mental-health issues affecting the elderly. A majority of the elderly people affected are women, in part because women constitute a larger percentage of the elderly population than men. Depression is widely underdiagnosed and undertreated in the elderly population. One of every 17 Americans age 65 or older has a diagnosable depressive illness in any given year. Older adults in the United States are also disproportion-

ately likely to commit suicide. For every 100,000 people age 65 or older, 14.3 died from suicide in 2004; this rate is about 40% higher than the national average.[6]

Poor physical health, limited independence, loss of privacy and freedom, and loss of one's partner or friends all contribute to stress and poor mental health in older women. Cognitive impairments in the elderly are often the result of some form of dementia, but may also result from severe depression. In many cases, depression occurs concurrently with chronic medical conditions such as heart disease, diabetes, cancer, and dementia. Because of the common occurrence of depression in the elderly, many health-care providers as well as patients and caregivers believe that depression is a normal part of aging or a normal consequence of chronic disease. Depression in older women can lead to disorientation, loss of short-term memory, verbal difficulty, and inappropriate reasoning skills. Personality changes also may result from dementia or depression or from a decrease in overall physical health.[7]

Discrimination—being singled out by others based on sexual, ethnic, or physical characteristics, including the presence of a mental disorder—is another risk factor for mental illness that women of all age groups experience. Discrimination can affect any aspect of a woman's life, including her work, marriage, and social status. Discrimination is one form of abuse, which in turn is a risk factor for mental illness. Abuse, whether physical or mental, puts women at high risk for developing depression, post-traumatic stress disorder, or obsessive-compulsive disorder. Many people with mental disorders suffered from childhood abuse or traumas, and their disorders represent a response to their repressed emotions. This factor may partly account for women's increased incidence of certain mental disorders, because women are at a higher risk of being victimized through rape, abuse, and sexual harassment.

Other reasons that women suffer from mental disorders may relate to their individual personality traits. Women who are prone to pessimistic thinking, have low self-esteem, feel they have little control over life events, and worry excessively are at higher risk for depressive and anxiety disorders. Many women also have a heightened sense of sympathy and empathy, which leaves them more vulnerable to suffering from depression after tragic events, even if they were not directly affected by the events themselves.

Stress

Stress is the physical, mental, or emotional response that a person experiences when subjected to any type of stressor, a situation that produces tension or requires a difficult

It's Your Health

Methods of Coping

Maintain a good support system.

Make time for pleasurable activities.

Avoid using food, drugs, or alcohol for mood enhancers. Use physical activity instead.

Develop positive thinking techniques.

Learn to control anger but not suppress it.

Practice body acceptance.

Get a good night's sleep.

Say NO to excessive responsibilities.

Use relaxation techniques to control stress.

decision. Stressors can range from daily hassles to life-altering events, and people experience and react to them in different ways. Today's women face special stressors. More women, especially those with young children, are becoming members of the paid workforce. However, women are still more likely than men to do the majority of work in taking care of dependent family members and in doing housework, often creating a "second shift" after a woman returns from her day job. Domestic chores, child care, and running errands can sap women of their energy and cause stress that affects both their home life and their work life.

Acute stress can be helpful for energizing and motivating a person, but chronic stress can overload a person and cause emotional symptoms such as edginess and distorted thinking. Chronic stress also can lead to physical symptoms such as increased heart rate and blood pressure, and lowered immune defense to common colds and other illnesses.[8] Women and men often perceive, evaluate, and respond to stress in different ways. Men may respond positively with physical activity, but negatively through aggression and substance abuse. In contrast, women often internalize their stress, which can cause feelings of failure and self-blame.

People adopt different strategies to cope with the stress in their lives. Because stress levels change over time, individuals may adjust their coping mechanisms accordingly. Positive ways of coping with stress include relaxation techniques; supportive, positive interactions with friends and family; and exercise (see the **It's Your Health** boxes on pages 338 and 353). People with better coping skills are less distressed overall and suffer from less pain, anxiety, depression, illnesses, and "burnout."

Nutrition

The food that people eat can also affect their mental health. The Food and Mood project out of the United Kingdom found that certain foods tend to increase stress levels whereas others help to calm the physiological effects of stress. "Food stressors" include chocolate, caffeine, sugar, and alcohol. Foods that can provide a calming effect include water, vegetables, fruit, and oil-rich fish. The study also found that eating regular meals and eating healthy snacks has a positive effect on mental health. The effects of nutrition on mental health are considered secondary, however, to other physiological and environmental factors.[9]

Perspectives on Mental Health

Epidemiological Data

More than one out of four American adults—about 58 million people—experience a diagnosable mental disorder in a given year.[10] About 13 million, or 1 out of 17 American adults, will suffer from a severe mental illness that seriously disrupts their day-to-day activities, and about half the people who have one mental disorder also have at least one other. Taken together, mental illnesses are responsible for 4 of the top 10 causes of disability, and among adults ages 15–44, cause more disease and injury than cancer.[10]

Men and women are equally likely to suffer from mental disorders, but the prevalence of specific mental disorders varies by gender. Gender differences exist not just in the prevalence of specific mental health disorders among women and men, but also in the way diseases manifest themselves in the two genders; men and women may experience the same disorder in different ways, including the average age that disorders appear, frequency of psychotic symptoms, course of disease progression, social adjustment, and long-term outcome.[11] Variations in mental illnesses may be partially a result of distinct brain structures and the presence of different brain hormones in males and females, which cause neurons to act differently. Evidence shows that the development of brain hemispheres differs by gender, possibly resulting in males and females using their brains in different ways when decoding words, deciphering emotion, and performing other basic tasks. The Gender Dimensions text box lists gender differences in common mental health disorders.

Economic Dimensions

In addition to their harmful effects on individual health, mental illnesses carry a great economic cost. One major study found that lost earnings from serious mental illnesses alone cost Americans $193 billion a year.[12] This estimate does not include the billions of dollars spent on medical care such as medications, clinic visits, and hospital visits; nor does it include the time and resources spent by families and caregivers of people with mental illnesses, or the cost of social problems such as increased crime and threats to public safety.

Treating mental illness is often a costly undertaking. Prescription drugs can be very expensive, especially for people who don't have health insurance or who are **underinsured**. Because individual responses to medications vary and medications sometimes have serious side effects, time and medical care must often be spent on determining, often by trial and error, the correct medication and dosage for a person's individual needs. Inpatient and outpatient mental health-care services are also expensive and require commitments of time and resources for patients and facilities providing care. Because people with serious mental illnesses sometimes have difficulty holding down jobs for long periods of time, they are at increased risk for being both uninsured and economically vulnerable.

Legal Dimensions

Most people with mental disorders are law-abiding citizens. If they have access to proper treatment, people with mental disorders are not more likely to commit crimes than the general population. However, if mental illnesses are left untreated or are not treated properly, a correlation between mental illness and crime does exist, especially among individuals with psychotic and mood disorders. Many people are not identified as suffering from a mental disorder during the legal and criminal process. A 2006 study by the Bureau of Justice Statistics found that more than half of prison and jail inmates suffered from at least one mental disorder, most often mania, depression, and psychotic disorders. Female inmates are more likely to have some form of mental illness than male inmates: 73% of women in state prisons, 61% of women in federal prisons, and 75% of women in jails had a significant mental disorder. Less than one-third of prisoners who had a mental health problem had received treatment since they were incarcerated.[13] These numbers likely reflect both a link between untreated mental disorders and crime as well as increased rates of mental illness that result from the trauma related to committing a crime, going to trial, and adjusting to a life in prison.

Mentally ill homeless people also create legal and ethical dilemmas for society. Many of these people became homeless years ago after cuts in federal and state funding to inpatient mental facilities and outpatient mental health clinics. These funding cuts forced facilities to release thou-

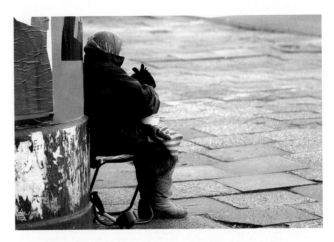

Mentally ill homeless people present a host of legal and ethical dilemmas for society.

sands of patients who were not capable of caring for themselves, and also removed a source of mental health care for thousands of others who were caring for themselves but were economically vulnerable. Without appropriate care and access to consistent medications and treatment, and with continued exposure to the stress of living on the street, over time many mentally ill homeless people have become less healthy, both mentally and physically. For this and other reasons, homeless people with mental disorders have a high incidence of arrests and encounters with the law for threatening behavior, substance abuse, or other disorderly conduct. They also face numerous health problems that develop from their unhealthy living conditions. The connection between the inability of many mentally ill people to access appropriate care and the incidence of criminal behavior underscores the continued need for social programs that improve the quality of life for the mentally ill in the United States.

Political Dimensions

The National Institute of Mental Health (NIMH) is the largest research organization in the world dedicated to improving mental health. Part of the National Institutes of Health, which itself is part of the federal government, the NIMH researches new ways to understand the mind, brain, and behavior; examine, treat, and prevent mental disorders; and promote and maintain good mental health. The Substance Abuse and Mental Health Services Administration (SAMHSA), another agency of the federal government, is responsible for preventing death and preventing, treating, and rehabilitating disability caused by mental illness and substance abuse. Whereas the NIMH tends to focus more on research and furthering scientific understanding, SAMHSA focuses on aid and research that more directly helps people who suffer from poor mental health or substance abuse.

Federal, state, and local policies and laws have enormous, far-reaching effects on mental health. The connections between the two are not always obvious. If stronger or more effective drug-enforcement laws are enacted they could reduce rates of drinking and illegal drug use among pregnant women, which in turn could prevent cases of mental illness resulting from fetal exposure to drugs and alcohol. A president's decision to send U.S. armed forces into combat will inevitably increase rates of post-traumatic stress disorder (PTSD), as those troops react to injuries and their experiences on the battlefield. It is even possible that a program offering low-interest loans to small businesses could reduce rates of depression if it lifted large numbers of people out of poverty and reduced the stresses and risk factors associated with living under the poverty line.

Laws and policies affect the affordability of mental health care. For years, people who had health insurance often found that the plans charged more for mental health services than for other services, or that the plans did not cover mental health services at all. This discrepancy often resulted in people being unable to afford mental health care and contributed to the false idea that mental health services are either unimportant or a luxury. In October 2008, Congress passed new legislation that required health insurance plans that offered mental health services to give those services the same coverage they offer for other physical health services; however, this law only affected insurance plans that offered mental health coverage to begin with.[14]

Preventing mental illnesses can minimize suffering and loss of productivity associated with the disorders, and eliminate the costs of diagnosing and treating the disorders after they develop. Simple, cost-effective ways to prevent mental illness include enacting policies to reduce head injuries by mandating the use of motorcycle helmets, reducing childhood exposure to lead by replacing old plumbing in public schools, and preventing fetal exposure to alcohol, tobacco, and other drugs by offering rehabilitation programs. Programs that support good parenting, such as ample maternity and paternity leave programs, or providing classes and support to new parents, have especially powerful mental-health-promoting effects for both children and parents.

Clinical Dimensions of Mental Illness

Mood Disorders

Mood disorders (also known as **affective disorders**) are mental disorders characterized by extreme disturbances of mood, the dominant emotion (or emotional tendency) a person feels at any given moment. Many factors including genetics, out-of-balance neurotransmitters, a person's life experiences, and other environmental factors can contribute to a mood disorder or influence how a given disorder progresses. Depression and dysthymia are associated with persistent sadness, whereas bipolar disorder is associated with rapid mood changes or sustained elevations in mood.[2]

Depression

Depression is a medical illness affecting the mind as well as the body that is usually triggered by stressful life events. Depression is characterized by persistent, inescapable feelings of sadness. These feelings are often accompanied by feelings of inadequacy and hopelessness, physical exhaustion, and other symptoms (**Table 12.1**). These symptoms are so intense they usually disrupt a person's basic activities, including eating, sleeping, maintaining relationships, and taking pleasure in life.[15] People with depression often feel undesirable and inadequate. They anticipate rejection and dissatisfaction from their interactions and experiences, and they blame themselves when their negative expectations are fulfilled. People with depression often know their feelings are unhealthy and unproductive, and want desperately to feel better, but are unable to do so. This inability to "snap

Table 12.1   **Symptoms of Depression**

Persistent sad mood
Constant feelings of sadness
Excessive crying
Low energy
Feelings of worthlessness or hopelessness
Difficulty concentrating or making decisions
Loss of interest in pleasurable activities
Sleep disturbances
Appetite and weight changes
Thoughts of death or suicide
Physical symptoms that do not respond to treatment

out of it" makes them feel even more weak and inadequate.[16] Feelings of hopelessness and worthlessness also make people with depression unlikely to seek professional help. Less than one-third of people with depression seek help from a mental health professional.[17]

Depression may coexist with other physical and mental illnesses or may be mistaken for Alzheimer's disease in the elderly. Certain medical conditions, such as thyroid disease, multiple sclerosis, and cancer, can result in depression. Depression also may arise as a response to a serious illness, a consequence of substance abuse, or a side effect of certain medications. In addition, depression frequently accompanies a number of chronic diseases, including coronary heart disease, diabetes, stroke, cancer, and HIV/AIDS.

Hormonal shifts during reproductive-related events and their link to mental illness have been the subject of much controversy. For example, it was previously believed that hormones were solely responsible for depression during premenstrual syndrome (PMS); however, research now shows that hormones may trigger, but are not solely responsible for, PMS-related depression. Severe depression during PMS, called premenstrual dysphoric disorder (PMDD), affects 3% to 7% of menstruating women.[18]

Postpartum depression is a type of depression that affects 10% to 15% of all new mothers.[15] This condition is different from the "baby blues," or postpartum blues, which occurs in the first 10 days after delivery and is quite common and typically mild. Postpartum depression typically begins three to six months after delivery and is much more severe (**Table 12.2**), although less severe than postpartum psychosis. Postpartum depression is more common in women with a history of depression, marital issues, lack of social support, or a history of negative life experiences. Although it often goes unnoticed and untreated, postpartum depression can greatly affect the mother and child as well as damage the relationship between the parents. For

women who are already at risk, menopause can be another hormone-related event that can trigger depression.

Research has shown that levels of the neurotransmitter **serotonin** are lower in people with major depression. Medications that boost levels of serotonin, called selective serotonin reuptake inhibitors (SSRIs), have proven able to relieve symptoms of depression. One study found that men's brains make 52% more serotonin than do women's brains, possibly explaining why depression can manifest differently in men and women.[19]

Genetics also play a major role in depression. Someone with a family history of depression is significantly more likely to develop depression than someone with no family history of the disease. Studies have shown that children with one depressed parent are two to three times more likely to experience depression by age 18 than are children without depressed parents. The risk doubles if both parents suffer from depression.[20]

A particular form of depression called **seasonal affective disorder (SAD)** is caused by seasonal shifts in daylight hours, which affect a person's circadian rhythm or sleep–wake cycle. SAD often affects women in their reproductive

Table 12.2	Symptoms of Postpartum Depression
Anxiety	
Feelings of hopelessness and guilt	
Panic attacks	
Insomnia	
Lack of interest in the baby	
Thoughts of suicide	
Thoughts of hurting self or baby	

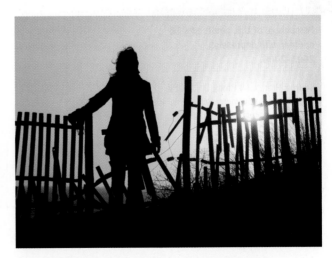

■ Therapeutic doses of bright light in the morning can help relieve depression caused by seasonal affective disorder (SAD).

years. Its symptoms include some of the atypical symptoms of depression, such as increased appetite, lethargy, and carbohydrate cravings. Researchers believe the cause of SAD may be related to melatonin disturbances. Therapeutic doses of bright light in the morning can help to relieve this condition.

Depression is the most common mood disorder among women and is about twice as common in women as it is in men. About 1 in 20 women has depression at any given moment, but more than 1 in 5 women will experience at least one depressive episode during their lives.[17] Adolescent females have an unusually high rate of depression. Before puberty, boys are more likely than girls of the same age to be diagnosed with depression or depressive symptoms, but this changes after puberty so that girls are far more likely to be diagnosed with depression.[17] Between the ages of 30 and 44—typically the years of childbearing and childrearing—rates of depression are three times greater for women than they are for men. Elderly women, especially women who are widowed, are in poor physical health, or have lost some or all of their independence, are also at risk for developing depression. Medical illness and the effects of multiple medications in the elderly make it even more difficult to diagnose depression. Yet another risk factor for depression is poverty. People living below the poverty level have a 13% chance of being depressed—three times the rate of people living above the poverty line.[17] **Figure 12.1** shows rates of depression in the United States by age, gender, and race/ethnicity.

Researchers are examining whether the higher rates of depression in women truly represent a greater incidence of depression or whether the rates reflect gender-based differences in the acknowledgment of mental illness or ability to recognize symptoms. The rate of depression in men may be underestimated because women are more likely than men to discuss feelings associated with being depressed, to admit to feeling depressed, and to seek help. Men are also more likely to direct negative feelings outward rather than inward, toward the self. (These same tendencies make men more likely to engage in self-destructive behaviors such as substance abuse and violent destructive behavior directed at others.) In Amish culture, where women's roles as mothers and homemakers are more highly valued than in U.S. society as a whole, and society frowns on self-destructive "macho" behaviors and alcohol consumption, rates of depression are equal for men and women.[16] Women also have higher rates of victimization from physical abuse, sexual harassment, and rape. Acts of violence such as these not only cause trauma, but foster low self-esteem, a sense of helplessness, social isolation, and, ultimately, depression. Being a caregiver for young children, aging parents, or ill family members—roles often filled by women—also has been noted as a risk factor for depression.

Dysthymia

Dysthymia is a milder, yet more chronic, form of depression. Even though dysthymia's symptoms are less severe than other forms of depression, dysthymia is still a serious, debilitating disease. It is diagnosed when symptoms last at least two years in adults or one year in adolescents and children. People with dysthymia exhibit a depressed mood

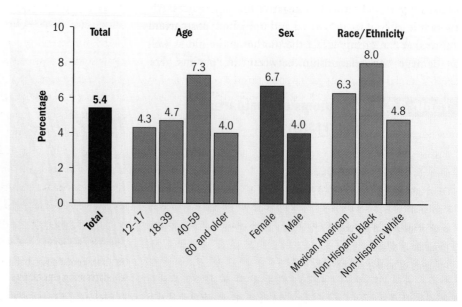

Figure 12.1

Percentage of U.S. adults age 12 or older with depression, 2005–2006.

Source: Pratt, L., & Brody, D. (2008). Depression in the *United States Household Population, 2005–2006*. Washington, DC: USDHHS.

and at least two other symptoms of depression, such as poor appetite or overeating, sleep difficulties, or low self-esteem. Dysthymia often begins in childhood or adolescence, but can occur at any age. Because it often develops at a young age, the depressed state becomes integrated within the woman's personality, often not only affecting her self-esteem and motivation, but also her ability to live a satisfying life and function normally. Dysthymia affects about 1.5% of the adult population (about 3.3 million adults) in any given year.[10]

Bipolar Disorder

Bipolar disorder, sometimes also referred to as **manic depressive disorder**, is somewhat like depression in that it affects a person's emotions and ability to function. But bipolar disorder is characterized by shifts in emotion, not by a single mood.[21] A person with bipolar disorder experiences episodes of both mania ("highs") and depression ("lows"). During manic episodes a person with bipolar disorder typically has an excess of energy, activity, and restlessness. At this point, a person could feel wonderful and euphoric, or overly stimulated and easily irritated. Other symptoms of a manic phase include racing thoughts, extreme distractibility, overconfidence, and an increased sex drive. People experiencing depressive episodes typically have deep, persistent feelings of sadness, anxiety, hopelessness, or guilt; they might also have low energy, a reduced sense of pleasure and a lowered sex drive, and thoughts of suicide.[21] In between manic and depressive episodes, a person with bipolar disorder could have extended periods of being within the normal range of moods. People with bipolar disorder are at great risk for abusing alcohol and other drugs and engaging in other self-destructive behaviors.

About 2.6% of the adult population (5.7 million people) will be affected by bipolar disorder in any given year. Bipolar disorder typically first appears during a person's twenties.[10] Gender differences are apparent in the manifestation of the disease, however, with women typically having more depressed episodes and more rapid cycling between depression and mania than do men.

Treatment

The good news is that treating mood disorders can provide great benefits, allowing people to live satisfying, functional, and healthy lives. The bad news, however, is that mood disorders have no "quick fix." Between 70% and 80% of people who experience one episode of depression will experience depression again at some point in their lives[22]; bipolar disorder typically requires ongoing treatment for a

The medications I take for depression make me sleepy—I need about an extra hour a day—and dull my sex drive. But I'd still much rather have those symptoms than the alternative. If you have ever been seriously depressed, you'd understand.

22-year-old woman

person to stay within a stable mood range. Short-term treatments for either of these illnesses are unlikely to be effective.[2] For both depression and bipolar disorder, the earlier a person decides to seek treatment, the better chance that person will have of making a recovery and of preventing further episodes.

Mood disorders can be treated with either medications or psychosocial treatment (some form of "talk therapy"). A combination of both of these forms of treatment usually works better than either form used alone.[15,21] Medications are a powerful, yet imperfect tool to treat people with mood disorders. Medications can gradually bring a person with depression or bipolar disorder back into a normal range of moods, but they may take days or even weeks to have any noticeable effects. Individuals respond differently to treatments and treatments may have side effects, so a person with a mood disorder taking medications should work with his or her psychiatrist to find the specific pharmaceutical drug and dosage that provides the most benefit while reducing side effects to a low, or at least acceptable, level. Because some medications for depression or bipolar disorder may affect fetal development, a woman with a mood disorder should talk with her psychiatrist about her medication routine if she is pregnant or wishes to conceive.

Antidepressant medications attempt to restore a depressed person's levels of **neurotransmitters**, particularly serotonin, norepinephrine, and dopamine, to a normal level. There are several types of antidepressant medications. The two newest, most commonly used types are called selective serotonin reuptake inhibitors (SSRIs) and serotonin and norepinephrine reuptake inhibitors (SNRIs). Older forms of antidepressants, including tricyclics or monoamine oxidase inhibitors (MAOIs), are more likely to have side effects, though these medications may be best for some individuals. Possible side effects of antidepressant medications include headaches, nausea, insomnia, constipation, and reduced sexual desire and function.

Bipolar disorder is usually treated with one or more of several kinds of medications known as "mood stabilizers." Mood-stabilizing drugs include lithium and several classes of anticonvulsant drugs. These drugs help to keep a person's mood within a consistent, central range. To work most effectively, these drugs should be taken on a regular basis. Sometimes a person with bipolar disorder can "feel" a mood shift approaching; if a person notices this and talks with his or her psychiatrist, a temporary change in his or her treatment plan can often prevent an episode from occurring.[21]

Psychosocial treatment for depression can provide benefits on either a short-term (around 10–20 weeks) or a continuous basis, depending on the individual's needs and desires. The two most popular forms of psychotherapy used to treat depression are cognitive-behavior therapy (CBT) and interpersonal therapy (IPT). CBT teaches a depressed person to recognize patterns of thinking and behaving that contribute to depression, and helps that person find new thoughts and behaviors that support recovery. IPT helps people to understand and improve their own personal relationships and interactions with other people. Psychotherapy is often the best treatment option for people with mild to moderate depression; for people with major depression, psychotherapy can be combined with antidepressant medications.[15]

For people with bipolar disorder, psychosocial treatment includes:

- Cognitive behavioral therapy, which helps patients to recognize and change harmful thought patterns and behaviors associated with the disorder

- Psychoeducation, which teaches patients (and sometimes relatives or loved ones) about the effects, treatment, and management of bipolar disorder

- Family therapy, which works on improving family relationships to improve harmful relationships or patterns of interaction that contribute to or result from the patient's symptoms

- Interpersonal and social rhythm therapy, which helps patients improve their personal interactions and establish regular daily routines[21]

Anxiety Disorders

Anxiety is an adaptive mental function that helps us live safe, productive lives. At healthy levels, anxiety can motivate a person to study for a test, look both ways before crossing the street, double-check that the front door is locked, or refrain from stealing or committing some other crime. **Anxiety disorders** occur when anxiety grows to unhealthy levels, or when it appears in situations in which no risks exist. People with anxiety disorders often know that the worries, fears, or behaviors caused by the disorders are unhelpful and unrealistic, but this knowledge does not eliminate the symptoms (see **Table 12.3**). Anxiety disorders include generalized anxiety disorder (GAD), social

Table 12.3 Symptoms of Anxiety Disorder
Feelings of terror and dread
Feelings of apprehension and uncertainty
Nervousness
Irritability
Rapid heartbeat
Chest pain
Fainting
Difficulty breathing
Sweating
Belief that feelings are signs of a heart attack

phobias (also known as social anxiety disorder), specific phobias, panic disorder, obsessive-compulsive disorder (OCD), and post-traumatic stress disorder (PTSD).[23]

Anxiety disorders affect about 40 million American adults (about one out of five adults) during a given year. Women are two to three times more likely than men to suffer from anxiety disorders. People with an anxiety disorder are disproportionately likely to experience some form of depression, another anxiety disorder, or engage in substance abuse in efforts to self-medicate. Anxiety disorders usually appear early compared to other mental illnesses: Three-fourths of people with an anxiety disorder will have their first appearance of that disorder before they turn 21.[10]

Generalized Anxiety Disorder

Generalized anxiety disorder (GAD) is characterized by chronic and exaggerated worry and tension that lasts for at least six months. People with GAD may worry about possible disasters involving themselves or their loved ones, or they may worry about the issues involving the routines of everyday life. This constant worrying eventually affects the body in many ways, producing symptoms such as an inability to relax, nausea, muscle tension or pain, trembling, or having to go to the bathroom frequently. The worrying can also interfere with concentration and memory. The severity of GAD varies from person to person: It can be relatively mild, or the anxiety can be intense and disabling enough to prevent a person from carrying out daily activities, holding a job, or interacting with others. GAD currently affects 6.8 million adults in the United States, two-thirds of whom are women.[23]

Social Phobia

Phobias are intense fears of something that poses little or no threat. A person with social phobia, or social anxiety disorder, experiences a powerful, lasting fear of interacting with other people. People with this mental disorder become very self-conscious in social settings, often imagining that they are being watched or judged, or that they are doing something embarrassing. A social phobia may create anxiety surrounding all human interactions, or it may be limited to specific situations, such as eating or drinking in public, or speaking in front of a group. Anxiety can last for days or weeks before a social event and can continue after. Fifteen million U.S. adults experience social phobia; about half of them are women.[10]

Other Phobias

People can develop phobias about other specific animals, objects, places, or events other than social interactions. Phobias may involve heights, closed spaces, flying, spiders, elevators, the sight of blood, or other things or situations. A phobia involves more than a moderate level of fear—a person can be afraid of any of the previously mentioned things without having a phobia. Phobias involve powerful, overwhelming fear that occurs not only when the object of the phobia appears, but also often when it is merely even thought about. Phobias can be especially disabling if the object of the phobia is common or difficult to avoid in a person's daily life. About 20 million U.S. adults, including 14 million women, have a specific phobia of some kind.[23]

Panic Disorder

Panic disorder affects about 6 million U.S. adults and is twice as common in women as in men. This disorder is characterized by panic attacks—periods of intense fear accompanied by physical and emotional distress that may last anywhere from 5 to 20 minutes.[23] The panic attack often strikes without warning. Its symptoms have often been mistaken for a heart attack, and include a pounding heart, sweating, faintness, dizziness, chest pain, nausea, and emotional symptoms such as a feeling of impending doom or of losing control. In many cases the intensity of the symptoms, as well as their unexplainable nature, makes the panic attacks themselves a major source of anxiety.

An initial panic attack usually occurs in a person's twenties during transition periods, times of considerable stress, or crises and often sends the individual to the emergency room. Some women have an isolated attack without ever developing the disorder; nevertheless, repeated panic attacks are a definitive sign of panic disorder. Panic attacks can be extremely disabling if they occur on a regular basis.

Obsessive-Compulsive Disorder

Obsessive-compulsive disorder (OCD) is an anxiety disorder in which a person develops intense, persistent fears, worries, or superstitions (obsessions), and uses specific rituals (compulsions), often repeated over and over again on a daily basis, for relief. One of the classic obsessions in OCD is an overwhelming fear of germs; a woman with this obsession might wash her hands dozens of times a day, or be afraid to touch a doorknob or any item that someone else has touched. Other obsessions include fear of social embarrassment, thoughts about having harmed a loved one, worries about having forgotten something or left something out of place, and intrusive sexual thoughts. The ritual adopted to find relief varies from person to person, but some common themes emerge. Rituals often involve repeatedly checking things, counting things, or touching things in a specific pattern or order. The rituals are distracting and time-consuming and do not actually bring pleasure, but, at most, short-lived relief from symptoms.[23]

Just over 2 million adults in the United States have OCD, which affects men and women in equal numbers. OCD usually appears in the first 20 to 30 years of a person's life, often appearing in childhood. OCD also runs in families, suggesting that genetics can predispose a person to the disorder.[23]

Post-Traumatic Stress Disorder

Post-traumatic stress disorder (PTSD) is an extremely debilitating disorder that occurs after an exposure to a terrifying event involving violent harm or the threat of violent harm. PTSD can result from situations such as armed combat, a car accident, sexual assault, mugging, or natural disaster. A person can develop PTSD if he or she was threatened directly, or if he or she witnessed a threat to a friend or family member. People with PTSD may become startled easily or may be constantly anxious and hypervigilant. Situations that remind them of the traumatic event can trigger "flashbacks" in which they relive part or all of their experience. Flashbacks can also occur in dreams or for no apparent reason while the person is awake. People with PTSD can also become emotionally numb, unable to maintain personal relationships or take pleasure from daily life. People with PTSD may also become violent or aggressive. They may also become depressed, or turn to substance abuse for relief.

PTSD was originally identified in male Vietnam veterans, but recent research has revealed that PTSD is a major public health concern for women as well. PTSD tends to last longer in women than it does in men. Women are more than twice as likely as men to develop PTSD after exposure to a traumatic event, in part because they are more likely to blame themselves. Women are also more likely than men to be victims of sexual assault, a major trigger

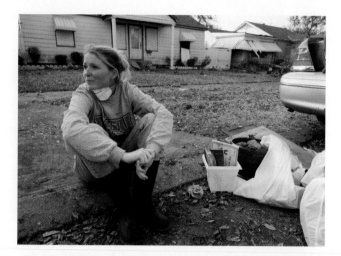

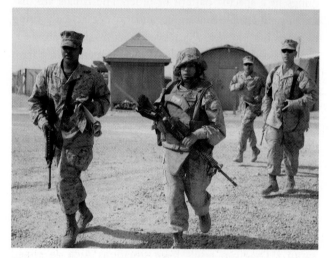

■ Professional counseling helps many people suffering from mental disorders.

event for PTSD. Women are more likely to experience PTSD if they have more than one traumatic experience, had or have a mental disorder before the trauma, or do not have good social support.[24] One bit of good news for women, however, is that they tend to recover from PTSD more easily than men, because they are more likely to be comfortable talking about their feelings and difficult personal issues. At least 7.7 million U.S. adults have PTSD,[23] but this number may be an underestimate.

The growing numbers of veterans trying to cope with daily life after returning from the wars in Iraq and Afghanistan, and the millions of Americans affected by the flooding of (and slow government response to) New Orleans and surrounding areas after Hurricane Katrina have brought new attention to PTSD as a serious illness that causes lasting harm. One study found that almost one in four residents of Mississippi directly affected by Hurricane

Katrina exhibited some signs of PTSD.[25] About one out of seven military personnel who have experienced combat in Iraq are women.[24] Women soldiers are much more likely than men to be victims of sexual assault or violence from their fellow soldiers and from superior officers. Although a male soldier may have to deal with significant stress from fighting enemy combatants but might be able to have a deep sense of trust around his fellow troops, a woman who has been sexually assaulted not only has to deal with the direct trauma of the experience, but can never fully relax.

Treatment

Like many other mental illnesses, anxiety disorders can be treated with medications, psychotherapy, or a combination of the two, depending on individual needs and preferences. Without treatment, people with anxiety disorders may find themselves making serious life decisions based on their likelihood of encountering a phobic or anxiety-producing object or situation. Treatment can provide great benefits for people living with anxiety disorders, but time and effort are necessary to see improvements; people sometimes believe that they can't be treated, or that the treatment doesn't work for them, when more time or an adjustment to the treatment is all that is needed.[23] Commonly prescribed medications for anxiety disorders include antidepressants, antianxiety medications, and beta blockers, a type of drug originally developed to treat heart conditions. Cognitive-behavioral therapy can help people with anxiety disorders learn to recognize and change thoughts and behaviors associated with the disorder. Another form of therapy used for anxiety disorders is called exposure/response therapy. Exposure/response therapy aims to desensitize sufferers to their fears by supporting them in staying calm while gradually confronting more and more anxiety-producing situations. Certain forms of group therapy can also help people with anxiety disorders, especially people with PTSD or social phobia. If a person with an anxiety disorder is experiencing another form of mental illness or has a substance-abuse problem, these issues will also need to be treated.

Eating Disorders

Eating disorders are serious mental illnesses characterized by dysfunctional eating patterns. But an eating disorder is much more than an unhealthy eating habit or a desire "not to eat." Like other mental illnesses, eating disorders have biological and environmental causes, distinct symptoms, and harmful consequences for the body.[26] People with eating disorders are also likely to have mental illnesses, including depression, anxiety disorders, and substance-abuse problems. At some point in their lives, between 0.5% and 3.7% of women will have anorexia, and between 1.1% and 4.2% of women will have bulimia.[27] Eating disorders are treatable, but success requires the person to acknowledge the seriousness of the issue and seek professional medical help.

There is no single explanation for why an eating disorder evolves. Eating disorders often begin with dieting; however, before dieting, other factors have already affected a person's mindset. Women may have a biological vulnerability to eating disorders. Levels of neurotransmitters and hormones that affect one's mood, appetite, and eating behavior may be altered in women with eating disorders. For example, the hormone serotonin creates feelings of satiety after eating and may be present at lower levels in women with bulimia. Therefore, these individuals tend to not feel as satisfied and may binge as a result. Poor self-image, depression, anxiety, loneliness, and certain family and personal relationships may contribute to the development of an eating disorder, too. The stresses associated with adolescent and adult life also can precipitate anorexia or bulimia.[28]

Our culture, with its unrelenting idealization of thinness, "the perfect body," and its presentation of weight loss as an accomplishment is also partly to blame. Consider the rise in pro–eating disorder Web sites that share information among those with eating disorders on how to better meet their disordered goals of weight loss and behavior control. Referred to as "pro-ana" for "pro-anorexia" and "pro-mia" for "pro-bulimia," the authors of these sites see them as a way to create a sense of support and community among people of like thinking. Many health professionals, however, see them as very dangerous and have mounted campaigns with Internet service providers to have the sites removed.

Eating disorders have harmful consequences for the mind and the body. People with eating disorders are more likely to suffer from other mental illnesses; they can also develop health complications including dental problems, kidney failure, and heart conditions.[26]

The *female athlete triad*—the interrelationship between disordered eating, **amenorrhea**, and **osteoporosis**—usually begins with disordered eating. Poor nutrition and intense athletic training cause weight loss and a decrease in or shutdown of estrogen production. Consequently, amenorrhea occurs. The final condition in the triad, osteoporosis, may follow if estrogen levels remain low and the

woman's diet is lacking in calcium and vitamin D. Although the triad can occur in any athlete, those at greatest risk are endurance athletes such as distance swimmers and runners, and athletes in sports where slim appearance is highly valued, such as gymnasts and figure skaters.

Anorexia Nervosa

Anorexia nervosa is characterized by deprivation of food and a body weight of at least 15% below the normal weight for a person's height and age. The DSM-IV classifies anorexia as an eating disorder associated with the following factors:

- Refusal to maintain an adequate weight
- Intense fear of gaining weight
- Distorted body image
- In women, three consecutive missed periods without pregnancy (amenorrhea)

Physical symptoms of anorexia nervosa include a significant loss of weight, a refusal to eat, amenorrhea, and a denial of unusual eating behaviors or weight change. As an anorexic person's metabolism slows down to adjust to the lack of nourishment, other symptoms, such as muscle weakness, constipation, brittle hair and nails, lethargy, and a lowering of the body temperature, which causes a constant feeling of coldness and slowness, occur. Psychological symptoms of this eating disorder include a distorted body image, confusion of self-image, a sense of being incompetent, depression, and withdrawal from others.[26] Individuals also tend to become socially withdrawn as the disorder progresses. Researchers note that the most notable belief shared by women with anorexia is that weight, shape, or being thin is the predominant reference for establishing personal value or self-worth.[29] Other identified psychological features of the illness include:

- A frustration over becoming overweight
- A fear of losing control over eating
- A loss of judgment relative to the requirement of food as a basic need for the body
- An unrealistic sense of body image

I look in the mirror and see myself as grotesquely fat—a real blimp. My legs and arms are really fat and I can't stand what I see. I know that others say I am too thin, but I can see myself and I have to deal with this my way.

100-pound anorexic girl

Women with anorexia often display obsessive-compulsive behaviors, such as obsessing about becoming fat and, consequently, compulsively exercising or practicing odd eating rituals to avoid becoming fat. Other compulsive activities may include constant weighing, looking in the mirror, and taking body measurements. Women with anorexia also are obsessed with food and eating, and will often cook, prepare, and shop for food for others. They will eat in secret and reject food in public.

Anorexia nervosa usually strikes in early to late adolescence. A general characteristic of the anorectic personality is a feeling of overall ineffectiveness as a person. The typical anorexic woman is highly critical of herself, has poor self-esteem, and believes that she is quite inadequate in most areas of personal and social functioning. She often feels powerless and unable to control many areas of her life, so she establishes power over her food intake and weight. Because of her perfectionist tendencies, the woman with anorexia believes that the ultimate sign of control is a "perfect" body. Symptoms of depression, with large mood swings, are commonly seen in individuals with the disorder. The increased risk for heart and kidney failure, suicide, and other serious consequences makes people with anorexia about 10 times more likely to die early than people without this condition.[26]

Bulimia Nervosa

Bulimia nervosa is an eating disorder characterized by cyclic binge eating (**bingeing**) followed by purging. Prevalence rates for bulimia range from 1% to 16%, with the highest rates occurring in adolescents and young adults.[24]

The DSM-IV associates four distinguishing characteristics of bulimia:

- Recurrent episodes of binge eating (at least two episodes per week for at least three months)
- A feeling of lack of control over eating behavior during the binge
- Regular engagement in purges
- Persistent over-concern with body shape and weight

Bulimia is a progressive disorder that usually begins with extreme hunger as a result of long periods of food deprivation from fasting or dieting. This hunger is followed by attempts at eating while still trying to control weight. Women with this eating disorder often maintain normal body weight but are extremely dissatisfied with their bodies. Some bulimics have reported that in their preadolescent years, they gained feelings of self-control and power

through this self-denial. The situation progresses to out-of-control binges/purges because the artificial elimination methods have relieved the feeling of being "stuffed," and the bulimic believes it is a good way to lose weight.

Binges often occur when bulimics feel that they have passed a self-imposed limit on acceptable food intake. Consequently, they feel defeated and generally gorge until they are interrupted or the food runs out. During such binges, the caloric intake may range from 2,000 to 3,000 calories and generally lasts for less than two hours but has been reported to last as long as eight hours. The binge foods of choice are usually high-calorie, easily ingested "junk" food that requires little preparation and can be obtained while keeping the binge secret from others. Bulimics have been known to use several modes of purging, including induced vomiting, diuretics, laxatives, fasts, enemas, diet pills, chewing for hours and then spitting out the food, and excessive exercise. The number of different methods of purging is a stronger index of the severity of the woman's condition than is the frequency of use of any one type.

The binge–purge cycle may occur anywhere from once or twice weekly to several times daily. The cycle often begins in response to a strong emotion, either positive or negative; this can be a food craving, stress, sleeplessness, anxiety, joy, excitement, physical or emotional pain, helplessness, hopelessness, loneliness, or sadness. After the binge, some women say they initially feel relaxed and soothed, but then these feelings turn to shame, guilt, and self-hatred. The women then feel the need to purge to relieve the fear of weight gain and to regain a sense of control and purity. After the purge, bulimics may feel relieved that they have controlled their weight but guilty and negative about succumbing to the cycle again. These feelings of guilt invariably lead the bulimic to perpetuate the behavior.

The victims of bulimia often appear to be independent high achievers and are of normal weight. Bulimia has traditionally afflicted adolescent and young adult females from middle-class backgrounds, but it affects other groups of women and men as well. Bulimics are often perfectionist, obsessive-compulsive, depressed, intense, insecure, sensitive to rejection, anxious to please, and dependent on others. They may be socially isolated as a result of their all-consuming preoccupation with food and weight and their struggle to hide their eating behavior. The majority of women who suffer from bulimia are aware that their eating habits are abnormal, but may believe that they have the ultimate weight control secret of being able to "have their cake and eat it, too." Other factors thought to contribute to the development of bulimia include family problems, maladaptive behavior, self-identity conflicts, history of sexual abuse, and cultural overemphasis on physical appearance. In addition to the psychological problems, bulimia nervosa can cause a variety of physical problems, including hypoglycemia, a slowed metabolism, spontaneous regurgitation, erosion of tooth enamel or tooth loss, bleeding and sores in the mouth and esophagus, and mineral deficiencies. **Table 12.4** compares the symptoms of anorexia nervosa with those of bulimia nervosa.

Binge Eating Disorder

Binge eating disorder (BED) is characterized by compulsive overeating without attempting to purge. Defining factors of BED include recurrent episodes of binge eating at least two days per week for a minimum of six months, as well as an overall sense of loss of control over the binges. Women with BED also have a preoccupation with food and weight, as well as a distorted body image.

Binge eating disorder is different from non-purging bulimia nervosa, because people with non-purging bulimia binge after periods of fasting and use excessive exercise as a way to compensate for their binges. Most people who suffer from BED are obese and have a long history of weight fluctuations. Women who suffer from BED are at high risk for medical problems associated with obesity, as well as depression and anxiety due to guilt and feelings of self-disgust. Many people with BED have reported histories of major family dysfunction and childhood abuse.

Table 12.4 Symptoms of Anorexia Nervosa/Bulimia Nervosa

Symptoms of Anorexia Nervosa

Loss of at least 15% of body weight

Intense fear of weight gain

Distorted body image (feeling fat even when too thin)

Absence of three consecutive menstrual periods (amenorrhea)

Insistence on keeping weight below a healthy minimum

Symptoms of Bulimia Nervosa

Repeated (usually secretive) episodes of bingeing and vomiting

Feeling out of control during a binge

Purging after a binge (vomiting, use of laxatives or diuretics, excessive exercise)

Frequent dieting

Extreme concern with body weight and shape

My friends confronted me about my anorexia in my senior year of high school. By that point it had gotten so bad that even I had to admit it—I got lost on the way to school because I couldn't think straight. It was really tough for the first year, and was still difficult after that, but now I'm really okay with it. In fact, I'm eating a healthier diet than I ever was before, even though I don't think about food nearly as much.

22-year-old woman

Treatment

People who have eating disorders are intensely secretive about them in most cases. Due to the nature of either not eating enough, bingeing and purging, or excessive exercise behaviors, however, friends and family members of girls affected by these disorders often have an idea that they are occurring. Many try to ignore their suspicions so as to protect the privacy of their friend or family member or out of a wish not to interfere. Women with bulimia and BED are often able to identify themselves. In contrast, women with anorexia are often in denial about their condition and usually are brought to treatment by concerned family members. Many women enter therapy to treat an eating disorder only after being persuaded to do so by people in their lives. It thus becomes extremely important for people to confront the women in their lives when they suspect disordered eating, and to provide them with support in finding the appropriate help. As with all health interventions, sensitivity and care need to be taken when discussing eating disorders with individuals, and one needs to have an understanding of the very central and painful role the disorder may play in an individual's life.

Several approaches are used to treat eating disorders, including motivating the patient, enlisting family support, and providing nutrition counseling and psychotherapy. Behavior modification therapy and drug therapy, such as antidepressants, may also be used. Hospitalization may be required for those patients with life-threatening complications or extreme psychological problems. If the patient's life is not in danger, treatment may be provided on an outpatient basis and may last for a year or longer.

Treatment is often a lengthy and difficult process, with many women suffering from relapses. Stopping the pattern of dysfunctional eating is essential for successfully treating an eating disorder, but this is not the only requirement. Healthful eating habits must be learned and established to replace the harmful behaviors. Additionally, people with eating disorders also need professional help to develop a realistic body image, develop positive self-esteem, and re-solve the underlying control issues that may have con-tributed to the eating disorder.

Other Disorders

Personality Disorders

Personality disorders are characterized by distorted and inflexible thoughts and behaviors that make it impossible for a person to live a productive life or establish fulfilling relationships. These types of disorders have created contro-versy in the field of psychiatry because it is often difficult to decide when the personality style of a person becomes deviant. For a woman to be diagnosed with a personality disorder, she must be experiencing long-term patterns of the distorted thoughts and behaviors and these behaviors must cause interpersonal trouble. Several personality disor-ders exist (**Table 12.5**), with histrionic and borderline per-sonality disorders being the most commonly diagnosed in women.

People with histrionic personality disorder are deeply emotional, have low self-control, and feel a strong need for attention. People with this mental disorder feel uncom-fortable and unappreciated unless they are constantly the center of attention. Because people with this disorder are very sensitive, they can be easily hurt by real or imagined slights. People with histrionic disorder often have a diffi-cult time maintaining stable jobs, living arrangements, and relationships. Additionally, their suggestibility, and need for attention and approval, can lead people with histrionic disorder to engage in risky sexual behaviors.[30] Borderline personality disorder (BPD) is also characterized by insta-bility in moods, relationships, identity, and behavior. Peo-ple with BPD may develop intense feelings of anxiety, anger, or depression that appear and disappear within sev-eral hours. The intensity of these feelings makes people with BPD more likely to hurt themselves, engage in sub-stance abuse, and commit suicide. The same intense, changing emotional pattern also makes it very difficult for people with BPD to build and maintain stable relation-ships.[31] A combination of environmental and genetic fac-tors likely play a part in whether a person develops histri-onic personality disorder or BPD.

Many people with personality disorders never enter treatment, although those who do usually seek help for de-pression or anxiety. Treatment can be beneficial, and it of-ten involves long-term psychotherapy, cognitive-behavioral therapy, and/or family or group therapy. Medications may

Table 12.5 Types and Symptoms of Personality Disorders
Antisocial: disrespectful of others; often in trouble with authorities
Avoidant: extremely inhibited socially; low self-esteem; intense fear of rejection
Borderline: poor self-image; unstable relationships; mood swings; impulsive behavior; extreme fear of being abandoned; self-destructive behaviors such as drug abuse, casual sex, and binge eating
Dependent: submissive; feelings of worthlessness; allows others to make important decisions; common in women who have suffered domestic abuse
Histrionic: seeks attention; acts overly emotional to attract desired attention; constantly seeks approval; is demanding and needy in re-lationships
Narcissistic: needs constant admiration and attention; has low self-esteem and an exaggerated sense of her own importance; con-stantly worried what others think of her
Obsessive-compulsive: obsessive about certain areas of life, includ-ing work; perfectionist tendencies; controlling personality
Paranoid: extremely distrustful; suspicious of others; extremely jeal-ous, unforgiving, and quick to anger
Passive-aggressive: passively resists taking on responsibilities; consistently fails to live up to demands placed on her; often is irri-table and complaining, resulting in problems in relationships
Schizoid: cannot form close relationships; has a very limited range of emotions; may lead to schizophrenia
Schizotypal: cannot form close relationships; eccentric in behavior; experiences distorted thinking and strange speech and behavior pat-terns; suffers from extreme social anxiety; often suspicious of others

be given with psychotherapy to relieve symptoms of depres-sion or anxiety.

Schizophrenia

Psychosis is a severe mental disorder characterized by loss of contact with reality and severe personality changes. Al-though mood disorders primarily affect how a person feels, psychosis disorders primarily affect how a person thinks and perceives the world. **Schizophrenia**, a type of psychosis, rep-resents an extraordinarily complex group of disorders and is the most chronic and disabling of the severe mental disor-ders. Many subtypes of schizophrenia exist, each of which is characterized by specific symptoms and a certain degree of disease severity. Although the word "schizophrenia" comes from the Greek word for "split," it does not mean that a schizophrenic person has a "split" or multiple personality. Instead this meaning describes the splitting of coherent thoughts in those who suffer from the illness.

Schizophrenia afflicts about 2.4 million U.S. adults (about 1% of the adult population), with men and women being affected equally. Gender differences are apparent in the development of the disease, however. Men are more likely to be affected between the ages of 16 and 25, whereas women are more likely to have a disease onset between the ages of 25 and 30. Women typically start with a milder form of the disease, experiencing more mood symptoms than psychoses. A significant proportion of women with schizophrenia experience an increase in symptoms during pregnancy and the postpartum period.

Living with schizophrenia can be terrifying. People with schizophrenia experience hallucinations (sensory perceptions, such as sights, voices, or smells, that are not there) and delusions (beliefs that are not true, such as that people are reading the person's mind, planning to harm or trap the person, or controlling the person's thoughts). To the person experiencing them, these hallucinations and delusions appear utterly real.[2] These and other symptoms can appear suddenly or gradually over a period of years. Other symptoms of schizophrenia include disordered thinking, difficulty interacting with others, and difficulty thinking clearly. Some women with schizophrenia may experience symptoms for years or decades at a time, whereas others may experience random episodes of symptoms throughout life. Treatments for schizophrenia are improving and can relieve many symptoms, but most people with schizophrenia continue to experience some degree of symptoms throughout their lives.[32]

Fewer than half of people with schizophrenia get adequate treatment. New medications that cause fewer side effects have been developed over the last decade. A newly developed class of drugs, the atypical antipsychotics, are more effective than older types of drugs, but have much more severe side effects. Psychotherapy and support groups also may be helpful for some patients. Schizophrenia is a difficult disease; only one in five people recovers completely and one in 10 takes his or her own life.[32]

Dissociative Disorders

Dissociative disorders develop as an unconscious way to protect oneself from emotional traumas by detaching from a part of one's personality. These disorders occur as a response to a severe childhood trauma. The created defense appears helpful to the individual, but is actually detrimental to the process of recovery.

Several types of dissociative disorders exist, with the most common being dissociative identity disorder, also known as multiple personality disorder. Dissociative identity disorder is associated with early childhood abuse and usually has its onset in late adolescence or early adulthood. The disorder is progressive in nature and often coexists with personality disorders. Women with this disorder are unable to process their thoughts, feelings, memories, and actions into a complete and single state of consciousness. Signs of dissociative identity disorder include amnesia, detachment from reality, and detachment from oneself through depersonalization. People with dissociative identity disorder often hurt themselves intentionally in acts of self-mutilation. Treatment includes psychotherapy to integrate the various personalities and to resolve feelings surrounding the traumatic event.

Dissociative amnesia, another form of a dissociative disorder, is loss of memory resulting from trauma. Depending on the form of dissociative amnesia, either some or all of the experiences from various time periods are blocked out. Therapy is used to help the person adjust to the current situation rather than to resolve the past.

Suicide

The taking of one's own life can be considered the most harmful symptom of mental illness. There are almost always warning signs that a person is at risk of suicide. More than 90% of people who kill themselves have depression or another diagnosable mental or substance abuse disorder. Adverse life events like a death in the family, a relationship breakup, or financial ruin, along with other risk factors, also may make a person more likely to take his or her own life. However, suicide is not a normal or acceptable response to stress. Many people have considered suicide at some point in their lives when they were depressed or experienced something very bad. Most would never act on these thoughts, and are thus not considered suicidal.

Risk factors for someone being suicidal include the following:

- Adverse life events in combination with other factors such as depression
- Prior suicide attempt
- Family history of mental disorder or substance abuse
- Family history of suicide
- Family violence, including physical or sexual abuse
- Firearms in the home
- Incarceration
- Exposure to suicidal behavior of others, including family members, peers, and even the media

Although more women than men report attempts at suicide, more men complete the act. Suicide is the eleventh leading cause of death in the United States—the ninth leading cause of death for males, and the sixteenth leading cause of death for females.[33] For many people, an attempt at suicide is a "cry for help." In adults, the strongest risk factors for attempting suicide are depression, substance abuse, and separation or divorce. Risk factors for children and adolescents include depression, substance use, and aggressive behavior. Friends and family members of people with known depression or with one of the risk factors mentioned earlier should pay close attention to their loved ones. If they demonstrate suicidal behaviors or discuss suicidal wishes, it is important to seek professional psychiatric, social work, or medical help immediately.

Suicide has become a major problem in many developing countries and Eastern European countries. Among rural communities in China and many former Soviet bloc countries, it is one of the leading causes of death for young women.

Preventive interventions for suicide are often intensive. They typically require learning new coping skills, recognizing the underlying factors causing distress, and receiving appropriate treatment for existing mental and substance abuse disorders.

■■■■

Informed Decision Making

Different people have different vulnerabilities to mental disorders based on their genetic inheritance, physical condition, social situation, and life experiences, but mental health is a concern for everyone. No one is immune to mental disorders, and even if you are fortunate enough to

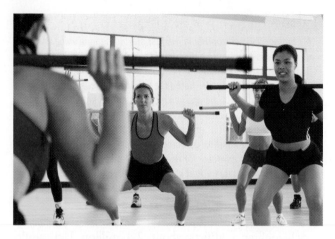

■ Women can improve their mental health by integrating physical activity into their day.

never experience one, it is almost certain that you will know and care for someone who has experienced one, has one now, or will have one.

Good mental health is more than merely the absence of mental illness, just as good physical health is more than just the absence of disease. There may be no perfect definition of good mental health, but being able to engage in rational thought and decision making; feeling a variety of emotions without being controlled by those emotions; being able to maintain stable, fulfilling relationships; and being able to cope with difficult circumstances are all signs of a healthy mind.

To maintain emotional well-being, it is essential to take care of oneself. Some women tend to put other people's needs before their own. If a woman does this on a consistent basis, it can put her under great stress and make her more likely to experience and suffer from mental illness. Finding appropriate coping mechanisms can help women deal with stressful situations and difficult circumstances. Some good coping mechanisms include taking time to relax, and having a trusted friend, family member, or mentor to talk to. Other basic healthy behaviors, like getting a good night's sleep, eating a nutritious diet, and integrating physical activity into one's daily routine, benefit the mind as well as the body. In particular, regular exercise yields enormous benefits for people suffering from depression and anxiety disorders. The **It's Your Health** text box lists healthful activities that evidence has shown as being specially beneficial in relieving stress and promoting good mental health.

If a woman does notice a pattern of disturbing thoughts, finds herself unable to cope with life's daily challenges, or finds herself anxious or unhappy most of the time, she

It's Your Health

Helpful Ways to Promote Good Mental Health and Relieve Stress

Here is a list of common activities that can provide relief from stress, anxiety, and depression, as well as promote good mental health.

- Watching a funny movie or show, telling and listening to jokes, or other activities that bring laughter
- Exercise (regular activity is best, but any amount of exercise brings benefits—for more information, see Chapter 9)
- Meditation or prayer
- Gardening
- Spending time with a pet or pets
- Getting a massage
- Visualization (imagining yourself on a calm beach, in a quiet meadow, or in some other peaceful, relaxing situation)
- Listening to music
- Napping or simply lying down, closing one's eyes, and relaxing
- Creative endeavors (writing, drawing or painting, dancing, singing, etc.)

should seek professional help. Seeking help is not always easy. Many people who could benefit from mental health services decide not to seek care out of fear that they will be labeled "crazy" or "unstable." Other people believe either that "things will get better on their own" or that treatment would be useless. It is important to remember that millions of Americans already benefit from (or would benefit from) some form of mental health treatment. And although some mental disorders may go away on their own, others do not, and treatment can often dramatically shorten the course of a disorder. **Self-Assessment 12.1** can help a woman determine whether she, or someone she cares about, needs to seek help.

Psychiatrists, clinical psychologists, and social workers are all trained, certified practitioners who have been educated in helping people with mental health problems. Many colleges and universities have some professional mental health services available, or at least can give referrals to nearby services. A good match between a patient and provider that includes mutual trust is key. Asking a mental health provider questions about his or her training, number of years in practice, experience treating someone with a similar problem, fees, types of insurance accepted, and methods of therapy can all help a woman decide whether that provider is best for her.

Many studies have proved the benefit of combining therapy and medication. Often, a combination of therapy with medication works better at treating mental illness than either medication or therapy alone. There are four basic forms of therapy:

- Traditional psychotherapy, which deals with psychosocial aspects of depression and is often referred to as "talk therapy"
- Psychodynamic psychotherapy, which deals with experiences from childhood to resolve rooted problems
- Cognitive-behavioral therapy, which works to identify and correct patterns of thinking and behaviors
- Interpersonal psychotherapy, which focuses on present problems and helps with improving relationships, communication skills, and coping skills

New medications have made it easier to bring relief to people with mental disorders. However, although medications can be of great benefit, they should not be thought of as a "magic bullet" that can instantly fix or eliminate mental illness. Medications can take days to weeks to have any effects, may require professional help and personal observation to determine the correct choice of medication and

Self-Assessment 12.1

Determining One's Need to Seek Professional Help

Experiencing any of the following symptoms for several weeks may be an indication that a person needs to seek professional help.

_____ Feelings of sadness, hopelessness, or worthlessness

_____ Loss of energy and drive

_____ Behavioral changes, such as restlessness, irritability, or self-destructive behavior

_____ Physical symptoms, such as headache, nausea, backache, or unexplained pain

_____ Prolonged worry or anxiety without any identifiable cause or reason

_____ Sudden episodes of intense and overwhelming fear for no apparent reason

_____ Irrational and uncontrollable fear or panic when exposed to a particular object or situation

_____ Frequent thoughts or talk about death or suicide

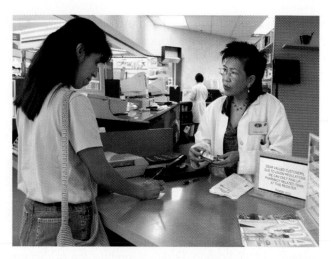

■ New medications have made it easier to bring relief to people with mental disorders.

dosage, and may cause unpleasant or dangerous side effects. Medications for mental illness include antidepressants, lithium (used for bipolar disorder), antianxiety medications, and antipsychotic medications.

■■■■
Summary

Mental health is a difficult concept to define, yet it is nevertheless essential for both individuals and societies to function. Mental health measures a person's ability to find peace in life, feel emotions without being controlled by them, build and maintain stable relationships, and cope with difficult circumstances. Biological, social, psychological, and environmental factors all influence mental health.

Mood disorders, anxiety disorders, and eating disorders are three kinds of mental disorders affecting women. These and other mental disorders affect the way people feel, think, perceive reality, and interact with the world. Left alone, mental disorders can cause a variety of harmful effects, perhaps the worst of which is suicide. Treatment for mental disorders may involve psychotherapy, medications, or a combination of both. Mental health should involve not just avoiding and treating mental disorders, but also practicing behaviors that reduce stress and promote good mental health.

■■■■
Topics for Discussion

1. Freud defined mental health as "the ability to love and to work." What do you think of this definition? Can you create a better one?

2. If you were president of the United States, what laws would you change to promote better mental health?

3. Why does stigma around mental illness exist? What can be done to reduce this stigma?

4. What are some of the advantages and disadvantages of prescribing medication for a mental disorder?

5. A young woman suspects that her friend has an eating disorder. What can she do? What if her friend denies the disorder in spite of overwhelming evidence?

6. A young woman suspects that her grandfather is depressed. What can she do? What if her grandfather tells her he doesn't know what "being depressed" means?

7. What are steps that you can take (as a class or as individuals) to promote good mental health?

Profiles of Remarkable Women

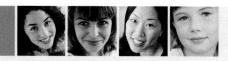

Dorothea Lynde Dix (1804–1887)

Dorothea Lynde Dix was a nurse and humanitarian who was instrumental in the reform of treatment of the mentally ill. Dix became interested in this issue when she visited a prison in Massachusetts that housed a number of mentally ill people. She saw naked prisoners in chains being kept in filthy quarters, with visible signs of harsh treatment and abuse. Dix spent the next two years researching the situation and then reported her findings to the Massachusetts legislature. Responding to her plea for humane care for the mentally ill, Massachusetts took action and moved the mentally ill people to an asylum. Dix sought change all over the United States through legislative reform, and her work prompted the establishment of 32 mental health hospitals across the United States. Dix also made an international impact, recommending reforms for prisons in Italy, France, Russia, Scotland, and Turkey.

Profiles of Remarkable Women

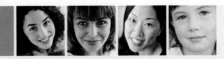

Tipper Gore (1948–)

Mary Elizabeth Aitcheson, nicknamed "Tipper" by her mother, grew up in Arlington, Virginia. Tipper met her future husband, Albert Gore, at his high school prom when she was 16, and they soon began dating. Gore headed north to study at Harvard University, and Tipper followed one year later to attend Boston University, where she majored in psychology. They were married in 1970, following Tipper's graduation, when she was just 21 and Gore was 22.

In 1975, Tipper received her master's degree in psychology from George Peabody College at Vanderbilt University in Tennessee, while she raised their first child and worked part-time as a newspaper photographer. Upon her husband's decision to run for Congress, Gore quit her job to help with his campaign and eventually moved to Washington, D.C., upon his election. As a Congressional spouse, she helped form the Congressional Wives Task Force, serving as Chair in 1978 and 1979. The task force sought to draw attention to the violence that children are exposed to through the media. She subsequently co-founded the Parents' Music Resource Center (PMRC) in 1985 to promote parental and consumer awareness of issues in popular entertainment marketed to children. Ultimately, the PMRC was successful in gaining a voluntary agreement between the Recording Industry Association of America and the National Parent-Teacher Association to place consumer labels on music with violent or explicit lyrics. Those warning labels are still in use today and have served as a model for labeling efforts for television and other media. In 1987, Gore authored her first book, *Raising PG Kids in an X-Rated Society,* which detailed her efforts to seek responsibility from the entertainment industry. Gore later generated considerable controversy for her stands against sexually explicit lyrics and violent references in popular music.

A major advocate for the homeless, Gore co-founded and chaired Families for the Homeless in 1986, a nonpartisan partnership of families that raises public awareness of homeless issues. She forged a partnership with the National Mental Health Association (NMHA) to produce a major photographic exhibit entitled "Homeless in America: A Photographic Project," which toured the nation. During her husband's vice presidency, Gore shifted her focus to mental health and children's issues, supporting the Children's Health Initiative and the Mental Health Parity Act. As Mental Health Policy Advisor to President Clinton, Gore was committed to eradicating the stigma associated with mental illness. Throughout her tenure, she worked to educate Americans about the need for quality, affordable mental health care. In 1989, her son Al was hit by a car and nearly killed. It took him a year to recover from his injuries. Gore later revealed she had suffered from clinical depression and had undergone treatment for depression following the accident. She was motivated to publicly speak about her personal struggle with depression by her desire to help eliminate the stigma attached to mental illness.

■■■■
Web Sites

American Psychological Association: http://www.apa.org

Anxiety Disorders Association of America: http://www.adaa.org

Depression and Bipolar Support Alliance: http://www.dbsalliance.org

Medline Plus: Mental Health: http://www.nlm.nih.gov/medlineplus/mentalhealth.html

National Association of Anorexia Nervosa and Associated Disorders: http://www.anad.org

National Eating Disorders Association: http://www.nationaleatingdisorders.org

National Institute of Mental Health: http://www.nimh.nih.gov

National Mental Health Information Center: http://www.mentalhealth.org

Substance Abuse and Mental Health Services Administration: http://mentalhealth.samhsa.gov

Swamp Nurse: What's the best hope for the first child of a poor mother? (article): http://www.newamerica.net/publications/articles/2006/swamp_nurse

■■■■
References

1. Kellogg, R. (2008). Quoted in *What Is Mental Health?* [Press Release]. Available at: http://www1.dshs.wa.gov/mediareleases/2008/pr08057.shtml.

2. U.S. Department of Health and Human Services. (1999). *Mental Health: A Report of the Surgeon General.* Rockville, MD: U.S. Department of Health and Human Services. Available at: http://www.surgeongeneral.gov/library/mentalhealth/home.html.

3. Pomerantz, E., Rydell Altermatt, E., & Saxon, J. (2002). Making the grade but feeling distressed: gender differences in academic performance and internal distress. *Journal of Educational Psychology* 94(2): 396–404.

4. Stewart, W. F., et al. (2003). Cost of lost productive work time among U.S. workers with depression. *Journal of the American Medical Association* 289(23): 3135–3144.

5. Vitiello, B., & Lederhendler, I. (2000). Research on eating disorders: current status and future prospects. *Biological Psychiatry* 47(9): 777–786.

6. Centers for Disease Control and Prevention, National Center for Injury Prevention and Control. (2007). *Web-Based Injury Statistics Query and Reporting System (WISQARS)*. Available at: http://www.cdc.gov/ncipc/wisqars.

7. Nadien, M. (1996). Aging women: issues of mental health and maltreatment. *Annals of the New York Academy of Sciences: Women and Mental Health* 789: 129–145.

8. Brydon, L., et al. (2008). Synergistic effects of psychological and immune stressors on inflammatory cytokine and sickness responses in humans. *Brain, Behavior, and Immunity* doi:10.1016/j.bbi.2008.09.007.

9. Lawson, W. (2003). Eat right to fight stress. *Psychology Today*. Available at: http://www.psychologytoday.com/articles/pto-2633.html.

10. National Institute of Mental Health. (2008). *The Numbers Count: Mental Disorders in America*. Washington, DC: NIMH. Available at: http://www.nimh.nih.gov/health/statistics/index.shtml.

11. Lapine, J. P. (2001). Epidemiology, burden and disability in depression and anxiety disorders. *Journal of Clinical Psychology* 62(suppl 13): 148–160.

12. Kessler, R.C., et al. (2008). Individual-level and societal-level effects of mental disorders on earnings in the United States: results from the National Comorbidity Survey Replication. *American Journal of Psychiatry* 165(6): 703–711.

13. James, D., & Glaze, L. (2006). *Mental Health Problems of Prison and Jail Inmates*. Bureau of Justice Statistics. Available at: http://www.ojp.usdoj.gov/bjs/abstract/mhppji.htm.

14. 110th Congress of the United States. (2008). *Mental Health Parity and Addiction Equity Act of 2008*. Available at: http://www.govtrack.us/congress/bill.xpd?bill=h110-1424.

15. National Institute of Mental Health. (2008). *Depression*. Washington, DC: NIMH. Available at: http://www.nimh.nih.gov/health/publications/depression/complete-index.shtml.

16. O'Connor, R. (1997). *Undoing Depression*. New York: Brown, Little and Company.

17. Pratt, L., & Brody, D. (2008). Depression in the United States Household Population, 2005–2006. *NCH Data Brief* 7. Rockville, MD: U.S. Department of Health and Human Services.

18. Halbreich, U., Borenstein, J., Pearlstein, T., & Kahn, L. S. (2003). The prevalence, impairment, impact, and burden of premenstrual dysphoric disorder (PMS/PMDD). *Psychoneuroendocrinology* 28(3): 1–23.

19. Nishizawa, S., Benkelfat, C., Young, S. N., et al. (1997). Differences between males and females in rates of serotonin synthesis in the human brain. *Proceedings of the National Academy of Science* 94(10): 5308–5313.

20. Silberg, J., Pickles, A., Rutter, M., et al. (1999). The influence of genetic factors and life stress on depression among adolescent girls. *Archives of General Psychiatry* 56: 225–232.

21. National Institute of Mental Health. (2008). *Bipolar Disorder*. Washington, DC: NIMH. Available at: http://www.nimh.nih.gov/health/publications/bipolar-disorder/complete-index.shtml.

22. Scott, J. (2006). Depression should be managed like a chronic disease. *British Medical Journal* 332: 985–986.

23. National Institute of Mental Health. (2008). *Anxiety Disorders*. Rockville, MD: U.S. Department of Health and Human Services. Available at: http://www.nimh.nih.gov/health/publications/anxiety-disorders/summary.shtml.

24. Vogt, D. (2006). *Women, Trauma and PTSD*. National Center for Posttraumatic Stress Disorder, U.S. Department for Veteran's Affairs. Available at: http://www.ncptsd.va.gov/ncmain/ncdocs/fact_shts/fs_women_lay.html.

25. Galea, S., Tracy, M., Norris, F., & Coffey, S. (2008). Financial and social circumstances and the incidence and course of PTSD in Mississippi during the first two years after Hurricane Katrina. *Journal of Traumatic Stress* 21(4): 357–368.

26. National Institute of Mental Health. (2007). *Eating Disorders*. Washington, DC: NIMH. Available at: http://www.nimh.nih.gov/health/publications/eating-disorders/nimheatingdisorders.pdf.

27. American Psychiatric Association Work Group on Eating Disorders. (2000). Practice guideline for the treatment of patients with eating disorders. *American Journal of Psychiatry* 157(1 Suppl): 1–39.

28. Vitiello, B., & Lederhendler, I. (2000). Research on eating disorders: current status and future prospects. *Biological Psychiatry* 47(9): 777–786.

29. Blank, S., Zadik, Z., Katz, I., et al. (2002). The emergence and treatment of anorexia and bulimia nervosa. A comprehensive and practical model. *International Journal of Adolescent Medicine and Health* 14(4): 257–260.

30. American Psychiatric Association. (2000). *Diagnostic and Statistical Manual of Mental Disorders* (4th ed.). Washington, DC: American Psychiatric Association.

31. National Institute of Mental Health. (2008). *Borderline Personality Disorder: Raising Questions, Finding Answers.* Washington, DC: NIMH. Available at: http://www.nimh.nih.gov/health/publications/borderline-personality-disorder.shtml.

32. National Institute of Mental Health. (2006). *Schizophrenia.* Washington, DC: NIMH. Available at: http://www.nimh.nih.gov/health/publications/schizophrenia/schizophrenia-booket---2006.pdf.

33. Heron, M. (2007). Deaths: leading causes for 2004. *National Vital Statistics Reports* 56: 5.

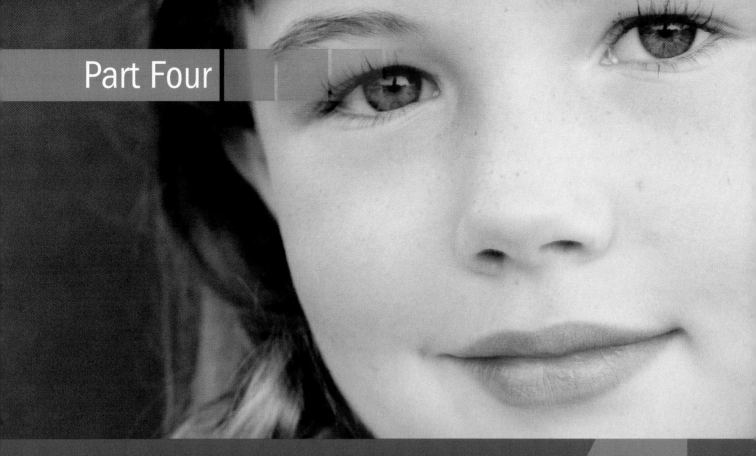

Part Four

Interpersonal and Social Dimensions of Women's Health

4

Chapter Thirteen

Substance Abuse

Chapter Objectives

On completion of this chapter, students should be able to discuss:

1. Substance use and abuse in women from sociocultural, legal, and economic perspectives.

2. Various dimensions of smoking.

3. The effects of smoking on a global scale.

4. Health consequences of smoking, including cardiovascular disease, cancer, other chronic diseases, and risks during pregnancy.

5. The significance of involuntary smoking from a health perspective.

6. Nicotine's role as an addictive drug and the reasons why women continue to smoke.

7. Basic strategies for quitting smoking and smoking cessation methods.

8. Epidemiological trends and various perspectives on alcohol use and abuse.

9. The physiological effects of alcohol on the body.

10. Alcoholism, the symptoms of alcoholism, and approaches to understanding alcoholism.

11. The basic treatment dimensions of alcoholism and special issues for women.

12. The mechanisms for drug entry into the body.

13. Abuse and misuse of legal and illegal drugs.

14. The risks and effects of various types of drugs.

15. The development of drug dependency and basic approaches to drug abuse treatment.

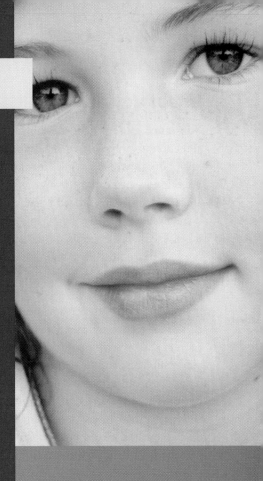

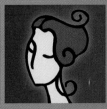

womenshealth.jbpub.com

Women's Health Online is a great source for supplementary women's health information for both students and instructors. Visit

http://womenshealth.jbpub.com

to find a variety of useful tools for learning, thinking, and teaching.

Introduction

Substance abuse is defined as the overuse of, misuse of, or addiction to any chemical substance such as tobacco, alcohol, or drugs (which includes over-the-counter [OTC] and prescription medications, as well as illicit drugs). Substance abuse and problems related to substance abuse are among society's most pervasive health and social concerns. Smoking tobacco, for example, is the single most preventable cause of death, disability, and disease in the United States and contributes significantly to the two leading killers in the United States, cardiovascular disease and cancer. Alcohol is associated with personal health consequences as well as alcohol-related injuries, fatalities, and crime. Over-the-counter and prescription drug abuse and misuse affect people of all ages, and are especially dangerous when combined with other medications or alcohol. Illicit drug use has profoundly affected the health of men, women, and children in the United States. Drug abuse is related to cardiac illness and death, neurological damage, fetal and infant morbidity and mortality, and infection with HIV and hepatitis.

Women are significantly affected by the entire spectrum of drug issues. An understanding of drugs, medications, dependency, and treatment issues within biological, social, and cultural contexts provides a foundation for understanding how drugs influence the quality of women's health.

Substance Use and Abuse

A **drug** is any chemical other than food that is purposely taken to affect body processes. Throughout history, people have used natural and manufactured drugs to alter their moods and serve as health aids. Opium, first cultivated in the Middle East and Asia, was used both therapeutically to induce calm and relieve pain and recreationally to induce euphoric dream states. Native Americans have used peyote, a potent hallucinogenic drug, as part of their religious practices for hundreds of years. Ancient Greek culture documented the use of many medicines, including perhaps the first hypodermic needle–like device for drug administration.

Today, drugs are consumed for legitimate health reasons, such as fighting off infections, as well as for illegal reasons, such as taking them for "fun" or pleasure. **Recreational drugs** are those drugs taken purely for fun. Although most people associate this term with illegal substances, legal substances such as alcohol, tobacco, caffeine,

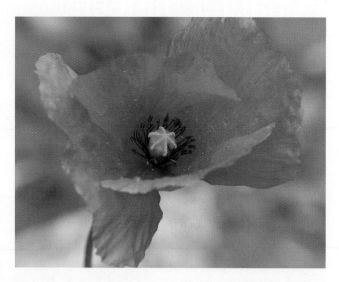

■ Opium, used both therapeutically and recreationally, is made from the sap of the seed pods of the opium poppy flower.

and many prescription drugs (such as amphetamines and tranquilizers) are also considered to be recreational drugs. All drugs, whether legal or illegal, prescribed by a doctor or purchased over-the-counter, are complex compounds that affect the body's activities.

Drugs are generally defined in terms of their legal or illegal status. The legal status of drugs, however, changes with time, and varies by country or state. In the 1920s and 1930s, for example, alcohol was illegal and marijuana was legal. Today, the reverse is true. In the early 1900s, opium, morphine, and cocaine were openly advertised and sold as "remedies" in the form of tonics, syrups, and elixirs. Coca-Cola was originally sold as both a remedy and a refreshing beverage; it contained cocaine until 1906, when the cocaine was replaced by caffeine. Today, marijuana use is tolerated in the Netherlands and in small amounts in most of Europe. Medical marijuana is legal in some countries, and a number of states in the United States have passed laws permitting marijuana use by patients with a doctor's approval. In 2005, the U.S. Supreme Court ruled that doctors can be blocked from prescribing marijuana, meaning the federal government can override state laws on patient use. Examples of illegal (illicit) drugs in the United States include marijuana, cocaine, and heroin. Despite a declared "war on drugs," drug availability continues to grow. No sector of U.S. society is immune to illegal drugs.[1] (See **Table 13.1.**)

Currently, legal drugs in the United States include alcohol, nicotine, caffeine, OTC drugs, and drugs obtained with a medical prescription. Prescribed medications are le-

Table 13.1 Illicit Drug Use in Lifetime, Past Year, and Past Month Among Persons Age 12 or Older, by Demographic Characteristics: Percentages, 2006 and 2007

| Demographic Characteristic | TIME PERIOD | | | | | |
| | Lifetime | | Past Year | | Past Month | |
	2006	2007	2006	2007	2006	2007
Total	45.4	46.1	14.5	14.4	8.3	8.0
Age						
12–17	27.6	26.2	19.6	18.7	9.8	9.5
18–25	59.0	57.4	34.4	33.2	19.8	19.7
26 or older	45.5	46.8	10.4	10.6	6.1	5.8
Gender						
Male	50.3	50.6	17.4	17.4	10.5	10.4
Female	40.9	41.8	11.8	11.6	6.2	5.8
Hispanic origin and race						
Not Hispanic or Latino	47.1	48.0	14.8	14.8	8.5	8.2
White	49.0	50.3	14.8	14.9	8.5	8.2
Black or African American	42.9	43.1	16.4	16.0	9.8	9.5
American Indian or Alaska Native	58.8	54.6	20.1	18.4	13.7	12.6
Native Hawaiian or other Pacific Islander	40.9	*	13.4	13.3	7.5	*
Asian	23.7	22.8	8.9	7.2	3.6	4.2
Two or more races	55.4	51.5	18.1	22.1	8.9	11.8
Hispanic or Latino	35.0	34.2	13.1	12.2	6.9	6.6

*Low precision; no estimate reported.

NOTE: Illicit drugs include marijuana/hashish, cocaine (including crack), heroin, hallucinogens, inhalants, or prescription-type psychotherapeutics used nonmedically, based on data from original questions not including methamphetamine items added in 2005 and 2006.

Source: SAMHSA, Office of Applied Studies, *National Survey on Drug Use and Health*, 2006 and 2007.

gal drugs that can be obtained only through the authorization of a licensed physician or dentist.

Using a drug for a purpose other than that for which it was originally intended constitutes **drug misuse**. Drug misuse includes taking more or less of a prescribed or OTC drug or using an outdated or a friend's prescribed medication. Frequently misused OTC drugs are sleep aids, antihistamines, and cough suppressants, containing dextromethorphan (DXM).

Excess drug use that is inconsistent with accepted medical practice constitutes **drug abuse**. The most frequently abused prescribed medications include pain relievers, tranquilizers, stimulants, and sedatives.

The dangers of misusing or abusing a particular drug are often associated with the drug's ability to cause addiction, or physical dependence. Many legal drugs—including barbiturates, tranquilizers, analgesics, opiates, alcohol, and tobacco—are addictive and can cause physical dependence. Besides physical dependence, drugs can create a **psycho-**

logical dependence, called habituation. Habituation is the repeated use of a drug because the user finds that each use increases pleasurable feelings or reduces feelings of anxiety, fear, or stress. Habituation becomes detrimental when the person becomes so consumed by the need for the drugged state of consciousness that all energies are directed to compulsive drug-seeking behavior.

Drugs can enter the body through several modalities:

- *Oral administration.* Taking a drug in capsule, tablet, or liquid form in the mouth and swallowing it is the most common way of consuming a drug. Drugs taken orally do not reach the bloodstream as quickly as those taken by other means.

- *Through the lungs.* The user sniffs a powder, such as cocaine; inhales gases, aerosol sprays, or fumes from solvents or other compounds that evaporate quickly; or smokes a substance. Inhaling drugs can produce serious, even fatal consequences.

■ *Use of a syringe.* Drugs may be injected subcutaneously (under the skin), intramuscularly (into the muscle tissue), or intravenously (directly into a vein). An intravenous injection results in the drug getting into the bloodstream immediately. Intramuscular and subcutaneous injections are slower in action.

Each person responds differently to different drugs at different times and in different settings. Several factors influence the effects of a drug:

■ A woman's underlying emotional state may be intensified by taking a drug. For example, a woman who is feeling depressed may feel more depressed.

■ Generalized physical conditions such as a cold, pregnancy, or menstruation may make the body more vulnerable to the effects of a drug.

■ Genetic differences among individuals may account for varying drug responses.

■ Mindset has been shown to play a role in drug effects. Someone who snorts cocaine to enhance sexual pleasure may feel more stimulated simply because that is what she expects to happen.

■ Social setting may influence drug effects. Drug effects at a noisy, crowded party are different from the effects produced at an intimate, subdued event.

Tolerance is the body's ability to withstand the effects of a drug. Continued use of certain drugs results in increased tolerance and decreased responsiveness, so increasingly larger doses become necessary to achieve a constant effect. Larger doses increase the risk of toxicity—the level at which a drug becomes poisonous to the body. Toxicity may result in damage to the body that is either temporary or permanent, minor or major, and can cause death.

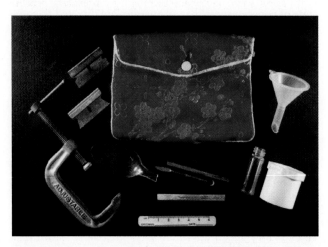

■ There are several ways that drugs can enter the body.

The use of several drugs at once is known as polyabuse. The average user who enters treatment is on five different drugs. The more drugs used, the greater the chance of side effects, complications, and possible life-threatening situations.

Sociocultural Dimensions of Women and Drug Use

The path toward drug abuse is believed to be complex, yet patterned, for women. The typical pattern begins with a breakdown of protective factors, such as family or environment, and results in an increase in fears, anxieties, phobias, and failed relationships. Studies indicate that several factors increase the likelihood of drug abuse in women:

■ Significant life stresses, such as divorce, loneliness, and dissatisfaction with a career[2]

■ Sexual abuse and physical abuse, beginning before the age of 11 and occurring repeatedly[3]

■ Issues such as low self-esteem, self-deprecation, anxiety, and conflict

Society's double standard for women prevails in drug use. A harsher stigma has always been placed on the addicted woman than on the addicted man. The greater social sanctions against addiction in women make some women less willing to seek help and their friends and families less willing to recognize the addiction and intervene.

Females also have a higher rate of substance abuse co-occurring with other psychiatric disorders, such as depression, anxiety, post-traumatic stress disorder, eating disorders, and borderline personality disorder.

Legal Dimensions of Substance Abuse

Criminalizing drug use disproportionately affects people of color. For example, whereas African Americans constitute 14% of marijuana users in general, they account for nearly one-third of all marijuana arrests. Hispanic and African American drug offenders both have a greater chance of being sentenced to prison than white drug offenders (40% and 20% greater, respectively). African Americans also receive longer prison terms for drug offenses than whites do, serving nearly as much time in prison for a drug offense as whites do for a violent offense.[4]

According to the U.S. Surgeon General's Office, since 1980 the number of women in prison has increased at nearly double the rate for men. There are now nearly seven times as many women in state and federal prisons as in 1980; in particular, the number of women incarcerated for drug offenses has risen 888% since 1980, and minority women (African American and Hispanic) represent a disproportionate share of this increase. Minority women are also least likely to receive effective drug treatment. Once arrested, many addicts are incarcerated where their addiction is either left untreated or worsens due to the widespread (albeit underground) availability of drugs in many prisons.

In addition to the legal status of the drugs themselves, some unique legal considerations are associated with drug use among women. Of particular concern is drug use during pregnancy. Pregnant drug users are at increased risk for miscarriage, ectopic pregnancy, stillbirth, low weight gain, anemia, hypertension, low-birthweight babies, and other medical problems. HIV infection, a possible consequence of intravenous drug use, is another risk among pregnant drug users. Approximately 5% of pregnant women between the ages of 15 and 44 reported being current users of illicit drugs in 2006–2007; this number represents roughly half the rate found among nonpregnant women in the same age group (9.7%). The rate of drug use among pregnant girls ages 15 to 17 was 22.6%, significantly higher than the rate among nonpregnant girls (13.3%).[1]

A number of states are now dealing with prenatal substance abuse through their legal systems. Some states require health-care professionals to report prenatal drug exposure; others have amended their child welfare laws to include prenatal substance abuse, using this as evidence of child abuse to end or diminish parental rights. This approach shifts the focus to punishment and away from the urgent need to provide appropriate drug treatment programs for women. Only a few states have viewed drug use by pregnant women as a sign of the need for treatment, forcing pregnant users into inpatient treatment programs. According to the Women's Law Project, punitive reproductive health policies have an especially negative effect on low-income women and women of color. About 80% of pregnant women charged with crimes for drug abuse are women of color, and drug testing of newborns is implemented almost exclusively by public hospitals that predominantly serve low-income women.[5] Such policies may have the effect of discouraging women from seeking needed prenatal care or drug treatment. The threat of criminal punishment fosters a climate of fear and mistrust between doctors and patients, potentially causing harm to the health of both women and their future children.

Economic Dimensions of Substance Abuse

According to the Office of National Drug Control Policy, drugs lead to 52,000 deaths and cost $110 billion per year in the United States.[6] The effects of drug use can be considered on both an individual and a societal level. Individual effects include:

- Physiological changes
- Mental dependence
- Conflicts in relationships

Societal costs include:

- Burden of drug-related crime
- Creation of treatment facilities
- Loss of individual productivity
- Care for children of drug-dependent parents
- The policing of illicit drug availability
- Treatment of medical complications resulting from inappropriate drug use

The federal government spends more than $13 billion on three areas of focus: (1) stopping drug use before it starts, (2) healing America's drug users, and (3) disrupting the market for illicit drugs. This number does not include over $385 million requested for counternarcotics support to Mexico and Central America.[7] Around the world, illicit drugs are one of the most lucrative exports for many countries.

The economic and social forces that come into play between drug users and drug sellers are significant. Across the board, drug use is more prevalent among people of lower socioeconomic status. Use of certain drugs, such as crack cocaine, is much more common among poorer people than among affluent people. These drugs tend to be relatively affordable on a per-dose basis. Most often drugs are exchanged for money, but frequently they are exchanged for sex. This practice is most common among poor female drug users, with crack addiction being a prevalent precursor to such behavior. Exchanging drugs for sex puts women at heightened risk for acquiring a sexually transmitted disease, such as HIV infection, and for becoming a target for sexual violence.

Regular tobacco use also imposes serious economic costs. Today, the price of a pack of cigarettes averages around $5 to $6, with state and city taxes bringing the cost up to as high as $10 per pack. State, federal, and local taxes often make up half or more of the price of cigarettes sold in stores. New York raised its state cigarette excise tax in early 2008 by $1.25 to $2.75 per pack, giving it the highest tax in the nation in 2008. As a result, a pack-a-day smoker may spend anywhere from $1,650 to more than $3,200 annually to fund her habit. In response to the price increase, an underground trade of cigarettes is thriving. Black-market cigarettes are being sold by street vendors for lower prices or market prices, with the vendor pocketing the tax money. Untaxed cigarettes are available on Indian reservations, in countries outside of the United States, and on the Internet for as little as $2.30 a pack. Organized crime and large-scale smugglers are now participating in the underground cigarette market. In addition to the cost of purchasing a pack of cigarettes, smokers are required by many employers to pay higher premiums for their health insurance coverage. Some companies have even implemented policies against hiring smokers in states where it is legal to do so.

Tobacco

Cigarette smoking is a major preventable cause of premature morbidity and mortality in the United States today. Tobacco causes more death and suffering than any other human-made material. Half of all Americans who smoke will die of a smoking-related disease. Lung cancer is the leading cause of cancer death among U.S. women and men. Roughly 90% of all lung cancer deaths and 30% of all cancer deaths are attributable to smoking.[8] Clearly, the health consequences of smoking are devastating to women's health.

Smoking is a complex addictive behavior, but smokers are not the only individuals affected by their tobacco use. Involuntary smokers—the nonsmoking spouses, partners, co-workers, children, and even pets of smokers who inhale either the exhaled smoke from smokers or the wafts from their cigarettes—experience significant smoking-related morbidity and mortality as well.

Epidemiological Trends and Issues

Tobacco was one of the New World "discoveries" of Spanish explorers 450 years ago, although archaeological and historical evidence suggests that the use of tobacco by women antedated European consumption of the products. Tobacco became an accepted component of early colonial life, and New England colonial women reputedly smoked while performing routine domestic duties. Through the next century, tobacco was also snuffed (inhaled), dipped, and chewed.

Cigarette smoking gradually increased in popularity. Technological "improvements" to cigarettes enhanced the ease of inhalation and modified their flavor and aroma. The 1920s were a critical period of change for women, characterized by radically altered social and cultural patterns. During this period, the tobacco industry began its portrayal of smoking as a form of rebellion, romance, and emancipation for women. Women began to smoke openly in public settings, and female cigarette smoking prevalence rates rose from 2% in 1930 to 34% in 1965.

Today, about one in four women younger than age 25 and one in five women in general in the United States smoke cigarettes. Smoking rates among adults have declined by nearly half since 1965.[9,10] The decline does not seem to affect all groups of women equally, however. Current smoking rates vary based on education and race/ethnicity (see **Figure 13.1** and **Table 13.2**).

Figure 13.1

Cigarette use, by race/ethnicity and age, 2004.

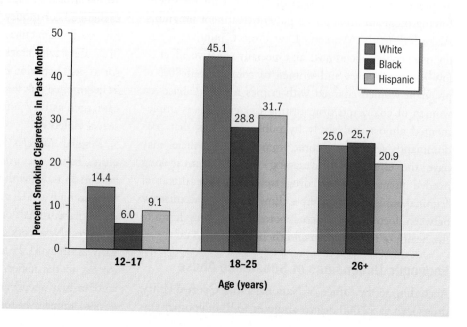

| **Table 13.2** | Percentage of Persons Age ≥ 18 Years Who Were Current Smokers,* by Sex and Selected Characteristics—National Health Interview Survey, United States, 2004 |

Characteristic	Men	Women	Total
Race/Ethnicity			
White, non-Hispanic	24.1	20.4	**22.2**
Black, non-Hispanic	23.9	17.2	**20.2**
Hispanic	18.9	10.9	**15.0**
American Indian/ Alaska Native	37.3	28.5	**33.4**
Asian[†]	17.8	4.8	**11.3**
Education[‡]			
< 8 years	23.5	10.5	**16.7**
9–11 years	38.3	29.8	**34.0**
12 years (no diploma)	29.9	21.9	**25.5**
GED[§] diploma	42.1	36.6	**39.6**
High school graduate	27.2	21.2	**24.0**
Associate degree	24.6	18.0	**20.9**
Some college	24.6	20.3	**22.2**
Undergraduate degree	13.5	10.1	**11.7**
Graduate degree	7.9	8.1	**8.0**
Age Group (years)			
18–24	25.6	21.5	**23.6**
25–44	26.3	21.4	**23.8**
45–64	25.0	19.8	**22.4**
≥ 65	9.8	8.1	**8.8**
Total	**23.4**	**18.5**	**20.9**

*Persons who reported smoking ≥ 100 cigarettes during their lifetime and at the time of interview reported smoking every day or some days.
[†]Does not include Native Hawaiians or other Pacific Islanders.
[‡]Persons aged ≥ 25 years.
[§]General Educational Development.

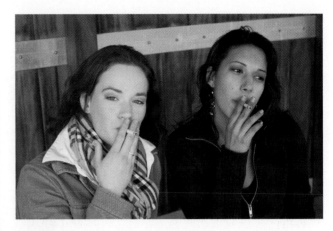

■ Females are beginning to smoke at younger ages, increasing their risk for suffering from smoke-related deaths.

More than half of all high school students have tried smoking, establishing a pattern for becoming smokers as adults. As with adults, rates of current cigarette smoking varied among high school students by race/ethnicity (see **Figure 13.2**). In addition, about 14% of high school students in the United States reported smoking cigars, with males being more likely to do so than females (19.4% compared to 7.6%).[11,12]

Other tobacco products, such as chew or dip, are popular in certain geographic regions and among athletes. Many young athletes falsely consider the nonsmoking form of tobacco to be safer and less likely to negatively affect their athletic performance.

Waterpipes, also known as hookahs, have become popular among some adolescents, college students, and young professionals. An old custom among some cultures in the Middle East, hookahs became popular throughout Europe and eventually made their way to the United States. Hookahs can now be found in fashionable clubs, restaurants, and cafes in many cities throughout the United States. A hookah works differently than an ordinary pipe; tobacco is indirectly heated with burning embers or charcoal and then the tobacco smoke filters through the water. The smoker inhales the filtered smoke through a mouthpiece attached to a rubber hose coming from the base. Although most people believe the water filtration and the long hose help to lessen or eliminate the dangers of smoking, the truth is that hookah smoking appears to be just as dangerous as cigarette smoking.[13] In fact, it may be even more dangerous because the waterpipe is used over a longer period of time than smoking a cigarette (about 40 to 45 minutes compared to 5 to 10 minutes). This longer period of inhalation and exposure may lead a smoker to

Among adults in the United States, American Indian/ Alaska Natives have the highest prevalence of tobacco use. Asian Americans and Hispanic women have the lowest prevalence. Among African Americans, Asian Americans, Pacific Islanders, Hispanics, American Indians/Alaska Natives, and whites, a higher percentage of men than women are cigarette smokers.

Among high school girls, smoking rates peaked in the mid-1990s but have since dropped rather dramatically.

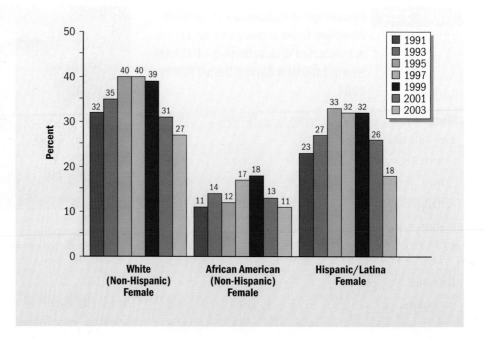

Figure 13.2

Current* cigarette smoking among female high school students, by race/ethnicity, 1991–2003.

Source: American Cancer Society, Surveillance Research. (2004). Youth Risk Behavior Surveillance System. *Morbidity and Mortality Weekly Report* 53(23): 499–502.

*Smoked cigarettes on one or more of the 30 days preceding the survey.

inhale as much smoke as consuming 10 or more cigarettes during a single hookah session.[14]

Societal Costs of Smoking

The human costs are the greatest toll associated with smoking. Annual tobacco-related deaths exceed the number of deaths from alcohol, cocaine, heroin, homicide, suicide, car accidents, fire, and AIDS combined. Each year, approximately 438,000 deaths in the United States are attributed to cigarette smoking.[13] Passive smoking, or involuntary smoking, causes thousands of deaths each year as well. The economic costs of smoking in the United States are estimated at $167 billion per year, including mortality-related productivity costs and medical expenditures for both adults and newborns.[15]

Smokers pay a human cost before dying as well. The smoking-related diseases of cancer, emphysema, and cardiovascular disease exact a toll measured in terms of suffering and disability. The estimates of costs are probably low, considering the costs for burn care from smoking-related fires and medical care costs associated with diseases from secondhand smoke are difficult to measure.

Legal Dimensions of Tobacco Use

All 50 states and the District of Columbia have placed some sort of restriction on where people can smoke. The laws range from restrictions in designated areas to sweeping prohibitions in all public places and workplaces. Examples of recent smoking legislation include the following:[16]

■ **Taxes.** All 50 states and the District of Columbia impose a cigarette excise tax. New York has the highest tax at $2.75 per pack and South Carolina has the lowest at $0.07 per pack. The national average for state cigarette excise taxes is $1.18 per pack.

■ **Youth access.** All 50 states and the District of Columbia prohibit the sale of tobacco products to minors. Age restrictions vary by state; in most states, tobacco sales to youths younger than 18 are banned. Alabama, Alaska, New Jersey, and Utah prohibit sales to minors younger than age 19. Nineteen states and the District of Columbia require a photo ID from purchasers who appear to be younger than 18. Penalties for purchasing tobacco vary by state as well. Nine states may suspend a minor's driver's license; 16 states require attendance of a smoking education/cessation program; and 25 states order minors to pay a fine and perform community service.

■ **Tobacco product vending machine sales.** Forty-eight states and the District of Columbia have restrictions on where vending machines can be placed; only Alabama and New Jersey do not. Seventeen states prohibit tobacco vending machines everywhere except for bars and taverns; some states include restrictions on machines in workplaces. Two states, Idaho and Vermont, prohibit tobacco vending machines altogether.

Advertising is clearly effective in perpetuating and promoting specific products to selected groups. Cigarette advertising is especially effective in increasing cigarette consumption by recruiting new smokers, enticing former smokers to relapse, making it more difficult for current smokers to quit cigarettes, and acting as an external cue or reminder to smoke. In the past, tobacco companies have targeted specific audiences and promoted specific brands with a calculated strategic effort. Minority communities and young women have been aggressively singled out, for example. Several brands are specifically targeted to the African American community and are heavily advertised in African American–oriented media. Other advertising and promotional campaigns have sought to introduce "feminine" cigarettes, which are slim or "ultra-slim" and characterized by decorative borders and sophisticated designer packaging.

Cigarette marketing campaigns have also targeted children. Cartoon characters, such as the Joe Camel cartoon figure, were one of the earlier methods to appeal to a younger audience. But after the use of cartoon characters was prohibited, companies started creating new flavors of cigarettes, such as Kauai Kolada (pineapple and coconut) and Winter Mochamint (chocolate and peppermint). In an attempt to control the purchase of these products, a number of states have introduced legislation specifically prohibiting the sale of flavored cigarettes.[17]

Cigarette manufacturers have responded to legal restrictions by increasing their advertising budgets. In 1998, the year that national advertising restrictions took effect, the combined marketing budget of the four largest cigarette manufacturers was $6.7 billion. By 2003, it had increased to more than $15 billion. These extra funds have been invested in new and innovative promotional campaigns.[18]

Smoking and Women Worldwide

Around the world, nearly one-third of all adults (approximately 1.3 billion people) are estimated to be smokers.[19] This high prevalence makes involuntary inhalation of tobacco smoke almost unavoidable throughout much of the world. Because tobacco smoking has primarily been a custom and addiction of men, women and children represent the majority of the world's passive or involuntary smokers.

The World Health Organization (WHO) estimates that approximately 700 million, or almost half, of the world's children are exposed to environmental tobacco smoke (ETS). Because the home is a predominant location for smoking, women and children are exposed to tobacco smoke most often as they carry out the tasks and pastimes of their daily lives—doing chores at home, eating, entertaining, and even sleeping. The exposures at home may be

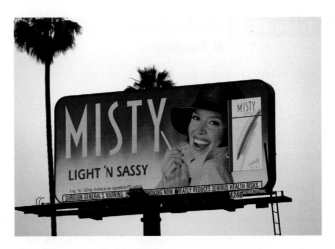

Tobacco companies are savvy in the ways they lure new smokers, particularly women.

compounded for many women and children by additional exposures at work and school.[20]

Tobacco companies are savvy in the ways they lure new smokers, particularly women. According to WHO, many tobacco companies cleverly link the emancipation of women in the developing world with smoking, similar to methods that were used in Western countries decades ago. According to the Institute for Global Tobacco Control, governments in developing countries may be less aware of the harmful effects of tobacco use on women and children and are preoccupied with other health issues; they mostly see tobacco as a problem confined to men. If no dramatic changes in prevention and cessation occur, the prevalence of smoking among women in developed and developing countries could rise to 20% by 2025.[20] To counter this trend, international non-governmental organizations are banding together to address smoking as a global health crisis, especially among women. Specific research and programs are being initiated around the globe to halt women's initiation of smoking and to address the harmful effects of exposure to ETS.

Health Consequences for Women Who Smoke

Tobacco use is the single most important preventable cause of death and disease in the United States (see **Table 13.3**). Almost half of all smokers between the ages of 35 and 69 die prematurely. Health risks to smokers depend not only on their smoking status, but also on specific smoking behaviors and the duration of such behaviors. Morbidity and mortality rates vary directly with the amount smoked, the depth of cigarette inhalation, the "tar" and nicotine content of cigarettes, and the duration of smoking. Inhalation patterns and puffing behavior determine exposure to carbon

Table 13.3 Women's Health Consequences of Smoking

Increased risk for cancer—lungs, larynx, oral cavity, esophagus, kidneys, and cervix

Increased risk for chronic obstructive pulmonary disease (COPD)—chronic bronchitis, emphysema

Increased risk for cardiovascular disease—myocardial infarction, chronic ischemic heart disease, arteriosclerotic vascular disease, subarachnoid hemorrhage, malignant hypertension

Complications of pregnancy and infant health—increased risk for low-birthweight babies, fetal growth retardation, preterm babies, ectopic pregnancy, spontaneous abortion, fetal death, SIDS, and neonatal death

Other risks—osteoporosis, urinary incontinence, decreased fertility, earlier menopause, peptic ulcer disease, and migraine headaches

monoxide and other toxic compounds. Mortality rates also vary inversely with initiation of smoking—in other words, the earlier a woman begins to smoke, the shorter her life. On average, women who smoke will lose 14.5 years of life from smoking.

Symptoms of smoking-related illness usually take years to develop, although irritation symptoms such as watery eyes, nasal irritation, squinting, and coughing develop fairly soon after a woman starts smoking. Smoking affects not only the smoker, but also others in the smoker's environment, including unborn babies (**Figure 13.3**). In addition, smoking causes premature signs of aging including wrinkles, blotchy skin, and discolored teeth.

Cardiovascular Disease

Coronary heart disease is the major cause of death among both men and women in the United States. Cigarette smoking doubles a woman's risk of myocardial infarction (heart attack) and doubles to quadruples her risk of sudden cardiac death. The use of oral contraceptives by women smokers, especially women older than age 35, increases the risk of myocardial infarction, stroke, and blood clots. Oral contraceptive users over the age of 35 who smoke are advised to stop smoking or change their method of contraception. Young and middle-age women who smoke have substantially higher rates of both fatal and nonfatal stroke than nonsmokers. Each year, more than 8,800 deaths from

Figure 13.3

Physiological effects of cigarette smoking.

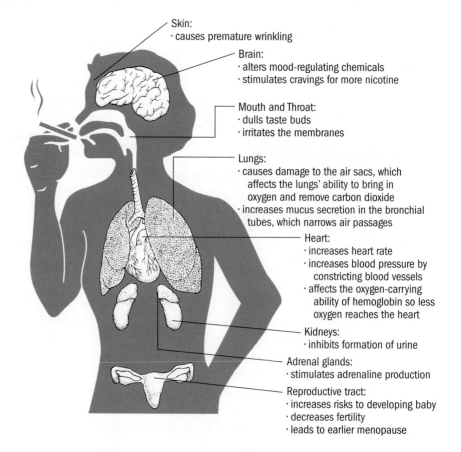

Skin:
· causes premature wrinkling

Brain:
· alters mood-regulating chemicals
· stimulates cravings for more nicotine

Mouth and Throat:
· dulls taste buds
· irritates the membranes

Lungs:
· causes damage to the air sacs, which affects the lungs' ability to bring in oxygen and remove carbon dioxide
· increases mucus secretion in the bronchial tubes, which narrows air passages

Heart:
· increases heart rate
· increases blood pressure by constricting blood vessels
· affects the oxygen-carrying ability of hemoglobin so less oxygen reaches the heart

Kidneys:
· inhibits formation of urine

Adrenal glands:
· stimulates adrenaline production

Reproductive tract:
· increases risks to developing baby
· decreases fertility
· leads to earlier menopause

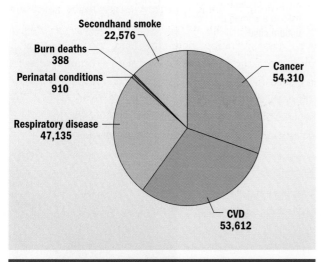

Figure 13.4

U.S. male and female deaths attributable to cigarette smoking.

Source: Centers for Disease Control and Prevention. (2005). *Morbidity and Mortality Weekly Report* 54(25): 625-628.

stroke and 40,000 deaths from coronary heart disease are attributed to smoking in women (see **Figure 13.4**).[15] Smoking is also a major risk factor for arteriosclerosis and peripheral vascular disease.

Cancer

Cigarette smoking has been shown to be a major risk factor for cancers throughout the body. More than 150,000 cancer deaths in the United States are associated with smoking each year, with 50,000 of these deaths occurring in women.[15] Smoking is associated with an increased risk of at least 15 types of cancer, including cancer of the lung, larynx, pharynx, mouth, esophagus, kidney, pancreas, and bladder in women (see **Figure 13.5**). Cigarette smoking and possibly exposure to passive smoke increase a woman's risk of cervical cancer as well.

Lung cancer death rates for women have increased by 400% over the past 30 years, and lung cancer is now the leading cause of cancer-related deaths among women.[20] Smoking accounts for more than 80% of lung cancer deaths in women.

Cigar smoking, like cigarette smoking, is associated with cancer of the lung, oral cavity, and esophagus.

Other Health Consequences

Cigarette smoking severely damages the respiratory system. About 8.6 million people will suffer smoking-related chronic conditions of the respiratory system. **Chronic obstructive pulmonary disease (COPD)**, also known as chronic lower respiratory disease (CLRD) or chronic

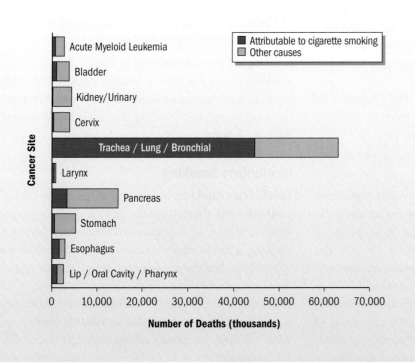

Figure 13.5

Annual number of cancer deaths attributable to smoking in females, by site—United States, 1997-2001.

Source: Centers for Disease Control and Prevention. (2005). Annual smoking-attributable mortality, years of potential life lost, and productivity losses—United States, 1997-2001. *Morbidity and Mortality Weekly Report* 54(25): 625-628.

obstructive lung disease (COLD), is characterized by permanent airflow obstruction and extended periods of disability and restricted activity. COPD encompasses many conditions, including emphysema and chronic bronchitis, which usually occur together:

■ With **emphysema**, the limitation of airflow results from irreversible disease changes in the lung tissue after years of assault on the lung tissue. The air sacs in the lungs are destroyed, which compromises the lungs' ability to bring in oxygen and remove carbon dioxide from the body. As a result, breathing becomes labored, and increased demand is placed on the heart.

■ **Chronic bronchitis** is characterized by constant inflammation of the bronchial tubes. The inflammation thickens the walls of the bronchi, and the production of mucus increases, resulting in a constricting or narrowing of the air passages.

Cigarette smoking is the major risk factor for developing COPD, with 80% to 90% of COPD deaths being attributed to smoking. Over the past few years, more women than men have died from COPD (66,000 females compared to 61,000 males).[21] Females who smoke also are nearly 13 times more likely to die from COPD than are female nonsmokers.

Women who smoke face an increased risk of osteoporosis and early menopause, with smokers reaching spontaneous menopause one to two years earlier than nonsmoking women. The age differences in menopause appear to be smoking-dose dependent. Women smokers also appear to have prematurely wrinkled skin and facial aging, and they often look older than their stated age.[22] Associations also have been made between smoking and infertility as well as smoking and frequent back pain.

Cigarette smoking also can worsen the symptoms or complications of allergies, asthma, and existing disorders of the pulmonary and circulatory system.

Smoking and Pregnancy

Quitting smoking may be one of the most significant things a pregnant woman can do to optimize the well-being of her baby. It is estimated that if all pregnant women stopped smoking, there would be an 11% decreased in stillbirths and a 5% decrease in newborn deaths.[23] Smoking is believed to be associated with 17% to 30% of low-birthweight babies, 14% of preterm deliveries, and 10% of all infant deaths. Although the prevalence of smoking during pregnancy has declined steadily in recent years, substantial numbers of pregnant women continue to

■ Smoking presents many risks to a woman and her unborn child.

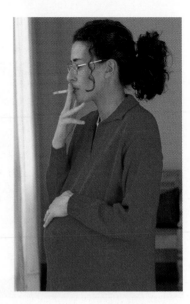

smoke, and only one-third of women who stop smoking during pregnancy are still abstinent one year after the delivery.[24]

Cigarette smoking during pregnancy retards fetal growth and is associated with miscarriage, stillbirth, sudden infant death syndrome (SIDS), and infant mortality. These risks increase directly with increasing doses of smoking. Nicotine and carbon monoxide are considered the two most important components in cigarettes that constitute major hazards to the fetus.

■ Nicotine reduces fetal breathing movements and uterine blood flow, and increases fetal heart rate.

■ Carbon monoxide reduces the amount of oxygen available to the fetus by as much as 25%.

Maternal prenatal smoking is not the only detrimental smoking source for infants. Studies suggest that paternal smoking may present a risk for babies as well. Women can continue to transmit smoking effects via breast milk after the baby is born.

Involuntary Smoking

Involuntary smoking, also known as "passive smoking" or environmental tobacco smoke (ETS), occurs when non-smokers breathe air contaminated by smokers. Involuntary smoking is not benign—it causes increased morbidity and mortality in healthy nonsmokers, young infants and children, and possibly even the family pet. Each year, as many as 35,000 to 40,000 deaths from heart disease, 3,000 deaths from lung cancer, and 150,000 to 300,000 lower respiratory infections in infants are estimated to occur due to ETS exposure.[15]

ETS is of special concern for babies and young children, for whom the major source of smoke exposure is the home. Involuntary smoking increases a child's risk of low birthweight; sudden infant death syndrome (SIDS); acute lower respiratory tract infections, such as bronchitis and pneumonia; induction and exacerbation of asthma; chronic respiratory symptoms; and middle-ear infections. In adults, ETS increases the risk of lung cancer, heart disease, and nasal sinus cancer. Studies also suggest a link between ETS exposure and the following conditions:

- Spontaneous abortion
- Adverse effects on cognition and behavior
- Exacerbation of cystic fibrosis
- Decreased pulmonary function in adults
- Increased risk of cervical cancer

For adults living in households where no one smokes, the workplace is the greatest source of exposure to ETS. The separation of smokers and nonsmokers within the same airspace may reduce, but does not eliminate, the exposure of nonsmokers to ETS. In 2008, 32 states prohibited smoking in government buildings, and 23 states, the District of Columbia, and Puerto Rico prohibit smoking in almost all public places and workplaces, including restaurants and bars.[16] Legislation in many states has mandated that many workplaces follow a nonsmoking policy.

Smoking as an Addiction

Although tobacco smoke contains literally thousands of compounds, the most significant from a health perspective are nicotine, tar, and carbon monoxide.

- **Nicotine** is the addictive element in cigarettes. It has several effects on the body, including increasing blood pressure, increasing heart rate, and negating hunger.

- Tar is a thick, sticky, dark fluid produced when tobacco is burned. It actually consists of hundreds of compounds, many of which are **carcinogenic** (capable of promoting growth of cancerous cells) in their own right. Through inhalation, tar settles and accumulates throughout the oral cavity and pulmonary system. The combination of tar and smoke further compromises the cardiopulmonary system.

- Carbon monoxide is another deadly by-product of cigarettes. This gas interferes with the ability of the blood to carry oxygen, impairs normal functioning of the nervous system, and contributes to degradation of the cardiopulmonary system.

Smoking addiction is defined as dependence on tobacco such that stopping smoking results in withdrawal symptoms. Smoking is clearly an addictive behavior, with nicotine being the primary addictive pharmacological component. **Self-Assessment 13.1** provides an opportunity to assess whether an individual is addicted to cigarette smoking.

Smoking cessation results in withdrawal, an adverse reaction characterized by unpleasant symptoms and an intense psychological and physiological demand for nicotine. Symptoms of withdrawal usually include the following:

- Cigarette craving
- Irritability
- Restlessness
- Anxiety
- Difficulty in concentrating
- Headache
- Drowsiness
- Varied gastrointestinal disturbances such as diarrhea and constipation

Are You Addicted to Cigarettes?

Carefully read and answer each of the following questions honestly.

1. Have you ever failed in an attempt to give up cigarettes?	yes	no
2. Have you ever failed in an attempt to cut back on cigarettes?	yes	no
3. Have you ever failed in an attempt to switch to a lower-tar and lower-nicotine cigarette?	yes	no
4. When you have not smoked a cigarette for a while, do you feel any withdrawal symptoms, such as an urge for a cigarette, irritability, anxiety, difficulty concentrating, or drowsiness?	yes	no
5. Have you developed any smoking-related side effects, such as a morning cough or a hoarse voice, yet continue to smoke?	yes	no

If you answered "yes" to any of these questions, you are probably hooked on cigarettes and have an addiction to tobacco. It is time to quit cigarettes, and seek help from your health-care provider if necessary.

It's Your Health

Strategies to Quit Cigarettes Gradually

Wait 15 minutes after the initial urge for a cigarette. This delay gives a feeling of control, and sometimes the urge will simply go away.

When an urge for a cigarette presents, use a distraction such as drinking water, making a phone call, taking a short walk, or brushing teeth.

Avoid the places where the smoking habit has thrived—a favorite chair, lingering after a meal, a coffee break.

Establish nonsmoking hours and gradually extend them.

Buy cigarettes only by the pack and never buy the same brand twice in a row.

Try to buy cigarette brands with successively lower levels of tar and nicotine.

Make it harder to get your cigarettes. Keep them in a locked drawer or with a friend.

Declare former smoking areas to be nonsmoking areas, such as the car, house, and office.

Don't empty ashtrays.

Collect cigarette butts and take a deep breath of the collection every day as a reminder of how dirty and smelly the smoking habit is.

Keep a daily record to document and reinforce progress with quitting.

The wide range of withdrawal symptoms that occur with cigarette smoking cessation, both physical and psychological, show considerable variability in their duration and intensity. For heavy smokers, withdrawal symptoms may occur within two hours of the last cigarette. The peak period of physiological symptoms from smoking cessation is usually 24 to 48 hours into abstinence, but many smokers report "craving" cigarettes for as long as a year. Withdrawal symptoms include depression, feelings of frustration and anger, irritability, troubled sleep, difficulty in concentrating, restlessness, headache, tiredness, and increased appetite.

Why Women Smoke

Women often initiate cigarette smoking in adolescence in the context of social interactions with peers. Adolescents are more likely to be smokers if their parents, older siblings, or peers smoke. Many smokers report that their primary reason for smoking is to give them something to do in social situations and/or to "fill time." Smoking dependence in females appears to be controlled less by the actual nicotine and more by the social situations in which smoking occurs. (See **It's Your Health** on page 375.)

Nicotine may have several different effects, sometimes acting as a relaxant and at other times functioning as a stimulant. This compound in itself reinforces and strength-

ens the desire to smoke. It also may facilitate short-term memory, help in performing certain tasks, reduce anxiety, negate hunger symptoms, temporarily relieve feelings of depression, and increase pain tolerance.

Fear of unwanted weight gain is a reason that many women have cited for not quitting smoking. Even many pregnant women who smoke indicate that their reason for doing so is to avoid weight gain. Smokers do tend to weigh less than nonsmokers. There is no scientific consensus yet regarding the physiological or biochemical mechanism that is responsible for this relationship between weight regulation and smoking behavior. Some evidence indicates that nicotine elevates the body's basal metabolic rate (BMR). The average person gains between 4 and 10 pounds upon quitting smoking, but exercise combined with a smoking cessation program can decrease this weight gain and increase rates of abstinence from smoking.

Women's concerns about weight gain and the maintenance of their smoking behavior sadly reflect their willingness to risk long-term detrimental—and potentially catastrophic—consequences in exchange for dealing with body image and weight-control issues. Teenage girls, in particular, often believe that smoking helps them control their weight, and this belief dissuades many from quitting this behavior. Health professionals, educators, mothers, and other female role models must strike a balance between recognizing that girls have concerns about their weight, while trying to refocus them on healthy behaviors, self-esteem, and safer coping strategies.

Quitting Smoking

Quitting smoking is the most significant personal behavior that one can undertake to improve one's health. Although the recovery from smoking takes time, cessation of smoking results in a gradual decrease in cancer and cardiovascular disease risk. For example, after 10 to 20 years of cessation, lung cancer rates for former smokers approach the rates of lifetime nonsmokers. Unfortunately, no such relationship exists between smoking cessation and lower risk of COPD. With cessation of smoking, the rate of functional pulmonary loss declines, but the previously lost function cannot be regained. Overall, however, timely cigarette smoking cessation is the best prevention of symptomatic pulmonary disease.

Quitting smoking is not an easy process. The woman who wants to quit smoking on her own has two options:

- **Gradual reduction** is a process of not only gently tapering the number of daily cigarettes smoked, but also

**Common Rationalizations
of Women Smokers**

It can't be as bad as they say.

The government wouldn't let them sell cigarettes if they were that harmful.

My aunt lived to be 80 and she smoked.

We all have to die sometime.

I have so much stress in my life.

I really need cigarettes to make things better.

I DON'T want to gain weight.

It is okay if I smoke because I eat well and exercise every day.

I only smoke at work, not at home.

I only smoke low-tar cigarettes.

I am too busy to eat, and smoking helps me to control my hunger.

I had smoked for years before I became pregnant with my first child. I quit smoking while I was pregnant, but as life became more stressful, I started again—just having a cigarette after a bad day or if my friends were over. Gradually, I began to smoke more and more. Four years later, my daughter told me that my mouth smelled bad, like I "lit a fire in it." I knew then that I had to quit this disgusting habit. Although I don't smoke anymore, I still want one after lunch, when I have a drink, just at certain times of the day. I will always be addicted.

32-year-old woman

cutting back on the relative amount of tar and nicotine by changing brands to those with lower and lower levels of these substances. Many strategies can be used in the process of gradual reduction, all of which serve to modify traditional smoking behavior and reinforce progress toward total cessation.

- Going "cold turkey" means making a decisive, sudden break from cigarettes. Some people find that they are able to go cold turkey if they do it one day at a time. They promise themselves to be smoke free for 24 hours; at the end of that day, they reaffirm their commitment to another smoke-free day. It may take several weeks or months for a former heavy smoker to become confident about the newly acquired nonsmoking status.

Smoking cessation programs have evolved since 1964, when the first Surgeon General's Report on Smoking and Health was published. Intervention strategies for smoking cessation now include a variety of treatment modalities. They may be individualized or group based, formal or informal in design. Multicomponent, behaviorally oriented programs seem to elicit the most favorable results for short-term and long-term cigarette cessation. These programs often incorporate several treatment modalities, including aversive conditioning, contracting, self-control, stimulus control, group support, and cessation maintenance. Pharmacological agents, such as nicotine gum and transdermal nicotine patches, are often used with multicomponent treatment programs as well. Although not all studies have produced consistent results, a number of investigations have shown that use of nicotine gum, in conjunction with sessions of counseling to deal with psychological issues, can help some people stop smoking. Transdermal nicotine patches are proving to be a more effective alternative than the gums. Other forms of treatment for smoking cessation that are available by prescription include nasal sprays, lozenges, and a special inhaler. Two medications also have been used for smoking cessation—Chantix® and Zyban. Neither product contains nicotine. Chantix is believed to work by blocking the receptors that nicotine targets. A public health advisory was issued on Chantix in early 2008 for side effects related to changes in behavior, agitation, depressed mood, suicidal ideation, and actual suicidal behavior. Zyban, also known as the antidepressant Wellbutrin, is believed to work by reducing nicotine cravings and, consequently, reducing interest in smoking. Although the option has not yet been proven effective by scientific studies, some people find hypnosis or acupuncture to be helpful in their quest to stop smoking. Research efforts to develop a vaccine for the prevention and treatment of tobacco addiction are currently under way.

Alcohol

Pure **alcohol** is a colorless liquid obtained by fermentation of a sugar-containing liquid. Ethyl alcohol (ethanol) is the type of alcohol found in alcoholic beverages. The amount of alcohol varies from beverage to beverage (**Table 13.4**). Nearly the same amount of alcohol is present in a 12-oz bottle or can of beer (4% alcohol), 5 oz of table wine (10% alcohol), and 1.25 oz of distilled spirits (40% alcohol). The National Institute on Alcohol Abuse and Alcoholism recommends that individuals who choose to drink and are not specifically at risk for alcohol-related problems should not exceed the one to two drinks per day limit recommended by the U.S. dietary guidelines.

Table 13.4 Alcohol Content in Beverages

Serving Size	Beverage	Alcohol by Volume (%)
12 oz	Light beer	2.4
12 oz	Beer	4.0
5 oz	Wine	10.0
1.25 oz	Vodka (80 proof)	40.0
	Whiskey (86 proof)	43.0

Each contains approximately 0.5 oz of alcohol.

Table 13.5 Blood Alcohol Concentrations

BAC	Effects
0.02–0.04	No overt effects; feelings of muscle relaxation and slight mood elevation
0.05–0.06	Relaxation and warmth; slight decrease in reaction time and slight decrease in fine muscle coordination
0.08–0.10	Balance, speech, vision, and hearing slightly impaired; euphoric feelings; increased loss of motor coordination
0.11–0.12	Difficulty with coordination and balance; distinct impairment of mental facilities and judgment
0.14–0.15	Major impairment of mental and physical control; slurred speech, blurred vision, and lack of motor skill
0.20	Loss of motor control; substantial mental disorientation
0.30	Severe intoxication with minimum conscious control of mind and body

Greater levels lead to unconsciousness, coma, and death from respiratory failure.

Source: Substance Abuse and Mental Health Services Administration.

Blood Alcohol Concentration

Blood alcohol concentration (BAC) is a physiological indicator used by clinicians and law enforcement officials to determine whether a person is legally "drunk." BAC represents the percentage of alcohol in the blood. A BAC of 0.10 (which is technically 0.10%) indicates the presence of approximately one part of alcohol per 1,000 parts of other blood components. As seen in **Table 13.5**, a BAC of 0.10 results in significant compromise of mental and psychomotor capabilities. In all 50 states, driving with a BAC of 0.08 or higher is illegal. The punishment for violating this limit, as well as the number and kinds of other laws related to driving while intoxicated, vary from state to state.

Many factors affect BAC and an individual's response to alcohol. For example, BAC is increased when greater amounts of alcohol are consumed at a faster rate and are consumed without food. Stronger drinks, smaller body size, older age, and being Asian or Native American also lead to increased BAC levels when drinking. In Asians and Native Americans, the metabolic process is unable to break down alcohol as quickly as the corresponding mechanism in whites. In addition to higher BACs, many Asians and Native Americans experience effects such as nausea, headaches, and flushing of the skin when they drink.

With regular alcohol consumption, more and more alcohol is required to achieve the same desired psychological effect, although motor coordination and judgment are impaired at the same level. After several years of drinking, some individuals develop "reverse tolerance" and actually become intoxicated after drinking only a small amount of alcohol.

Epidemiological Trends and Issues

Although alcohol consumption is generally considered a personal and private issue, its effects permeate all sectors and dimensions of society. Alcohol has been a constant component of American life since colonial days. Attempts to control, restrict, or abolish alcohol in the United States have all met with failure. In 1919, the 18th Amendment to the Constitution was ratified in an attempt to stop the rapid growth of alcohol addiction. During the Prohibition era, illegal sales of bootlegged beverages and prescription "medications" prevailed as people sought ways around the ban. Prohibition was officially repealed in 1933 by the ratification of the 21st Amendment.

During the nineteenth and early twentieth centuries, most people who opposed alcohol consumption believed that alcoholics were morally weak. Today, there is a greater awareness of the highly complex nature of alcoholism. The public admissions of alcoholism by well-known women such as Betty Ford, Drew Barrymore, Lindsay Lohan, Elizabeth Taylor, and Nicole Richie have reinforced the fact that alcoholism is a personal and pervasive health problem that affects women from all walks of life.

According to the U.S. Department of Health and Human Services, 46% of females age 12 or older report current (past-month) alcohol use; 57% of women ages 18 to 25 report current drinking; and 16% of girls ages 12 to 17 report alcohol use.[1] American Indian/Alaska Native women are most likely to have alcohol dependence or abuse issues (13.7%), as compared with white women (5.6%), black women (3.5%), Latina women (3.8%), or Asian women (2.3%).[25] In general, women not only are less likely to drink than men, but they also generally drink less and are less likely to become alcohol dependent.

Cultural factors influence the prevalence of alcoholism because the perception of drunken behavior as deviant depends on the culture in which it occurs. It has been suggested that when drinking is a part of family rituals or ceremonies and when there is great disapproval of public drunkenness, there is a corresponding lower prevalence of heavy drinking. Gender-based social norms often contribute to alcohol consumption patterns. For example, in some cultures, men are drinkers while women generally abstain.

Alcohol consumption rates also vary by region and by level of education. Alcohol use is higher in the Northeast (56.0%), Midwest (54.6%), and West (50.8%) than in the South (46.8%); the rate of alcohol use is also higher in large metropolitan areas (53.5%) as compared with small metropolitan and nonmetropolitan areas (50.9% and 44.0%, respectively). Higher levels of education are associated with greater prevalence of current use of alcohol. Individuals with higher levels of education tend to be moderate drinkers more so than those who are less educated; 68.5% of college graduates and 36.5% of adults with less than a high school degree are current drinkers.[1]

Psychosocial Dimensions of Alcohol Use and Alcoholism

Social phenomena contribute to alcohol consumption by women and influence their access to recovery services. Society's double standard for women certainly prevails where alcoholism is concerned. The popular media and folklore portray a male drunk as comical and lovable, but a drunken woman as loose, weak, and immoral. This double standard extends into the treatment arena. The greater social sanctions applied to alcoholism in women make some women less willing to seek help and others less willing to recognize that they need help. Because alcoholic women violate the stereotype of feminine behavior, they often distress their families and friends and even the health professionals who might support them.

Depression has been found to be associated with alcohol consumption and has been suggested as a factor in the alcohol drinking behavior of women. As in the age-old question of "which came first, the chicken or the egg?", it is difficult to establish whether alcohol is a symptom of depression or a consequence of it.

Victimization is another factor associated with alcohol-related problems. Studies have found that women who reported being sexually abused in childhood or physically abused as adults were more likely to experience alcohol-related problems as adults. The relationship between vic-

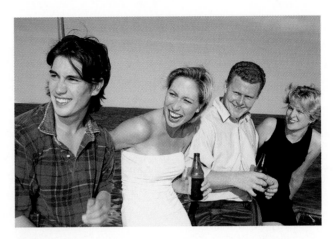

Alcohol is an accepted and often traditional part of many social events.

timization and alcohol may be confounded by the fact that victimization often leads to depression, which in turn is associated with alcohol use.

Although the literature includes few studies on alcohol and drug use among lesbians, it has been suggested that lesbians consume more alcohol for longer periods and are more likely than heterosexual women to use alcohol in combination with other drugs.[26] Lesbian women may be at greater risk of alcohol problems because of the social disapproval directed at their sexual orientation.

Societal Costs of Alcohol Use and Alcoholism

With more than 126 million Americans reporting current use of alcohol and 17 million calling themselves heavy drinkers, the economic, social, and personal costs of alcohol-related crimes, accidents, illnesses, and deaths are profound.[27] It has been estimated that the cost of alcohol abuse and alcoholism in the United States is $148 billion, including $19 billion for health-care expenditures.[28] Almost 70% of the costs of alcohol abuse are related to lost productivity—45% to alcohol-related illness and 21.2% due to premature death. In addition, underage drinking costs Americans more than $58 billion per year.[29]

The costs to society from alcohol cannot be measured just in terms of dollars; the human costs of drinking are incalculable. Alcohol contributes to significant morbidity and mortality among Americans (**Table 13.6**). In 2001, an estimated 75,766 death were attributed to alcohol; about 21,000 of these deaths were women. About half of the deaths were a result of chronic conditions, while the other half were a result of falls, homicides, motor vehicle accidents, suicides, and other acute conditions.[27] Alcohol contributes to several often-fatal illnesses, most notably liver disease, cancer, and cardiovascular disease.

Complications from Chronic Alcohol Consumption

Cancer:
    Cancer of the liver, larynx, esophagus, stomach, colon, breast, and skin (malignant melanoma)
Cardiovascular effects:
    Hypertension, stroke, and cardiovascular disease
Organ damage:
    Brain, stomach, colon, pancreas, and kidneys
Diabetes
Fetal alcohol syndrome
Impotency and infertility
Diminished immunity
Sleep disturbances

Legal Issues of Alcohol Use and Alcoholism

There are many legal issues related to drinking. During the Prohibition era, alcohol was illegal in the United States. Although a constitutional amendment made it legal again, both states and the federal government have since enacted laws that limit its use. Nationally, alcohol use is limited to people older than age 21. In some other countries, no such age limit exists. In many Muslim countries, such as Saudi Arabia, alcohol use is illegal.

In addition to setting age limits on alcohol use, states have enacted other laws governing drinking and driving, drunk and disorderly behavior, purchase of alcohol for a minor, and driving with an open container of alcohol; all of these laws limit how and when individuals can consume alcohol. Most of the penalties associated with alcohol abuse or misuse involve misdemeanor charges or fines, but some —for example, drunk driving violations—entail mandatory jail time in many states.

Effects of Alcohol

Alcohol functions as a central nervous system depressant that effectively impairs all major body systems. When consumed in small quantities, it has a mild, relaxing effect. Consumption of larger quantities results in compromised sensory motor coordination, judgment, emotional control, and reasoning capabilities. As seen in **Figure 13.6**, because alcohol circulates throughout the body, nearly all bodily functions can be affected by increased alcohol consumption. It usually takes about 15 minutes for alcohol to reach the bloodstream, and the peak effect occurs in one hour. Once in the bloodstream, alcohol is quickly carried to the liver, heart, and brain.

Figure 13.6

Physiological effects of alcohol.

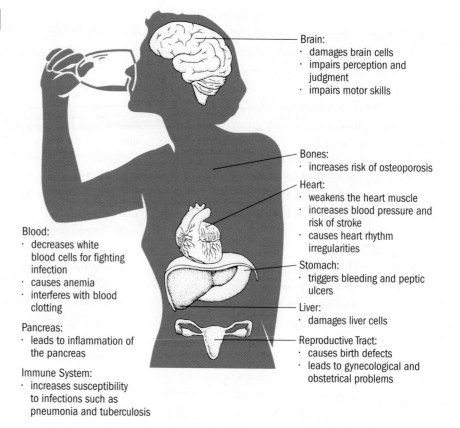

The liver is the organ most vulnerable to alcohol because it metabolizes alcohol. Heavy drinking may lead to alcoholic hepatitis, which is characterized by inflammation and destruction of liver cells, and **cirrhosis**, which produces progressive scarring of liver tissue. More than 90% of heavy drinkers develop fatty liver, a type of liver disease; 20% will develop liver cirrhosis.[30] Compared with men, women develop alcohol-induced liver disease over a shorter period of time and after consuming less alcohol.[31]

Chronic heavy alcohol consumption is also associated with cardiovascular damage. Consuming one or two alcoholic drinks per day appears to lower the death rate from coronary heart disease; however, heavier drinking increases the risk of alcohol-associated heart muscle disease. In response to the evidence that one or two drinks per day may prevent heart attacks and stroke, researchers are investigating the effects of light alcohol consumption on the liver. Alcohol also is associated with various cancers, although there is still controversy surrounding the association between alcohol and breast cancer (Chapter 10).

Perhaps the most dramatic effects of alcohol are on the brain and behavior. As a central nervous system depressant, alcohol alters the activity of brain neurons, impairing sensory, motor, and cognitive function. Moderate amounts of alcohol also have disturbing effects on perception, judgment, and psychomotor skills. Alcohol's anesthetic effect may cause diminished perception of pain and temperature, possibly leading to serious injury or exposure to extreme temperatures. Although drinking may decrease judgment, increase interest, and reduce inhibitions in sex, it also impairs a man's ability to achieve or maintain an erection and a woman's ability to achieve orgasm. Additional drinking results in a progressive reduction in behavioral activity, which may lead to sleep, general anesthesia, coma, and even death.

Alcohol is particularly dangerous when combined with other drugs, such as depressants and antianxiety medications. Of the 100 most frequently prescribed drugs, more than half contain at least one ingredient that interacts adversely with alcohol. Combining alcohol with drugs may produce an effect greater than that expected with either substance taken alone (**Table 13.7**). Acetaminophen (brand name Tylenol) can be especially toxic to the liver when taken in combination with many drinks, in rare cases leading to acute hepatic failure.

Heavy alcohol consumption typically leads to several nutritional problems for the chronic user. Because alcohol dulls the senses of taste and smell, heavy drinkers often

Table 13.7 Alcohol and Drug Interactions

Type of Drug	Examples	Possible Effects
Analgesics (narcotic)	codeine, Demerol, Percodan	Increased CNS* depression possibly leading to respiratory arrest and death
Analgesics (nonnarcotic)	aspirin, acetaminophen, ibuprofen	Gastric irritation and bleeding Increased susceptibility to liver damage
Antidepressants	Tofranil, tricyclics (Elavil)	Increased CNS depression, decreased alertness
Antianxiety drugs	Valium, Librium, Xanax, Ativan	Increased CNS depression, decreased alertness
Antihistamines	Actifed, Dimetapp, cold medications (prescribed and over-the-counter)	Increased drowsiness
Antibiotics	penicillin, erythromycin	Nausea, vomiting, headache Some antibiotics are rendered less effective
CNS* stimulants	caffeine, Dexedrine, Ritalin, Adderall	Somewhat counter depressant effect of alcohol but do not influence level of intoxication
Diuretics	Lasix, Diuril, Hydromox	Reduction in blood pressure with possible lightheadedness
Psychotropics	Tindal, Mellaril, Thorazine	Increased CNS depression possibly leading to respiratory arrest
Sedatives	Dalmane, Nembutal, Quaalude	Increased CNS depression possibly leading to respiratory arrest and death
Tranquilizers	Valium, Miltown, Librium	Increased CNS depression, decreased alertness and judgment

*CNS: Central nervous system.

skip meals and develop nutritional deficiencies. Alcohol consumption also has been associated with osteoporosis due to alcohol's ability to block the absorption of calcium. Chronic consumption disrupts normal digestive processes, resulting in gastritis (inflammation of the stomach lining), stomach ulcers, and intestinal lesions, which interfere with the metabolism of vitamins and minerals. In addition, alcoholism has been associated with thiamine (vitamin B_1) deficiency, which is believed to play a critical role in diseases of the nervous, digestive, muscular, and cardiovascular systems.

Physiologically, women appear to have less body water than men of similar body weight and produce lower levels of alcohol dehydrogenase, the enzyme responsible for ethanol metabolism. As a result, women absorb about 30% more alcohol than men do into the bloodstream before it can be metabolized in the liver.[32] The alcohol reaches women's brains and other organs more quickly, resulting in more rapid intoxication than in men as well as more organ-specific ethanol toxicity. For a woman of average size, one drink has the same effect as two drinks have on the average-sized man. Women alcoholics also are more likely to suffer liver damage than men.

Hormone levels affect alcohol metabolism. Studies have indicated that both the menstrual cycle and the use of oral contraceptives influence blood alcohol levels. The rate of alcohol metabolism and peak BAC attained with a standard dose of alcohol may vary depending on estrogen levels. Moderate alcohol consumption may increase the risk of breast cancer in postmenopausal women taking hormone replacement therapy.[33] These variances may help explain why some women have difficulty predicting their response to alcohol and their feelings of loss of control over their responses.

Alcohol can also harm reproductive health and pregnancy. Although alcohol crosses the placental barrier, its effects on the developing fetus vary because of differences in the degree and timing of exposure, genetic differences in maternal metabolism of alcohol, maternal nutritional status, and possible interaction with other drug compounds. Women who are alcoholics or who drink heavily during pregnancy have a higher rate of spontaneous abortion. A direct effect of alcohol in pregnant women is fetal alcohol syndrome (FAS). This syndrome is distinguished by specific physical and mental abnormalities in infants born to mothers who drank alcohol during pregnancy (see Chapter 6). FAS has the following symptoms:

- Small body size and weight
- Slower than normal development and failure to catch up

- Skeletal deformities
- Facial abnormalities
- Organ deformities
- Central nervous system handicaps[34]

Alcohol consumption may inhibit the release of oxytocin and prolactin, two hormones that are important for initiation and maintenance of lactation. It also may alter the composition of a woman's breast milk and inhibit milk production.[35]

Alcohol plays an indirect role in many unwanted pregnancies and sexually transmitted infections (STIs). Because of impaired judgment and reasoning from intoxication, contraception may be forgotten or ignored, judgment may be distorted, and danger may not be perceived. In addition to unwanted pregnancies and STIs, alcohol is often a factor in acquaintance rape cases and incidents of pressured sex.

Chronic heavy drinking also may be associated with menstrual disorders, infertility, and possibly early menopause.

Alcoholism

Alcoholism has officially been recognized as a disease for more than 25 years. The traditional definition of an alcoholic is a person whose consumption of alcohol interferes with a major aspect of her life. Alcoholism has since been redefined as a primary, chronic disease with genetic, psychological, and environmental factors influencing its development and manifestations. Alcohol has a generational cyclic effect. Children of alcoholics are more likely to suffer abuse, to have psychological or emotional problems, to become alcoholics, and to marry alcoholics. Approximately one in five U.S. adults have lived with an alcoholic while growing up.[36]

Chronic alcohol abuse usually manifests itself as one of the following patterns:

- Daily intake of large amounts of alcohol
- Regular heavy drinking on weekends
- Periods of sobriety between binges of daily heavy drinking that may last for weeks or months

Alcoholism generally appears between ages 20 and 40, but can present in childhood or early adolescence. Alcohol becomes a problem when an individual is no longer able to control when and how much drinking takes place. Clinical diagnosis of alcoholism is based on the presence of at least three of the following symptoms, persisting for

I used to think that I couldn't be an alcoholic. I had a good job and I drank only wine. I certainly don't look like an alcoholic, whatever that look is. It took a long time for me to admit that I really was dependent on that wine. I needed it every day just to dull the world.

30-year-old woman

a month or more or occurring repeatedly over a longer period of time:

- Alcohol taken in large amounts (5 or more drinks per day)
- Persistent desire to quit drinking or one or more unsuccessful attempts to cut down or quit alcohol
- Considerable time spent obtaining, using, or recovering from alcohol
- Continued drinking despite social, psychological, or physical symptoms such as ulcers that are caused or worsened by alcohol
- Withdrawal symptoms, such as physical trembling, sweating, high blood pressure, delusions, and hallucinations, when alcohol intake is curbed
- The avoidance or relief of withdrawal symptoms by drinking
- Desire or need for a drink to start the day
- Denial of an alcohol problem
- Sleep problems
- Attempts to control drinking by changing brands or going on the wagon
- Depression and paranoia
- Failure to recall what happened during a drinking episode
- Dramatic mood swings
- Participation in behaviors or activities while drinking that are regretted afterward
- The experience of the following symptoms after drinking: headaches, nausea, stomach pain, heartburn, gas, fatigue, weakness, muscle cramps, irregular or rapid heart rate

Risk Factors for Alcoholism

Family history of alcohol problems, early initiation of drinking, and victimization may increase a woman's risk for alcohol abuse or alcoholism. Studies on identical twins as compared with fraternal twins, for example, show that identical twins are more likely to have similar rates of al-

cohol dependence, abuse, and heavy consumption, suggesting a genetic component to alcoholism. There is also a significant association between alcoholism in people who were adopted and their biological parents, further reinforcing this hypothesis.[37] Women who were sexually, verbally, or physically abused also reported more alcohol-related problems.

Many psychiatrists believe that alcohol abuse can be a symptom of a personality disorder and that drinking alcohol is the person's way of seeking relief from stress. The act and the effects of drinking reinforce drinking behavior, and the cycle of abuse begins. Traits associated with alcoholism, such as history of antisocial behavior, high levels of depression, and low self-esteem, have been identified.

Treatment Dimensions of Alcoholism

The most difficult and significant step for an alcoholic is admitting to an alcohol problem. Often well-intended friends or family members, out of fear, embarrassment, loyalty, or hope, shield the alcoholic from the truth. Confrontation—either personal or via an accident or drunk-driving conviction—that makes the individual acknowledge the alcohol problem is often a turning point in seeking assistance (**Self-Assessment 13.2**). Recovery from alcoholism is enhanced when the person has a strong emotional support system, including concerned family, friends, and employer.

Alcoholism is a complex problem, and each case must be treated with sensitivity and recognition of its unique situation and contributing factors. Standard treatment programs focus on the relief of physiological dependence but do not eliminate the underlying disease. Individual personality, psychological factors, and sociocultural factors must be addressed to help the alcoholic regain control of her life. Alcohol treatment programs often follow three steps in the treatment of alcoholism:

1. Managing acute intoxication episodes
2. Correcting chronic health problems associated with alcoholism
3. Changing long-term behavior

The most successful treatment modalities combine different approaches and provide ongoing support for people who are learning to live without alcohol. Many alcohol treatment facilities assist clients in overcoming their physical addiction to alcohol and helping them deal with their withdrawal symptoms (**Table 13.8**) through detoxification programs. Detoxification programs are generally available in medical or psychiatric hospitals. Psychological addiction

Self-Assessment 13.2

National Council on Alcoholism Self-Test: Do You Have a Drinking Problem?

1. Do you occasionally drink heavily after a disappointment or a quarrel, or when your parents give you a hard time?   yes   no

2. When you have trouble or feel pressured at school, do you always drink more heavily than usual?   yes   no

3. Have you noticed that you are able to handle more liquor than you did when you were first drinking?   yes   no

4. Did you ever wake up on "the morning after" and discover that you could not remember the evening before, even though your friends tell you that you did not pass out?   yes   no

5. When drinking with other people, do you try to have a few extra drinks that others DON'T notice?   yes   no

6. Are there certain occasions when you feel uncomfortable if alcohol is not available?   yes   no

7. Have you recently noticed that when you begin drinking you are in more of a hurry to get the first drink than you used to be?   yes   no

8. Do you sometimes feel a little guilty about your drinking?   yes   no

9. Are you secretly irritated when your family or friends discuss your drinking?   yes   no

10. Have you recently noticed an increase in the frequency of your memory blackouts?   yes   no

11. Do you often find that you wish to continue drinking after your friends say that they have had enough?   yes   no

12. Do you usually have a reason for the occasions that you drink heavily?   yes   no

13. When you are sober, do you often regret things you did or said while drinking?   yes   no

14. Have you tried switching brands or following different plans for controlling your drinking?   yes   no

15. Have you often failed to keep the promises you've made to yourself about controlling or cutting down on your drinking?   yes   no

16. Have you ever tried to control your drinking by changing jobs or moving to a new location?   yes   no

17. Do you try to avoid family or close friends while you are drinking?   yes   no

18. Are you having an increasing number of financial and academic problems?   yes   no

19. Do more people seem to be treating you unfairly without good reason?   yes   no

20. Do you eat very little or irregularly when you are drinking?   yes   no

21. Do you sometimes have the shakes in the morning and find that it helps to have a little drink?   yes   no

22. Have you recently noticed that you cannot drink as much as you once did?   yes   no

23. Do you sometimes stay drunk for several days at a time?   yes   no

24. Do you sometimes feel very depressed and wonder whether life is worth living?   yes   no

25. Sometimes after periods of drinking, do you see or hear things that aren't there?   yes   no

26. Do you get terribly frightened after you have been drinking heavily?   yes   no

Those who answer "yes" to two or three of these questions may wish to evaluate their drinking in these areas. "Yes" answers to several of these questions indicate the following stages of alcoholism:

Questions 1–8: Early Stage: Drinking is a regular part of your life.

Questions 9–21: Middle Stage: You are having trouble controlling when, where, and how much you drink.

Questions 22–26: Beginning of the Final Stage: You no longer can control your desire to drink.

Source: National Council on Alcoholism and Drug Dependence, Inc. http://www.ncadd.org.

is usually addressed immediately after the detoxification process is completed. Programs such as Alcoholics Anonymous (AA), which is entirely run by volunteers who are recovering alcoholics, provide support for people trying to maintain their abstinence from alcohol. Studies conducted by Alcoholics Anonymous show that the average length of sobriety for its members is more than eight years; 50% of members have been sober for more than five years, 24% for between one and five years, and 26% for less than one year. Since the organization began in 1935, Alcoholics Anonymous has supported more than 100,000 groups and had over 2 million members in 150 countries.[38] AA meetings can now be found in towns and cities across the country almost every day of the week.

Table 13.8 Alcohol Withdrawal Symptoms

Irritability	Dry mouth
Agitation	Elevated blood pressure
Depression	Headache
Lack of concentration	Anxiety
Body tremors	Puffy, blotchy skin
Nausea and vomiting	Fitful sleep with nightmares
Generalized weakness, achiness	Brief hallucinations
Sweating	Delirium tremens (DTs)
Fever	

Table 13.9 Number of Female Emergency Department Drug Mentions, 2000–2002

Drug Type	2000	2001	2002
Alcohol in combination	80,948	85,328	79,957
Cocaine	59,314	65,713	69,852
Heroin	30,146	30,023	31,173
Marijuana	33,334	37,781	41,707
Methamphetamine	4,841	6,680	6,565
MDMA (Ecstasy)	2,011	2,331	1,987
LSD	948	820	112
PCP	1,720	1,683	2,738
Total mentions	513,271	538,166	553,874

Source: Substance Abuse and Mental Health Services Administration. (2004). Emergency Department Trends from the Drug Abuse Warning Network.

Women alcoholics who enter treatment programs have special needs. Their treatment programs must be culturally sensitive and incorporate issues such as age, socioeconomic status, drug use, and sexual orientation into their format. Strategies that can assist women in addressing their alcohol problems include use of culturally appropriate, non-stigmatized language; development of supportive case management; implementation of a mentoring or buddy system; expansion of childcare services; and creation of a multimedia campaign that educates women.

Drugs

No drug use is completely benign. At a minimum, all psychoactive drugs affect the central nervous system. Many habitual drug users end up in the emergency room as a result of overdosing, accident, or injury related to the drug use (see **Table 13.9**). In addition to the direct physiological effects and risks of drug use, additional risks may be associated with the administration of drugs to the body. For example, the process of using needles to inject drugs presents serious risks beyond those of using drugs. Many diseases, including hepatitis and HIV, can be transmitted from one person to another via contaminated injection equipment. The effects and risks of drugs are summarized in **Table 13.10**.

Epidemiological Trends and Issues

According to the National Survey on Drug Use and Health, the rate of current illicit drug use is 5.8% for females and 9.1% for girls ages 12 to 17. Males and females had similar current rates of most illicit drugs, including cocaine, crack, hallucinogens, and inhalants.[1]

Drug overuse and misuse are particular problems among older women. Although they are generally not users of illicit drugs, older women may be likely to be consumers of high levels of medications. Women age 65 or older represent 12% of the general population, but they receive more than 25% of all written prescriptions.[39] Medications such as sedatives, hypnotics, antianxiety drugs, antihypertensive drugs, vitamins, analgesics, diuretics, laxatives, and tranquilizers are prescribed for elderly women at a rate that is 2.5 times the prescription rate for elderly men. Women are diagnosed with anxiety and depression disorders more often than men are, so they are prescribed drugs more often to treat these disorders. Gender differences in weight, body composition, gastric emptying time, cerebral blood

■ There is no particular stereotype of a drug-dependent woman.

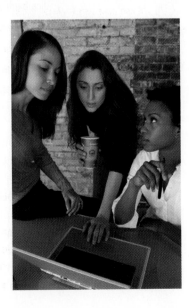

Table 13.10 Summary of Effects and Risks of Drugs

Cocaine and Crack

Names	"Coke," "snow," "lady," "rock," "blow"
Physiological effects	Speed up physical and mental processes; create sense of heightened energy and confidence
Health effects	Headaches, exhaustion, shaking, blurred vision, nausea, seizures, loss of appetite, loss of sexual desire, impotence, impaired judgment, hyperactivity, babbling, paranoia, violence
Long-term risks	Nasal damage (if snorted); lung damage (if smoked); hepatitis and HIV (if injected); damage to heart and blood vessels; chest pain; heart attack; disruptions in cardiac rhythm; stroke; damage to liver
Special risks to women	Increased danger of miscarriage and physical and mental impairment of the fetus; increased risk of congenital malformations, fetal deaths, and SIDS

Amphetamines

Names	Benzedrine ("bennies"), dextroamphetamine (Dexedrine, "dex," Adderall), methamphetamine (Methedrine, "meth," "crank"), Desoxyn ("copilots"), methylphenidate (Ritalin), pemoline (Cylert), phenmetrazine (Preludin), "black beauties"
Physiological effects	Speed up physical and mental processes; lessen fatigue; boost energy; sense of excitement
Health effects	Loss of appetite; blurred vision; headache and dizziness; sweating; sleeplessness; trembling; anxiety and paranoia; delusions and hallucinations
Long-term risks	Cardiovascular damage—hypertension, stroke, heart failure; malnutrition, vitamin deficiencies; skin disorders; ulcers; sleeplessness; fever; brain damage; depression; violent behavior; fatal overdose
Special risks to women	Not yet determined

Barbiturates

Names	Pentobarbital (Nembutal, "yellow jackets"), secobarbital (Seconal, "reds"), thiopental (Pentothal), amobarbital (Amytal, "blues," "downers"), phenobarbital (Luminal, "phennies"), methaqualone ("love drug," Quaalude, "ludes," "Q"), sopor ("Sopors")
Physiological effects	Mild intoxication, drowsiness, lethargy, decreased alertness
Health effects	Drowsiness, poor coordination, slurred speech, impaired judgment, hangover, confusion, irritability; cold skin; depressed respirations; rapid heart rate
Long-term risks	Disrupted sleep; impaired vision; increased risk of fatal overdose with increased use
Special risks to women	Risk of birth defects and subsequent behavioral problems if used during pregnancy

Antianxiety Drugs

Names	Benzodiazepines: chlordiazepoxide (Librium), diazepam (Valium), oxazepam (Serax), flurazepam (Dalmane); dicarbamates: meprobamate (Equanil, Miltown), alprazolam (Xanax), lorazepam (Ativan)
Physiological effect	Slows down central nervous system
Health effects	Slurred speech, drowsiness, stupor
Long-term risks	Physical and psychological dependence; possible fatal overdose; withdrawal can lead to coma, psychosis, and death
Special risks to women	Menstrual irregularities and failure to ovulate have been reported

flow, and use of hormones in contraception and hormone replacement therapy can influence the effect these drugs have in women.

Although many use prescribed medication appropriately, some older women develop a dependency on sleeping pills, muscle relaxants such as Valium, or diet pills. In the 1950s and 1960s, a high percentage of middle-class women were prescribed these medicines, which were widely viewed as acceptable coping tools. Today, many of these women continue to see the use of these drugs as an acceptable way to dull emotions, anxiety, or stress caused by the demands of everyday life.

Stimulants

Stimulants affect the central nervous system and increase heart rate, blood pressure, strength of heart contractions, blood glucose level, and overall muscle tension. Collectively, these effects place additional stress on the body.

Table 13.10 Summary of Effects and Risks of Drugs (continued)

Marijuana and Hashish

Names	Marijuana ("pot," "grass," "weed," "Mary Jane"), hashish ("hash")
Physiological effects	Relaxes the mind and body; heightens perceptions
Health effects	Increased heart rate; dry mouth and throat; impaired perceptions and reactions; lethargy; nausea; disorientation, possible hallucinations, heightened anxiety
Long-term risks	Psychological dependence; impaired thinking, perception, memory, and coordination; increased heart rate and hypertension; compromised immunity
Special risks to women	Prenatal use may lead to fetal effects, including small head, poor growth, lower birthweight

Psychedelics

Names	LSD ("acid"), mescaline, PCP ("angel dust," "peace pill")
Physiological effects	Alters perceptions and produces hallucinations
Health effects	Increased heart rate, hypertension, fever, headache, nausea, sweating, and trembling; delusions and unpredictable violence
Long-term risks	Possible flashbacks, psychological dependence; stupor, coma, convulsions, heart and lung failure; brain damage
Special risks to women	Effects on fetus unknown

Inhalants

Names	Depends on specific product
Physiological effects	Temporary feelings of well-being; giddiness; hallucinations
Health effects	Nausea, sneezing, coughing, nosebleeds, loss of appetite, decreased heart and breathing rates; impaired judgment; loss of consciousness
Long-term risks	Hepatitis, liver and kidney failure; respiratory impairment; blood abnormalities; possible suffocation
Special risks to women	Not yet determined

Opiates/Synthetic Narcotics

Names	Opium, morphine, codeine; heroin ("horse," "junk," "smack," "downtown"); methadone (Dolophine, "meth," "dollies"); hydromorphone (Dilaudid, "little D"); oxycodone (Percodan, "perkies"); meperidine (Demerol, "demies"); propoxyphene (Darvon)
Physiological effects	Relaxation of the central nervous system; pain relief; temporary sense of well-being
Health effects	Nausea and vomiting; restlessness; reduced respirations; lethargy; weight loss; slurred speech; mood swings; sweating
Long-term risks	Physical dependence; malnutrition; compromised immunity; hepatitis; HIV; skin lesions; fatal overdose
Special risks to women	Higher risk for preterm labor, intrauterine growth retardation, and preeclampsia

Caffeine, one of the most widely used stimulants in the world, is found in many different sources. It has a variety of effects:

- Relief of drowsiness
- Help in the performance of repetitive tasks
- Improved mental capacity for work
- Increased basal metabolic rate

In addition, caffeine has been shown to trigger anxiety, insomnia, irregular heartbeat, faster breathing, upset stomach and bowels, dizziness, and headaches in some women. Women who drink a lot of caffeine and then suddenly stop their consumption may experience headaches, irritability, and fatigue.

Cocaine is a popular stimulant drug that is ingested by approximately 2.1 million Americans, approximately 0.8% of the population.[1] The immediate effects of cocaine last 5 to 15 minutes because the drug is rapidly metabolized by the liver. With repeated use, the brain becomes tolerant to cocaine, and users need more of it to get high.

Crack is a smokable mixture of cocaine and baking soda. Because it sets off rapid ups and downs, this drug produces a powerful chemical and psychological dependence. Crack users often need another "hit" within minutes of the previous one. Smoking cocaine in its "freebase" form also delivers a concentrated high that can disappear within seconds.

Cocaine and crack are dangerous for both pregnant women and their unborn babies, causing miscarriages, premature labor, low-birthweight babies, and babies with small head circumferences. Women who use cocaine while pregnant are more likely to miscarry in the first three months of pregnancy than other groups of women are, including those who do not use drugs and those who use heroin or narcotics. Infants born to cocaine and crack users suffer major complications, including drug withdrawal and permanent disabilities. Because cocaine affects blood pressure, it can deprive the fetal brain of oxygen or cause brain vessels to burst, so that the fetus experiences the prenatal equivalent of a stroke, resulting in permanent physical and mental damage. In addition, cocaine babies have higher-than-normal rates of respiratory and kidney problems. Visual problems, low birthweight, seizures, depression, lack of coordination, and developmental retardation are common among cocaine babies as well.

Amphetamines are manufactured chemicals sold under a variety of names. Generally found in pill form, they may also be ground and sniffed or made into a solution for injection. Amphetamines were once widely prescribed for weight control because they suppress the appetite and stimulate the central nervous system. A serious side effect of these drugs is the strain placed on the cardiovascular system, which can lead to severe cardiovascular damage. Use of methamphetamine, a form of amphetamine often referred to as "meth," "crank," or "ice," has skyrocketed in recent years as the drug has become cheaper and more widely available.

Anabolic steroids are synthetic derivatives of the male hormone testosterone. These powerful compounds are legitimately prescribed for treatment of burns and injuries, but athletes and others who want to appear muscular and athletic have increasingly illegally misused them. Women who take anabolic steroids risk development of a deepened voice, breast reduction, enlargement of the clitoris, changes in or cessation of the menstrual cycle, and growth of facial hair. Other potential effects include an increased risk of heart disease or stroke, liver tumors and jaundice, acne, bad breath, aching joints, and increased aggression. Both men and women run a risk of HIV transmission when needles are shared for steroid injection. Anabolic steroid users can become increasingly aggressive and paranoid. Studies have shown steroids to be addictive substances that create the same problems with dependence and withdrawal as cocaine.

Depressants and Antianxiety Drugs

Drugs that relax the central nervous system are called depressants, sedatives, or hypnotics. The most widely used depressant is alcohol. Depressants have a synergistic effect when they are mixed together. As the user builds up tolerance, the likelihood of a potentially fatal overdose increases.

Barbiturates are depressants that are used medically for inducing relaxation and sleep, relieving tension, and treating seizures. They may also be administered intravenously as a general anesthetic. Low doses of barbiturates produce mild intoxication and euphoria and decrease alertness and muscle coordination. With a higher dose, the person may suffer slurred speech, decreased respiration, cold skin, weak and rapid heartbeat, and unconsciousness. Side effects of these drugs include drowsiness, impaired judgment and performance, and a hangover that may last for hours or days. Regular barbiturate use leads to physical dependence. Barbiturate addicts tend to be sleepy, confused, or irritable.

Barbiturates also present problems in pregnancy. These drugs easily cross the placenta and can cause birth defects and behavioral problems. Babies born to mothers who abused sedatives during pregnancy may be physically dependent on the drugs and are more prone to respiratory problems, feeding difficulties, disturbed sleep, sweating, irritability, and fever.

Barbiturate withdrawal is a time-consuming process and medically difficult to manage. Withdrawal symptoms include anxiety, insomnia, delirium, and convulsions. Systemic dependence is so critical that occasionally an abrupt ending of barbiturate use leads to death.

Antianxiety drugs, such as benzodiazepines, are primarily prescribed to treat tension and muscular strain. The most commonly used benzodiazepines are alprazolam (Xanax) and diazepam (Valium). Benzodiazepines are relatively fast-acting medications, creating effects in less than an hour. Drowsiness and loss of coordination are the most common side effects. When used in combination with other substances, such as alcohol, benzodiazepines can cause serious and possibly life-threatening complications. When taken with benzodiazepines, medications such as anesthetics, antihistamines, sedatives, muscle relaxants, and some prescription painkillers may increase central nervous system depression. Similar to the barbiturates, high doses of these drugs result in slurred speech, drowsiness, and stupor. Physiological and physical dependence on antianxiety drugs may occur within two to four weeks. Withdrawal symptoms from antianxiety drugs may include coma, psychosis, and death.

Cannabis (Marijuana)

Cannabis, known as marijuana, "pot," or "weed," consists of a mixture of crushed leaves and flower buds of the *Cannabis sativa* plant; this drug is usually ingested by smoking. **Hashish** also is an extract of cannabis, but is 2 to 10 times as concentrated as marijuana. Tetrahydrocannabinol (THC) is the primary psychoactive ingredient in both drugs.

When taken in low to moderate doses, the effects of marijuana are similar to the effects of alcohol and some tranquilizers. In contrast to alcohol, however, marijuana at low doses does not dull sensation, but rather may cause slight alterations in perception. Its immediate physical effects include an increased heart rate, bloodshot eyes, and dry mouth and throat. High doses diminish the ability to perceive and react and cause sensory distortion. Hashish users may experience vivid hallucinations and LSD-like psychedelic reactions, and some people experience acute panic attacks.

Chronic use of marijuana has been shown to suppress ovulation and alter hormone levels in women. Frequent use

I don't really know how I got into heroin. It started with friends and was fun. I was curious and thought it was something I could easily handle. It ran away with me. I didn't realize how desperate I had become until I was arrested for stealing. I couldn't believe that I was in jail.

22-year-old woman

of this drug during pregnancy may result in lower-birthweight infants and appears to be associated with impaired verbal, perceptual, and memory skills, as well as difficulties with decision making and sustained attention in children.[2] Studies show conflicting results regarding smoking marijuana and its relationship to cancer. Frequent marijuana use has been linked to cancer of the head and neck as well as bladder cancer.

Marijuana for medical use has been a subject of controversy for many years. The drug has been studied for its possible analgesic effect; its potential for reducing spasms and spasticity produced by multiple sclerosis and partial spinal cord injury; its use for chemotherapy-related nausea and vomiting; its ability to lower intraocular pressure to treat glaucoma; and its work as an appetite stimulant for wasting syndrome due to HIV infection, anorexia, and cancer.[40] Some believe that evidence for the prescription of marijuana remains inadequate and that other medications produce similar results without the side effects. Many others believe that marijuana is useful and find ways to obtain the drug for medical purposes.

Psychedelics and Hallucinogens

Hallucinogenic drugs create changes in perceptions and thoughts. A common feature of a hallucinogenic experience is the suspension of normal psychic mechanisms that integrate the self with the environment. Some of the more common effects induced by hallucinogenic drugs include changes in mood, sensation, perception, and relations. These drugs produce tolerance to the **psychedelic** effects, but do not create physical dependence or produce symptoms of withdrawal, even after long-term use. As with most psychoactive drugs, however, there is a danger of psychological dependence.

Peyote and lysergic acid diethylamide (LSD) are both hallucinogens. Mescaline is the active ingredient in peyote, a spineless cactus with a small crown, or button, that is dried and then swallowed. From earliest recorded time, natives in northern Mexico and the southwestern United States have used peyote as a part of traditional religious rites. LSD ("acid") also is ingested orally and produces hallucinations, including bright colors and altered perceptions of reality. The hallucinogenic experience, or "trip," is characterized by slight increases in body temperature, heart rate, and blood rate; sweating; chills; and sometimes headaches and nausea. A "bad trip" may result in an acute anxiety reaction that may trigger panic, depression, confusion, fear of insanity, and distorted thoughts and perceptions. The most common delayed reaction of LSD is a "flashback," in which individuals reexperience the perceptual and emotional changes originally produced by the drug.

Narcotics

Narcotics include the opiates—opium and its derivatives, morphine, codeine, and heroin—and some other non-opiate synthetic drugs. All narcotics have sleep-inducing and pain-relieving properties. They may be used medically for pain relief, but they have a high potential for abuse. Narcotics relax the user and, when injected, may produce an immediate rush. They also may result in restlessness, nausea, and vomiting. With large doses, the skin becomes moist, cold, and bluish, and the pupils become smaller. Respiration slows, and the user may become unresponsive. Death is possible. Over time, opiate users may develop heart infections, skin abscesses, and congested lungs. Infections from unsterile equipment increase the risk of hepatitis, tetanus, and HIV infection. Heroin use among young women has increased in recent years as availability of the drug has spread from urban to suburban environments. Among students surveyed, roughly 1.5% of eighth graders, tenth graders, and twelfth graders reported using heroin at least once during their lifetimes. More than 14% of eighth graders, 18% of tenth graders, and 30% of twelfth graders reported that heroin was "fairly easy" or "very easy" to obtain.[41]

Although narcotics such as heroin affect a woman's ability to conceive, many addicts still can become pregnant. Use of heroin during pregnancy is believed to affect the developing brain of the fetus and possibly cause behavioral abnormalities in childhood. A baby of a heroin addict is born an addict as well and often suffers severe withdrawal symptoms after birth.

Inhalants

Inhalants are chemicals that produce vapors with psychoactive effects and are predominantly abused by pre-adolescents and young adults. Many products that are used in this way are not meant for inhalation, such as solvents, aerosols, cleaning fluids, and petroleum products. Most

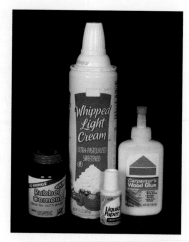

■ Many products that are used as inhalants are not meant for inhalation and are extremely dangerous.

inhalants produce the same effects as anesthetics—namely, they slow down bodily functions. At low doses, users may feel slightly stimulated; at higher doses, they may feel less inhibited. Regular use of inhalants leads to tolerance, so the user needs increasingly higher doses to attain the desired effects. Inhalants may cause serious medical complications, such as hepatitis with liver failure, kidney failure, respiratory impairment, destruction of bone marrow and skeletal muscles, blood abnormalities, and irregular heartbeat. Because many inhalants are widely available household products, inhalants are often tried by young people or those who cannot afford or do not have access to more illicit drugs.

Designer Drugs

Designer drugs are produced in chemical laboratories and then sold illegally. Such synthetic narcotics are particularly dangerous because they are more powerful than those derived from natural substances. The risk of brain damage or fatal overdose from ingestion is correspondingly higher.

MDMA (3,4-methylenedioxymethamphetamine), commonly known as "Ecstasy," is an example of a designer drug. It is somewhat related to mescaline and amphetamines. It has been identified as one of the "club drugs" that include GHB, Rohypnol, Ketamine, and methamphetamine. Ecstasy use is dramatically increasing among young women. In the United States, the drug has been associated with a predominantly white, middle-class population. Immediate effects of the drug include a feeling of warmth and openness. Delayed responses, usually within a day, include insomnia, muscle aches, fatigue, and difficulty concentrating. Chronic use of MDMA has been shown to cause brain damage in humans; the extent of damage is directly correlated with the extent of MDMA use. Heavy users also have significant impairments in visual and verbal memory.[42]

I had a knee injury from playing tennis and was given a prescription for Percocet. A few weeks later, after I had stopped taking the medicine, a friend and I decided to take some Percocet just for fun. The next night, we took more. Before I knew it, I was taking pills every night. I needed more each night to make me feel good. When I ran out of pills, I panicked and called the doctor for a refill. I didn't even realize how quickly I had become addicted.

28-year-old woman

Prescription Drugs

The three classes of prescription drugs most commonly abused are opioids prescribed for pain, which include morphine, codeine, and oxycodone (e.g., OxyContin, Percodan, Percocet); central nervous system depressants for anxiety and sleep disorders such as barbiturates and benzodiazepines (e.g., Valium, Librium, and Xanax); and stimulants for sleep disorders and attention-deficit hyperactivity disorder (e.g., Dexedrine and Ritalin). Any of these medications, when used improperly, can lead to serious health consequences and even death. Prescription drug use and abuse are on the rise in the United States, especially among older adults, adolescents, and women. In 2003, more than 6.3 million Americans reported currently using prescription drugs for nonmedical purposes (see **Figure 13.7**).[43]

Drug Dependency

Drug dependency refers to the attachment—physical or psychological (or both)—that a person may develop to a drug. *Physical dependence* occurs when physiological changes in the body's cells cause an overpowering, constant need for a drug. If the drug is not taken, the user develops withdrawal symptoms, such as intense anxiety, extreme nausea, and deep craving for the drug. Tranquilizers, painkillers, barbiturates, and narcotics may produce physical dependence. *Psychological dependence*, also referred to as habituation, results in a strong craving for a drug because it produces pleasurable feelings or relieves stress or anxiety. Physical and psychological dependence do not always coexist. For example, marijuana and LSD may not create physical dependence, but their continued use has been demonstrated to cause psychological dependence.

Cross-tolerance, or cross-addiction, often presents with drug dependency. In this condition, a state of physical dependence exists in which psychological need for one psychoactive substance leads to dependence on similar substances.

Treatment Dimensions of Drug Dependency

There are three basic approaches to drug-abuse treatment: detoxification, therapeutic communities, and outpatient drug-free programs. Different forms of intervention may help different people and be applicable to different dependencies.

- *Detoxification* is the supervised withdrawal from drug dependence, either with or without medication, in a hospital or outpatient setting.

- *Therapeutic communities* are highly structured, drug-free environments in which abusers live under strict rules while participating in group and individual therapy.

Figure 13.7

More than 6.3 million Americans reported current use of prescription drugs for nonmedical purposes in 2003.

Source: Office of Applied Studies, Substance Abuse and Mental Health Services Administration. (2004). *National Survey on Drug Use and Health.*

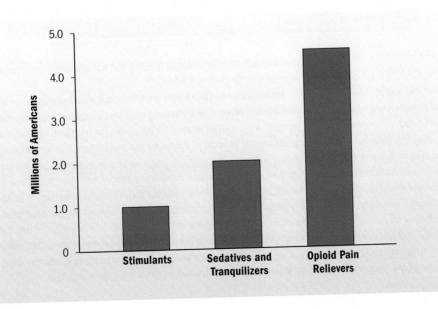

Do I Have a Drug Problem?

Carefully read and honestly respond to the following statements:

1. Sometimes I am preoccupied with getting and taking a drug.   yes   no

2. Sometimes I don't go to an important event at school or work, or a social or recreational event, so that I can get or take a drug instead.   yes   no

3. I continue to use a drug despite the fact that it makes things with my family or friends worse, or it interferes with school or work activities.   yes   no

4. I have developed a specific physical or mental condition from my drug use (example, irritated nose from cocaine).   yes   no

5. I have repeatedly tried to cut down or eliminate my use of a drug.   yes   no

6. I am sometimes unable to fulfill my obligations (to family, friends, work, or school) because of my drug use.   yes   no

7. I feel specific symptoms when I cut back or eliminate the drug.   yes   no

8. I sometimes take another drug to relieve withdrawal symptoms.   yes   no

9. I sometimes use the drug in larger doses or over a longer period than recommended.   yes   no

10. I need to take more of the drug now than I did before to get the same effect.   yes   no

If you answered "yes" to any of these statements, it is important to seek help now with your drug problem.

■ *Outpatient drug-free programs* are available through community and treatment facilities. Self-help programs include Narcotics Anonymous (NA) and Pills Anonymous (PA), which follow the philosophy of Alcoholics Anonymous. In these programs, users admit to their helplessness and put their faith in a "higher power." Many people do not recognize their own drug problems, and require intervention by friends and family before they will seek treatment (see **Self-Assessment 13.3**).

■■■■

Informed Decision Making

Although many outside factors affect whether a person eventually uses or becomes addicted to drugs, alcohol, or tobacco, personal responsibility is always an issue. Personal responsibilities include:

■ Understanding the breadth of impact that use of a particular substance can have on a person's physical and psychological well-being

■ Being aware of how the substance affects personal behaviors and the assessment of reality

■ Being able to ascertain and acknowledge that a problem with substance abuse may be present

Recognizing the warning signs of substance dependence or addiction and seeking early treatment intervention are signs of initial success in addressing the issue. Maintaining abstinence after treating the problem is an ongoing process.

Gender Dimensions

TREATMENT PROGRAMS

Drug dependency treatment programs must address the spectrum of physical and psychosocial issues that confront the addict. These challenges are especially difficult for female addicts, who experience concerns such as contraception, pregnancy, motherhood, childrearing, and health problems in addition to the underlying drug dependency. Women are generally less likely to seek treatment for drug abuse, and they respond differently than men to drug treatment. Female addicts often are caregivers and are reluctant to seek care for themselves because of the needs of others. In addition, they more often need specialty treatment than males. These types of services include prenatal treatment, mental health services, domestic violence counseling, and childcare assistance. In 2003, 35% of U.S. substance abuse treatment facilities provided special programs or services for women. Some programs also provided activities for children, housing and transportation assistance, and services for pregnant women.[44]

Psychosocial and behavioral treatment programs that emphasize increased self-esteem and choosing positive life options may be more successful with certain women. Unfortunately, few programs focus on the special needs of women or acknowledge the barriers that women must overcome to obtain treatment. These barriers may include, but are not limited to, lack of day care for children, lack of safe drug-free housing, fear of losing their children, financial and legal difficulties, lack of transportation, and health problems requiring services beyond drug treatment. In addition, treatment needs of women should be evaluated with the realization that women do not constitute a homogenous group, but rather run the gamut of pregnant women, adolescent users, older women, single professionals, and housewives, to name but a few subgroups.

Tobacco

Informed consumers are aware of the multidimensional and interdependent issues of smoking and realize that this problem has no immediate or simple solution. If a woman is a smoker, the single most significant step she can take to improve her chances of well-being is to quit smoking. Regardless of the difficulty—and breaking any addictive behavior is undeniably difficult—smoking causes serious damage to the body and shortens the life span, and quitting smoking brings serious health benefits.

Avoiding involuntary smoking is not always simple. Although legislation now restricts smoking in many areas, smoking still occurs in many restaurants, bars, and smoking lounges. Also, children are subjected to smoking in their own homes, cars, and even in the womb before birth. Non-smokers' desire for a "smoke-free" environment presents a potential threat to smokers, who feel that their rights to smoke are violated. The challenge for nonsmokers is to assert their right to a smoke-free environment in a nonviolent but assertive manner. Much of the resistance by smokers is defensive, as they are reminded of their own need to quit and their fear of failure and frustration with the process.

Women often do not consider tobacco to be a drug. In reality, tobacco can decrease the effects of certain medications such as acetaminophen, antidepressants, and insulin taken for diabetes. Smoking also increases the risk of heart and blood vessel disease when taking oral contraceptives. Tobacco should be identified as a drug when health-care providers inquire about medications or drug use.

Alcohol

If a woman chooses to drink, several suggestions can help provide her with a framework for decision making and skills development for responsible and safe drinking behavior. For those with a propensity toward excessive drinking, it is important to set a limit and stick to it. A limit of one or two drinks per day may be a reasonable amount for some; only drinking during social activities and only drinking on weekends are other possible limits. It is also critical to have healthy coping strategies to avoid turning to alcohol when upset or depressed. Alcohol neither fixes a problem nor provides an escape. When drinking becomes the primary focus of an activity, a significant risk for serious long-term alcohol problems arises.

Communication skills are an important component of responsible drinking. Learning to say, "No, thank you, I have had enough to drink," is an important step in exercising personal power and control over drinking behavior.

Pacing alcohol consumption is important as well. Drinking a week's worth of alcohol on a Friday night is not the same as moderately paced drinking throughout the week. Also, recognize that alcoholic beverages are not good or wise thirst quenchers, as alcohol leads to dehydration. Food should be consumed before drinking, so it is a good idea to eat something before going to a party or meeting someone for a drink.

Helping others to drink in moderation is also a personal responsibility issue. It is not wise to push drinks or refill empty glasses quickly. Food helps to slow the absorption of alcohol and should be encouraged first, particularly if guests have not eaten for a while. Nonalcoholic beverages should always be available as well. Perhaps the most important responsibilities are never to serve alcohol to a guest who seems intoxicated and never to permit an intoxicated person to operate a vehicle. Assuming responsibility includes making contingency plans for intoxication. The early identification of designated drivers helps ensure safe transportation home for guests. If intoxication occurs despite efforts to prevent it, assume responsibility for the health and safety of guests by providing transportation home or overnight accommodations. Stay with the person if he or she is vomiting. If the person is lying down, turn his or her head to the side and protect the person from swallowing the vomit. Monitor the breathing status. If there are any signs of unconsciousness or respiratory problems, seek immediate medical attention. Remember that the only thing that sobers a drunk person is time. (See **Table 13.11**.)

Table 13.11 How to Handle a Friend Who Is Intoxicated

- Try to find out what the person was drinking and if she took any other drugs or medicines.

- Help your friend get home safely; don't let her drive, get in a car with another friend who has been drinking, or walk home alone in an unsafe area.

- Encourage your friend to go to sleep; the only way to sober up is to give it time.

- Position your friend on her side to prevent her from choking if she vomits. Check on her regularly to be sure she is responsive and breathing.

- Avoid giving your friend any medication, including aspirin, ibuprofen, or acetaminophen.

- Call for help if she is unresponsive or vomiting while unconscious; call for help if you fear being alone with the intoxicated friend.

Source: Reprinted by permission of Julie Barnes, coordinator, Substance Abuse Services, University of Northern Iowa.

Other Drugs

Understanding the short- and long-term negative effects that drugs can have, while also developing personal strengths and self-confidence, is the foundation that enables a woman to resist drugs effectively. Knowing how to cope with stress in a healthy way can minimize the likelihood that a woman will turn to drugs as a coping mechanism. The enhancement of self-esteem is another significant personal strength that provides a foundation for drug avoidance.

Early identification and treatment offer hope to the person who is using drugs. Unfortunately, many people either fail or refuse to see the signs that a person is using drugs. Many treatment and counseling centers offer free telephone services that provide advice on assessing the situation and helpful resources for action. Confronting the substance abuser is sometimes best handled by a group of loved ones and in the presence of a trained counselor. Outlining how the abuse has affected each person in the abuser's life and how much each person cares about the abuser helps to balance the information. It is unrealistic to expect the abuser to quit without assistance. Although offering support is beneficial, the abuser needs to know that treatment and therapy are necessary.

Informed decision making is also an essential responsibility with prescribed and OTC medication use. Many women have little or no idea why they take certain prescribed medications, or they have multiple and vague reasons for using complex OTC medications. Drugs, whether prescribed or self-medicated, can have powerful adverse reactions with other drugs, certain foods, alcohol, tobacco, and caffeine. Older women are often subject to dangerous and possibly fatal drug interactions due to the numerous medications and supplements they are taking. Because many of the most serious effects of drugs are often wrongly attributed to "being depressed" or "growing old," women should know about possible adverse drug reactions and side effects so such events can be recognized and reported. They should also know which foods and other drugs interact with the medications being taken and whether specific dietary recommendations have been identified for the medications.

Co-dependency

The concept of co-dependency is important for many women who become embroiled within the chaos of another person's life. The term "co-dependent" is used to describe a person obsessed, tormented, or dominated by the

It's Your Health

Co-dependency

A person (friend, spouse, partner, parent) may, without meaning to, allow or help the addict to remain dependent on drugs through enabling behaviors. These enabling behaviors may include the following activities:

- Rescuing: displaying overprotective behavior that permits the addict to use drugs at home to avoid being discovered or at risk elsewhere.
- Rationalizing: accepting and explaining the addict's behavior; making excuses for the behavior.
- Shielding: covering up for addicts; running interference for them at work, school, and for obligations.
- Controlling: personally attempting to control the addict's use of drugs with bribes or rewards (money, favors, sex).
- Covering: taking over chores, assuming job responsibilities, paying bills, or giving/loaning money to the addict so that he or she can buy drugs.
- Cooperating: becoming involved in buying, selling, testing, preparing, or using the drug.

behavior of others. Growing out of the older notion of "co-alcoholic," a term once applied to the wives of heavy drinkers, the premise of co-dependency is that everyone in a user's or abuser's family is diseased. Consciously or unconsciously, and to their lifelong detriment, co-dependents interact with the user and "enable" this person to partake in her addiction. Co-dependents often feel helpless, miserable, hopeless, and angry as they accept the victim role. A woman may be co-dependent in a relationship with a lover, spouse, parent, child, or friend. A co-dependent typically feels responsible for the behavior and mood of the other.

The co-dependent must learn how to separate her own life from that of the addicted person's. The recovery from co-dependence is similar to recovery from alcohol or drug dependence in that only the co-dependent can take the necessary steps toward her own recovery. A co-dependent must learn not to try to control someone else's life and to stop playing the victim role. Many co-dependents have received useful support and encouragement from various

I feel responsible for [my husband] Joe's drinking. He really has no one else who understands and helps him. I try to be patient each time he is drunk and clean up the mess. I keep thinking that if I just try harder in understanding maybe he won't have this problem.
35-year-old woman

programs, such as the Twelve-Step Program of Al-Anon, a support group for family and friends of alcoholics.

■ ■ ■ ■
Summary

Despite the overwhelming evidence of their detrimental effects, tobacco, alcohol, and other drugs continue to harm women, their children, and others in their environment. Eliminating smoking is a cornerstone of the improvement of women's health in the United States. Smoking cessation is often the single greatest decision a woman can make toward improving her health. Women also must exercise caution and wisdom with alcohol and legal drug use. Knowing the consequences of drinking alcohol, being "alcohol wise," and assuming personal responsibility are the first steps in controlling alcohol use. Reducing the kinds and amounts of drugs taken—recreational drugs, prescribed medications, OTC medications, and substances such as caffeine—should also be an important health goal.

■ ■ ■ ■
Topics for Discussion

1. Should pregnant women be permitted to drink alcohol, use drugs, or smoke? Should states intervene in cases of maternal substance use?

2. Is it a sign of personal weakness or strength for a woman to admit that she has a problem with alcohol or drugs?

3. What should a woman do or say when she knows her friend has a problem with drugs or alcohol, but the friend does not think that she has a problem?

4. Can smokers' rights and nonsmokers' rights both be protected at the same time?

5. How can young girls be educated to resist peer pressure and advertising pressure to initiate cigarette smoking?

6. Discuss how the abundance of drugs in a neighborhood affects a community. What type of social action is needed to help keep this community safe and become drug free?

7. List all chemicals and substances that you use to change your state of consciousness, such as caffeine, tobacco, alcohol, prescription drugs, over-the-counter drugs, and illegal drugs. Try to give up one or more of these substances for a period of time, and replace it with a healthy behavior such as exercise. Keep a record of how you feel and any changes that you notice in your health or behavior.

8. Should natural substances and over-the-counter medicines be regulated in the same way that prescription drugs are?

Profiles of Remarkable Women

Drew Barrymore (1975–)

Drew Barrymore was born into an acting family; her kin include the legendary actors Lionel, John, and Ethel Barrymore. Drew Barrymore began her career at the age of just 11 months, appearing in a Puppy Choice dog food commercial. She got her first movie role at the age of two, playing a boy in *Suddenly Love.* At age five, she appeared in *Altered States,* and she was turned into a household name when she starred in the blockbuster *E.T.: The Extraterrestrial.* She continued her appearance in films, including Stephen King adaptations *Firestarter* (1984) and *Cat's Eye* (1985).

Soon after, Barrymore tried alcohol for the first time at age 9 and marijuana at age 10. She then turned to cocaine, stirred controversy with her near-nude appearances in *Far from Home,* and was forced into ASAP Family Treatment Center, a drug rehabilitation clinic. Following rehab, Barrymore published a memoir entitled *Little Girl Lost* and made a comeback in Hollywood in the early 1990s.

Barrymore's persistence and energy have helped her recover from the difficulties of growing up in front of the camera and in the public eye, and have shaped her into a strong and determined woman. She has not only appeared in numerous successful movies, but has also produced her own films, including *He's Just Not That Into You, Never Been Kissed, Charlie's Angels,* and a remake of *Donnie Darko.* A dedicated philanthropist, Barrymore often donates her time and resources to a number of charities. She is actively involved in volunteering for and supporting animal rights issues and anti-fur campaigns, urging young people to vote, and advocating for children's rights.

9. Is it better to put drug addicts in jail or to send them to mandatory drug treatment programs?

10. Is there any validity to the arguments to legalize marijuana? What about other illicit drugs? Discuss the pros and cons of a change in policy in this area.

■ ■ ■ ■

Web Sites

Alcoholics Anonymous: http://www.aa.org

College Drinking: Changing the Culture:
http://www.collegedrinkingprevention.gov

National Institute on Alcohol Abuse and Alcoholism:
http://www.niaaa.nih.gov

National Institute on Drug Abuse:
http://www.nida.nih.gov

Recovery Services: http://www.soberrecovery.com

SAMHSA's National Clearinghouse for Drug and Alcohol Information: http://www.health.org

Substance Abuse and Mental Health Services Administration: http://www.samhsa.gov

Surgeon General's Guide to Quitting Smoking:
http://www.surgeongeneral.gov

■ ■ ■ ■

References

1. Substance Abuse and Mental Health Services Administration, Office of Applied Studies. (2008). *Results from the 2007 National Survey on Drug Use and Health: National Findings* (NSDUH Series H-34, DHHS Publication No. SMA 08-4343). Rockville, MD.

2. Substance Abuse and Mental Health Services Administration, U.S. Department of Health and Human Services. (2002). *2001 National Household Survey on Drug Abuse*. Rockville, MD: DHHS.

3. National Center on Addiction and Substance Abuse, Columbia University. (2003). *The Formative Years: Pathways to Substance Abuse Among Girls and Young Women Ages 8–22*. New York: Columbia University.

4. The Sentencing Project. (2005). *Briefing: The Federal Prison Population: A Statistical Analysis*. Washington, DC: The Sentencing Project.

5. Center for Women Policy Studies. (2001). *Women, Pregnancy and Substance Abuse*. Washington, DC: Center for Women Policy Studies.

6. Office of National Drug Control Policy. (2003). *Drug Fact Sheet*. U.S. Department of State. Washington, DC: Office of National Drug Control Policy.

7. Office of National Drug Control Policy. (2008). *National Drug Control Strategy FY2009 Budget Summary*. Washington DC: Office of National Drug Control Policy.

8. American Cancer Society. (2008). *Cancer Facts & Figures 2008*. Atlanta, GA: American Cancer Society.

9. National Center for Health Statistics. (2003). *Health, United States, 2003 with Chartbook on Trends in the Health of Americans*. Hyattsville, MD: Public Health Service.

10. Centers for Disease Control and Prevention. (2004). Cigarette smoking among adults—United States, 2002. *Morbidity and Mortality Weekly Report* 53(20): 427–431.

11. American Cancer Society. (2008). *Cancer Facts and Figures, 2008*. Atlanta, GA: American Cancer Society.

12. Centers for Disease Control and Prevention. (2008). Youth risk behavior surveillance—United States. *Morbidity and Mortality Weekly Report* 57(SS04).

13. American Lung Association. (2007). *An Emerging Deadly Trend—Waterpipe Tobacco Use*. Available at: http://slati.lungusa.org/reports/TrendAlert_Waterpipes.pdf.

14. World Health Organization. (2005). *Waterpipe Tobacco Smoking: Health Effects, Research Needs and Recommended Actions by Regulators*. Geneva: WHO.

15. Centers for Disease Control and Prevention. (2005). Annual smoking-attributable mortality, years of potential life lost, and economic costs—United States, 1997–2001. *Morbidity and Mortality Weekly Report* 54: 625–628.

16. American Lung Association. (2008). *State Legislated Action on Tobacco Issues*. Available at: http://slati.lungusa.org.

17. American Lung Association. (2006). *From Joe Camel to Kauai Kolada—The Marketing of Candy-Flavored Cigarettes*. Available at: http://slati.lungusa.org/factsheets.asp.

18. Alexander, W. (2006). *The New Face of Cigarette Advertising: Cigarette Marketing Strategies After the MSA*. Chapel Hill, NC: UNC-Chapel Hill.

19. World Health Organization. (2003). *World Health Report 2003: Shaping the Future.* Geneva: World Health Organization.

20. Samet, J., & Yoon, S. Y. (Eds.). (2001). *Women and the Tobacco Epidemic: Challenges for the 21st Century.* Geneva: World Health Organization.

21. Centers for Disease Control and Prevention. (2007). Deaths: final data for 2004. *Vital Statistics Report* 55(19).

22. Matikainen, T. (2001). Aromatic hydrocarbon receptor-driven Bax gene expression is required for premature ovarian failure caused by biohazardous environmental chemicals. *Nature Genetics* 28: 355–360.

23. U.S. Department of Health and Human Services. (2004). *The Health Consequences of Smoking: A Report of the Surgeon General, 2004.* Atlanta, GA: Centers for Disease Control and Prevention, Office on Smoking and Health.

24. U.S. Department of Health and Human Services. (2001). *Women and Smoking: A Report of the Surgeon General.* Rockville, MD: DHHS.

25. Substance Abuse and Mental Health Services Administration, Office of Applied Studies. (August 2, 2007). *The NSDUH Report: Gender Differences in Alcohol Use and Alcohol Dependence or Abuse: 2004 and 2005.* Rockville, MD: SAMHSA.

26. Gruskin, E. P., Hart, S., Gordon, N., & Ackerson, L. (2001). Patterns of cigarette smoking and alcohol use among lesbians and bisexual women enrolled in a large health maintenance organization. *American Journal of Public Health* 91(6): 976–979.

27. Centers for Disease Control and Prevention. (2004). Alcohol-attributable deaths and years of potential life lost—United States, 2001. *Morbidity and Mortality Weekly Report* 53(37): 866–870.

28. National Institute on Alcohol Abuse and Alcoholism (NIAAA). (1998). Drinking in the U.S.: Main findings from the 1992 National Longitudinal Alcohol Epidemiologic Survey (NLAES). *U.S. Alcohol Epidemiologic Data Reference Manual.* (1st ed., vol. 6). NIH Publication No. 99-3519. Rockville, MD: NIAAA.

29. Levy, D. T., Stewart, K., & Wilbur, P. M. (1999). *Costs of Underage Drinking.* Pacific Institute. U.S. Department of Justice, Office of Juvenile Justice and Delinquency Prevention.

30. National Institute on Alcohol Abuse and Alcoholism (NIAAA). (2007). *Alcohol Alert No. 72: Cirrhosis.* Rockville, MD: NIAAA.

31. Caithers, R. L., & McClain, C. (2006). Alcoholic liver disease. In: Feldman, M., Friedman L. S., & Brandt, L. J. *Feldman: Sleisinger & Fordtran's Gastrointestinal and Liver Disease* (8th ed.). Philadelphia, PA: Saunders Elsevier, Chapter 81.

32. National Institute on Alcohol Abuse and Alcoholism. (2002). *Alcohol Research & Health*, Volume 26, Number 4.

33. Nelson, H. D., Humphrey, L. L., Nygren, P., et al. (2002). Postmenopausal hormone replacement therapy: scientific review. *Journal of the American Medical Association* 288: 872–881.

34. Bertrand, J., Floyd, R. L., Weber, M. K., et al. (2004). *Fetal Alcohol Syndrome: Guidelines for Referral and Diagnosis.* Atlanta, GA: U.S. Department of Health and Human Services, CDC. Available at: http://www.cdc.gov/ncbddd/fas/documents/FAS_guidelines_accessible.pdf.

35. American Academy of Pediatrics. (2005). Breastfeeding and the use of human milk. *Pediatrics* 115(2).

36. American Academy of Child and Adolescent Psychiatry. (2002). *Facts for Families: Children of Alcoholics.* No. 17. Available at: http://www.aacap.org/cs/root/facts_for_families/children_of_alcoholics.

37. National Institute on Alcohol Abuse and Alcoholism (NIAAA). (2003). *Alcohol Alert No. 60: Genetics of Alcoholism.* Rockville, MD: NIAAA.

38. Alcoholics Anonymous (AA). (2004). *Alcoholics Anonymous 2004 Membership Survey.* Washington, DC: AA.

39. National Center for Health Statistics. (1999). *Health, United States, 1999, with Health and Aging Chartbook.* Hyattsville, MD: National Center for Health Statistics.

40. American Medical Association. (2001). *Medical Marijuana.* Presented by AMA Council on Scientific Affairs as CSA Report 6 at the 2001 AMA Annual Meeting.

41. National Institute on Drug Abuse & University of Michigan. (2004). *Monitoring the Future. 2004 Data from In-School Surveys of 8th-, 10th-, and 12th-Grade Students.* Dearborn, MI: University of Michigan.

42. McCardle, K., Luebbers, S., Carter, J., Croft, R., & Stough, C. (2004). Chronic MDMA (ecstasy) use, cognition and mood. *Psychopharmacology* 173(3,4): 434–439.

43. National Institute on Drug Abuse. (2005). *Prescription Drugs: Abuse and Addiction.* NIDA Research Report. NIH Publication Number 05-4881.

44. Brady, T. M., & Ashley, O. S. (Eds.). (2005). *Women in Substance Abuse Treatment: Results from the Alcohol and Drug Services Study (ADSS)* (DHHS Publication No. SMA 04-3968, Analytic Series A-26). Rockville, MD: Substance Abuse and Mental Health Services Administration, Office of Applied Studies.

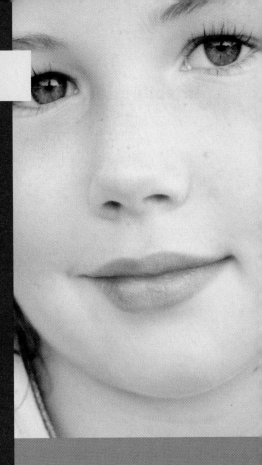

Chapter Fourteen

Violence, Abuse, and Harassment

Chapter Objectives

On completion of this chapter, the student should be able to discuss:

1. The different forms of violence.

2. Violence from a sociocultural, historical, and economic perspective.

3. The influence of poverty, alcohol and drugs, and the media on violence.

4. Violence as a global issue.

5. Types of family and intimate violence.

6. The definition of stalking and actions a woman can take to protect herself.

7. Forms of battering, including physical, sexual, property, psychological, and social violence.

8. Violence in lesbian relationships.

9. Concerns with battering during pregnancy.

10. Battering in women with disabilities.

11. Concepts and issues of child abuse.

12. Concepts and issues of elder abuse.

13. Differences between stranger and intimate rape.

14. Effects of rape on physical health, mental health, sexual intimacy, and relationships.

15. Prevalence of violence toward women by strangers.

16. Sexual harassment as a form of social control and its effects on women in the workplace.

17. Strategies for effective communication to deal with intimate violence and sexual harassment.

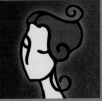

womenshealth.jbpub.com

Women's Health Online is a great source for supplementary women's health information for both students and instructors. Visit

http://womenshealth.jbpub.com

to find a variety of useful tools for learning, thinking, and teaching.

Introduction

Violence takes place throughout modern society, and it occurs in many forms. In 2002, the World Health Organization (WHO) compiled the first comprehensive summary of the problem of violence on a global scale in *The World Report on Violence and Health*.[1] The typology in the *World Report* classifies violence into three categories according to who commits the violent act: self-directed violence, interpersonal violence, and collective violence.

Self-directed violence includes suicidal behavior and **self-mutilation** (see **It's Your Health**). Suicide is discussed in further detail in Chapter 12.

Interpersonal violence includes family/partner violence toward a child, partner, or elder and community violence toward an acquaintance or a stranger. Family and intimate violence—including stalking, domestic battering, child abuse, elder abuse, and rape in many cases—are major facets

of the violence epidemic. Although most intimate violence qualifies as a crime, historical and cultural traditions to a large extent have condoned violence within the family setting. Violence by strangers—such as robbery, carjackings, aggravated assault, rape, and homicide—affects women as either the victims of the crime itself or the victims of the situation through loss of a partner or family member. Sexual harassment is considered a form of violence as well, because it also involves an unjust use of power.

Collective violence is an act of violence by people as a group in an effort to achieve social, political, or economic objectives. It can take a variety of forms, including armed conflicts; genocide, repression, and other human rights abuses; terrorism; and organized violent crime. Many acts of violence toward women evolve as a result of women's subordinate status in society. Forms of abuse affecting women as a group in certain populations include female genital mutilation, female infanticide, trafficking of women and girls for sexual exploitation, and acts of rape during war. These acts of abuse have traditionally been associated with countries other than the United States; recent evidence shows that these offenses against women occur worldwide.

Violence often has mental and physical consequences for its victims, including long-term disability or death. Each year, more than 1.6 million people worldwide lose their lives to violence. Indeed, violence is among the leading causes of death for people ages 15 to 44 years old.[1] Women are disproportionately victims of violence throughout the world. More than 2.5 million females experience some form of violence each year. On average, one in three females is abused by an intimate partner during her lifetime. Several global studies suggest that half of all women who die from homicide are killed by current or former husbands or partners.[2]

This chapter provides an overview of violence, focusing on interpersonal violence and the issues that contribute to violence and victimization. Informed decision-making criteria for women are reviewed as well.

It's Your Health

Self-Harm or Self-Injury

Self-harm, self-injury, self-inflicted violence, or self-mutilation is any self-directed, repetitive behavior that causes physical injury. These acts are not usually suicide attempts but rather behaviors meant to express or release emotional turmoil. They are often referred to as para-suicidal behaviors. Examples include the following acts:

■ Skin cutting with razors or knives (the most common pattern)

■ Burning, branding, or biting oneself

■ Picking one's skin or hair

■ Hitting with hammer or other object; bone breaking

■ Extreme injuries such as auto-enucleation (self-removal of the eye), castration, or amputation

There are several known risk factors for self-injury:

■ Female gender

■ Adolescence and college age

■ Substance abuse or personality disorders

■ History of parasuicidal behavior

People who self-harm are unable to indentify or express difficult feelings in a healthy way. They use self-harm as a coping mechanism. They often feel increasing tension or physical arousal before the act and release of pleasure or gratification after the act. Little is known about the cause of self-mutilation, but studies are looking at biological, psychological, and social contributions to the disease. Medications, psychotherapeutic approaches, and crisis interventions are all forms of treatment. See the Web sites at the end of this chapter for more information.

Source: Adapted from Fong, T. (2003). Self-mutilation: impulsive traits suggest new drug therapies. *Current Psychiatry* 2(2).

Perspectives on Violence, Abuse, and Harassment

Sociocultural Issues

Cultural differences in values, attitudes, and behavioral norms across ethnic and racial groups must be considered in any examination of violence. Unfortunately, data are scarce in this area. Overall, it has proved difficult to assess

I feel like it was my fault that I was raped. I had a little too much to drink and I went back to my apartment with him. I wanted to kiss him, but I didn't want to have sex. When he started forcing me to do more than kiss, I asked him to stop. But he wouldn't listen. I probably shouldn't have invited him back with me and I feel guilty for leading him on.

19-year-old college sophomore

attitudes toward rape and other violent crimes. Some studies indicate that the public tends to blame victims of rape, rather than those who commit the violent act. In some cases, people believe the violence was justified.

Cultural attitudes about violence toward women may be based on societal acceptance of male dominance. In many cultures, both men and women believe that a man has the right to control his wife's and daughters' behaviors and that a disobedient woman should be punished. By legitimizing these acts of violence, cultures perpetuate violence against women. Women are particularly vulnerable to abuse by their partners in societies where there are marked inequalities between men and women, rigid gender roles, weak sanctions against violent behavior, and cultural norms that support a man's right to sex regardless of a woman's feelings. Violence in intimate relationships can be triggered by a number of factors, including a woman not obeying her husband, not having food ready for him, refusing him sex, or simply being a woman.[3]

Society's tolerance of rape between intimate partners, especially married partners, is an important dimension of violence. Many people believe that marriage affords men the right to have sex with their wives at any time. In these settings, if the wife refuses, the husband can force her to have sex or punish her through violent means. "Blaming the victim" is a key concept in relationship violence from a women's health perspective. Women who feel they are at fault or that they "deserved" punishment may not report a rape. Certain factors, including a woman's style of dress, her relationship with the assailant, evidence of resistance, presence of alcohol or drugs, and location of the incident, may affect a third party's attitude toward the rape and contribute to his or her belief that the rape may actually be "excusable" or "understandable."

Cultural differences in reporting of rape may lead to further insight regarding society's view of rape and differing views among people of different racial and ethnic backgrounds. One large national survey found that American Indian/Alaska Native women were significantly more likely to report rape and physical assault than were women of other backgrounds. Asian/Pacific Islander women were least likely to report rape victimization. Hispanic women were less likely to report rape victimization than were non-Hispanic women in regard to non-intimates; however, in a more recent survey, Hispanic women were significantly more likely than non-Hispanic women to report that they were raped by a current or former intimate partner at some time in their lifetime (**Figure 14.1**).[4] The explanation for these differences is unclear. More research is needed to determine whether the reporting of incidents of violence is based on the existence of less violence in certain racial and ethnic groups or on social, demographic, and environmental factors that keep a woman from reporting an incident.

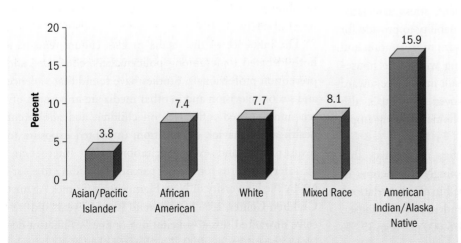

Figure 14.1

Percentage of women reporting rape in their lifetime by race/ethnicity of victim.

Source: Tjaden, P., and Thoennes, N. (2000). *Extent, Nature, and Consequences of Intimate Partner Violence.* Washington, DC: National Institute of Justice, Office of Justice Programs, U.S. Department of Justice.

Historical Trends

Historically, it has been socially acceptable for a husband to physically discipline his wife. The United States followed English law and allowed physical discipline of wives by their husbands until U.S. courts criminalized wife beating in the twentieth century.[5]

Rape also has been documented in American history since the arrival of the Europeans. Spanish explorers used female Native American captives for sexual services and raped Native American women whose tribes they conquered. Native American cultures, however, prohibited rape, and it had rarely occurred until the arrival of the explorers. Fears of brutal rapes by Native American men were found to be unsubstantiated during colonial-era "Indian" wars. Indeed, English women who had been held captive reported no such treatment.[6]

In seventeenth-century New England in particular, female servants were at high risk of rape and sexual harassment. During that era, an estimated one-third of rape victims were female servants, even though that group represented only 10% of the total population.[6] Later, in the South, where slave labor was increasingly used instead of indentured servants, African female servants found themselves victimized by white owners and overseers who viewed them as property—available for service of their sexual needs. Some historians assert that rape was used to dominate female slaves in a system that otherwise treated them as equals to male slaves.[7]

Poverty Influences

Poverty has been identified as an extremely important factor in many aspects of violence, including family violence. The relationship between violence, poverty, and joblessness may be a result of feelings of inadequacy and low self-esteem brought on by unemployment, stress associated with financial instability, and/or an inability to provide for one's family. Often, these emotions turn to frustration and anger, and eventually lead to fighting within the household. In turn, displaced anger can result in violence toward one's partner or children. Unemployed individuals also spend significantly more time in the home, allowing ample opportunities for tensions to rise.

The feminization of poverty refers to the fact that women and children are overwhelmingly the victims of poverty. Women often remain trapped in abusive relationships because of their financial dependence on the abuser. In households with incomes under $15,000 per year, 35.5% of women suffered violence from an intimate partner.[8] Living in circumstances of stress and poverty can also lead

some women to become perpetrators of violence against their children, spouses, or family members.

Alcohol and Drug Influences

Substance use and abuse consistently have been found to be associated with all forms of relationship violence. It is unclear whether a direct cause-and-effect relationship exists between the use of drugs or alcohol and violence or whether this situation involves two overlapping social epidemics. Violence in a home may cause depression and lack of self-esteem, possibly leading to an increased use of alcohol abuse. Conversely, conflicts in interpersonal relationships may arise as a consequence of substance use and abuse and lead to violent behavior.

Data from the National Crime Victim Survey highlight the strong association between interpersonal violence and substance use. Among victims able to tell whether there was substance use by the perpetrator, 30% reported alcohol use by the offender at the time of the crime. Two-thirds of victims who suffered violence by a curent or former partner, reported alcohol use by the offender.[9] American Indians, who are victimized at rates twice as high as the national average, are more likely to experience violence by an offender of a different race. Alcohol can play a significant role in violence, especially among certain groups. For example, 62% of American Indian victims report an offender who was under the influence of alcohol, compared to 42% for the national average.[10]

Media Influences

Media access through television, movies, video and computer games, and the Internet is a major influence in the lives of Americans, especially for children and adolescents. Media can be a powerful tool for positive learning and entertainment, but can also pose a threat to emotional and physical safety.

The influence of the media in U.S. culture remains a hotly debated topic among policymakers, educators, and prevention professionals. Studies have found that violence and sex on television and in other media are important, often unrecognized influences on children and adolescent health and behavior. In addition, unwanted exposure to sexual pictures and sexual solicitations on the Internet create safety concerns for today's parents. According to a survey by the University of New Hampshire's Crimes Against Children Center, 13% of children (10 to 17 years old) receive unwanted sexual solicitations online.[11] This is a decrease from 19% in 2000. The Internet has made it easier for pedophiles to gain access to pornographic collections as

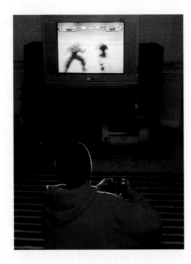
Gaming violence has been shown to influence children and adolescents.

I cannot describe how I felt when it was over. I was wondering if it would have been better if I had died. I was humiliated, angry, hurt, and so violated. He had been someone I had trusted—I thought that he was a friend. Looking back, though, there were clues to his violent nature. I had ignored them. It was a mistake for which I paid dearly.

18-year-old student

well as to solicit children online. Child pornography has devastating effects on children, both on those who are exploited in the actual pictures and on those who view it. To counter this problem, the National Center for Missing and Exploited Children, in partnership with the Federal Bureau of Investigation, Bureau of Customs Immigration Enforcement, U.S. Secret Service, U.S. Postal Inspection Service, and state and local law enforcement in Internet Crimes Against Children Task Forces, operates the national CyberTipline and the national Child Pornography Tipline. These tiplines allow people to report suspicious behavior to a reliable source that can follow up on a possible danger.

Costs of Victimization

The cost of crime is great, with crime victims experiencing a number of losses relating to the crime. The financial burden to the victim includes health-care costs for treating any physical and mental injuries, as well as lost wages for missed workdays. It is estimated that the annual health-related costs of rape, physical assault, stalking, and homicide by intimate partners are more than $5.8 billion. Victims of intimate partner violence lose nearly 8 million days of work as a result of violence.[12] Other costs may include stolen property in burglaries and expenses for repairing or replacing damaged property. There are costs that impose a burden on society as well, such as police services, fire services, and state victims' services. In the United States, all levels of government combined spent $167 billion for police protections, corrections, and judicial and legal activities in 2001.[13] Victims of violent crime and their families received $445 million in compensation benefits in 2003. This compensation was mainly for medical and dental expenses, lost wages and lost support, and mental health counseling.[14]

But the cost burden of violence includes much more than just financial losses. Intangible losses, such as long-term pain and suffering and reduced quality of life, are much more difficult to quantify. Studies show a significant relationship between intimate partner violence and chronic pain, headaches, vaginal infections and bleeding, digestive problems, depression, low self-esteem, and substance abuse.[15] All of these findings lead to even higher direct medical costs and consequently more losses for the victim. Many studies have found that the intangible loss of quality of life exceeds the tangible losses for victims of all crimes.

Legal Dimensions

The number of violent crimes by intimate partners against females has significantly decreased over the past decade. This decrease has been attributed to the Violence Against Women Act (VAWA) of 1994, which was reauthorized in 2000 and again in 2005 to continue existing programs and increase funding. Important aspects of VAWA include these provisions:

- Making it a crime to cross state lines to continue to abuse a spouse or partner
- Creating tough new penalties for sex offenders
- Prohibiting anyone facing a restraining order for domestic abuse from possessing a firearm
- Providing a substantial commitment of federal resources for police, prosecutors, and prevention service initiatives in cases involving sexual violence or domestic abuse
- Requiring sexual offenders to pay restitution to their victims
- Requiring states to pay for rape examinations
- Providing funds for federal victim-witness counselors
- Extending rape shield laws to protect crime victims from abusive inquiries into their private conduct
- Requiring that released offenders report to local enforcement authorities

Global Issues

Violence is a global issue. According to a 2005 World Health Organization study, 20% to 71% of the female population of the world have been victims of domestic violence.[16] Partner violence accounts for a significant number of deaths among women; studies from a range of countries show that about half of female murder victims were killed by a husband or a boyfriend, often during an ongoing abusive relationship. In many countries, deaths are concealed as accidents. For example, it is suspected that many deaths of women in India that are recorded as "accidental burns" were actually murders where women were doused with kerosene and set on fire.[1]

In some countries, nearly one in four women reports sexual violence by an intimate partner and for one out of three women, her first sexual experience will be forced. Even in health-care settings, tens of thousands of women each year are subjected to sexual violence, including sexual harassment by providers, genital mutilation, forced gynecological exams, and obligatory inspections of virginity. Rape is also used as a documented weapon of war. During the Bosnia–Herzegovina conflict, estimates of the number of women raped by soldiers range from 10,000 to 60,000.[1]

Worldwide data on child abuse are scarce; nevertheless, it is estimated that 57,000 homicides occurred among children younger than 15 years of age worldwide in 2000. Nonfatal child abuse also occurs in virtually every country. In a study conducted in the Republic of Korea, for example, 67% of parents admitted whipping children to discipline them and 45% reported hitting, kicking, or beating their children. In Ethiopia, 21% of urban schoolchildren and 64% of rural schoolchildren reported bruises or swelling from parental punishment.[1]

In Southeast Asia, hundreds of thousands of children are involved in the sex trade, and poverty in those countries continually drives more boys and girls into this arena. Although the demand is driven mostly by local clients, sex tourism continues to grow and fuel the market in countries such as Thailand, Cambodia, and Vietnam. In Cambodia, almost all of the girls in prostitution are the main providers for their families. Children as young as age 12 from poor families are sold by parents or agents into the sex trade.

Elder abuse also occurs around the world. In some countries, rapid socioeconomic change weakens family networks that once supported older generations. For example, countries of the former Soviet Union have a growing number of elderly who are left to fend for themselves, resulting in numerous cases of elder neglect. Theft of agricultural products and livestock has been identified as a type of abuse endured by older people in rural areas of the Caribbean.

Family and Intimate Violence

Family and intimate violence refers to violence between individuals in a significant relationship; it can be directed toward former or current spouses or partners, dates, elders, and children.

Violence against women is primarily intimate violence. In the United States, one out of every four women will experience violence by an intimate partner at some point during her lifetime. Family and intimate violence includes many forms of mental and physical crime, as well as threatening with injury (see **Self-Assessment 14.1**).

Self-Assessment 14.1

Recognizing a Potentially Abusive Partner

1. Did the person grow up in a violent family? Was he or she abused as a child?

2. Is the person jealous of your friendships and does he or she try to control the time you spend with other people?

3. Does the person lose his or her temper frequently and overreact to minor problems and frustrations?

4. Does the person abuse alcohol or drugs?

5. Does the person control the finances and make all the decisions within the household?

6. If male, does he have a distorted concept of manhood? Does he have traditional ideas about women's roles versus men's roles?

7. Do you fear the person when he or she is angry?

8. Has the person used physical or psychological coercion to pressure you for sex? Has he or she ever physically assaulted you?

If you answer "yes" to one or more of these questions, you may be at risk of abuse. Talk to your health-care professional about ways to prevent abuse before it happens.

Stalking

Stalking, as defined by the National Institute of Justice, is a "course of conduct directed at a specific person that involves:

- Repeated visual or physical proximity (with 'repeated' meaning on two or more occasions);
- Nonconsensual communication;
- Verbal, written, or implied threats; or
- A combination thereof that would cause fear in a reasonable person."[18]

Stalkers are frequently a current or former spouse, cohabitating partner, or date at some point in the stalked women's lives.[3] There is also often a strong association between stalking and other forms of violence in intimate relationships. One survey found 81% of women stalked by a current husband, former husband, or cohabitating partner were physically assaulted by that partner; 31% also were sexually abused by that partner.[4]

Although every stalking case is different, a stalker's behavior typically becomes increasingly threatening, serious, and violent. The behavior may begin with the stalker making harassing calls, watching or following someone, sending unwanted mail, or making verbal threats. The activity generally escalates from what initially may be bothersome and annoying, to the level of obsessive, dangerous, violent, and potentially fatal acts. Some stalkers may not have a violent motive, but still may cause harm if jealousy or anger is involved.

States have passed laws to prevent stalking and punish those who engage in acts of stalking. The first anti-stalking law was passed in California in 1990 in response to several high-profile cases in which the perpetrators stalked and eventually killed their victims. In each case, the victim had notified the police of the stalker's threatening behavior, yet the police were unable to do anything legally unless the stalker acted on the threats. The California law gave law enforcement officers the right to intervene in stalking cases before the stalker acted on his or her threats. Since then, all states have passed similar laws. Restraining or protection orders can be issued to protect citizens against stalking situations. A woman who believes she is being stalked should take action, as outlined in **Table 14.1**.

Another form of stalking, called **cyberstalking**, is defined as threatening behavior or unwanted advances directed at another using the Internet and other forms of online communications. Victims are targeted through chat rooms, e-mail, and message boards. The stalker may send obscene, threatening, or improper messages; a barrage of unwanted e-mails; or electronic viruses. Online stalking often turns into offline stalking, bringing a real threat of physical harm to the victim. Law enforcement agencies estimate that cyberstalking is a factor in 20% to 40% of all stalking cases. Although current state laws encompass any type of unwanted communication with the victim, many states are now further protecting their residents from cyberstalking by specifically including electronic transmission of communication.

Domestic Violence

Domestic violence, also referred to as **battering**, occurs when a person subjects a current or former romantic partner to forceful physical, social, and psychological behavior so as to coerce her, without regard to her rights. Battering includes five types of interpersonal violence: physical, sexual, property, psychological, and social. Physical violence includes slapping, choking, punching, kicking, pushing,

---

Table 14.1 Guidelines for Women Who Are Being Stalked

These guidelines provide practical information for a woman who believes she is being stalked, but is not in imminent danger. The guidelines do not guarantee her safety, but rather they should reduce her risk of harm.

- Record each incident of stalking with great detail. This record can be used as evidence against the perpetrator if necessary.
- Let family and friends know about the stalker. This protects not only the victim, but also those close to the victim.
- Be extremely alert when away from home; carry a whistle to alert others nearby, or a cellular phone to report suspicious behavior or to contact someone for help if necessary.
- Seek protection, restraining, or stay-away orders.
- Inquire about the state's stalking laws because each state's laws differ, and see how they apply to this specific case.
- Note any illegal acts by the stalker, such as entering the residence without permission, destroying property, and so on. By reporting these acts to the police, the acts are not only documented for future evidence, but also may require that the stalker be incarcerated or ordered to stay away from the woman.
- Create a safety plan. Keep a list of important numbers, such as law enforcement, legal representation, and safe places. Victims may want to keep important items and extra money in one place to grab in a rush if necessary.
- Other preventive measures include changing the locks on doors; adding extra outside light around the residence; maintaining an unlisted phone number; varying regular routes; staying in public places when out of the house; and informing neighbors so they can alert someone if they see something suspicious.

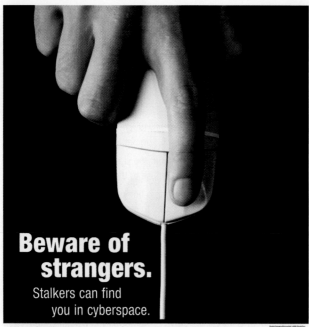

■ The Internet provides many perpetrators with opportunities to stalk. Reprinted with permission from the National Center for Victims of Crime.

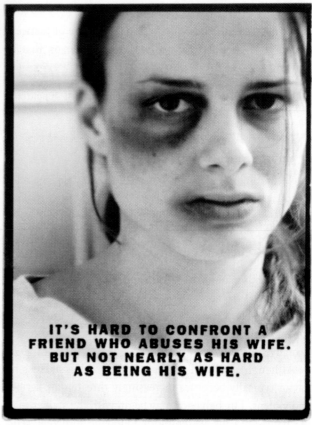

■ At least one out of every three murdered women is killed by her husband or boyfriend. Reprinted with permission from the Family Violence Prevention Fund.

and using objects as weapons. Forced sexual activity constitutes sexual violence. Property violence denotes threatened or actual destruction of property. Psychological and social forms of violence include threats of harm, physical isolation of the woman, extreme jealousy, mental degradation, and threats of harm to children, pets, or other loved ones.

Battering of women is a major health problem. It occurs in families of all racial, economic, educational, and religious backgrounds. Violence in a home often involves more than the adult couple. More than 15 million children in the United States live in families in which partner violence occurred at least once in the past year; nearly half of these families experienced severe partner violence.[18] Research suggests that almost all of these children are aware of the violence in their homes; even if they do not see it, they hear the screams and see the bruises, broken bones, and abrasions sustained by their mothers.[19]

Domestic violence is thought to be more prevalent among immigrant women than among U.S. citizens. Im-

migrants from some cultures condone the use of violence from a man toward his wife or other women in the family. Newly immigrated women are also often more vulnerable, with less access to legal and social services, as well as extended family or other support networks. Immigrant women also may not feel that they are protected by the U.S. legal system or may feel that they are unable to seek help from authorities if their immigrant status is unstable.[20] Studies involving Latina, South Asian, and Korean immigrants demonstrated that 30% to 50% of these women have been sexually or physically victimized by a male intimate partner.[21]

Although battering of women occurs at all socioeconomic levels of society, the rate of intimate violence against

My boyfriend always put me down when we were alone and when we were out without friends. He told me that I needed to lose weight, I should shave more often, and I should change my hair. I always tried to make him happy; but he would still find something that he didn't like about me. Even when he cheated on me, he blamed me for pushing him away. I didn't even realize how abusive he was until he finally left me for another woman.

24-year-old woman

women generally increases as household income levels decrease (**Figure 14.2**).[22] Spousal abuse perhaps appears more frequently under economically disadvantaged conditions because educated, middle-class, and affluent women tend to have more resources with which to avoid or leave violent relationships. For example, affluent women may seek confidential professional help and are more likely to be able to afford and get to a safe location to stay, such as a hotel or friend or relative's house in another city or state.

Relationship violence can and often does lead to death. In recent years, the mortality rate from relationship violence has been high: An intimate killed about 33% of female murder victims. In the United States, more than three women are murdered every day by an intimate partner.[23] Battering is often underdiagnosed during medical visits because both the patient and her health-care provider may be reluctant to initiate or discuss the topic. One study showed that 92% to 98% of women did not discuss their experiences of abuse with their health-care providers.[24] Al-

though most states have mandatory reporting requirements for child abuse or elder abuse, only a small number of states have a corresponding requirement for health-care providers to report battering of women.

Battering in Same-Sex Relationships

Although research on domestic violence has increased considerably in the last two and a half decades, only recently has attention been given to the problem of partner abuse among homosexual couples. Research in this area is especially difficult. In 2006, there were 3,534 reported incidents of domestic violence affecting lesbian, gay, bisexual, or transgender victims in major cities around the United States; about 35% of these victims who disclosed their gender identified themselves as female.[25]

Lesbian victims of partner abuse are doubly stigmatized—first because of their victimization and second because of their sexual orientation. Many lesbians perceive battering as a heterosexual phenomenon and therefore may not recognize the patterns of abuse within their own relationships. Additionally, fewer protective measures from the legal system are available to lesbians. Such victims of domestic violence often find it difficult to seek assistance from the courts and police when their relationships are not recognized in many states' legislatures. Most battering-related services are designed for heterosexual female victims and heterosexual male offenders, making it difficult for lesbians to find support. This lack of services is believed to be a major contributor to the lack of recognition of lesbian, bisexual, and gay domestic violence.

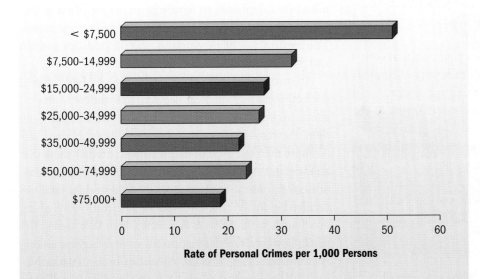

Rate of Personal Crimes per 1,000 Persons

Figure 14.2

Victimization rates for persons age 12 and older, by annual family income.

Source: Greenfield L. (2005). *Criminal Victimization in the United States, 2003 Statistical Tables. National Crime Victimization Survey* (NCJ 207 811). Washington, DC: U.S. Department of Justice.

Battering During Pregnancy

Women are not immune to battering during pregnancy. Each year, as many as 335,000 pregnant women experience intimate partner violence.[26,27] Battering during pregnancy has numerous consequences. Women who are battered may be less likely to seek prenatal care and gain sufficient weight. They also may be more likely to engage in harmful behaviors such as smoking or alcohol use. Battering during pregnancy is linked to an increased risk of miscarriage, premature labor, fetal distress, and low birthweight. Blunt abdominal trauma can lead to fetal death or low birthweight by provoking preterm delivery. Excessive stress and anxiety for the mother also may cause adverse effects.[28]

Battering in Women with Disabilities

Women with disabilities are about as likely as other women to experience physical, sexual, or emotional abuse at some point in their lives. Women with disabilities, however, were more likely to report multiple perpetrators, longer duration of abuse, and more intense experiences of abuse.[29]

Disabled women are most commonly abused by an intimate partner, followed by a family member, a personal care attendant, a stranger, or a health-care provider. The abuse often begins subtly, as the abuser tries to determine how much violence will remain unnoticed. Abuse may take the form of psychological, physical, or financial abuse, or it may involve neglect by withholding care, medication, or mobility devices.

Many people with disabilities are especially vulnerable to victimization because of their real or perceived inability to fight or flee, or to tell anyone about the abuse. Many battered women's shelters may be inaccessible or lack at-

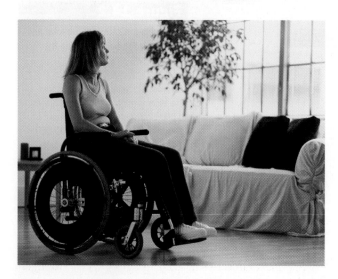

■ Women with disabilities face unique challenges with violence.

tendant care or personnel who are trained in working with specific conditions. A woman therefore may find herself trapped in an abusive situation. Consequently, health-care practitioners need to find ways to conduct at least part of their visit with a woman with disabilities in private. This opportunity allows a woman to answer questions and confide in her practitioner without a caretaker or family member being present.

Child Abuse

As defined by the Child Abuse Prevention and Treatment Act, **child abuse and neglect** includes any act or the failure to act on the part of a parent or caretaker that presents an imminent risk of serious harm or actually results in serious physical or emotional harm, sexual abuse, exploitation, or death of a child. A child is defined as a person younger than age 18, except in sexual abuse cases, in which the age is specified by the child protection laws of the child's state of residence. Included in the definition of child abuse and neglect is the withholding of medically indicated treatment that in a professional's medical judgment would be effective in improving or curing a life-threatening condition. The four major types of maltreatment of children include physical abuse, child neglect (failure to provide for a child's basic needs including physical, educational, or emotional needs), sexual abuse, and emotional abuse.

In the United States, an estimated 905,000 children were victims of abuse and neglect in 2006 (roughly 48% boys and 52% girls). More than 80% of these children were maltreated by one or both parents, most commonly the female parent; women represented nearly 60% of all perpetrators of such violence. The abuser's gender differed by type of maltreatment: Neglect and medical neglect were most often attributed to female perpetrators, whereas sexual abuse was most often attributed to male perpetrators. The median age of perpetrators was 31 years for women and 34 years for men.[30]

Approximately 66% of the maltreated children suffered neglect, including medical neglect; 16% suffered physical abuse; approximately 9% were sexually abused; and more than 6% were emotionally maltreated. Many children suffer more than one type of maltreatment. Studies show that an estimated 1,500 children died as a result of child abuse or neglect; only a small percentage of these child fatalities occurred in foster care. One-half of all victims were white, one-fourth were African American, and 18% were Hispanic; however, rates of victimization were highest among African American children, American Indian/Alaska Native children, and children of multiple races (see **Figure**

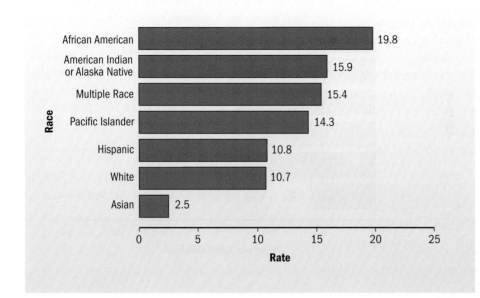

Figure 14.3

Race and ethnicity of victims, 2006.

Source: U.S. Department of Health and Human Services, Administration on Children, Youth and Families. (2008). *Child Maltreatment 2006.* Washington, DC: U.S. Government Printing Office.

14.3). Reasons for child abuse and neglect as reported by state agencies included substance abuse by one or both of the parents, poverty or other economic strain, parental capacity and skill, and other incidents involving domestic abuse.

In a survey by the National Center on Child Abuse Prevention Research, 85% of states reported substance abuse as a major problem in families with suspected child maltreatment.[31] Research also suggests that although children from all socioeconomic levels suffer from abuse and neglect, children from families with annual incomes of less than $15,000 were more than 25 times as likely to suffer maltreatment than were children from families with annual incomes of $30,000 or more.[32] Many problems associated with poverty contribute to child maltreatment, including more transient residence, poorer education, and higher rates of substance abuse and emotional disorders. Moreover, families at the lower socioeconomic levels have less adequate social support systems to assist parents in their childcare responsibilities.

Almost without exception, abusive parents were themselves abused or neglected as children. This underscores the resulting cycle of abuse: Battered children often grow up to become battering adults. Child abuse is frequently a symptom of family violence. One large study revealed that women who had both witnessed violence between their parents and been victims of parental abuse themselves were twice as likely to abuse their partner or children than were women who had been exposed to only one or the other type of violence. Women appeared to be most strongly influenced by their mother's behavior. With every witnessed incident in which the woman's mother had attacked her father, there was an increased likelihood that the woman would

- Abuse her child;
- Abuse her partner; or
- Become the victim of her current partner.[33]

Several psychological traits have been associated with child abusers:

- Immaturity and dependency
- A sense of personal incompetence
- Difficulty in seeking pleasure and finding satisfaction as an adult
- Social isolation
- A reluctance to admit the problem and seek help
- Fear of spoiling children
- A strong belief in the value of punishment
- Unreasonable and age-inappropriate expectations of children
- Low personal self-esteem

Any combination of these traits results in an inability to cope and problem-solve effectively when a problem or crisis evolves. In such cases, the outcome may ultimately be abuse.

The most largely victimized age group is the youngest (< 1 year of age), with victimization decreasing with age

Figure 14.4

Victimization rates by age group, 2006.

Source: U.S. Department of Health and Human Services, Administration on Children, Youth and Families. (2008). *Child Maltreatment 2006.* Washington, DC: U.S. Government Printing Office.

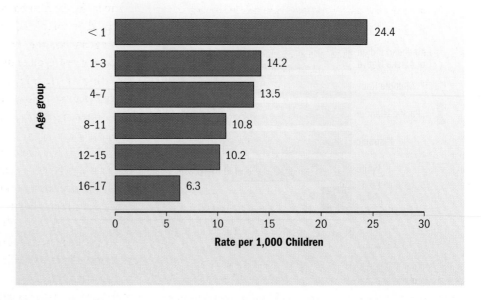

(see **Figure 14.4**). A history of child abuse can lead to behavioral and psychological problems, relationship problems, low self-esteem, depression, suicidal behavior, alcohol and substance abuse, sexual dysfunction, and sexual risk-taking later in life.[3]

Elder Abuse

As the number of people older than age 60 has rapidly grown, so has the number of abuse cases involving elderly victims. **Elder abuse** is a serious problem for women because they generally live longer than men. In most cases, elders become increasingly dependent on others for their care as they get older. It is estimated that 1 to 2 million Americans age 65 or older have been vicitmized by someone who provided care for them. Even after accounting for their larger share of the aging population, women still account for two-thirds of all elder abuse reports.[34] There are three major situations for abuse of the elderly:

- Domestic abuse (maltreatment by someone who has a relationship with the victim)
- Institutional abuse (maltreatment by staff in a residential facility)
- Self-neglect (failure to care for oneself)

Within these situations, the National Center on Elder Abuse defines seven types of elder abuse:

- *Physical elder abuse* is the use of physical force that results in bodily injury, physical pain, or impairment.
- *Sexual elder abuse* is nonconsensual sexual contact of any kind with an elderly person.

- *Emotional or psychological elder abuse* is the infliction of anguish, pain, or distress through verbal or nonverbal acts.
- *Financial or material exploitation* occurs when an elder's funds, property, or assets are misused or misappropriated by another.
- *Neglect* refers to the refusal or failure of a caretaker to perform his or her obligations or duties to an elderly person. Neglect can be active, when the failure or refusal to acknowledge an obligation is intentional, or passive, when the failure is unintentional.
- *Self-neglect* is the failure to provide oneself with adequate food, water, clothing, shelter, safety, personal hygiene, and medication, thereby threatening the elderly person's own health or safety.
- *Abandonment*, also known as "granny dumping," occurs when an elderly person is deserted by an individual who has physical custody of the elder or by a person who has assumed responsibility for providing care to the elder.

Elder abuse has been discovered in people of all racial, ethnic, and economic backgrounds in the United States. In general, elders who are unable to care for themselves are more likely to suffer abuse. Researchers have found that in 90% of substantiated cases, perpetrators of elder abuse were family members, with two-thirds being adult children or spouses. Men were more likely to be perpetrators of abuse in cases of abandonment, physical abuse, emotional abuse, and financial and material exploitation. Women were slightly more likely to be perpetrators in cases of neglect. In self-neglect cases, approximately two-thirds of elders were female, 75 or older, and white.[35]

In one survey conducted in the United States, 36% of nursing-home staff reported having witnessed at least one incident of physical abuse of an elderly patient in the previous year, 10% admitted having committed at least one act of physical abuse themselves, and 40% said that they had psychologically abused patients.[34] Abusive acts within institutions include physically restraining patients, depriving them of dignity and choice over daily affairs, and providing insufficient care (allowing them to develop pressure sores, for example).

Several factors have been identified that contribute to a high stress level for relatives of a dependent older person and, therefore, may contribute to elder abuse. These factors include caregiver stress, impairment of the dependent elder, and resentment of dependency, especially as the level of dependency increases. In many cases of abuse, caregivers are unprepared, unable, or unwilling to provide the necessary care. Elder abuse is also related to emotional problems, such as alcohol or drug use by the abuser, social isolation of the abuser and the abused, and lack of community support. It has also been hypothesized that the abuser may be repeating a cycle of violence, similar to the cycle identified in cases of child abuse and neglect. That is, the abuser of an elderly parent may have been abused by the parent in childhood, or the abuser may have witnessed the same type of elder abuse by the parent against the abuser's grandparent.

Rape and Sexual Assault

Rape and sexual assault are violent crimes of aggression. Rape is a nonconsensual event, involving the use of force or the threat of force to sexually penetrate the victim's vagina, mouth, or rectum.[4] Sexual assault often refers to forced sexual contact, but this term is frequently used as an all-encompassing descriptor for any type of unwanted sexual advances, including rape. A large survey conducted by the National Institute of Justice and the Centers for Disease

Control and Prevention found that 1 of 6 women and 1 of 33 men in the United States have been the victim of attempted or completed rape as a child or an adult.[4] Determining an accurate estimate of the number of women raped per year is quite difficult given the significant underreporting of the crime. In 2004, there were 204,370 reported victims of rape, attempted rape, or sexual assault in the United States. Of these individuals, 95,420 were victims of sexual assault, 43,440 were victims of attempted rape, and 65,510 were victims of completed rape.[36] Nine out of every 10 rape victims were female.[36]

Rape may occur among strangers or intimates. Acquaintance rape, or **date rape**, is defined as rape in which the victim and the rapist were previously known to each other and may have interacted in some socially appropriate manner. About two-thirds of rape victims in the United States know their assailant. Approximately 47% were raped by a friend or acquaintance, 17% by an intimate, and 3% by another relative; 31% of victims were raped by a stranger; and in 2% of the cases, the relationship could not be identified (see **Figure 14.5**).[36] Rape by a co-worker, teacher, professor, a husband's friend, or boss—anyone the individual knows—is considered acquaintance rape.

Many victims of rape are children and adolescents; about 44% of rape victims are younger than age 18 and about 15% are younger than age 12.[36] Although physical abuse and neglect account for the greatest portion of child abuse incidents, child sexual abuse is another tragic dimension of child abuse in general. Of the substantiated child abuse cases in 2000, 10% comprised sexual abuse cases.[37] It is difficult to determine the incidence rate of sexual abuse among children. One recent report found that 13% of girls and 3.4% of boys had been sexually abused.[38] In reported cases, three-fourths of adolescent sexual assault victims knew their attackers—21.1% were family members and 32.5% were acquaintances or friends.[38] Males are reported to be the abusers in most sexual abuse cases involving children.

Figure 14.5

Perpetrator relationship to victim in cases of sexual assault/rape.

Source: Catalano, S.M. (2005). *Criminal Victimization, 2004.* Washington, DC: Bureau of Justice Statistics, U.S. Department of Justice.

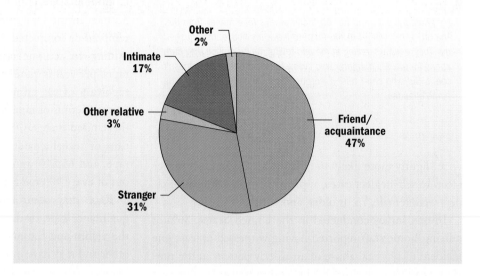

Other 2%

Intimate 17%

Other relative 3%

Friend/acquaintance 47%

Stranger 31%

In many cases of date or acquaintance rape, the rape has been facilitated by the use of drugs to render the victim unconscious or incapacitated. Flunitrazepam, commonly known as Rohypnol, is one type of "date rape drug." This drug is 10 times as strong as Valium and is tasteless and odorless. It dissolves in liquid, takes effect quickly, and produces memory loss for as long as eight hours. Rohypnol is especially popular on high school and college campuses, as well as in nightclubs. Many women have been raped after consuming a drink with the drug dissolved in it. The use of the drug is extremely dangerous and can cause death. Gamma hydroxybutyrate (GHB) and gamma butyrolactone (GBL) are found in liquid form and have also been associated with sexual assault. Abuse of GHB and GBL can lead to coma and seizures. Ketamine, used as a tranquilizer in cats, is another common date rape drug that is snorted. It is referred to as "special K" and can cause death.

Rape also can happen in a marriage, during a legal separation, or after a divorce. Rape in marriage is often called spousal rape or marital rape. Historically, husbands had unlimited sexual access to their wives and, therefore, rape within marriage was not recognized as a crime. In 1993, marital rape became a crime in all 50 states. Many states provide exemptions for certain situations, such as mental or physical impairment of a woman rendering her unable to consent, that protect husbands from being prosecuted for rape. In addition, rape can occur between people of the same sex. The National Violence Against Women Survey found that 10.8% of women rape or sexual assault victims were assaulted by a female.[4]

Rape is often characterized as not being a "clear-cut" crime such as murder. Societal pressures and norms have reinforced beliefs that rape is sometimes justifiable, depending on the circumstances. For various reasons, most rapes go unreported. In fact, an estimated 58% of rapes are never reported to the police.[36] These unreported rapes may be perceived as a threat to public safety, because if the rapists are not dealt with in the criminal justice system, their violent behavior may continue. The underreporting of rape is due to a number of factors, including the pattern of "blaming the victim." Many women fear unwanted publicity from making a formal complaint, and others distrust hospital and law enforcement agencies. Reasons for women not reporting rape include feelings of shame or guilt, fear that they would not be believed, and fear of reprisal or punishment if the rapist is an acquaintance or employer.

Around the world, countless women in prisons and jails are at risk of rape and other forms of sexual violence. Re-

■ Most rapes go unreported.

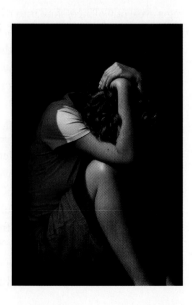

It's Your Health

Information About "Date Rape Drugs"

Rohypnol (roofies, ruffies, roach, R2, rophies, la roche, rib, mind eraser, the forget pill, the date rape drug)

■ **Characteristics:** small white pill (often has "ROCHE" on one side for Hoffmann-La Roche, its manufacturer, and a circled "1" or "2" on one side); can be swallowed as a pill, dissolved in a drink, or snorted; tasteless and odorless

■ **Effects:** may feel dizzy, disoriented, nauseated, sleepy, extremely relaxed, or drunk; can cause difficulty speaking or moving, unconsciousness, and loss of memory; effects may last from two to eight hours.

Gamma Hydroxybutyrate (GHB, liquid ecstasy, easy lay, liquid X, energy drink, somatomax, scoop, Georgia Home Boy, grievous bodily harm, goop)

■ **Characteristics:** white powdered material or liquid form

■ **Effects:** may feel drowsy, dizzy, or nauseated; may cause unconsciousness, seizures, severe respiratory depression, and coma

Ketamine (special K, vitamin K, cat tranquilizer, k)

■ **Characteristics:** white powdered material, similar to cocaine; can be snorted, smoked with marijuana, or dissolved in beverages

■ **Effects:** short-acting hallucinatory effects; can affect the senses, judgment, and coordination for 18 to 24 hours

Ways to Protect Yourself

■ Don't leave a beverage unattended or accept a drink from an open container.

■ Don't drink from someone else's drink.

■ Don't drink any beverage with a funny taste, odor, residue, color, or consistency.

■ Go to parties with trusted friends; watch out for each other and leave together.

---

porting procedures in prisons are often ineffectual, and complaints are routinely ignored. To make matters worse, punishment for the crime is rare and some inmates face retaliation from the offender if a report is made.

Reducing Risk of Rape/Sexual Assault

Risk reduction for rape entails taking actions—by both women and society as a whole—to eliminate the inappropriate use of physical and sexual force. These strategies include measures to reduce one's susceptibility to physical assault. This does not mean that women are "at fault" if communication attempts fail and a rape subsequently occurs; it does mean that women owe it to themselves to communicate explicitly their intent, or lack thereof, in sexual matters.

An important concept in reducing the risk of rape, particularly date and marital rape, is formalized preparation and training. Four critical components should be included in any risk reduction program for rape:

1. Discussion and understanding of the facts of rape and dispelling the myths of rape

2. Skills training in developing honest and direct communication about dating and sexual needs and desires

3. Practical interventions (combination of audiovisual presentations, group discussions, and role playing)

4. Preparation for what to do when rape occurs, with an emphasis on early support and counseling

These measures are valuable in improving a woman's self-esteem and self-confidence as well as for providing practical rape intervention strategies and a heightened awareness of local supportive resources and services.

Response to Rape/Sexual Assault

In the event that rape or sexual assault occurs, a woman's first concern should be finding safety and calling the police. The police will assist the victim in seeking medical attention, which is important for treating any physical injuries, testing

It's Your Health

Reducing the Risk of Date Rape

Be wary of a relationship that is operating along classic stereotypes of dominant male and submissive, passive female. The dominance in ordinary activities may extend to the sexual arena.

Be wary when a date tries to control behavior or pressures others in any way.

Be explicit with communication. Don't say "no" in a way that could be interpreted in any way as a "maybe" or "yes."

Avoid ambiguous messages with both verbal and nonverbal behavior. Saying "no" and permitting heavy petting implies confusion or ambiguity.

First dates with an unknown companion may be safer in a group.

Avoid remote or isolated spots where help is not available.

Limit alcohol and illegal drug use.

It's Your Health

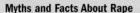

Myths and Facts About Rape

Myth: Rape only occurs in the "bad part of town," not in nice neighborhoods.

Fact: Six out of 10 sexual assaults take place at the victim's own home or at the home of a friend, neighbor, or relative.

Myth: Rape occurs only late at night, in the dark.

Fact: Forty-three percent of rapes occur between 6 P.M. and midnight; 24% of rapes occur between midnight and 6 A.M.; and the other 33% take place between 6 A.M. and 6 P.M.

Myth: If a person pays for a date, he or she has the right to expect something back, such as sex.

Fact: No one ever owes anyone sex.

Myth: If a person returns to his or her date's apartment or house, the date has the right to expect sex.

Fact: Consent for sexual contact is not defined by one's willingness to enter someone else's home or inviting someone into his or her home, including a date.

Myth: People who commit rapes are unable to control their sexual urges.

Fact: Rapists are not driven by uncontrollable sexual urges, but rather by the need to feel powerful and in control. Forcing someone to engage in sexual intercourse against her or his will is an act of violence and aggression. Sex is the weapon used to humiliate and control the victim.

Myth: Rapists are always strangers to the victim.

Fact: Approximately 66% of rape victims know their assailant.

Myth: All rapists are African American men who rape white women.

Fact: In approximately 88% of rapes, the victim and the offender are members of the same race. Whites tend to rape whites; blacks tend to rape blacks.

Myth: All rapists are men.

Fact: Although men commit 99% of forcible rapes, women do commit rape and other sexual assault offenses. In 2000, 300 women were serving time for rape and 900 more for other sexual assaults in the United States.

Myth: Only promiscuous women or women wearing provocative clothing are victims of rape.

Fact: Neither provocative dress nor promiscuous behavior is an invitation for unwanted sexual activity. Forcing someone to engage in non-consensual sexual activity is sexual assault, regardless of the way the person dresses or acts.

Myth: All rape victims are women.

Fact: In 2001, 1 in every 10 rape victims was male.

Myth: Women who are raped were asking for it.

Fact: No one deserves to be raped. A victim should never be blamed for the actions of the perpetrator.

Sources: National Crime Victimization Survey, 1999; National Crime Victimization Survey, 2000; Sex Offenses and Offenders. Bureau of Justice Statistics, U.S. Department of Justice, February 1997.

---

for sexually transmitted infections (STIs) and HIV/AIDS, and collecting medical evidence for prosecution. It is important to report the assault to the police immediately; the decision about whether to prosecute the offender can be made later. A woman also should contact her local rape crisis center to inquire about counseling and support.

Reactions to and recovery from rape show considerable variability among individuals. Victims of rape often suffer from mental health problems, gynecological issues, negative health behaviors, chronic health conditions, and even fatal outcomes. Rape also may lead to unwanted pregnancies and STIs, including HIV/AIDS. Being tested immediately after the incident for STIs may help a woman prevent long-term consequences from disease. Post-exposure prophylactics, including antibiotics, emergency contraceptive pills, hepatitis B vaccination, and antiretroviral drugs, can be administered.

A common psychological reaction to violent encounters, such as rape, is post-traumatic stress disorder (PTSD; see Chapter 12). At some point during their lifetimes, 32% of all rape victims develop PTSD, compare with 9% of victims of non-crime-related trauma, such as car accidents.[39]

Rape trauma syndrome is another condition associated with rape victims. It is usually described as having two phases. The first phase, or acute phase, includes the immediate emotions following the event. These emotions can vary and include, but are not limited to, shock, anger, numbness, guilt, disbelief, embarrassment, shame, feelings of being unclean, anxiety, denial, fear, self-blame, or restlessness. This phase is often characterized by significant disruption in a woman's life. The second phase of rape trauma syndrome includes attempts at reorganizing one's life and lifestyle, and learning to cope again. Victims may decide to change schools, jobs, or routes to school or work in an attempt to remove reminders of the event from their daily lives. Overwhelming feelings often develop that the victim may not directly link to the rape. Often the rape is repressed and not acknowledged (sometimes for years), but the feelings do not disappear. Depression, guilt, and loss of self-esteem are common reactions during this phase. Other psychological problems include suicide attempts, eating disorders, substance abuse, social phobia, and other anxiety disorders. Being a victim of rape can also affect a woman's sexual health and intimacy. Mediating factors that may influence how a woman reacts to a rape experience include individual coping and reaction patterns, demographic variables, characteristics of the assault, historical variables, and social supports.

Violence by Strangers

Although relatives or acquaintances of the victim commit most violent offenses against women, the number of crimes committed by strangers is increasing. These crimes include such acts as carjacking, robbery, murder, gang violence, sexual assault, and rape. Victimization rates of men exceed those of women in all types of violent crimes, except rape and sexual assault. In general, women are more likely to be victimized by an intimate than by a stranger, except in cases of robberies. Strangers also commit roughly two-thirds of the aggravated assaults against females.[36]

Another aspect of stranger violence is the concept of hate crimes, crimes that "manifest evidence of prejudice based on race, religion, sexual orientation, or ethnicity." In 2006, 7,722 hate crime incidents were reported to U.S. law enforcement. More than half of these crimes were motivated by race; religious bias accounted for about 1,400; sexual orientation for about 1,200; ethnicity for about 980; and disability for less than 100.[40]

Although stranger victimization cannot always be avoided, people can take a number of measures to protect themselves. When alone, women should avoid isolated areas and carry a whistle or cellular phone, if possible, in case of emergency. Flashy jewelry and large sums of money should be worn or carried using discretion when visiting high-crime areas. Women who are aware of their surroundings and use common sense can greatly reduce their risk of victimization; this does not mean, however, that women who are victimized are at fault. The circumstances and characteristics of each violent crime and each victim are unique, and it is not practical or realistic to imagine that these strategies alone could prevent all types of violence. Prevention is just the best—albeit limited—tool currently available to women.

Sexual Harassment

Although **sexual harassment** can occur in any setting, it has been most commonly reported in the workplace. The stereotype of sexual harassment, as in many forms of violence, involves a male harasser and a female victim. In reality, sexual harassment recognizes no gender boundaries—the victim and the harasser may even be the same sex. Three types of harassment have been defined:

- *Gender harassment* constitutes behavior that conveys a degrading or hostile attitude toward women.

- *Unwanted sexual attention or advances* include behaviors such as staring, commenting, touching, or repeated requests for dates or sexual favors.

- *Sexual coercion*, also referred to as quid pro quo (defined as an "equal" exchange or substitution), is the use of threats or bribery to obtain sexual favors.

The offensive conduct may interfere with a woman's ability to perform her regular duties at work and often creates an intimidating or hostile working environment. Women who are at the greatest risk for sexual harassment are those in careers traditionally considered to be male occupations. Sexual harassment can be initiated by anyone, but it is more likely to be used by someone with more power or authority than the recipient. In addition to suffering physical and emotional victimization, the threat of economic vulnerability often leaves the victim with the feeling that she has few real options in the situation.

Sexual harassment is often trivialized and not recognized as a violation of rights or personal dignity. Harassers may offer excuses for their behavior, but these excuses perpetuate power disparities and further dehumanize women. As with other forms of sexual victimization, harassment operates as an instrument of social control.

It's Your Health

Common Excuses for Sexual Harassment

"Sexual harassment is a trivial distraction from the real work."
Sexual harassment can have long-term emotional impact on the victim. The emotional and economic impact of sexual harassment is not trivial in nature or form.

"I didn't mean any harm. I was just having fun."
Sexual harassment is similar to poking someone with a stick. The fun is one-sided and unfair.

"She should take it as a compliment that we like her when we say things like that."
Unwanted and unsolicited sexual advances and innuendoes, particularly from others in positions of power, can be frightening. The victim can hardly feel "complimented" when she feels threatened and put down.

"She just wanted to make trouble here with a complaint."
Women are caught between the proverbial rock and a hard place. If they accept the harassment, they perpetuate the behavior and risk further, and perhaps worse, harassment. If they file a complaint, they are labeled as troublemakers, with no guarantees that the situation will be corrected. Filing a complaint may also place a woman's job security or career in jeopardy.

Sexual harassment on the job can appear in many forms, and its ramifications can be devastating. A common situation involves a boss or supervisor who requires sexual services from an employee as a condition for keeping a job or getting a promotion. Less blatant forms of workplace sexual harassment include being subjected to obscenities or being made the target of sexual jokes and innuendoes. Personal humiliation and degradation are outcomes of workplace sexual harassment, and the financial consequences of not complying with sexual coercion on the job may be devastating. Many victims, especially if they are supporting families, cannot afford to be unemployed. Also, many find it difficult to seek other work while they are employed. If they are fired for refusing to be victimized, unemployment compensation is not always available. When it is available, the amount usually represents just a fraction of the person's regular salary. Thus, a person who quits or is fired as a result of sexual harassment faces the prospect of severe financial difficulties.

Employers are becoming increasingly more sensitive to this issue, perhaps motivated in part by court decisions that have awarded large payments to victims. It is an employer's responsibility to maintain a workplace that is free of sexual harassment by educating employees about which behaviors constitute harassment and taking appropriate measures if these behaviors occur. The U.S. Department of Labor Employment and Training Administration can provide training guidelines for the workplace.

A new report from the American Association of University Women found that nearly two-thirds of college students have encountered some type of sexual harassment while at college. More than half of female students have been subjected to sexual comments and jokes, and about 35% have experienced physical harassment by being touched or grabbed in a sexual manner. Students who are lesbian, gay, bisexual, or transgender are more than twice as likely to be harassed as heterosexual students. Only 7% of students reported the harassment. Many students actually admit to sexually harassing other students; the reason more than half gave for the harassment was "I thought it was funny."[41]

Victims of sexual harassment may experience a range of adverse emotional and physical effects, including anger, humiliation, shame, embarrassment, nervousness, irritability, and lack of motivation. Guilt is another common feeling, as if the victim has done something wrong to encourage the harassment. The sense of alienation and helplessness reported by many victims of sexual harassment is similar to that experienced by many rape victims. Sexual

A guy I worked with would always come up behind me and start rubbing my shoulders. When I asked him to stop, he told me that I needed to relax, that he was just trying to help by giving me a massage. I didn't know who to tell, but it made me really uncomfortable, especially because he continued to do it even after I asked him to stop. Eventually, I went to our Human Resources department and it turned out that another co-worker had just reported him for making lewd comments to her. Within a week, he was fired. Although I felt bad at first for turning him in, it just made me too uncomfortable and nervous to work with him. I think I did the right thing.
26-year-old computer programmer

harassment victims may also experience psychosomatic effects, including headaches, stomach ailments, back and neck pain, and a variety of other stress-related ailments.

Dealing Effectively with Harassment

Individuals who have been sexually harassed have several options. First, the victim should recognize that criminal charges can be filed against the perpetrator. If the coercion falls short of attempted rape or assault, it is often wise to confront the person responsible for the harassment. The confrontation should be stated in clear terms, and the specific behaviors should be identified as sexual harassment. The victim should make it clear that the behavior is unwelcome and will not be tolerated and that, if it continues, charges will be filed through appropriate channels. Some victims carefully document what has occurred and provide a written confrontation rather than undertake a verbal discussion. Others may choose to seek out the assistance of their human resources department if the sexual harassment occurs within a work setting.

If the behavior does not stop, the next step is to discuss it with the supervisor of the person responsible for the harassment. It is often helpful to talk to other employees—many times there is more than one victim. Discussing the matter with other employees provides peer support and pressure for the behavior to stop. Official complaints can be filed with local or state Human Rights Commissions or Fair Employment Practice Agencies.

If legal action is necessary, victims can file lawsuits in federal courts under the Civil Rights Act. Lawsuits can also be filed under city or state laws prohibiting employment discrimination. One lawsuit can be filed in a number of jurisdictions. A person who has been the victim of sexual harassment is more likely to receive a favorable court ruling if attempts were made to resolve the problem within the organization before taking the issue to court.

Informed Decision Making

Knowing the facts about violence can lead to a certain level of paranoia and anger, both unhealthy conditions. Identifying the factors that contribute to violence and working to eliminate them are much more constructive reactions to potential or perceived threats of violence. For example, although miscommunication is clearly not the only or major cause of rape, it is often a factor. Misinterpretation of communication is frequently cited as a reason for the high prevalence of date rape and courtship violence. Women and men need to communicate more effectively, both in terms of their feelings and in explicitly stating their needs in the relationship, each person's responsibility within the family, and personal preferences and wishes regarding sexual behavior.

Many people still believe that men should be aggressive and that women should be passive, compliant, and pleasing to others. When people—whether male or female—buy into these stereotypes, it sets the stage for problems. For example, women who have been socialized to be passive may not think that they have a right to express their opinions openly and freely. Men who have been socialized to live up to a "macho" image may think that they need to "score" with women or control women to be "real" men. They may expect women to go along with their need to prove themselves or believe that a woman means "yes" when she says "no."

To address these stereotypes, a woman must take several steps:

- Recognize the inherent limitations in any stereotype
- Be open in discussing values with respect to relationships and sexuality
- Decide for herself and be explicit about when she will or will not have sex
- Understand that coercion and violence are never acceptable or deserved within a relationship
- Avoid situations where inebriation by one or both parties makes open and clear communication difficult

Many women find it difficult to talk openly about relationships and sexuality. Instead of using clear communication, they rely on assumptions, hints, innuendoes, and considerable hope that their partner understands. Unfortunately, such indirect communication is highly unreliable. Expectations and values about relationships and sexuality should be explicitly expressed. Communication is bidirectional: In a relationship, each person must carefully listen to the other person and confirm what has or has not been said.

Finally, "no" means "no."

Sources of Help

Women in abusive relationships first need to identify and acknowledge the presence of the problem. Denial, avoidance, and protection of the abusive partner often prevent or delay such acknowledgment, particularly for women who may have grown up in a dysfunctional family situation.

Professional counseling and support are needed when the problem has been identified. Most communities have services and facilities to support female victims of violence, including local crisis hotlines. Hotline counselors can provide callers with phone numbers of facilities that provide counseling, supportive services, and emergency shelter. Shelters provide physical safety, psychological counseling, and referral services. Many local organizations have been organized by women who have been battered themselves and recognize

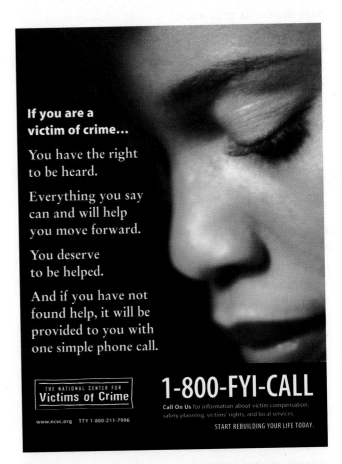

If you are a victim of crime...

You have the right to be heard.

Everything you say can and will help you move forward.

You deserve to be helped.

And if you have not found help, it will be provided to you with one simple phone call.

THE NATIONAL CENTER FOR
Victims of Crime

www.ncvc.org   TTY 1-800-211-7996

1-800-FYI-CALL

Call On Us for information about victim compensation, safety planning, victims' rights, and local services.

START REBUILDING YOUR LIFE TODAY.

■ Reaching out for help can be the most important step. Reprinted with permission from the National Center for Victims of Crime.

Profiles of Remarkable Women

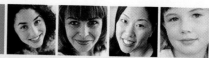

Yvette Cade (1974–)

Yvette Cade is a survivor. In 2005, three weeks after a judge dismissed her protective order against her husband in a district court in Maryland, Cade's husband showed up at her place of employment, doused her with gasoline, and set her on fire. She suffered third-degree burns over 60% of her body. After undergoing multiple surgeries, Cade pulled through and has become an advocate for domestic violence victims. She has spoken out numerous times about her abusive relationship, including telling her story to a national audience on *Montel Williams* and *Oprah*.

Yvette and her family have used her personal tragedy to encourage other sufferers of domestic violence to leave their abusive partners and find freedom. She and her family speak about the importance of family support to get through a tragedy such as this. Yvette's situation resulted in significant changes in several states, including her home state of Maryland, regarding enforcement of protection orders and the court's responsibility to treat domestic violence as a serious crime.

Yvette was honored in 2007 by the U.S. Congressional Victim's Rights Caucus for being a survivor and offering hope to victims of domestic violence. She and her family started the Yvette Cade Fund to help fund Yvette's continued need for medical treatment and further surgeries, as well as raise money for domestic violence awareness activities.

the need for sensitive and protected outreach services. Support groups provide the opportunity for women to share common concerns, fears, and information. For many women, the most important step in taking control of a violent situation is admitting there is a problem and reaching out for help.

Summary

Women bear a disproportionate burden as victims of violence. Violence affects women not only as the actual victims of crimes, but also as the wives, girlfriends, mothers, and daughters of male victims or male perpetrators, and as the perpetrators themselves. Many women are left alone to raise children; girls are raised without fathers; and some women lose their sons. These women, as well as women as victims of violence, are all at risk of psychological reactions, such as a general loss of self-esteem, depression, anxiety disorders, and suicide. Children in battering households may experience illness, emotional problems, increased fears, increased risk of abuse, injuries, and death. They also may learn to accept abusive behavior as a normal part of life, and may grow up to abuse their own children or someone else's. In addition, battering leads to high societal costs, such as increased crime; legal, medical, and counseling costs; and an overall decrease in quality of life. Efforts are urgently needed to address and reduce the full spectrum of violence against women.

Topics for Discussion

1. How does style of dress serve as a form of nonverbal communication? How can this communication be interpreted or misinterpreted?
2. How do sociocultural values and attitudes contribute to the continuing victimization of women?
3. What can a woman do to reduce her risk of assault?
4. What should a woman do if she believes that a friend is in an abusive relationship?
5. Do cultural practices and rituals that involve body modifications qualify as self-mutilation? What are some examples of these practices?
6. What are some steps that may be involved during a rape exam? What evidence may be collected to help in making a case against a rapist?

Web Sites

Children's Defense Fund:
   http://www.childrensdefense.org
Family Violence Prevention Fund:
   http://www.endabuse.org
National Center for Missing and Exploited Children:
   http://www.missingkids.com

National Center on Elder Abuse:
http://www.ncea.aoa.gov

National Committee for the Prevention of Elder Abuse:
http://www.preventelderabuse.org

NYC Gay and Lesbian Anti-Violence Project:
http://www.avp.org

Rape, Abuse and Incest National Network (RAINN):
http://www.rainn.org

Self-Abuse Finally Ends (SAFE):
http://www.selfinjury.com

U.S. Department of Justice, Office on Violence Against Women: http://www.ovw.usdoj.gov

References

1. World Health Organization. (2002). *World Report on Violence and Health: Summary.* Geneva: World Health Organization.
2. United Nations Department of Public Information. (2008). *Unite to End Violence Against Women Fact Sheet.* DPI/2498. Geneva: UN.
3. Population Information Program, Johns Hopkins University School of Public Health. (1999). Ending violence against women. *Population Reports.* XXVII(4).
4. Tjaden, P., & Thoennes, N. (2000). *Extent, Nature, and Consequences of Intimate Partner Violence: Findings from the National Violence Against Women Survey.* Washington, DC: National Institute of Justice, Office of Justice Programs, U.S. Department of Justice.
5. Attorney General's Family Violence Task Force. (1989). *Domestic Violence: A Model Protocol for Police Response.* Harrisburg, PA: Attorney General's Family Violence Task Force.
6. D'Emilio, J., & Freedman, E. B. (1988). *Intimate Matters.* New York: Harper and Row.
7. Davis, A. Y. (1983). *Women, Race, and Class.* New York: Vintage Books.
8. Centers for Disease Control and Prevention. (2005). *Behavioral Risk Factor Surveillance System Survey Data.* Atlanta, GA: U.S. Department of Health and Human Services, Centers for Disease Control and Prevention.
9. Greenfeld, L. A., & Henneberg, M. A. (2001). Victim and offender self-reports of alcohol involvement in crime. *Journal of the National Institute on Alcohol Abuse and Alcoholism* 25(1): 20–31.
10. Bureau of Justice Statistics. (2004). *American Indians and Crime, 1992–2002.* Washington, DC: Bureau of Justice Statistics, U.S. Department of Justice.
11. Wolak, J., Mitchell, K., & Finkelhor, D. (2006). *Online Victimization of Youth: Five Years Later.* Concord, NH: Crimes against Children Research Center, University of New Hampshire.
12. Centers for Disease Control and Prevention. (2003). *Costs of Intimate Partner Violence Against Women in the United States.* Atlanta, GA: U.S. Department of Health and Human Services.
13. Bureau of Justice Statistics. (2004). *Justice Expenditure and Employment in the United States, 2001.* Washington, DC: U.S. Department of Justice.
14. National Association of Crime Victim Compensation Boards. (2004). *Compensation to Victims Continues to Increase.* Alexandria, VA: NACVCB. Available at: http://www.nacvcb.org.
15. Campbell, J., Jones, A. S., Dienemann, J., et al. (2002). Intimate partner violence and physical health consequences. *Archives of Internal Medicine* 162: 1157–1163.
16. García-Moreno, et al. (2005). W*HO Multi-country Study on Women's Health and Domestic Violence Against Women. Initial Results on Prevalence, Health Outcomes and Women's Responses.* Geneva: WHO.
17. Greenfield, L., et al. (1998). *Violence by Intimates: Analysis of Data on Crimes by Current or Former Spouses, Boyfriends and Girlfriends.* Bureau of Justice Statistics Factbook. Washington, DC: U.S. Department of Justice.
18. McDonald, R., Jouriles, E. N., Ramisetty-Mikler, S., et al. (2006). Estimating the number of American children living in partner-violent families. *Journal of Family Psychology* 20(1): 137–142.
19. Family Violence Prevention Fund. (2003). *The Effects of Domestic Violence on Children.* Available at: http://www.endabuse.org.
20. Voices for Change: Immigrant Women and State Policy Center for Women in Government and Civil Society. (2004). *Building Bridges to Stop Violence Against Immigrant Women: Effective Strategies and Promising Models for Reaching and Serving Immigrant Women.* Albany, NY: University at Albany.
21. Raj, A., & Silverman, J. (2002). Violence against immigrant women: the roles of culture, context, and legal immigrant status on intimate partner violence. *Violence Against Women* 8(3): 17–20.
22. Greenfield, L. (2005). *Criminal Victimization in the United States, 2003 Statistical Tables. National Crime*

Victimization Survey (NCJ 207811). Washington, DC: U.S. Department of Justice.

23. Bureau of Justice Statistics Crime Data Brief. (February 2003). *Intimate Partner Violence, 1993–2001.* Washington, DC: USDOJ.

24. Wijma, B. (2003). Gynecologists could help identify sexual, physical, and emotional abuse. *Lancet* 361: 2107–2113.

25. National Coalition of Anti-Violence Programs. (2007). *Lesbian, Gay, Bisexual, and Transgender Domestic Violence in the United States in 2006.*

26. Peterson, R., Saltzman, L., Goodwin, M., & Spitz, A. (2004). *Key Scientific Issues for Research on Violence Occurring Around the Time of Pregnancy.* National Center for Chronic Disease Prevention and Heath Promotion, and the National Center for Injury Prevention and Control, Centers for Disease Control and Prevention. Atlanta, GA: CDC.

27. Lipsky, S., Holt, V., Easterling, T., & Critchlow, C. (2003). Impact of police-reported intimate partner violence during pregnancy on birth outcomes. *Obstetrics and Gynecology* 102: 557–564.

28. Liebschutz, J., Frayne, S., Saxe, G., & Charney, P. (2003). *Violence Against Women: A Physician's Guide to Identification and Management.* Philadelphia, PA: American College of Physicians/American Society of Internal Medicine.

29. Nosek, M. A., Hughes, R. B., Taylor, H. B., & Howland, C. A. (2004). Violence against women with disabilities: the role of physicians in filling the treatment gap. In: S. L. Welner & F. Haseltine (eds.), *Welner's Guide to Care of Women with Disabilities* (pp. 333–345). Philadelphia, PA: Lippincott, Williams and Wilkins.

30. U.S. Department of Health and Human Services, Administration on Children, Youth and Families. (2008). *Child Maltreatment 2006.* Washington, DC: U.S. Government Printing Office.

31. National Center on Child Abuse Prevention Research. (2001). *Current Trends in Child Abuse Prevention, Reporting, and Fatalities: The 1999 Fifty State Survey.* Chicago: Prevent Child Abuse America.

32. U.S. Department of Health and Human Services, National Center on Child Abuse and Neglect. (1996). *Third National Incidence Study of Child Abuse and Neglect: Final Report* (NIS-3). Washington, DC: U.S. Government Printing Office.

33. Heyman, R. E., & Slep, A. M. S. (2002). Do child abuse and interparental violence lead to adulthood family violence? *Journal of Marriage and Family* 64: 864–870.

34. Toshia, T., & Kuzmeskus, L. M. (1999). *Types of Elder Abuse in Domestic Settings—Elder Abuse Information Series,* no. 1. Grant No. 90-am-0660. Washington, DC: National Center on Elder Abuse, Administration on Aging.

35. National Center on Elder Abuse. (1998). *The National Elder Abuse Incidence Study: Final Report.* National Center on Elder Abuse at the American Public Health Services Association in Collaboration with Westat. Washington, DC: National Center on Elder Abuse, Administration on Aging.

36. Catalano, S. M. (2005). *Criminal Victimization, 2004.* Washington, DC: Bureau of Justice Statistics, U.S. Department of Justice.

37. Snyder, H. (2000). *Sexual Assault of Young Children as Reported to Law Enforcement: Victim, Incident, and Offender Characteristics.* Washington, DC: Bureau of Justice Statistics, U.S. Department of Justice.

38. National Institute of Justice. (2003). *Youth Victimization: Prevalence and Implications.* Washington, DC: U.S. Department of Justice.

39. Kilpatrick, D. G., et al. (2007). Rape-related PTSD: issues and interventions. *Psychiatric Times,* 24(7): 315–318.

40. U.S. Department of Justice. (2006). *Hate Crime Statistics, 2006: Uniform Crime Reports.* Washington, DC: Federal Bureau of Investigation, Criminal Justice Information Services Division.

41. American Association of University Women. (2006). *Drawing the Line: Sexual Harassment on Campus.* Washington, DC: AAUW.

Chapter Fifteen

Women in the Workforce

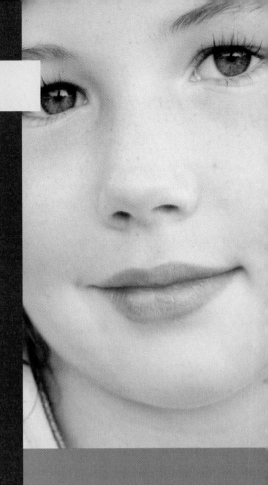

Chapter Objectives

On completion of this chapter, the student should be able to discuss:

1. Historical trends related to women in the workforce.

2. Occupational trends of women.

3. Work issues for special populations.

4. Work-related barriers specific to low-income women and women on welfare.

5. The wage gap between the two genders and the concepts of the "glass ceiling" and the "sticky floor."

6. The connection between work, family, and personal life.

7. The lack of basic benefits and family-friendly work policies for a significant number of women.

8. The effects of housework, child care, elder care, and the work environment on a woman's general well-being.

9. Work-related stress and the comparison of mental well-being of employed women versus nonworking women.

10. Musculoskeletal injuries in the workplace and ways to protect against these injuries.

11. Chemical, biological, and physical hazards in the workplace and their effects on women's reproductive health.

12. Global dimensions of women in the workforce.

13. Ways for employers and employees to increase productivity and satisfaction.

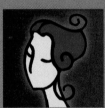

womenshealth.jbpub.com

Women's Health Online is a great source for supplementary women's health information for both students and instructors. Visit

http://womenshealth.jbpub.com

to find a variety of useful tools for learning, thinking, and teaching.

Introduction

Over the past century, women have gone from being a workplace rarity to an essential part of the workforce. In 1900, women made up roughly one-fifth (18.3%) of the labor force with 5.3 million women working. These numbers rose to 29.6% of the labor force in 1950 (18.4 million women) and increased further to 46% of the labor force in 2008 (67.7 million women).[1-3] Women, however, are still not reaching the highest echelons of the work world in great numbers. In 2007, 13 *Fortune* 500 companies had female CEOs and only 10% had women holding at least one-fourth of their officer positions.

The rising number of women in the workforce has highlighted many new issues, including pay differentials between genders, the balancing of work and family, health and safety in the workplace, and the struggle for many women between choosing a career and choosing to stay home. On average, full-time women employees with the same job responsibilities who are performing at equal levels as their male counterparts now earn $0.81 for every $1 earned by men (**Figure 15.1**).[4] Greater awareness of the problem and legislation have failed to solve this problem. Women also typically shoulder more of the burden of family and household responsibilities than men do, often working at their paying jobs and then taking on a "second shift" of responsibilities when they return home. Some women who choose to stay home feel conflicted by their choice, as do some women who choose to pursue a career and leave their child with a surrogate provider.

As women have increased their presence in the workforce, general health and safety issues have arisen. Workstations, tools, and protective equipment have traditionally been designed for men and therefore may compromise the health and safety of women. Health hazards from biological, chemical, and disease-causing agents are significant in

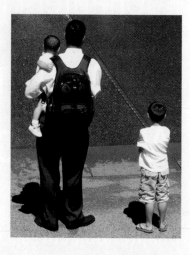

■ Men and women are redefining traditional roles and responsibilities for their families.

many predominantly female occupations, including the textile, laundry, and meat industries; health care; and food preparation. Additionally, physically intense activities or exposure to certain substances while on the job can harm working women who are pregnant.

In this chapter, gender differences in the workplace, the balancing of work and family, and occupational safety issues are discussed. In addition, the chapter presents strategies for decreasing job stress and increasing workplace satisfaction.

Trends and Issues

Historical Issues

In colonial times, all members of the family worked together as an economic unit. Although the majority of women's paid jobs outside the home appeared to be extensions of their household duties—making clothing, cleaning house, teaching, or cooking—women also worked as blacksmiths, silversmiths, shopkeepers, and operators of grist mills. When their husbands were off at sea or at war, women continued to operate the family businesses until the husbands returned; other women accompanied troops to war and served as nurses and cooks. Some women even became spies or posed as men and entered battle.

The Industrial Revolution brought women into the factories, providing many with new skills, educational opportunities, and social outlets. Many European women immigrated to the United States to work as indentured servants, with hopes of a more promising future. Workplace violence, sexual harassment, and unfair pay were issues for a number of these women, who were often physically and sexually abused on the job, and deprived of personal freedom and financial compensation. Because many women's positions were viewed as temporary, working women typically earned enough wages to help make ends meet, but not enough to make a comfortable living.

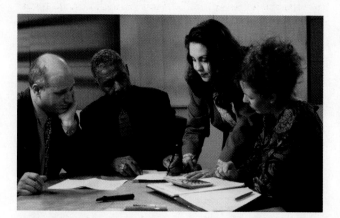

■ While women make up half of the workforce, they continue to earn less than their male counterparts for the same responsibilities.

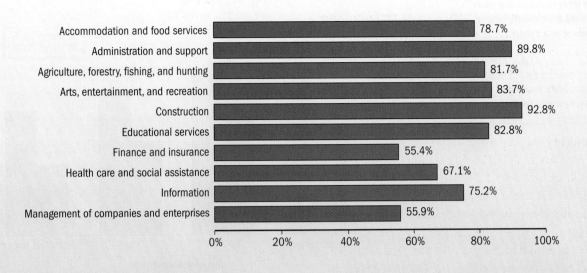

Figure 15.1

Women's earnings as a percentage of men's earnings.

Source: U.S. Census Bureau, 2006 American Community Survey. Available at: http://www.factfinder.census.gov

In the mid-1800s, Charlotte Woodward campaigned to change laws to give women rights to their earnings, as opposed to the custom of husbands having ownership of their wives' money. The New York Married Women's Property Act, which was passed in 1848, represented a major step for women's rights; by 1860, other states had passed similar laws.[5] It was not until 1974, however, that Congress passed the Equal Credit Opportunity Act, which made it unlawful for creditors to discriminate against women on the basis of sex or marital status, thereby enabling women in the United States to establish their own credit lines.

Women continued to find opportunities to earn wages, with many working to build professional careers as lawyers, journalists, physicians, and teachers. Wyoming was the first state to provide equal pay for female teachers under a law passed in 1869, followed soon thereafter by California.[5] Although exceptions did arise, most women continued to work in occupations traditionally associated with women—for example, nursing, clerical work, and domestic servant positions.

When World War II began, the types of jobs available to women increased dramatically. "Rosie the Riveter" became the symbol for women workers in the U.S. defense industries. More than 6 million women, from all backgrounds and from all over the country, worked at industrial jobs that challenged traditional notions of women's capabilities and ensured U.S. productivity that helped win the war. During the war years, women became streetcar con-

ductors, taxicab drivers, machine operators, business managers, and railroad workers. They unloaded freight, worked in lumber mills and steel mills, and made munitions. In essence, women occupied almost every aspect of industry. This trend led to a rise in salaries and an overall commitment by women to their jobs, though many women lost their new positions when the men returned from war.

Over the past 60 years, the number of women in the workforce has continued to grow. Today, women are more likely than men to attend college, a major change from 30 years ago. The desegregation of college majors has led more women into fields such as architecture, business, and the sciences.[6] Many women are postponing childbearing and marriage, having smaller families, and, in turn, focusing on building their careers and developing themselves as individuals before taking on the roles of wife and mother. Women have opened up numerous opportunities for themselves by attending college, fighting for equal rights in the workplace, and breaking barriers in many occupations traditionally associated with men. Despite all of the advances, however, gender discrimination in jobs persists.

Occupation Trends of Women

The realities of women in the workforce can be better understood by looking at the rates of participation in the workforce according to age and educational level, the professions in which women are concentrated, and the

Figure 15.2

Labor force participation rates increased dramatically among mothers over 31 years.

Source: Bureau of Labor Statistics. (2006). *Charting the U.S. Labor Market in 2005*. Washington, DC: U.S. Deparment of Labor.

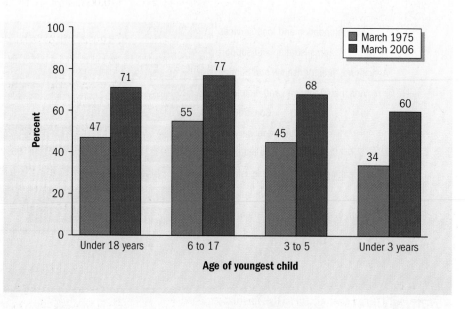

percentage of women-owned businesses. Such statistics begin to paint a more complete picture of women's opportunities and persistent hurdles, and they show how solving the dilemma of child care would affect many women's ability to work.

Of the 120 million women age 16 or older in the United States, approximately 60% are in the labor force either working or looking for work.[3] Women ages 35 to 44 represent the highest percentage of working women (**Figure 15.2**).[7] This may be partly due to the fact that women are

more likely to participate in the workforce as their children get older. More than three-fourths of women age 25 years or older who are employed are college graduates. Most working women (75%) are employed full time (**Table 15.1**). In addition, nearly 50% of multiple jobholders are women.[8]

Although women work in all industries and contribute in multiple ways to the economy, their participation is often concentrated in certain sectors. The majority of employed women work in technical, sales, and administrative support occupations (**Table 15.2**). Nearly one of every five employed women works as a teacher (excluding post-secondary positions), secretary, manager or administrator, or cashier.[9]

Table 15.1 Employment Status of Women, Ages 25–64, by Educational Attainment, 2005

	Participation Rate	Unemployment Rate
Total	68.6%	4.2%
Less than high school	43.8%	10.0%
High school graduate, no college	64.8%	4.9%
Some college or associate's degree	72.8%	4.0%
College graduates, total	78.0%	2.4%
Bachelor's degree	76.4%	2.5%
Master's degree	80.9%	2.1%
Professional degree	81.2%	1.9%
Doctoral degree	85.0%	2.3%

Source: U.S. Department of Labor. (February 2006). *Women in the Workforce: A Databook*.

Table 15.2 Employed Women by Occupational Group, 2005

Occupation	Percentage of Total That Are Women
Medical and health service managers	71.2%
Computer software engineers	21.9%
Chief executives	23.8%
Chemical engineers	14.3%
Psychologists	67.3%
Social workers	80.1%
Lawyers	30.2%
Pre-school and kindergarten teachers	97.7%

Source: U.S. Department of Labor. (2006). *Women in the Labor Force*. Bureau of Labor Statistics.

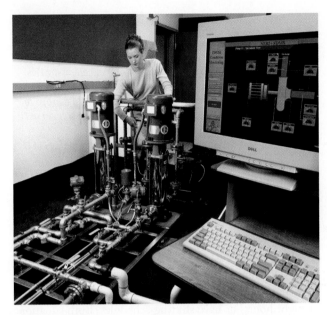

■ By breaking the barriers of traditionally male-dominated fields, women have created greater opportunities for themselves in the workplace.

According to the U.S. Census Bureau's Survey of Business Owners and Self-Employed Persons, women own 28.8% of all nonfarm businesses, totaling nearly 6.5 million businesses.[10] (Women-owned businesses are defined as privately held firms in which women own 51% or more of the firm.) More than half of such firms were in the services industry, particularly business services and personal services. Women cite a variety of reasons for starting their own businesses:

- Flexibility
- Independence
- Outlet for creativity
- Relief from sexual harassment in the workplace
- An exit from poverty[10]

In recent years, the number of women in the workforce who have young children has significantly increased. Today, 54.2% of mothers with infants and toddlers (younger than age 2), 62.8% of mothers with children ages 3 to 5, and 73.7% of mothers with children ages 6 to 17 are in the workforce.[11,12] The number of dual-earner families also has increased. Before World War II, less than 10% of the workforce was from a dual-earner family. Today, more than 57% are dual-earner families. In nearly 75% of dual-earner families, both partners work full time.[13] What is surprising is that many two-parent families with young children are having difficulty making ends meet. Fifty percent of young

children are members of families with incomes less than $40,000; 25% are in families making less than $20,000.[14]

Special Populations

Women with Disabilities in the Workplace

Women with disabilities confront many barriers in the workplace:

- Lack of job opportunities or appropriate jobs
- Inaccessible work environments
- Lower wages than people without disabilities
- Discouragement by family and friends
- Fear of losing health insurance or Medicaid
- Little or no accessible parking or public transportation nearby

In addition, once a job has been secured and other barriers worked through, there still may be a need for adaptations to workstations, special work arrangements or hours, handrails or ramps, or communication access for hearing or visually impaired individuals. The severity of a woman's disability has the greatest influence on her employment status. According to the National Institute of Disability and Rehabilitation Research, only 24.7% of women with a severe disability have a job, as compared with 68.4% of women with a nonsevere disability (74.5% of women with no disability had jobs).[15] Women with disabilities are employed in a variety of occupations, including the service industry, managerial and professional occupations, and middle management positions. In terms of pay, women with disabilities earn, on average, less than women with no disabilities. Women with disabilities that directly affect their work are

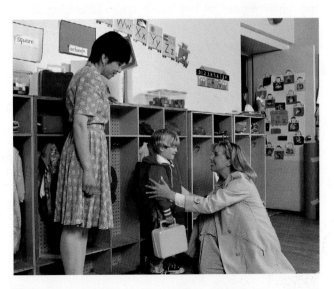

■ Child care remains a major challenge for working parents.

more likely to live below the poverty level than those people without work disabilities. Approximately 40% of women with a severe work disability are living in poverty.[15]

Older Women

Women have increasingly been participating in the part-time labor force during the traditional years of retirement. This trend is largely attributable to the fact that individuals are living longer and healthier lives and/or finding their retirement savings are not adequate to make ends meet. Older women may have special health needs as members of the workforce, including the need for easy or disabled access to a work site, close proximity to restrooms, and seats with supportive backs or armrests to assist in getting up and down. Employers should be aware of the special needs of older workers, as they provide a valuable and often highly educated supplement to the workforce.

Socioeconomic Issues

Although many women face the difficult task of finding and keeping a job that is rewarding both mentally and financially, low-income women—particularly welfare recipients—face even greater obstacles. For these women, the consequences of not finding employment or the inability to maintain a job can have devastating consequences. Welfare recipients and low-wage workers are disproportionately women and minorities with family responsibilities. Women heads of household represent a high percentage of this group. Welfare-to-work programs that were supported by the dramatic welfare reform passed in 1996 have helped many of these women move from welfare into paid employment. Most of these individuals work in service industries characterized by low hourly wages (averaging about

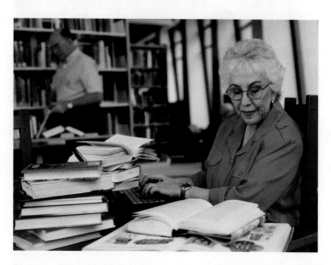

■ Older workers have unique needs in their workplace environments.

I have a high school degree and a few college-level courses, but I can't get a job that pays enough to cover child care and bills. I'm now living with my mom, and she basically takes care of my kids. But I want to make it on my own! How can I afford to go back to school and take care of my kids at the same time? If I don't go to school, how can I get a job to make enough money to support us? I feel like I'm stuck in a situation that I'll never get out of.

26-year-old woman with two children under the age of 5

$8 per hour), however, and are at significant risk for layoffs or work-hour reduction in a down economy.

Work opportunities for low-income women or women on welfare are often limited because many persons in this situation lack education, training, transportation, or child care. Many jobs available to low-income women or women on welfare either are available at odd hours (such as evening or night hours) or have shifting schedules. Both situations make transportation and childcare options even more difficult. Low-income women who live in rural areas with little or no public transportation often have trouble getting to and from job training centers, let alone to jobs. Other women are caught between taking a job to put food on the table and leaving young children at home alone because of lack of child care. For many women, even when they are able to find transportation and child care, their low wages are eaten up by the costs for those transportation and childcare services.

Low-wage jobs often provide few or no benefits, such as health-care coverage, paid sick leave, or paid family leave. Furthermore, because the positions do not require advanced skills, employers are typically quick to replace a woman who may have to miss work because her child is sick.[16] A recent study reported that women who left welfare to work were less likely than other working women to have jobs that offered paid sick days, family leave, or flexible job schedules, even though they were more likely to have children with chronic health problems.[17]

Equal Pay for Equal Work

A great challenge for working women has been the battle of receiving equal pay for performing equal work. Men in the same jobs as women often earn more than women with the same education and years of experience.

In 2006, women who worked full time, regardless of age, race, or educational attainment, earned a median weekly salary of $600 compared with $743 for men—that is, they earned approximately four-fifths (81%) of what men make (**Table 15.3**).[4] Earning differences between genders varied by demographic features, with the greatest contrast arising between men and women ages 45 to 64, with women earning about 73% as much as men in this age range. The narrowest gap between earnings was among workers 16 to 24 years old; in this demographic group, women earned 95% of what men earned (**Figure 15.3**).[4] As a result of these differences, the average 25-year-old woman who works full time, year-round, until retiring at age 65 will earn more than half a million dollars less over her lifetime than the average working man.[18] To elucidate this point even further, men with a professional degree have average annual incomes of more than $70,000, while women with the same degree average $40,000 per year. In other words, these women work Monday through Friday to earn what a man in a comparable position has earned by noon on Wednesday.[19]

The pay gap is closing in some fields, but not in others and not quickly enough. For example, in comparison to men in the same occupation, on a weekly average:

- Women lawyers make almost $500 less
- Women bartenders make about $70 less
- Women engineers make about $150 less
- Women doctors make nearly $500 less
- Women registered nurses make about $100 less
- Women professors make nearly $300 less[3]

Not only do women make less money than men in virtually every profession, but women are clustered in low-paying professions. In 2006, women earned 80.7% of what men

earned.[20] Less than 2% of all working women earn more than $75,000 per year.[21] Many women are worried about the "sticky floor"—employment practices that keep full-time,

Table 15.3	Women's and Men's Median Weekly Earnings by Selected Characteristics, 2006

Characteristic Age	Women ($)	Men ($)
Total, 16 years or older	600	743
16 to 19	395	348
20 to 24	305	435
25 to 34	583	661
35 to 44	644	836
45 to 54	659	897
55 to 64	658	902
65 or older	510	658
Race/Ethnicity		
White	609	761
Black	519	591
Hispanic	440	505
Asian	699	882
Educational Attainment		
Less than a high school diploma	358	469
High school graduate, no college	500	678
Some college or associate degree	602	796
College graduate	905	1,205

Source: Bureau of Labor Statistics. (2007). *Highlights of Women's Earnings in 2006.* U.S. Department of Labor.

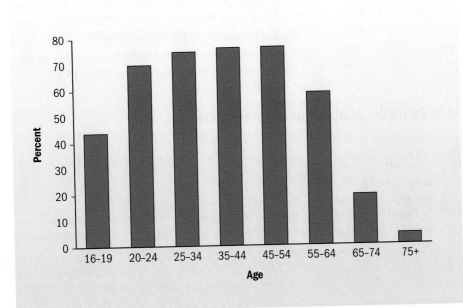

Figure 15.3

Percentage of women in the labor force.

Source: U.S. Deparment of Labor Statistics, 2008.

working women right at the poverty threshold level. One-fourth of women who work full time do not earn enough to move their families above the federal poverty threshold. At the other extreme, women continue to fight against the "glass ceiling" phenomenon—employment practices that effectively keep working women out of top-ranking positions. For example, according to a 2002 report, women held only 15% of corporate officer positions in the *Fortune* 500 companies, and there were only six women chief executive officers in all *Fortune* 500 firms. Changes are occurring, although the rate of change is slow.

Besides lower wages, a grim reality for working women is the lack of paid sick or family leave, childcare benefits, flexibility of schedule associated with employment, and employer-provided health insurance, pension plans, or retirement benefits. According to a survey conducted by the AFL-CIO:

- 54% of women reported no paid leave to care for a baby or an ill family member
- 74% say their employers do not offer childcare benefits
- 34% have no flexibility or control over their schedule[22]

In addition, two-thirds of the approximately 60 million women working outside of the home in the United States do not have pension plans; those who do receive half the benefits enjoyed by their male counterparts.[19]

Although gender discrepancies in income are often thought of as a woman's issue, it is clearly a family issue. With more women in the workforce, more families are depending on dual incomes. In the AFL-CIO's Ask a Working Woman Survey, almost two-thirds of working women and more than half of married women said that they provided half or more of their family's incomes.[23] In 1970, women maintained 5.6 million families in the United States, meaning that there was no other provider in the household; in 2004, women were the head of household with no

spouse present in 12.3% of households. Women maintained 14% of white families, 47% of black families, and 24% of Hispanic-origin families. Given the large number of women who are the sole providers for their families and work in low-paying jobs, it comes as no surprise that 28.3% of all families maintained by women were below the poverty level in 2007.[25]

Race/Ethnicity Issues

In general, women occupy proportionally more of the lower-paying jobs than men do, and they receive fewer benefits and less flexibility in their working conditions than men do. Minorities—and especially minority women—are even more likely to be in these less desirable positions. While white workers of either gender earned more than their black and Hispanic counterparts, for white women age 16 or over average weekly earnings ($626) were 17% higher than black women's ($533) and 32% higher than those of Hispanic women ($473).[4]

In 1999, women were one-third more likely than men to be among the working poor, and African American and Hispanic women were two to three times more likely than white women to be members of the working poor group.[24] Less than 2% of white women, 1% of African American women, and 1% of Hispanic women earn more than $75,000 per year; meanwhile, 70% of white women, 73% of African American women, and 82% of Hispanic women earn less than $25,000 per year.[21]

Achieving Equal Pay

One key factor for women who are seeking to help themselves is education. Completing high school is the first step in increasing one's potential income. The median income for women increased by 35% for those with a high school degree, another 8.6% for those with an associate's degree, and 24.5% for a bachelor's degree (see **Table 15.4**).

Table 15.4 Women's Income by Educational Attainment Level, 2004

Elementary/Secondary			College					
Less than 9th Grade	9th to 12 Grade, No Completion	High School, Completion (includes equivalency)	Some College, No Degree	Associate's Degree	Bachelors's Degree	Master's Degree	Professional	Doctorate
$17,023	$19,162	$26,029	$30,816	$33,481	$41,681	$51,316	$75,036	$68,875
	+12.56%	+35.83%	+18.39%	+8.6%	+24.49%	+23.11%	+46.22%	+34.21% (from master's)

Source: Center for Labor Statistics, 2007.

To achieve fair compensation for their work, women should learn what fair and equitable pay is for their position and experience, be aware of the laws that prohibit pay discrimination against women, and support efforts to bring "pay equity" to their workplaces. Employees should encourage their employers to implement a pay equity policy, along with a way of creating a grading system to categorize jobs based on education, skills, and experience. Pay rates should be adjusted so that jobs of equal value are paid equally.

Balancing Work and Family Life

Thirty-four percent of women say that the biggest problem facing women today is combining family and work.[25] Women continually juggle many tasks in an effort to perform well at work, run a household, provide a loving home for their children, spend quality time with their partners, and provide care for their elders. Women who have multiple roles, as mother and provider for example, have a lower incidence of depression and other mental health problems than women who have only one role; however, in many cases, having multiple roles can contribute to strain and stress.

One in five working parents is a member of the "sandwich generation," meaning that the individual is caring for both children and elderly relatives. More than one-third of those with elder responsibilities—men and women alike—reduced their work hours or took time off to provide the necessary care.[13] Fifty-four percent of Americans say they will probably be responsible for the care of an elderly parent or other relative in the next 10 years. Women account for 70% of the unpaid people caring for the elderly; they also constitute the majority of paid workers, including nurses, nurse's aides, and home health-care workers.[25]

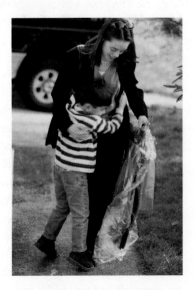

■ Many women who have entered the workforce continue to work on household chores and child care when they return home from work.

Child Care

Childcare facilities, relatives, and nannies have become a necessity for working families with children. More than three-fourths of preschool-age children with employed mothers are regularly cared for by someone other than their parents. In 2005, 61% of children from birth to age 6 spent some time in non-parental child care.[30] A babysitter or nanny regularly cares for 6% of children in the child's home. Families with children between the ages of three and five say that child care is their third greatest expense after housing and food.[25] The cost of full-day child care can range from $4,500 to $20,000 per year per child. In addition to the high costs, 9 out of 10 Americans describe finding quality child care as "difficult."[25,30] Only 12 states require childcare providers to have any early childhood training prior to minding children in their homes.[31]

Child care does not always ease the stress for working women. In fact, 52% of women say that childcare problems affect their ability to perform well at work.[25] Eighty percent of employers reported that childcare problems force employees to lose work time. In addition, only 9% of sampled workers with children in daycare facilities report feeling "very successful" in balancing work and family.[32]

The Current Situation

Working Mother magazine rates the 100 best companies for working mothers every year, based on various measures of flexibility within the workplace, such as flextime, telecommuting, and job sharing. Companies also are rated on their propensity to listen to employees by surveying them on work–life topics and, in response to the survey results, adding features such as lactation rooms. The top-rated companies do not just offer policies, but market them as well.[33] *Ms.* magazine has reported, however, that some of these companies officially offer flextime to employees but do not necessarily practice what they preach. In many organizations, workers in low-wage jobs are half as likely as managers and professionals to have flextime; low-wage workers are also more likely to lose a day's pay when they must stay home to care for a sick child.[34]

Within many companies, only 20% of employees have access to childcare information and referral services; 25% are provided with access to eldercare information and referral services. Only 12% of employees with children younger than age six have childcare services on or near their work site that are operated or sponsored by their employers, and these facilities are usually located at headquarters where managers and executives work.[14] Even those lower-paid employees who have access to referrals or

Gender Dimensions

MOTHERHOOD

Motherhood is often a woman's principal source of stress; she may enjoy this role and be committed to it, but nevertheless may feel strained by it. Her stress may be exacerbated by society's normative expectation of "good mothering," which does not usually encompass full-time employment.[26,27] Although being in the workforce increases a woman's opportunities for obtaining resources, power, social identity, positive self-esteem, and involvement with others, involvement in paid employment may also be a source of stress. The benefits of work depend on the woman's working conditions, her marital status, her stability in her job, and her ability to handle many roles at once. The more demanding and difficult the job and the less supportive the workplace, the greater the negative spillover from one's work life to one's personal life.

Working mothers often feel the stresses of work significantly more than working fathers do. Mothers, for example, often must juggle the multiple responsibilities of maintaining high job performance and being the primary caregiver for children. Single mothers frequently carry this double burden, resulting in them being even more stressed than married working women. Although men are performing more household responsibilities than they did 20 years ago, women continue to spend more time than men doing housework on top of increasing their workloads outside the home. This trend has led to an increase in the work-family life conflict experienced by these parents.

One study showed that women spend 30.8 hours per week doing paid work and 25.6 hours on family care. By comparison, men spend 39.7 hours per week doing paid labor and 14.3 hours on family care or housework.[28] Housework and family care tend to be more unbalancing to a person's sense of well-being because the tasks are thought to be more repetitive, dirtier, menial, unending, and relatively inflexible. Even when men do housework, it is often work that can be scheduled, such as lawn maintenance or repairs. In contrast, women are often responsible for cleaning, cooking, and caring for children—duties that cannot be postponed.[26] Married men are more likely to have partners who are willing to take care of tasks at home, making men's lives more balanced. On the other hand, men in general do not adjust their time in response to their wives' employment status.[29]

Besides doing more housework, mothers spend more time on average with their children than fathers do. Mothers spend an average of 3.2 hours per workday with their children, whereas fathers spend an average of 2.3 hours with their offspring. Seventy percent of parents feel that they do not have enough time to spend with their children. In fact, both parents have less time for themselves than they did 20 years ago; fathers have 1.2 hours during the workday, whereas mothers have 0.9 hour.[13] Couples also have less time together. Nearly 46% of married women or women living with someone work different schedules than their partners do.[22]

---

nearby childcare facilities usually find the fees too high for their earnings. Many of the company-operated daycare centers are open only during regular business hours, such as 8 A.M. to 6 P.M.; however, close to one-third of employees with young children have unpredictable or erratic work schedules, and these are the employees who are most likely to earn less than $25,000 per year.[14,22]

The Future

Many women suffer from job- and family-related stress, but do not feel they have any options that would relieve that stress. Some women aspire to the "superwoman" ideal—for example, being a high-powered executive while keeping a clean house, preparing home-cooked meals, spending quality time with her children, and being a loving and supportive wife. Women need to find their individual balance of work and family responsibilities and make changes if they are dissatisfied with their situation. For women with partners, open communication about the sharing of responsibilities can help couples to establish a good balance within their home. In situations where both partners work, sharing of chores is essential to minimize stress and maximize quality family time.

For single women, it is important to find balance between work and home responsibilities, too. This may mean reviewing policies at work that allow for job sharing or flextime, or advocating for these options if they are not provided by one's employer. Women without these options need the power and support of other women, employers, and politicians to fight for them. Women who own businesses should set examples for pay equity, fair workplaces, supportive work environments, and family-friendly policies.

Health and Safety in the Workplace

Women's work-related stress has been linked to factors such as lack of supportive workplace policies, unfair pay, concerns for quality child care, inflexible scheduling, and lack of support and help at home. In times of economic upheaval, concerns over downsizing and layoffs create added pressures. Other stressors revolve around lack of control at work, such as high workload demands, unreasonable deadlines, role ambiguity and conflict, repetitive and boring work, and strained relationships with co-workers or supervisors.[35] The stress from this type of work often produces little job satisfaction and a poor sense of well-being. The following jobs are associated with high stress because of the need to respond to others' demands and timetables with little control over events:

- Secretaries
- Waitresses
- Middle managers
- Police officers
- Editors
- Medical interns[36]

Long-term exposure to job stress can lead to higher levels of depression, anxiety, and other mental illnesses. In one survey, 60% of employed women cited stress as their number one problem at work.[36] As jobs become more demanding and less rewarding, employees often feel more stressed by the end of the workday and have less time and energy for their families. Twenty-five percent of employees reported feeling stressed often or very often over the past three months, and 25% described feeling emotionally drained often or very often. More than one-fourth of employees are not in as good a mood as they would like for their families; 28% of people feel they have no energy for their families or other important people upon returning from work. This in turn creates a negative sense of well-being and results in negativity that affects a person's performance at work.[36]

A person's work setting can create physical stress as well, because of noise, lack of privacy, poor lighting or ventilation, poor temperature control, or inadequate sanitary facilities. Physical stress on the body is a consequence of many different occupations. Jobs that require being on one's feet for long hours can result in leg pain, swelling, and varicose veins; secretarial and computer-related jobs are often accompanied by neck and back aches and eye strain; and women on production lines suffer from musculoskeletal injuries resulting from repetitive motions. These types of difficulties are not restricted to gender, yet certain factors make women more susceptible to this type of injury. Typical designs of equipment and workstations accommodate the larger-on-average size of males as compared with females. For example, higher workstations and chairs that cannot be adjusted to the correct height for women promote poor posture, excessive reach, and strain on the neck, back, shoulders, and arms. Hand tools designed for larger hands may create unnecessary pain, stressed muscles, and calluses. Protective equipment and clothing that are too large have a greater likelihood of slipping off, getting caught in equipment, or creating gaps for harmful agents to seep through, thereby compromising a woman's safety.

Musculoskeletal injuries, also referred to as ergonomic injuries, disproportionately affect female workers. Although women account for only 33% of the people injured at work in the United States, they constitute 64% of repetitive motion injuries, which include the following conditions:

- **Carpal tunnel syndrome**—a condition that occurs when tendons in the wrist become inflamed after being aggravated
- **Tendonitis**—inflammation caused by friction from overuse of tendons
- Muscle strains from overexertion

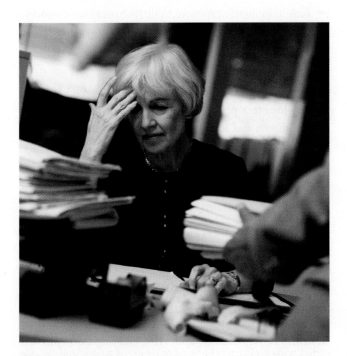

■ Long-term exposure to work-related stress can lead to higher levels of depression, anxiety, and other illnesses.

It's Your Health

Tips for Lifting Loads Safely

- Test the weight of the load before lifting. If too heavy or awkward, enlist a co-worker to help or use a cart or dolly.
- Figure out where you need to move the load and how you are going to get to your destination before you lift.
- Lift with your legs shoulder-width apart and bend at your knees and hips, not your waist.
- Lift with tightened stomach muscles and using your leg muscles to reduce strain on your back.
- Hold the load close to your body at waist height.
- Avoid twisting during the lift; pivot your body or move your feet if necessary.
- Stretch and strengthen your back and stomach with exercises if lifting is part of your daily occupation.

Self-Assessment 15.1

Symptoms of Repetitive Strain Injuries

- Do you have numbness and/or tingling in your hand that often feels worse when you lift your hand over your head?
- Do you often experience wrist weakness?
- Do you have numbness or tingling in the inside of your arm or into your fingers?
- Do you often feel numbness or tingling in multiple fingers and does your hand often "fall asleep" at night? Do you frequently drop objects?
- Do you have achiness, stiffness, tightness, or a burning sensation in your fingers, forearm, elbow, or shoulder?
- Do you experience muscle tightness at the side of your neck?

If you are experiencing one or more of these symptoms, you may have an overuse injury. Women should speak to their health-care provider about preventing, reducing, and/or treating these types of disorders.

It's Your Health

Tips for Preventing Injuries at Computer Workstations

- Reduce repetitive motions by alternating tasks throughout the day.
- Take frequent breaks, and stretch during the breaks if possible.
- Avoid bending or twisting your neck, or twisting your trunk.
- Keep shoulders relaxed and arms close by sides when working.
- Maintain good posture by keeping back and neck erect with shoulders relaxed.
- Keep your feet supported on the floor or on a footrest to reduce pressure on the lower back.
- Position your computer monitor so that it is centered directly in front of you and your neck is in a neutral or straight position when viewing it.
- Reduce glare on your screen by tilting the monitor, reducing overhead lights, and avoiding direct glare from windows.
- Rest your eyes every 30 minutes by looking away from the screen and focusing on various objects around the room or outside.

Repetitive motions can result in compressed nerves, often in the nerves from the neck to the hand. **Self-Assessment 15.1** discusses some of the common symptoms that nerve injuries can cause. Repetitive motion injuries account for more than half of all work time lost due to injuries and illness among women (**Table 15.5**).[38,39]

Women in lower-wage occupations and occupations employing large numbers of women are at significant risk of musculoskeletal disorders. Examples of these occupations include nursing aides, cashiers, maids, nurses, and assemblers. Many of these jobs employ a large number of minorities, such as Hispanic, Southeast Asian, and African American women. Back injuries are common among employees who need to lift large items or even people. Safe lifting can be accomplished with the correct lifting technique and awareness regarding the amount of weight being lifted.

Computer-related injuries have also become a significant concern in the workplace (**Self-Assessment 15.2**). Prolonged use of a computer keyboard or mouse, as well as sitting at a computer working intensively without stretching, can lead to frequent muscle aches and nerve pain in the hands, arms, shoulders, neck, and back. Another common complaint of computer workers is visual discomfort, which is accompanied by eyestrain and headaches. Being aware of these risks and correcting improper posture and techniques can help prevent discomfort and injury.

Almost two-thirds of injured workers were men in 2005, well above their 59% share of work time, according to NCLS. Women accounted for more injuries and illness than men in management, business, financial occupations, professional and related occupations, service occupations, and office and administrative support occupations (**Figure 15.4**).

Exposure to certain chemical, biological, and physical toxins, many of which are suspected carcinogens, allergens, or agents that cause respiratory illness, are also serious concerns for many working women. Occupational exposures occur in many industries that employ large numbers of women and minorities:[37]

- Meat industry: exposure to suspected carcinogenic fumes
- Laundry/dry-cleaning industry: exposure to carcinogenic solvents that increase risk of kidney, cervical, bladder, skin, and liver cancer
- Textile industry: exposure to dust that causes a variety of lung diseases
- Metal-working industry: exposure to various carcinogens that increase the risk of lung cancer
- Agriculture: exposure to pesticides and herbicides that may lead to a possible increased risk of non-Hodgkin's lymphoma and lung cancer
- Health-care industry: exposure to numerous toxic and allergenic substances, infectious diseases, and radiation
- Service industry: exposure to excessive cigarette smoke in bars or restaurants

Health-care workers face additional hazards, including needlestick injuries and latex allergies. Approximately 600,000 to 800,000 needlestick injuries occur annually in health-care settings, mostly involving nurses (more than 90% of whom are women). Needlestick injuries can cause serious infections from bloodborne pathogens, such as hepatitis B, hepatitis C, and HIV, creating both physical and emotional threats to workers. In addition, 8% to 12% of health-care workers who have frequent latex exposure

Table 15.5 Ergonomic Injuries Among Women

Description of Injury	Number of Lost-Worktime Injuries to Women	Percentage of All Workers Injured
Carpal tunnel syndrome	18,740	68%
Tendonitis	8,965	62%
Injured due to repetitive motion	43,671	64%
Due to repetitive typing or keyboard entry	10,890	89%
Due to repetitive placing/grasping	14,223	64%
Due to repetitive use of tools	4,682	46%

Source: Bureau of Labor Statistics. (2000). *Lost-Worktime Injuries and Illnesses, 2000.*

Self-Assessment 15.2

Computer Workstation Evaluation Checklist

Posture

- Are your hands, wrists, and forearms straight, in-line, and roughly parallel to the floor?
- Is your head level or bent slightly forward and balanced?
- Is your head in line with your torso?
- Are your elbows close to your body and bent at 90 to 120 degrees?
- Are your feet fully supported by the floor or a footrest?
- Is your back fully supported when sitting vertical or leaning back slightly?
- Are your shoulders relaxed?
- Thighs and hips should be supported by a well-padded chair.
- Knees should be at the same height as the hips with the feet slightly forward.

Keyboard/Mouse

- Is your keyboard directly in front of you at a distance that allows your elbows to stay close to your body with your forearms approximately parallel with the floor?
- If you have limited desk room, do you use a keyboard tray to ensure adequate positioning?
- Is your keyboard in a position that lets you avoid reaching with the arms, leaning forward with the torso, and using extreme elbow angles?
- Can you reduce awkward wrist angles by lowering or raising the keyboard or chair to achieve a neutral wrist posture?

Seating

- Does your backrest support your lower back (lumbar area)?
- Does your seat width and depth accommodate your body? Is the seat pan not too long?
- Does the seat front not press against the back of your knees and lower legs?
- Is the seat cushioning rounded with a waterfall front devoid of sharp edges?
- If there are armrests, do they support both forearms while you complete computer tasks?

Lighting

- Does your office have well-distributed diffuse lights that reduce glare on the computer screen?
- Does your office use light, matte colors and finishes on walls and ceilings to better reflect indirect lighting and reduce dark shadows and contrast?

Computer Screen

- Is your computer display screen at right angles to windows and light sources?
- Is the monitor clean and free of dust?
- Is the top of the screen at or below eye level?

Work Techniques

- Are your computer tasks organized in such a way that allows you to vary tasks with other work activities or take micro-breaks and recovery pauses?

If you answered "No" to one or more of these questions, you are putting yourself at risk of injury. Use the checklist guidelines to improve your workplace health and avoid injuries.

Source: Adapted from the U.S. Department of Labor's Office of Safety and Health Administration's eTool, Computer Workstation Evaluation. (http://www.osha.gov/SLTC/etools/computerworkstations/checklist.html)

Figure 15.4

Injuries and illnesses and hours worked, by gender of worker, 2005.

Source: U.S. Bureau of Labor Statistics. U.S. Department of Labor, November, 2005.

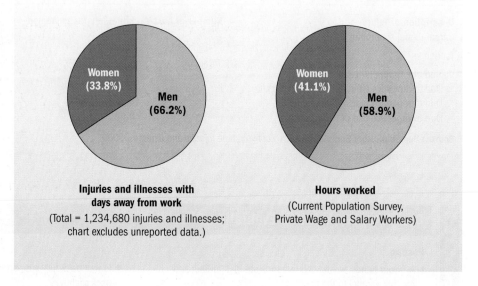

Injuries and illnesses with days away from work
(Total = 1,234,680 injuries and illnesses; chart excludes unreported data.)

Hours worked
(Current Population Survey, Private Wage and Salary Workers)

develop sensitivity to this material. Symptoms can be as mild as contact dermatitis or as severe as **anaphylactic shock** (a severe and possibly fatal allergic response to a foreign substance, characterized by difficulty breathing and low blood pressure). The hazard from latex use is recognized in many different industries, including people in the latex-manufacturing industry, police, food handlers, and sanitation engineers.[39] Pregnant women also appear to have a higher sensitivity to latex than does the general population.[40]

The causes of most reproductive health problems are still unknown, but certain harmful substances can affect the health of pregnant women. Approximately 75% of all women of reproductive age are in the workforce, and more than half of all children born in the United States are born to working mothers. Women can be exposed to many different types of health hazards at work during pregnancy. Hazards from environmental pollutants in the workplace can cause multiple effects, depending on when the woman is exposed (see **Tables 15.6 and 15.7**). Substances may cause fetal damage, such as birth defects, low birthweight, developmental disorders, miscarriages or stillbirths, infertility, menstrual cycle effects, and even childhood cancer. Other possible hazards to pregnant women include prolonged standing, lifting, and long work hours.[41]

Other Health Concerns

Many women work in the informal work sector, employed in jobs that are seasonal (like agriculture) or domestic (like housecleaning). Because many of these jobs employ women who may not have official work permits or are "paid under the table" (meaning that the women do not receive benefits or declare taxes), significant additional risks are associated with them. Injuries that occur during migrant crop picking, for example, often go untreated because the workers have few resources and are afraid of drawing the attention of authorities. Additionally, women who do odd jobs around the home, such as cleaning houses or painting, often do not have health coverage or disability coverage should an injury occur.

Hazardous work environments put many youths at risk of serious injuries (**Figure 15.5**). Young workers have been killed on construction sites, during robberies while tending retail establishments, and while working on farms. Common nonfatal injuries incurred by young workers include

■ Health-care workers face unique workplace hazards.

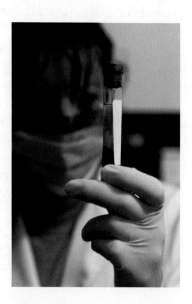

Table 15.6 Chemical and Physical Agents That Are Reproductive Hazards for Women in the Workplace

Agent	Observed Effects	Potentially Exposed Workers
Cancer treatment drugs (e.g., methotrexate)	Infertility, miscarriage, birth defects, low birthweight	Health-care workers, pharmacists
Certain ethylene glycol ethers	Miscarriage	Electronics and semiconductor workers
Carbon disulfide	Menstrual cycle changes	Viscose rayon workers
Lead	Infertility, miscarriage, low birthweight, developmental disorders	Battery makers, solderers, welders, radiator repairers, bridge repainters, firing range workers, home remodelers
Ionizing radiation (e.g., X rays and gamma rays)	Infertility, miscarriage, birth defects, low birthweight, developmental disorders, childhood cancers	Health-care workers, dental personnel, atomic workers
Strenuous physical labor (e.g., prolonged standing, heavy lifting)	Miscarriage late in pregnancy, premature delivery	Many types of workers

Source: National Institute for Occupational Safety and Health. (1999). *The Effects of Workplace Hazards on Female Reproductive Health.* Department of Health and Human Services: Publication No. 99–104.

Table 15.7 Disease-Causing Agents That Are Reproductive Hazards for Women in the Workplace

Agent	Observed Effects	Potentially Exposed Workers	Preventive Measures
Cytomegalovirus (CMV)	Birth defects, low birthweight, developmental disorders	Health-care workers, workers in contact with infants and children	Good hygienic practices such as handwashing
Hepatitis B virus	Low birthweight	Health-care workers	Vaccination
Human immunodeficiency virus (HIV)	Low birthweight, childhood cancer	Health-care workers	Practice universal precautions
Human parvovirus B19	Miscarriage	Health-care workers, workers in contact with infants and children	Good hygienic practices such as handwashing
Rubella (German measles)	Birth defects, low birthweight	Health-care workers, workers in contact with infants and children	Vaccination before pregnancy if no prior immunity
Toxoplasmosis	Miscarriage, birth defects, developmental disorders	Animal care workers, veterinarians	Good hygienic practices such as handwashing
Varicella-zoster virus (chickenpox)	Birth defects, low birthweight	Health-care workers, workers in contact with infants and children	Vaccination before pregnancy if no prior immunity

Source: National Institute for Occupational Safety and Health. (1999). *The Effects of Workplace Hazards on Female Reproductive Health.* Department of Health and Human Services: Publication No. 99–104.

sprains and strains, burns, cuts, and bruises. Homicide was the leading cause of death among youths in retail trade, accounting for nearly two-thirds of the youth fatalities in the industry. Most of these homicides were the result of robberies.[42]

Pregnant and lactating women may face additional stresses as they cope with sickness caused during preg-

I'm trying to get a permanent position in the United States as a research scientist so I don't have to go back to Russia. My boss makes me work long hours and always yells at me if I make a mistake. I was pregnant last year, and he still made me work with radiation in the lab. I was scared to complain for fear of losing my job. I didn't lose my job, but I ended up losing my baby.

32-year-old Russian scientist

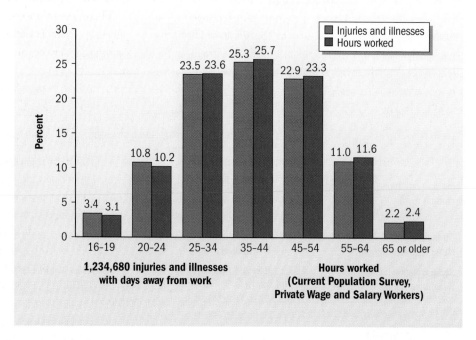

Figure 15.5

Injuries and illnesses and hours worked, by gender of worker, 2005.

Source: U.S. Bureau of Labor Statistics. U.S. Department of Labor, November, 2005.

(Legend: Injuries and illnesses; Hours worked)

16-19: 3.4, 3.1; 20-24: 10.8, 10.2; 25-34: 23.5, 23.6; 35-44: 25.3, 25.7; 45-54: 22.9, 23.3; 55-64: 11.0, 11.6; 65 or older: 2.2, 2.4

1,234,680 injuries and illnesses with days away from work

Hours worked (Current Population Survey, Private Wage and Salary Workers)

nancy, co-workers' responses to pregnancy, and the time and privacy needs of nursing or pumping breast milk. Sexual harassment in the workplace is also a major form of stress (see Chapter 14).

Global Dimensions

Around the globe, women are becoming more active in the workforce. Approximately 70% of women in developed countries and 60% of women in developing countries are engaged in paid employment. Worldwide, more women are participating in and completing their education, resulting in better job opportunities and consequently better status in their families and society. Although much progress has been made, however, millions of women remain unprotected by labor laws and poorly compensated for their work. They are not treated as equals and often experience discrimination and significant pay differences.

The proportion of informal work done by women has increased dramatically over the last decade. In some countries of sub-Saharan Africa, for example, nearly 90% of the female labor force is in the informal economy. This informal—and often invisible—work accounts for a significant amount of output, including the production of handmade goods, services such as laundry and sewing, and vast amounts of child care. In developing countries, a great effort has been made to quantify the amount of informal

work women do. By recognizing the role of the informal workforce, of which women represent the majority, the groups are helping to legitimize the work they do and help women gain access to key financial resources that could assist them in getting ahead. Examples of such efforts include micro-lending programs, where women are loaned small sums of money to further their businesses without the need for collateral and with reasonably low interest

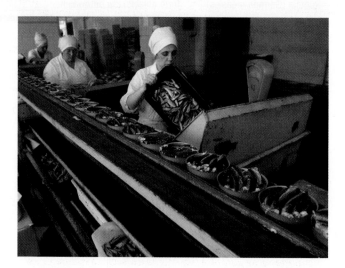

■ Women are becoming increasingly more active in workplaces across the globe.

rates. The rate of payback from these women-focused micro-lending programs has been higher than that observed with any other formal credit program that has been measured. Once women gain access to these loans, they have the ability to create sustainable and profitable business opportunities for themselves and their families. By having greater access to capital, women can better protect themselves from the significant workplace health hazards that present themselves in many formal and informal work environments. In addition, the money that women make from their work enterprises is overwhelmingly reinvested into the health and well-being of their families.

In terms of work and families, government policies around the world vary. It is interesting that the United States—one of the richest countries in the world—does not guarantee women any paid family leave, unlike many other countries. Worldwide, 128 countries mandate some sort of paid family leave. For example,

- In Germany, a new mother receives 14 weeks of leave at full pay.
- In Italy, a new mother receives 20 weeks of leave at full pay.
- In Canada, new mothers have the right to take a full year off from work at 60% pay.
- In Norway, new mothers can take one year off from work at 80% pay.

Informed Decision Making

Working women, with and without children, experience significant stress that affects their health, relationships, work productivity, and young children. Supportive companies produce workers who are less stressed, feel more successful in the balancing of work and family, are more satisfied with both their work and home lives, and are more loyal and committed to their employers.[25]

There are solutions. First, employers should help employees prepare to better balance parenthood and work life by offering services related to family planning, preconception health care and counseling, and parenting classes. Second, the Family and Medical Leave Act (FMLA) could be expanded to help families in crisis. The FMLA of 1993 provides 12 weeks of unpaid, job-guaranteed leave for employees who need to care for newborns or a seriously ill relative, or to recover from a serious illness of their own. This benefit is available to employees who have worked at least 1,250 hours over the past year for employers with 50 or more employees. Currently, the act covers only 57% of the country's private workforce.[34] Workers in entry-level, low-paying jobs are less likely to be offered a paid maternity leave than are managers and are less likely to get the time off after having a baby. Although the FMLA was originally envisioned as dealing with a women's issue, 42% of those who have requested family and medical leave since its passage are men.

Employers can also ease new mothers' return to the workplace by providing breastfeeding support through lactation assistance programs and private breastfeeding rooms. Only 10% of working mothers continue nursing for six months following birth, compared with 24% of at-home mothers. Thirty-seven percent of employers currently provide opportunities for women who are nursing to continue to do so; this provision cuts down on absenteeism and health-care costs for both mothers and infants.[14]

In addition, employers need to help employees find affordable quality child care and elder care, develop childcare programs, or offer employee assistance for childcare facilities. Childcare assistance programs need to include more flexibility, by allowing for the needs of employees who work night and weekend shifts (**Figure 15.6**). Flexible work schedules, job-sharing programs, and prorated benefits for part-time and temporary employees also need to be enforced—two-thirds of part-time workers and three-fifths of temporary workers are women.[19] Many employers have established flexible work policies and are promoting the idea of a family-friendly workplace. Unfortunately, the people who need the extra support are the people who are often the least likely to receive it.

Women also need to be aware of their rights in the workplace. Discrimination should not be tolerated, and actions can be taken if a woman suspects she is being treated unfairly because of her gender, race, age, religion, pregnancy, sexual orientation, or disabilities.

I just had my second child, and I have six months off to care for him. My two-year-old goes to day care at my firm's on-site child-care center. When I return to work, I'll work part time so I get to spend time with my children. The women of my firm have said that there's no problem with taking advantage of flextime and taking off six months to care for my newborn. I hope they're right! I feel very fortunate to be part of a firm that takes such good care of its employees.

30-year-old lawyer

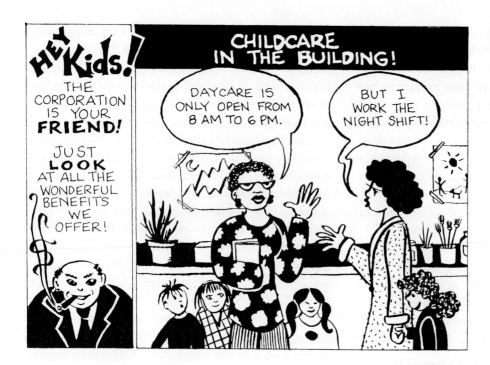

Figure 15.6

Childcare programs need to be developed with more flexibility to allow for night and weekend shifts.

Source: © Jennifer Camper.

Profiles of Remarkable Women

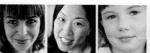

Patricia Ireland (1945–)

Patricia Ireland began her career by working as a flight attendant for Pan American World Airlines from 1967 to 1975. Upon being told that her medical benefits didn't apply to her husband even though wives of male employees were covered, Ireland sued her employer and won—a victory that marked the beginning of her activism. Ireland received her law degree from the University of Miami Law School in 1975, then worked as a partner in a major Miami law firm. She served as legal counsel to Dade County and Florida National Organization for Women (NOW) for seven years. From 1987 to 1991, Ireland served as executive vice president and treasurer of the national NOW organization.

In 1991, Ireland became president of NOW, the largest, most visible, and most successful feminist organization in the United States. Her major contributions included organizing NOW activists to defend women's access to abortion, elect a record number of women to political office, work more closely in coalitions with other social justice and civil rights groups, and champion international feminist issues.

Ireland developed NOW's Project Stand Up for Women; in 1992, she led NOW in organizing a crowd of 750,000 for the organization's March for Women's Lives. In the same year, she initiated the "Elect Women for a Change" campaign. This campaign provided feminist candidates with experienced organizers who trained and deployed volunteers to staff phone banks, distribute leaflets and posters, organize fundraisers, and get people to the polls.

As part of NOW's work with the Up and Out of Poverty Now! coalition, Ireland delivered testimony and organized lobby days, news briefings, and protests on behalf of poor women. She served on the board of the Rainbow/PUSH Coalition and, in 1993, was a co-convener and keynote speaker for the thirtieth anniversary march on Washington commemorating the legacy of Dr. Martin Luther King, Jr. She has put forth significant efforts on behalf of lesbian and gay rights, including serving as a speaker and major organizer for the 1993 March on Washington for Gay, Lesbian, and Bi Civil Rights.

Ireland was the prime architect of NOW's Global Feminist Program. In 1992, she brought together women from more than 45 countries to participate in the Global Feminist Conference. Although no longer president of NOW, Ireland continues to champion many international feminist issues.

■■■■
Summary

The workplace has emerged as the modern-day "community" for many people. It provides a social life, a support system, and opportunities for volunteering, and it affects people's moods and their values.

- Women are participating in all jobs and careers today, but inequities in pay and advancement persist.
- Women still shoulder the majority of the burden of children and home life, even when working.
- Women benefit greatly from quality, affordable, and accessible child care, enabling them to have choices about labor force participation.
- The stress of work and family, and the attempt to "do it all," is not an insignificant women's health issue.

Employers must continue to make an effort to create a more supportive and rewarding work environment. By promoting a healthy work–life balance, employers benefit, as do employees. At the same time, women should strive to find such a balance in their lives, by setting priorities, discussing options with their employers and partners, and advocating for fairness and support in the workplace.

As both genders become accustomed to a more equitable sharing of responsibilities inside and outside the home, women will be afforded a more balanced existence between work and family. As Arlie Hochschild so aptly states, "Up until now, the woman married to the 'new man' has been one of the lucky few. But as the government and society shape a new gender strategy, as the young learn from example, many more women and men will be able to enjoy the leisurely bodily rhythms and freer laughter that arise when family life is family life and not a second shift."[43]

■■■■
Topics for Discussion

1. What questions should a woman ask before taking a job to ensure that she will receive all of the benefits that she may need?

2. Discuss how the cycle of poverty creates additional barriers to employment opportunities for women.

3. What strategies could women use in the workplace to determine whether chemical, biological, or physical hazards are present?

Profiles of Remarkable Women

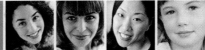

Angela Braly (1962–)

At the age of 46, Ms. Braly has become what some people refer to as "the most powerful woman in health care." Ms. Braly runs WellPoint—the 42,000-employee health insurance company that runs Blue Cross and Blue Shield plans in 14 states. WellPoint's annual sales of $56 billion are more than PepsiCo, Kraft, or Xerox. Ms. Braly assumed her responsibilities in June 2007, after serving as executive vice president, general counsel, and chief public affairs officer for WellPoint. In her previous role, she was responsible for public-policy development, government relations, legal affairs, corporate communications, marketing, and social-responsibility initiatives. She managed the nation's largest Medicare claims-processing business and the federal employee health-benefits business.

Previously, Ms. Braly was president and CEO of Anthem Blue Cross and Blue Shield in Missouri. In 2007 Ms. Braly was named one of *Modern Healthcare* magazine's "Top 25 Women in Healthcare," was ranked #16 on *Forbes* magazine's "World's Most Powerful Women" list, and was ranked #4 by *Fortune* magazine on its list of the "50 Most Powerful Women." Also in 2007, the *Wall Street Journal* named her #1 on its list of "Women to Watch." She is the only woman to lead a *Fortune* 50 company.

Ms. Braly has managed to have a family as well as a successful career. She is married with three children. Her husband is a stay-at-home dad, helping to run the home and family while she works. According to news reports, Ms. Braly is a skilled and tough negotiator and coalition builder.

Ms. Braly is a lawyer by training, having received her juris doctor from Southern Methodist University School of Law and her undergraduate degree from Texas Tech University.

4. What are some strategies women can use to find balance in their professional, educational, and personal lives?

5. What are some strategies women can use when seeking greater equity opportunities in specific workplaces?

■■■■
Web Sites

American Federation of Labor—Congress of Industrial Organizations: http://www.aflcio.org

Business and Professional Women/USA: http://www.bpwusa.org

Institute for Women's Policy Research: http://www.iwpr.org

National Institute for Occupational Safety and Health—Women: http://www.cdc.gov/niosh/topics/women/

National Organization for Women: http://www.now.org

U.S. Department of Labor: http://www.dol.gov

U.S. Department of Labor—Bureau of Labor Statistics: http://www.bls.gov

■■■■
References

1. U.S. Bureau of the Census. (1976). *The Statistical History of the United States—From Colonial Times to the Present.* Washington, DC: U.S. Department of Commerce.

2. U.S. Department of Labor. (1989). *Handbook of Labor Statistics.* Bulletin 2340. Washington, DC: Bureau of Labor Statistics.

3. U.S. Department of Labor. (2008). *Employment and Earnings.* Washington, DC: Bureau of Labor Statistics.

4. U.S. Department of Labor. (2007). *Highlights of Women's Earnings in 2006.* Report 1000. Washington, DC: Bureau of Labor Statistics.

5. Mofford, J. H. (Summer 1996). Women in the workplace. *Women's History Magazine,* pp. 10–13.

6. Parcel, T. L. (1999). Work and family in the 21st century: it's about time. *Work and Occupations* 26(2): 264–274.

7. U.S. Department of Labor. (2007). *Employment Projections: 2006–16.* Washington, DC: Bureau of Labor Statistics.

8. Business and Professional Women's Foundation. (2007). *101 Facts on the Status of Working Women.* Washington, DC: Business and Professional Women's Foundation.

9. U.S. Department of Labor. (2007). *Women in the Labor Force: A Databook.* Washington, DC: Bureau of Labor Statistics.

10. Lowrey Y. (August 2006). *Women in Business, 2006: A Demographic Review of Women's Business Ownership.* Washington, DC: Office of Advocacy, U.S. Small Business Association.

11. Organization for Economic Cooperation and Development (OECD). (May 2008). *Mothers in the Workforce.* OECD Family Database.

12. U.S. Department of Labor. (2007). *Women in the Labor Force: A Databook.* Washington, DC: Bureau of Labor Statistics, p. 16.

13. Lee, M., & Mather, M. (June 2008). *U.S. Labor Force Trends.* Washington, DC: Population Reference Bureau.

14. Galinsky, E., Bond, J., & Sakai, K. (2008). *2008 National Study of Employers.* New York: Families and Work Institute.

15. Jans, L., & Stoddard, S. (1999). *Chartbook on Women and Disability in the United States.* An InfoUse Report. Washington, DC: U.S. National Institute on Disability and Rehabilitation Research, p. 18.

16. National Partnership for Women and Families. (2007). *Where Families Matter: State Progress Toward Valuing America's Families.* Washington, DC: National Partnership for Women and Families.

17. London, A., Scott, E., Edin, K., & Hunter, V. (2004). Welfare reform, work-family tradeoffs, and child well-being. *Family Relations* 53(2): 148–158.

18. Weichselbaumer, D., & Winter-Ebmer, R. (2005). A meta analyis of the international gender wage gap. *Journal of Economic Surveys* 19(3): 479–511.

19. Blau, F. D., & Kahn, L. M. (2007). The gender pay gap. *The Economists' Voice* 4(4): 5–6.

20. U.S. Department of Labor, Bureau of Labor Statistics. (2006). *Overview of BLS Statistics on Wages, Earnings, and Benefits.* Washington, DC: U.S. Deparment of Labor.

21. AFL-CIO. (1999). *It's High Time—Past Time—for Women of Color to Earn Equal Pay.* AFL-CIO Working Women's Department.

22. AFL-CIO. (2000). *Ask a Working Woman Survey.* AFL-CIO Working Women's Department.

23. AFL-CIO. (1997). *Ask a Working Woman Survey.* AFL-CIO Working Women's Department.

24. AFL-CIO. (2003). *Fact Sheet: Equal Pay for Women of Color.* AFL-CIO Working Women's Department.

25. DeNavas-Walt, C., Proctor, B. D., & Smith, J. C. (2008). *Income, Poverty, and Health Insurance Coverage in the United States: 2007.* U.S. Census Bureau, Current Population Reports, P60-235. Washington, DC: U.S. Government Printing Office.

26. Milkie, M. A., & Petola, P. (1999). Playing all the roles: gender and the work–family balancing act. *Journal of Marriage and the Family* 61: 476–490.

27. Pilar Matud, M. (2004). Gender differences in stress and coping styles. *Personality and Individual Differences* 37(7): 1401–1415

28. Robinson, J. P., & Godbey, G. (1997). *Time for Life.* University Park: Pennsylvania State University Press.

29. Erickson, R. J. (2005). Why emotion work matters: sex, gender, and the division of household labor. *Journal of Marriage and Family* 67(2): 337–351.

30. Federal Interagency Forum on Child and Family Statistics. (2006). *America's Children: Key National Indicators of Well-Being, 2006.* Washington, DC: U.S. Government Printing Office. Available at: http://childstats.gov/americaschildren/tables.asp.

31. Wiggans, S., & Bergmann, B. (2003). *America's Child Care Problem: The Way Out.* New York: Macmillan.

32. Hochschild, A. R. (1997). *The Time Bind.* New York: Holt.

33. Cartwright, C. (2007). 100 best companies for working mothers. *Working Mother.*

34. Holcomb, B. (2000). Friendly for whose family? *Ms.* X(3): 40–45.

35. Wyn, R., & Soliz, B. (2004). Women's health issues across the lifespan. In *Health Policy: Crisis and Reform in the U.S. Health Care Delivery System.* Charlene Harrington, Carroll L. Estes, & Cassandra Crawford (Eds.), Sudbury, MA: Jones & Bartlett Publishers, pp. 148–159.

36. Judge, T. A., Jackson, C. L., Shaw, J. C., Scott, B. A., & Rich, B. L. (2007). Self-efficacy and work-related performance: the integral role of individual differences. *Journal of Applied Psychology* 92(1): 107–127

37. Centers for Disease Control and Prevention. (2001). *Women's Safety and Health Issues at Work.* National Institute of Occupational Safety and Health.

38. U.S. Department of Labor. (2006). *Lost-Worktime Injuries and Illnesses.* Washington, DC: Bureau of Labor Statistics.

39. AFL-CIO. (2003). *Women Workers Need OSHA's Ergonomic Standards.* Department of Occupational Safety and Health.

40. Cheng, L., & Lee, D. (1999). Review of latex allergy. *Journal of the American Board of Family Practitioners* 12(4): 285–292.

41. National Institute for Occupational Safety and Health. (1999). *The Effects of Workplace Hazards on Female Reproductive Health.* Department of Health and Human Services: Publication No. 99-104.

42. U.S. Department of Labor Statistics, U.S. Department of Labor. (2006). *Non-Fatal Workplace Injuries by Age and Hours Worked.* Available at: http://www.bls.gov/iif/oshwc/osh/os/osh05_24.pdf.

43. Hochshild, A. (1989). *The Second Shift.* New York: Avon Books.

GLOSSARY

A

Abortion   The spontaneous or induced expulsion of an embryo or fetus before it is viable or can survive on its own.

Abruptio placentae   A complication of pregnancy in which the placenta separates prematurely from the wall of the uterus.

Abstinence   In terms of sex, the practice of refraining from sexual activity.

Acquired immune deficiency syndrome (AIDS)   A progressive disease caused by HIV, which gradually destroys an infected person's immune system. AIDS is the final stage of HIV infection. Although there is no way for an infected person to get rid of HIV, modern medications can often slow the progress of the disease, or prevent AIDS from developing entirely.

Acute disease   A disease that begins and ends quickly. Examples include pneumonia and localized infection.

Adenocarcinoma   A cancer that originates from cells of the endocrine glands.

Adenomyosis   A benign condition caused by the development of tumors on the walls of the uterus, which can bleed and cause pain during menstruation.

Adjuvant therapy   Methods such as chemotherapy and radiation therapy that enhance the effectiveness of surgery in cancer treatment.

Aerobic bacteria   Bacteria that are oxygen dependent.

Aerobic exercise   Any physical activity in which the amount of oxygen taken into the body is slightly more than or equal to the amount of oxygen used by the body.

Afterbirth   The placenta and amniotic sac that are expelled from the womb after a baby is delivered.

Alcohol   A colorless liquid obtained by fermentation of a sugar-containing liquid. Ethyl alcohol (ethanol) is the type of alcohol found in alcoholic beverages.

Alcoholic   A person whose experiences interfere with normal life activities due to regular and continuous drinking of alcohol.

Alcoholism   Traditionally, the disease of an alcoholic, who is a person whose consumption of alcohol interferes with a major aspect of his or her life. Alcoholism has since been redefined as a primary, chronic disease with genetic, psychological, and environmental factors influencing its development and manifestations.

Allopathic school   A school that teaches a system of medical practice making use of all measures proved of value in treatment of disease (i.e., conventional medicine exclusive of homeopathic practices).

Alzheimer's disease   An irreversible, progressive brain disorder that occurs gradually and results in memory loss, behavior and personality changes, and a decline in cognitive abilities.

Amenorrhea   Absence of the menstrual period in a woman by age 16 (primary amenorrhea) or absence of the menstrual period for three to six consecutive months in a woman who has had regular periods since the onset of menstruation (secondary amenorrhea). It often is caused by stress, acute weight loss, or excessive strenuous exercise.

Amniocentesis   Procedure between the sixteenth and twentieth weeks of pregnancy intended to detect fetal defects. The amniotic sac is punctured with a needle and syringe, and amniotic fluid is obtained for analysis.

Amnion   The innermost membrane of the amniotic sac, which contains the amniotic fluid.

Amniotic fluid   Watery fluid that surrounds a developing embryo and fetus in the uterus.

Amphetamines   Synthetic stimulants that increase energy and alertness, produce euphoria, and suppress appetite. Excessive use can cause headaches, irritability, dizziness, insomnia, panic, confusion, and delirium.

Anabolic steroids   Synthetic derivatives of the male hormone testosterone usually taken to increase muscle mass. Their use often results in serious physiological and psychological side effects.

Anaerobic bacteria   Bacteria that are intolerant of oxygen.

Analgesic   Medication that relieves pain without inducing loss of consciousness.

Anaphylactic shock   A severe and sometimes fatal allergic reaction to a foreign substance that causes symptoms such as weakness, shortness of breath, and falling blood pressure.

Androgens   Any steroid hormone (hormone made in the outer layer of the adrenal gland) that increases the development and growth of male physical qualities. Testosterone is an androgen that stimulates the growth of male characteristics.

Androgyny   A blending of typical male and female qualities in an individual.

Aneurysm   A type of weakened blood vessel that can cause a stroke. This ballooning of a weakened region of a blood vessel may result from several factors, including a congenital defect, chronic blood pressure, or an injury to the brain. If left untreated, the aneurysm continues to weaken until it ruptures and bleeds in the brain.

Angina pectoris   Chest pain resulting from insufficient supply of blood (oxygen) to the heart muscle.

Anorexia nervosa   An eating disorder characterized by self-starvation, excessive weight loss, and a host of other physiological and psychological illnesses.

Antihistamine   A medication used to reduce the effects of histamine, a substance found in body tissues that plays a role in allergic reactions.

Antioxidants   Substances that prevent cells called "free radicals" from harming the body's tissues. Antioxidants are present in many fruits and vegetables. They work to neutralize free radicals and protect genes from damage, possibly decreasing the risk of cancer and heart disease and delaying the effects of aging.

Anxiety disorders   Group of conditions that share extreme or pathological anxiety as the principal disturbance of mood. Anxiety disorders include panic disorder, agoraphobia, generalized anxiety disorder, specific phobia, social phobia, obsessive-compulsive disorder, acute stress disorder, and post-traumatic stress disorder. Anxiety disorders are the most common mental disorder in the United States and affect a significant number of people worldwide.

Aorta   The great artery arising from the left ventricle of the heart; the largest artery.

Aortic valve   A valve located between the left ventricle and the aorta.

Arrhythmias   Erratic heartbeats.

Arteries   Vessels in the body that supply oxygenated blood to the tissues.

Arterioles   Small arteries.

Arteriosclerosis   Any arterial disease that leads to the thickening and hardening of the arterial walls, slowing the flow of blood.

Arthritis   Inflammation of the joints. Arthritis encompasses more than 100 diseases and conditions that affect joints, the surrounding tissues, and other connective tissues.

Artificial insemination   Introduction of semen into the uterus or oviduct by unnatural means close to the time of ovulation. It is most often used when the infertility problem is male related.

Assisted reproductive technology (ART)   Any treatment or procedure that involves the handling of human eggs and sperm with the purpose of helping a woman become pregnant.

Asymptomatic viral shedding   Most often associated with herpes simplex virus infections. Viral shedding occurs when active herpes virus, present in the nerve cells of an infected person, moves along the nerves to the surface of the skin. Shedding often occurs without any symptoms (asymptomatic), but the person may still be infectious, meaning that it can be passed on to others.

Atherosclerosis   A type of arteriosclerosis characterized by deposits of fatty substances or plaques on inner walls of arteries that narrow blood vessels.

Athletic amenorrhea   The cessation of regular menstrual periods due to excessive exercising.

Atrial fibrillation   A disorder in which the heart's two small upper chambers (the atria) quiver instead of beating effectively. Because blood is not pumped completely out of them, it may pool and clot. If a piece of a blood clot in the atria leaves the heart and becomes lodged in an artery in the brain, a stroke results.

Atrium   The left or right upper blood-receiving chamber of the heart.

Autoimmune disease   A disease caused by autoantibodies or lymphocytes that attack normal components of the body—molecules, cells, or tissues—by the organism producing them. It is more common among women than men.

Azoospermia   Complete absence of sperm in semen, which is often the cause of male infertility.

B

Bacteria   Single-celled organisms that multiply and cause disease by forcing the body to release poisons and germ-fighting antibodies. Unlike viral infections, bacterial infections usually can be treated by antibiotics.

Bacterial vaginosis   Inflammation of the vagina, caused by an overgrowth of the normal bacteria found in the vagina and resulting in an imbalance. The most common cause of vaginitis, this infection is sometimes, but not always, sexually transmitted.

Balloon angioplasty   A procedure used to open narrowed or blocked coronary arteries. A small, hollow tube called a catheter is inserted into an artery near the blockage. A balloon near the end of the catheter is then inflated, which helps to widen the vessel and allows blood to flow. A wire mesh stent is usually placed at the site of the narrowing to keep the artery open.

Barbiturate   A class of sedatives that have a depressant effect on the central nervous system.

Bariatric surgery   Gastrointestinal surgery for obesity that alters the digestive process. The operation promotes weight loss by closing off parts of the stomach to make it smaller.

Barrier contraception   A method of birth control that provides a physical or chemical barrier to prevent sperm from fertilizing eggs. All barrier methods (except plain condoms) are used with spermicide, a chemical that breaks down the cell walls of sperm. Most barrier methods are used inside the vagina to cover the cervix and prevent sperm from entering the uterus. Male condoms are protective sheaths that enclose the penis during intercourse and ejaculation.

Bartholin's glands Two small glands located just inside the vaginal opening that help lubricate the vagina.

Basal cell carcinoma A nonmelanoma skin cancer that begins in the basal cells of the epidermis (outer layer of skin). It usually develops in areas exposed to the sun, such as the head and neck.

Basal metabolic rate (BMR) The amount of energy needed to maintain essential body functions under resting conditions, usually expressed in terms of calories per hour per kilogram of body weight.

Battering Repeatedly subjecting a person to forceful and coercive physical, social, and/or psychological behavior.

Beneficiary In terms of insurance, an individual who is eligible to receive benefits under an insurance policy.

Benign tumor A noncancerous growth that does not spread to other parts of the body.

Bicuspid valve A valve that separates the left atrium and the left ventricle of the heart; also known as the mitral valve.

Bilateral salpingo-oophorectomy Surgical excision of the fallopian tube and the ovary.

Bile Fluid produced by the liver and stored in the gallbladder that plays a key role in the digestion of fats.

Binge eating disorder (BED) An eating disorder characterized by a lack of control in overeating and overeating in secret. Victims do not force themselves to vomit, however, as with bulimia nervosa.

Bingeing The consumption of large amounts of food that is characteristic of bulimia nervosa.

Biomedical research Studies relating to the activities and applications of science to clinical medicine.

Biopsy The removal and microscopic examination of a tissue sample to determine whether cancer cells are present.

Bipolar disorder (manic depression) A mental disorder that is characterized by wide mood swings that can occur within hours or days and that features abnormally euphoric or irritable moods.

Birth control Umbrella term that refers to procedures that prevent the birth of a baby, including all contraceptive measures, sterilization, and abortion procedures.

Bisexual A person having a sexual orientation to persons of both sexes.

Blastocyst A mass of embryonic cells that results from repeated divisions of the zygote.

Blood Liquid medium of the circulatory system composed of plasma (fluid), erythrocytes (red blood cells), leukocytes (white blood cells), and platelets.

Blood alcohol concentration (BAC) A physiological indicator used by clinicians and law enforcement officials to determine whether a person is legally "drunk." BAC is expressed in terms of the percentage of alcohol in the blood.

Blood pressure The pressure exerted against the walls of the arteries, veins, and heart chambers when the heart pumps, specifically when the left ventricle contracts.

Body composition Proportions of fat, muscle, and bone making up the body. Body composition is usually expressed as percentage of body fat and percentage of lean body mass.

Body mass index (BMI) Weight (in kilograms) divided by height squared (in meters). A value of 25 or greater indicates obesity-related health risks.

Bone remodeling The process that removes older bone (resorption) and replaces it with new bone (formation) so as to maintain a healthy skeleton.

Braxton-Hicks contractions The contraction of the uterus at irregular intervals throughout pregnancy. These contractions are not like "real" labor contractions in that they do not gradually increase in frequency, intensity, or duration.

Breast self-examination The systematic palpation of the breast tissue of each breast while lying on one's back.

Breech Birth presentation in which the feet, knees, or buttocks of the fetus present before the head.

Bulimia nervosa An eating disorder characterized by a secretive cycle of bingeing and purging.

C

Calcium A mineral found mainly in the bones and the teeth. Calcium is important for bone health throughout life. Sources include dairy products, canned fish, seeds and nuts, some green vegetables such as broccoli and kale, and calcium-fortified foods.

Calorie The amount of heat required to raise the temperature of 1 gram of water by 1 degree Celsius.

Cancer A general term for more than 100 diseases that are characterized by uncontrolled, abnormal growth of cells. Cancer cells can spread through the bloodstream and lymphatic system to other parts of the body.

Candidiasis A common inflammation of the vagina caused by an overgrowth of the normal bacteria found in the vagina; it is not usually sexually transmitted, but it can be. Also known as a yeast infection.

Cannabis A mixture of crushed leaves and flowers of the *Cannabis sativa* plant that is usually ingested by smoking. Also known as marijuana, "pot," or "weed."

Capillaries Minute, hair-like vessels connecting arterioles and venules.

Carbohydrates An organic compound such as starch, sugar, or glycogen, composed of carbon, hydrogen, and oxygen. Carbohydrates are a source of bodily energy.

Carcinogen   A substance or agent that is known to cause cancer. Examples of carcinogens include nicotine, asbestos, and ultraviolet radiation.

Carcinogenesis   The overall staging process by which normal cells become malignant. It may be induced by chemical, physical, or viral agents.

Carcinogenic   The ability to cause cancer.

Carcinoma   A cancer that is the most common of all tumors, accounting for approximately 85% of all cancers. This term generally refers to cancer that begins in tissues that line or cover an organ.

Carcinoma-in-situ   Cancer that involves only the top layer of the organ without invading deeper tissues.

Cardiovascular disease   A group of diseases that includes two major categories: diseases of the heart and cerebrovascular disease (primarily stroke).

Cardiovascular endurance   The ability of the body to perform aerobic activities for extended periods of time.

Cardiovascular system   The network of structures that pump and carry blood through the body, including the heart, arteries, veins, and capillaries.

Carpal tunnel syndrome   A common, painful problem in the wrist and hand that occurs in the tendon and the carpal tunnel (a channel in the wrist for the nerve that serves the palm and thumb side of the hand). It is caused by pressure on the nerve that causes weakness, pain when the thumb is bent toward the palm, and burning, tingling, or aching that may spread to the forearm and shoulder.

Cauterization   The use of heat to destroy abnormal cells.

Cephalopelvic disproportion   A complication of pregnancy in which the size of the baby's head is deemed too large or the mother's birth canal is too small to accommodate vaginal delivery. This condition is an indication for cesarean delivery.

Cerebral aneurysm   Abnormal outpouching of an artery in the brain, which, due to the stress of blood rushing through it, may weaken and rupture.

Cerebrovascular accident (stroke)   A condition in which blood vessel damage occurs in the brain.

Cervical cap   A contraceptive device made of latex and individually customized to fit snugly over the cervix.

Cervical dysplasia   Abnormal changes in the cells of the cervix. This benign condition is considered precancerous and can develop into cancer if left untreated.

Cervicitis   An inflammation of the cervix.

Cervix   The small end of the uterus extending into the vagina.

Cesarean delivery   The surgical procedure in which an infant is delivered through an incision made in the abdominal wall and uterus.

Chemotherapy   The treatment of disease with anticancer drugs or chemicals.

Child abuse and neglect   Physical or mental injury, sexual abuse or exploitation, negligent treatment, or maltreatment of a child by a person who is responsible for the child's welfare under circumstances that indicate that the child's health or welfare is harmed or threatened.

Chlamydia   A sexually transmitted infection (STI) that is caused by the bacterium *Chlamydia trachomatis*. Most people are asymptomatic and, therefore, are not aware of their infections. If left untreated, chlamydia can cause serious damage to a woman's reproductive system. Chlamydia is the most frequently reported infectious disease in the United States.

Chloasma   Darkening of skin pigment on the upper lip, under the eyes, and on the forehead; commonly linked to pregnancy or taking oral contraceptives.

Cholesterol   One of the steroids or fat-like chemical substances manufactured by the body and also consumed in foods of animal origin. It is essential for the manufacture and maintenance of cells, sex hormones, and nerves throughout the body.

Chorion   Outer membrane of the amniotic sac that expands around the fetus as it grows.

Chorionic villus sampling   A procedure performed to detect fetal abnormalities in which samples of chorionic villi are removed and examined.

Chromosomes   The structures in the nucleus of each cell composed of DNA and protein that contain the genes that provide information for the transmission of inherited characteristics.

Chronic bronchitis   Constant inflammation of the bronchial tubes. The inflammation thickens the walls of the bronchi, and the production of mucus increases, resulting in a constricting or narrowing of the air passages.

Chronic disease   A disease that lasts longer than several weeks, often for the length of a person's life; it may be ongoing or progress slowly. Examples include diabetes, heart disease, and lupus.

Chronic obstructive pulmonary disease (COPD; also known as chronic lower respiratory disease [CLRD] or chronic obstructive lung disease [COLD])   A disease characterized by permanent airflow obstruction and extended periods of disability and restricted activity.

Cirrhosis   Alcohol-induced liver disease.

Climacteric   Physiological changes that occur during the transition period from fertility to infertility in both sexes.

Clinical trial   A research study designed to answer specific questions about new vaccines, new therapies, or new ways of using known treatments. Clinical trials are used to determine whether drugs or treatments are both safe and effective.

Clitoridectomy   The removal of the clitoris; also known as female genital mutilation or female circumcision.

Clitoris   A highly sensitive structure of the female external genitalia, the only purpose of which is sexual pleasure.

Co-dependent   A person in a continuing relationship with a chemically dependent person whose actions enable the addiction to continue.

Cognitive-behavioral therapy   A short-term treatment, usually lasting several months, that teaches people to identify and change patterns of thinking that cause them to perceive certain situations or objects as dangerous.

Coitus   Technical term for penile–vaginal intercourse.

Colonoscopy   An examination of the colon using a flexible lighted instrument called a colonoscope.

Colostomy   A surgically created opening from the outside of the body into the colon that provides a new path for waste material to leave the body after part of the colon has been removed.

Colostrum   Early milk, or milk produced during the pregnancy and for three to five days after birth. Colostrum is yellowish in color, thicker than milk, and rich with protective antibodies and protein.

Colposcope   A lighted magnifying instrument used to examine the vagina and cervix.

Colposcopy   A procedure in which a colposcope is used to examine the vagina and cervix.

Complex carbohydrates   One of the main sources of fuel for the muscles. Complex carbohydrates are found in breads, cereals, pasta, rice, and vegetables such as potatoes and corn.

Conception   Formation of a viable zygote by the union of the male sperm and the female ovum; fertilization.

Conceptus   The products of conception or fertilization, including the fertilized egg and its enclosing membranes.

Condom   A barrier contraception method consisting of a sheath, preferably latex, that covers the penis during intercourse. It prevents pregnancy by collecting the semen in the receptacle tip.

Congenital heart disease   A heart condition present when a baby is born. It may include many different conditions, most of which can be surgically corrected.

Congestive heart failure (CHF)   A condition in which the heart loses its ability to contract properly or sufficiently to meet the demands placed on it.

Conization   The surgical removal of a cone-shaped piece of tissue intended to determine whether abnormal cells have invaded tissue beneath surface cells or to treat a precancerous lesion. Also called cone biopsy.

Contraception   Intentional prevention of conception or impregnation through the use of various devices, agents, drugs, sexual practices, or surgical procedures.

Contraceptive sponge   A contraceptive device that acts both as a cervical barrier by absorbing ejaculated sperm and as a source of spermicide. It is available without fitting or prescription.

Contraindication   A medical condition that renders a course of treatment inadvisable or unsafe that might otherwise be recommended.

Co-payment   A type of cost sharing whereby the enrollee or covered person pays a specified flat amount per unit of service or unit of time, and the health-care insurer pays the remainder of the cost.

Coronary artery bypass surgery   A type of surgery that creates a "bypass" around the blocked part of the coronary artery to restore the blood supply to the heart muscle.

Corpus luteum   A yellowish body that forms on the ovary at the site of the ruptured follicle where the egg has been released. It secretes progesterone to help prepare the body for pregnancy.

Corset   A close-fitting undergarment or outer garment worn to support and shape the waistline, hips, and breasts.

C-reactive protein   A protein produced by the liver during periods of inflammation that is detectable in blood in various disease conditions. The C-reactive protein blood test is used as an indicator of acute inflammation.

Crack   A highly addictive smokeable form of cocaine; also known as "rock."

Cryosurgery   Surgical procedure that freezes and destroys abnormal tissues.

Cryotherapy   Freezing of an infected area.

Cunnilingus   Oral stimulation of the clitoris or vulva.

Cyberstalking   Threatening behavior or unwanted advances directed at another person using the Internet and other forms of online communications.

Cystic fibrosis   An abnormality of the respiratory system and the sweat and mucous glands. Cystic fibrosis is the most common genetic disorder among whites in the United States.

Cystic mastitis   The most common breast disorder in women, resulting in tender and lumpy breast tissues. Also known as fibrocystic breast disease.

Cyst   An abnormal growth of cells consisting of a thin-walled sac filled with fluid.

Cystitis   Inflammation of the bladder.

Cytomegalovirus (CMV)   A viral infection that causes mild flu-like symptoms in adults but that can cause small birth size, brain damage, developmental problems, enlarged liver, hearing and vision impairment, and other malformations in newborns. Babies with CMV are infected in utero, although only 10% of those so infected have symptoms. Pregnant women often acquire CMV from young infected children with few or no symptoms. CMV is the most common prenatal infection today, and it is an opportunistic infection of HIV/AIDS.

D

Date rape   Rape in which the victim and the rapist were previously known to each other and may have interacted in some socially appropriate manner. Also known as "acquaintance rape."

Delirium tremens (DTs)   A condition induced by alcohol withdrawal and characterized by excessive trembling, sweating, anxiety, and hallucinations.

Dementia   Cognitive decline, often occurring in old age. This mental deterioration and decline in intellectual functioning is severe enough to interfere with routine daily activities.

Depression   A mental condition in which a person feels extremely sad, worthless, and hopeless. In more severe cases, the person may experience thoughts of suicide. Types of depression include clinical depression, bipolar depression, seasonal affective disorder (SAD), dysthymia, and postpartum depression.

Diabetes mellitus   A disease characterized by abnormal glucose production or metabolism. A person with diabetes has either a deficiency of insulin (the hormone produced by the pancreas needed to convert glucose to energy) or a decreased ability to use insulin. As a result, glucose builds up in the bloodstream and, without treatment, may damage organs and contribute to heart disease.

Diagnostic and Statistical Manual of Mental Disorders (DSM-IV-TR)   Currently in its fourth edition, a manual published by the American Psychiatric Association. It attempts to describe all mental health disorders for adults and children.

Diaphragm   A latex, dome-shaped cap inserted over the cervix to prevent conception.

Diastolic   The second reading of blood pressure that represents the amount of pressure the blood exerts against the wall of the artery when the heart rests between beats.

Diethylstilbestrol (DES)   A synthetic estrogen originally prescribed to prevent miscarriages. DES caused malformations of the reproductive organs in some women who were exposed to the drug during fetal development.

Digital rectal examination   An examination intended to detect colorectal cancer in which the physician inserts a lubricated gloved finger into the rectum to feel for abnormal areas.

Dilation and curettage (D&C)   A minor surgical procedure in which the cervix is expanded enough (dilated) to permit the cervical canal and uterine lining to be scraped with a spoon-shaped instrument called a curette.

Dissociative disorders   Disorders that develop as an unconscious way to protect oneself from emotional traumas by detaching from a part of one's personality. These disorders occur as a response to a severe childhood trauma.

Diuretic   A drug that expedites the elimination of fluid from the body.

Dizygotic twins   Two offspring developed from two eggs released from the ovary and fertilized at the same time. They may be the same or opposite sex and may differ physically and in genetic traits. Also called fraternal twins.

Domestic violence   Subjecting a spouse, partner, or family member to any forceful physical, social, and psychological behavior so as to coerce that person without regard to his or her rights. Also known as battering.

Double-contrast barium enema   A type of X-ray procedure in which a mixture containing barium is inserted into the rectum. The barium mixture outlines the lower part of the bowel, enabling any blockages or abnormalities in the lining of the bowel to be identified.

Down syndrome   A congenital condition characterized by various degrees of mental retardation and abnormal development. It is caused by the presence of an extra chromosome, usually number 21 or 22.

Drug   Any chemical other than food that is purposely taken to affect body processes.

Drug abuse   The excessive use of a drug that has dangerous side effects.

Drug dependency   The attachment—physiological or psychological (or both)—that a person may develop to a drug. Physical dependence occurs when physiological changes in the body's cells cause an overpowering constant need for a drug.

Drug misuse   The use of a drug for a purpose other than its original intent.

Dysmenorrhea   Pain or discomfort just prior to or during menstruation.

Dyspareunia   Painful intercourse that can stem from physical or psychological causes.

Dysplasia   Abnormal cells that are not cancerous; classified as mild, moderate, or severe.

Dysplastic nevi   Atypical moles.

Dysthymia   A form of depression that is milder and less disabling than major depression, but more chronic in nature.

E

Eclampsia   A life-threatening condition during pregnancy that causes convulsions and may lead to coma and death of the mother and baby. Eclampsia progresses from preeclampsia.

Ectoparasitic infections   Infections caused by tiny parasites that reside on the skin and survive on human blood and tissue. Infections include scabies and pubic lice ("crabs"). Parasites cause itching and may cause bumps or a rash, but are easily treated with a topical cream.

Ectopic pregnancy   The implantation of a fertilized egg outside the uterus.

Edema   An abnormal accumulation of fluid in body parts or tissues that results in swelling.

Effacement   The thinning of the cervix before delivery.

Egg donation   A type of assisted reproductive technology used when a woman is unable to produce eggs or has a genetic disorder that will be passed on to her child. Egg donors must be willing to dedicate an enormous amount of time to this effort because of the amount of drug treatment and monitoring that they must undergo.

Elder abuse   The injury, maltreatment, or neglect of an older person from a physical, psychological, or material perspective.

Electrocardiograph (ECG)   A device used to record the electric activity of the heart so as to diagnose heart problems.

Electrocautery   Electrical burning of an infected area.

Electrodessication   Tissue destruction by heat.

Embolism   A condition in which an embolus (clot) traveling in the bloodstream suddenly becomes lodged in a blood vessel.

Embolus   A clot circulating in the bloodstream.

Embryo   An organism in its early stage of development in humans. The embryonic period lasts from the second to the eighth week of pregnancy.

Embryo transfer   A fertility procedure in which the sperm of the infertile woman's partner are placed in another woman's uterus during ovulation. The fertilized egg is removed a few days later and transferred to the uterus of the infertile woman.

Emotional or psychological elder abuse   The infliction of mental or emotional anguish of an older person through such means as humiliation, intimidation, or threats.

Emphysema   The limitation of airflow as the result of irreversible disease changes in the lung tissue after years of assault on that tissue. The air sacs in the lungs are destroyed, and the lungs are compromised in bringing oxygen and removing carbon dioxide from the body. As a result, breathing becomes compromised, and increased demand is placed on the heart.

Endometrial hyperplasia   An overgrowth of the lining of the uterus (endometrium) resulting from lack of ovulation. Failure to ovulate leads to too much estrogen and not enough progesterone being produced by the body. When this occurs, the endometrium builds up but is not shed during the menstrual cycle.

Endometriosis   A benign condition in which tissue that looks like endometrial tissue grows in abnormal places outside the uterus.

Endometrium   The tissue that lines the inside of the uterine walls.

Environmental tobacco smoke (ETS)   Smoke resulting from others who are smoking cigarettes or cigars. Also referred to as passive or secondhand smoke.

Enzyme linked immunosorbent assay (ELISA)   Laboratory test used to detect antibodies produced in response to HIV infection. If HIV antibodies are found with this test, it is repeated. If antibodies are found on a second ELISA test, a Western blot test is performed.

Epidemiology   The study of patterns of disease in the population. Epidemiology is concerned with the frequency and type of a disease in groups of people and the factors that influence the distribution of the disease.

Epidural anesthesia   A type of anesthetic used during delivery that is injected through a catheter placed in a space beside the spinal cord. Epidurals are the most common choice of anesthesia made by pregnant women and allow the mother to be awake for the birth.

Episiotomy   An incision in the mother's perineum that enlarges the opening of the vagina to provide more room for the infant during delivery and to help prevent tearing of the vaginal tissues.

Epstein-Barr virus   One of the eight known types of human herpesviruses; causes mononucleosis.

Erythrocytes   Red blood cells. Erythrocytes carry oxygen and carbon dioxide.

Estrogen   A class of hormones that produce female secondary sex characteristics and affect the menstrual cycle.

Eugenics   The study of or belief in the possibility of improving the qualities of the human species or a human population by such means as discouraging reproduction by persons having genetic defects (or presumed to have inheritable undesirable traits) or encouraging reproduction by those presumed to have positive traits.

Exercise   Routine or structured physical activity that a person performs with the goal of improving his or her health.

F

Fallopian tubes   Tubes or ducts that allow for the passage of ova from the ovary to the uterus.

Familial adenomatous polyposis (FAP)   A condition in which polyps are inherited and affect the gastrointestinal tract. Individuals with FAP develop hundreds to thousands of polyps throughout the colon at a young age.

Family and intimate violence   Forms of violence that include child abuse, incest, courtship violence, date rape, battering, marital rape, and elder abuse.

Fat   A lipid with one, two, or three fatty acids, which is responsible for multiple body functions.

Fat-soluble vitamins   Vitamins absorbed with the aid of fats in the diet or bile from the liver through the intestinal membrane and stored in the body.

Fecal occult blood testing A simple procedure of smearing a small sample of stool on a slide containing a chemical that changes color in the presence of hemoglobin. Developing tumors cause minor bleeding, which results in the presence of occult blood (small amounts of blood in the stool).

Fecundity The physical ability of a woman to have a child. Women with impaired fecundity include those who find it physically difficult or medically inadvisable to conceive or deliver a child.

Fee for service A traditional method of health-care payment in which physicians and other providers receive payment that does not exceed their billed charges for each unit of service rendered.

Fellatio Oral stimulation of the penis or scrotum.

Female athlete triad The interrelationship between disordered eating, amenorrhea, and osteoporosis. Beginning with disordered eating, the combination of poor nutrition and intense athletic training causes weight loss and a decrease in or shutdown of estrogen production. Consequently, amenorrhea occurs. The final condition in the triad, osteoporosis, may follow if estrogen levels remain low and the woman's diet continues to lack calcium and vitamin D.

Female condom A form of barrier contraception that lines the entire vagina, preventing the penis and semen from coming in direct physical contact with the vagina.

Female genital mutilation Any of the three types of genital mutilation: removal of the prepuce and/or the tip of the clitoris; removal of the entire clitoris (both prepuce and glans) and the adjacent labia; or removal of the clitoris, the adjacent labia (majora and minora), and the joining of the scraped sides of the vulva across the vagina. Often referred to as female circumcision or female genital cutting.

Feminism The policy, practice, or advocacy of political, economic, and social equality for women. It is the principle that women should have rights equal to those of men.

Fertility The state of being fertile; capable of producing offspring.

Fertility awareness methods Several methods—including the calendar or rhythm method, the basal body temperature method, and the cervical mucus method—that can help a woman determine her most fertile time. These methods can be used to prevent pregnancy or to help a woman become pregnant.

Fertilization The union of an ovum and a sperm.

Fetal alcohol syndrome (FAS) Alcohol-related defects among infants due to prenatal maternal alcohol consumption. They are usually characterized by growth retardation, facial malformations, and central nervous system dysfunctions including mental retardation.

Fetal distress Signs of distress in the fetus such as slowing of heart rate or acid in the blood.

Fetus The unborn baby in the uterus from the eighth week of gestation until birth.

Fiber Plant parts that cannot be digested in the human digestive tract. High-fiber diets protect against certain cancers and heart disease.

Fibroadenoma A nonmalignant form of breast tumor.

Fibrocystic breast disease The most common breast disorder in women, resulting in tender and lumpy breast tissues. Also known as cystic mastitis.

Fibroid A benign uterine tumor composed of muscular and fibrous tissue.

Flexibility The range of motion permitted by joints.

Folate A B vitamin found in foods such as chickpeas, spinach, strawberries, kidney beans, and citrus fruits and juices.

Folic acid A form of folate used to fortify grain-based foods, such as bread, flour, rice, pasta, and cereal. It is vital for cell growth and function and for the development of a healthy neural tube in fetuses.

Follicle stimulating hormone (FSH) A pituitary hormone secreted by a female during the secretory phase of the menstrual cycle. It stimulates the development of ovarian follicles.

Food insecurity Lack of access to nutritionally balanced and safe foods or having limited access to nutritious and affordable food.

Forceps Surgical instruments used for grasping. Obstetric forceps may be used to extract a baby from the birth canal during delivery.

Formulary A list of drug products that a payer has identified as part of a given health insurance product's covered benefits.

Fornication Voluntary sexual intercourse between persons not married to each other.

G

Galactosemia Inherited disease characterized by lack of enzyme needed for processing galactose (sugar in milk products); can cause mental retardation if not treated promptly.

Gamete intrafallopian transfer (GIFT) A procedure for treating infertility that involves placing sperm and egg cells into the fallopian tubes.

Gangrene Localized tissue death due to inadequate blood supply or bacterial invasion.

Gastritis Inflammation of the stomach lining.

Gender The economic, social, and cultural attributes and opportunities associated with being male or female.

Gender dysphoria The overall psychological term used to describe the negative or conflicting feelings about one's sex or gender roles.

Gender identity   How one psychologically perceives oneself as either male or female.

Gender roles   The public expression of one's gender identity as well as the cultural expectations of male and female behaviors.

Generalized anxiety disorder (GAD)   An anxiety disorder that causes an ongoing general feeling of intense worry and fear, often for no apparent reason.

Generic drug   The chemical equivalent of a brand-name drug that is available once the brand-name drug goes off patent. Generic drugs are typically less expensive than their brand-name counterparts.

Genetic phenotype   The observable traits or characteristics of an organism—for example, hair color, weight, or the presence or absence of a disease.

Gestational diabetes   A form of the disease that develops in 2% to 5% of all pregnancies, but usually disappears when the pregnancy is over.

Glycemic index   A measure of how fast glucose enters the bloodstream after a carbohydrate is eaten and thus how quickly the carbohydrate increases a person's blood sugar.

Gonadotropin-releasing hormone (GnRH)   Hormone responsible for reproductive hormone control; stimulates release of follicle stimulating hormone at the beginning of the menstrual cycle.

Gonadotropins   Pituitary hormones that stimulate activity in the testes or ovaries.

Gonorrhea   A sexually transmitted bacterial infection that can cause dangerous complications leading to infertility, ectopic pregnancy, or persistent pain in the pelvic area. It can even spread to the bloodstream and cause arthritis or life-threatening heart or brain infections.

Group B streptococcus (GBS)   A type of bacterium that can cause illness in newborn babies and pregnant women. Pregnant women with GBS do not necessarily infect their babies; however, babies who develop signs and symptoms are at risk of sepsis, pneumonia, meningitis, long-term disabilities such as hearing or vision loss, and death. Obstetricians can test women for GBS and prevent disease by administering antibiotics intravenously during labor.

H

Hallucinogenic drugs   Drugs that create changes in perceptions and thoughts. A common feature of a hallucinogenic experience is that the drug suspends normal psychic mechanisms that integrate the self with the environment.

Hashish   An extract of cannabis that is 2 to 10 times as concentrated as marijuana.

Hate crime   A crime in which the defendant intentionally selects a victim or, in the case of a property crime, the property that is the object of the crime because of the actual or perceived race, color, national origin, ethnicity, gender, disability, or sexual orientation of the person or property.

HDL cholesterol   A type of lipoprotein in the blood that carries cholesterol and fats out of the body. Often referred to as "good" cholesterol.

Heart attack   Death of a certain portion of the heart.

Hemoglobin   The iron-containing protein in the red blood cell that carries oxygen from the lungs to the cells and carbon dioxide away from the cells to the lungs. It also is responsible for the red color of blood.

Hemorrhagic stroke   A condition in which blood vessels leading to and within the brain rupture, causing the brain to no longer receive blood and oxygen.

Hepatitis   Inflammation and destruction of liver cells.

Hepatoma   A cancer that originates from liver cells.

Herpes simplex virus (HSV)   A family of contagious viruses that infect humans. Viruses in the herpes family include HSV-1 and HSV-2, which can cause sores in the mouth or genital area (the latter infection is often referred to as "genital herpes") as well as the virus that causes chicken pox.

Heterosexual   A person with sexual orientation to persons of the opposite sex and/or sexual activity with another of the opposite sex.

High-density lipoprotein (HDL)   A type of lipoprotein in the blood that carries cholesterol and fats out of the body. It is often referred to as the "good" cholesterol.

Histoplasmosis   Infection caused by breathing in airborne spores of fungus; the disease primarily affects the lungs, but occasionally affects other organs. Histoplasmosis is an opportunistic infection of AIDS.

HIV (human immunodeficiency virus)   A virus that attacks and damages the white blood cells in the body's immune system that are needed to fight off infection. HIV eventually causes AIDS (acquired immune deficiency syndrome), when so many white blood cells have been destroyed that the immune system can no longer fight off illness.

Homeostasis   A constant environment within the body.

Homocysteine   An essential amino acid found in the blood. Increased levels of homocysteine can harm the artery lining and increase risk for coronary artery disease.

Homologous   Refers to parts that resemble one another or originate from the same tissue, such as the external genitals, gonads, and some of the internal structures of males and females.

Homophobia   Irrational fears of homosexuality, the fear of the possibility of homosexuality in oneself, or self-loathing toward one's own homosexuality.

Homosexual   A person whose primary social, emotional, and sexual orientation is toward members of the same sex.

Honor killings   The killing of a woman who has a (sexual) contact with a man outside the frame of marriage, even when she has been a victim of rape. It is intended to maintain and protect the honor of the family. Offenders often are younger than age 18 and are sometimes treated as heroes in their communities. Such killings have been reported in Pakistan, Jordan, Yemen, Lebanon, Egypt, the Gaza Strip, and the West Bank.

Hormone   Chemicals produced by one part of the body that influence activity, growth, or metabolism in another part of the body.

Host uterus   A procedure in which the sperm from a man and the egg from a woman are combined in a laboratory. The fertilized egg then is implanted into the uterus of a second woman, who agrees to bear the child that is not genetically related to her.

Hot flash   An uncomfortable sensation of menopause consisting of internally generated heat beginning in the chest and moving to the neck and head or spreading throughout the body. Also known as hot flushes.

Human chorionic gonadotropin (hCG)   A hormone produced by the chorionic villi in a pregnant woman.

Human genome   The DNA contained in an organism or a cell, which includes both the chromosomes within the nucleus and the DNA in mitochondria.

Human papillomavirus (HPV)   An extremely common sexually transmitted virus. There are many strains of HPV; some of them can cause genital warts in men or women, and other kinds can cause cervical dysplasia in women, which, if left untreated, can lead to cervical cancer.

Hunger   The painful or uneasy feeling caused by the continuous and involuntary lack of food.

Hymen   Tissue that partially covers the vaginal opening.

Hyperglycemia   High blood sugar levels, whereby a person may become very ill. Early signs of hyperglycemia include high blood sugar, high levels of sugar in the urine, frequent urination, and increased thirst.

Hyperplasia   A precancerous condition characterized by an increase in the number of normal cells.

Hypertension   A blood pressure that remains elevated above what is considered a safe level. Also known as high blood pressure.

Hyperthyroidism   Thyroid disease resulting from an overactive thyroid, most commonly caused by Graves' disease.

Hypoactive sexual desire disorder (HSDD)   A persistent lack of interest in or desire for sex. This disorder often reflects relationship problems but may be caused by other physical or personal difficulties.

Hypoglycemia   Low blood sugar levels that can cause a person to become nervous, shaky, and confused and can result in the person passing out.

Hypothyroidism   Thyroid disease resulting from an underactive thyroid, most commonly caused by Hashimoto's disease.

Hysterectomy   The surgical removal of the uterus, resulting in surgically induced menopause.

Hysteroscopy   A procedure used to view the inside of the uterus through a telescope-like device called a hysteroscope.

I

Iatrogenic   Induced in a patient by a medical treatment or procedure. Used to refer to an infection or other complication of treatment.

Immune system   The body's natural defense system, which works to protect the body from pathogens.

Implantation   The embedding of the fertilized ovum in the uterine lining six to seven days after fertilization.

In vitro fertilization (IVF)   A procedure for treating infertility that involves removing the ova from a woman's ovary. The ova and the sperm (from the woman's partner) are placed in a medium; if fertilization occurs, the conceptus is injected into the woman's uterus.

Incidence   The number of new cases of a disease or condition in a given period of time.

Indemnity health insurance   A form of health insurance in which a person prepays a premium in exchange for a specific amount of monetary coverage in the event of illnesses or accidents. If an illness or accident occurs, the enrollee or the care provider submits a claim to the insurance organization. The insurance organization then reimburses the party for all or, in most cases, a percentage of the incurred costs.

Infant mortality rate   The number of deaths of children less than 1 year old divided by the number of live births that year. The infant mortality rate is an important epidemiological indicator of the well-being of pregnant women, infants, and children.

Inferior vena cava   The major vein that carries oxygen-poor blood into the right atrium of the heart.

Infertility   The inability to conceive a child.

Infibulation   The removal of the clitoris, the labia majora and labia minora, and the joining of the scraped sides of the vulva across the vagina where they are secured with thorns or sewn with catgut or thread. A small opening is kept to allow passage of urine and menstrual blood. An infibulated woman must be cut open to allow intercourse on her wedding night and is closed again afterwards to secure fidelity to the husband. Infibulation is the most extreme form of female genital mutilation.

Inhalants Chemicals that produce vapors with psychoactive effects and are predominantly abused by pre-adolescents and young adults.

Insulin-dependent diabetes mellitus (IDDM) A type of diabetes that often appears in childhood or adolescence. It is considered an autoimmune disease because the immune system attacks and destroys the insulin-producing beta cells in the pancreas so that the pancreas produces little or no insulin. Also called type 1 diabetes or juvenile diabetes.

Intersexuality The sexual physiology of an individual in which the person is born with sex chromosomes, external genitalia, or internal reproductive organs that are not considered "standard" as male or female.

Intracytoplasmic sperm injection (ICSI) A procedure for treating infertility that involves the injection of a single sperm directly into a mature egg.

Intrauterine device (IUD) A small, flexible, plastic T-shaped device that contains either copper or the hormone progesterone and is inserted into the uterus by a clinician to prevent pregnancy. The IUD can be left in place for 1 to 10 years, depending on the type of device.

Intrauterine growth retardation Poor fetal growth for a given duration of pregnancy.

Involuntary smoking A situation in which nonsmokers have to breathe air contaminated by smokers. Also known as passive smoking or environmental tobacco smoke (ETS).

Iron A mineral that is needed to make hemoglobin (a compound in the blood).

Ischemic stroke A condition in which blood vessels leading to and within the brain become blocked, causing the brain to no longer receive blood and oxygen.

Isoflavone A phytoestrogen that is present in soybeans and soy-based products.

J

Jaundice A condition in which accumulation of pigments in the blood produces a yellowing of the skin and eyes.

K

Kegel exercises Exercises that help strengthen the vaginal and pelvic floor muscles to help prepare the muscles for delivery, aid in a speedy recovery from delivery, help prevent or treat urinary incontinence, and help prevent or treat the loss of pelvic support.

L

Labia majora The outer lips of the vagina.

Labia minora The inner lips of the vulva, one on each side of the vaginal opening.

Lactation The production and secretion of milk by the mammary glands.

Lactational amenorrhea method (LAM) A contraceptive method used by breastfeeding women that is effective only if all three of the following criteria are met: menstrual periods have not yet returned, the mother is fully breastfeeding, and the baby is younger than six months old.

Lamaze A method of childbirth preparation in which the expectant mother is prepared psychologically and physically through breathing exercises and concentration to control pain during childbirth while maintaining consciousness.

Laparoscopy Examination of a woman's abdominal cavity to view the ovaries, fallopian tubes, and other structures.

LDL cholesterol A type of lipoprotein that contains cholesterol and triglycerides and is considered harmful because it promotes fatty deposits on the inner lining of arteries. Also called "bad" cholesterol.

Left atrium One of the two upper chambers of the heart. It receives blood with oxygen from the lungs.

Left ventricle One of the two lower chambers of the heart. It pumps blood from the heart to the body tissues.

Lesbian A woman whose sexual orientation is to women; a female homosexual.

Leukemia A cancer that originates within the blood and blood-producing organs.

Leukocytes White blood cells. Leukocytes act as scavengers to rid the blood and body of bacteria and waste. Several types of white blood cells exist, each of which has its own role in fighting bacterial, viral, fungal, and parasitic infections.

Life expectancy The number of years a person born at a given point in time is expected to live from birth.

Lipoprotein A compound found in the bloodstream containing a core of lipids with a shell of protein, phospholipid, and cholesterol.

Lobectomy Removal of the lobe of a lung.

Long-term care Custodial care provided over a prolonged or indefinite period of time, required because of a person's disability or aging. Skilled nursing facilities, or nursing homes, are the most common types of long-term care facilities.

Low birthweight A birthweight of less than 5.5 pounds (2.5 kg). Low birthweight, along with how far along in pregnancy the baby is delivered, are the two biggest predictors of infant health and survival.

Low-density lipoprotein (LDL) A type of lipoprotein that contains cholesterol and triglycerides and is considered harmful because it promotes fatty deposits on the inner lining of arteries. Also called "bad" cholesterol.

Lp(a) A lipoprotein that, when present in elevated levels, may cause blockages to increase in size and blood to thicken. Lp(a) is an inherited factor and cannot be controlled by lifestyle choices.

Lumpectomy A procedure in which only the cancerous lump and a small amount of surrounding tissue are removed from the breast.

Lupus A complex chronic inflammatory disorder in which the immune system forms antibodies that target healthy tissues and organs. Lupus can be a mild, moderate, or severe disease.

Luteinizing hormone (LH) The hormone secreted by the pituitary gland that stimulates ovulation in the female.

Lyme disease A type of inflammatory arthritis that is caused by a tiny, tick-borne bacterium. If Lyme disease is not treated, it can lead to cardiac problems, neurological disorders, or infectious arthritis (usually of the knees).

Lymphoma A tumor, usually cancerous, that originates from lymph tissue that is part of the body's immune system.

M

Macromineral One of the six major minerals—calcium, chloride, magnesium, phosphorus, potassium, and sodium.

Macular degeneration Common eye disease associated with aging that gradually destroys sharp central vision.

Malignant tumor A tumor that is cancerous and capable of spreading to other tissues and invading adjacent areas.

Malnutrition An imbalance between the body's nutritional needs and the intake or digestion of nutrients, which may result in disease or death. Malnutrition can be caused by an unbalanced diet, digestive problems, or absorption problems.

Mammography A procedure in which a low-dose X ray of the breast is taken so as to detect tumors.

Managed care A system of health-care delivery that aims to manage utilization of services and cost of services, while measuring performance. The goal is a system that delivers value by giving people access to quality, cost-effective health care.

Mastectomy Removal of the entire breast tissue and possibly underarm lymph nodes to treat cancer.

Mastitis An infection in the breast, usually caused by bacterial infection. It results in localized pain, redness, and heat with symptoms of fever, nausea, and vomiting.

Masturbation Excitation of one's own or another's genital organs, usually to orgasm, by manual contact or means other than sexual intercourse.

Maternal morbidity and mortality Death or illness while pregnant or within a defined time period of the termination of pregnancy, irrespective of the duration and the site of the pregnancy, from any cause related to or aggravated by the pregnancy or its management but not from accidental or incidental causes.

Maternal serum alpha-fetoprotein screening A prenatal screening test that measures a substance produced by the baby's kidneys found in the mother's blood between the thirteenth and twentieth weeks of pregnancy.

Medicaid A joint federal/state health insurance program for low-income persons who receive public assistance or whose medical expenses "spend down" their income to qualify for the program. This program is administered by each state, and places fairly tight restrictions on payment for physician services and drugs. Also known as Title XIX.

Medical abortion The use of medications, often mifepristone and misoprostol, or misoprostol alone, to end a pregnancy.

Medicare A health insurance program providing benefits to approximately 30 million elderly (aged 65 or older) and disabled Americans. It is funded by the federal government and administered by the Centers for Medicare and Medicaid Services (CMS).

Melanocytes Pigment-producing cells in the skin.

Melanoma A cancer that originates within the melanocytes.

Melatonin A hormone that is important in regulating the body's response to biological rhythms, such as the light–dark cycle.

Menarche The initial onset of menstrual periods in a young woman.

Menopause The cessation of regular menstrual periods by surgical or natural means. Also known as the climacterium, the "change of life."

Menstrual cycle A recurring cycle (beginning at menarche and ending at menopause) in which the endometrial lining of the uterus prepares for pregnancy. If pregnancy does not occur, the lining is shed at menstruation. The average menstrual cycle is 28 days.

Metastasis The spread of cancer from one part of the body to another. Cells in the metastatic tumor (the second tumor) are like those in the original tumor.

Mineral A naturally occurring inorganic substance. These nutrients are essential in small amounts for regulating body functions.

Miscarriage A pregnancy that terminates before the twentieth week of gestation because of fetal defects or pregnancy problems.

Mitral valve The valve separating the left atrium and ventricle.

Modified radical mastectomy Removal of the breast. Modified radical mastectomy is a less extensive procedure than radical mastectomy because the underlying chest wall muscles and some of the nearby lymph nodes are not removed. Also known as total mastectomy.

Monounsaturated fat A type of fat that comes from both plant and animal sources and is liquid at room temperature and solid or semi-solid when refrigerated. Monounsaturated fats help to lower blood cholesterol.

Monozygotic twins   Two offspring developed from one fertilized egg that splits into equal halves. Monozygotic twins are of the same sex, share the same genes, and look nearly identical. Also called identical twins.

Mons veneris   A triangular mound over the pubic bone above the vulva.

Mood disorders (affective disorders)   Conditions characterized by extreme disturbances of mood.

Morbidity rate   The rate of illness in a given population over a period of time.

Mortality rate   The rate of death in a given population over a period of time.

Multiple sclerosis (MS)   An autoimmune disease that is characterized by the loss of the myelin covering of the nerve fibers of the brain and spinal cord.

Muscular endurance   The ability to withstand the stress of physical exertion.

Muscular strength   Physical power, such as the amount of weight one can lift, push, or press in a single effort.

Mycobacterium avium complex (MAC)   An infection contracted through contaminated food, soil, or water and affecting only those with weakened immune systems. MAC is an opportunistic infection of HIV/AIDS.

Myocardial infarction   Heart attack.

Myomectomy   Surgical removal of a uterine fibroid.

Myometrium   The smooth muscle layer of the uterine wall.

N

Narcotics   A class of drugs that includes the opiates—opium and its derivatives, morphine, codeine, and heroin—and some non-opiate synthetic drugs. All narcotics have sleep-inducing and pain-relieving properties.

Natural menopause   The failure of the ovaries to respond to the luteinizing and follicle-stimulating hormones that are produced in the anterior pituitary, which is under the control of the hypothalamus. As a result of this failure, ovulation becomes somewhat erratic. The mechanisms for these changes are not well understood. Menopause is considered complete once monthly periods have ceased altogether.

Neoplasm   A type of tumor that is a new growth of tissue serving no physiological function. The growth may be benign or malignant.

Neural tube defects   Defects of the spine and brain caused by failure of the neural tube to close during pregnancy.

Neuroblastoma   A cancer that originates from cells in the nervous system.

Neurotransmitter   A group of chemical found in the brain and nervous system that transmit and modulate communication between neurons.

Nicotine   The addictive element in cigarettes. Nicotine has several effects on the body, including increasing blood pressure, increasing heart rate, and negating hunger.

Non-governmental organizations (NGOs)   According to the World Bank, "private organizations that pursue activities to relieve suffering, promote the interests of the poor, protect the environment, provide basic social services, or undertake community development." This term can be applied to any non-profit organization that is independent from government, including a large charity, community-based self-help group, research institute, church, professional association, and lobby group.

Noninsulin-dependent diabetes mellitus (NIDDM)   The most common type of diabetes. Approximately 90% to 95% of all people with diabetes have NIDDM. In this type of disease, the pancreas usually produces insulin but the insulin is not used effectively. Also referred to as type 2 diabetes or adult-onset diabetes.

Nonmelanoma   The most common cancers of the skin (usually basal cell and squamous cell cancers). Nonmelanoma cancers include all skin cancers except malignant melanoma.

Norplant   A hormonal method of birth control that prevents ovulation and is administered by implanting capsules of hormones under the skin of the inside part of the upper arm. The manufacturing of Norplant has been discontinued.

Nutrient   A substance essential to life that the body cannot produce on its own. Nutrients are provided by food and assist in the growth and development of the body.

Nutrition   The science studying the need for and the effects of food on an organism.

O

Obesity   The excessive accumulation of fat in the body; a condition of being 20% or more above ideal weight.

Obsessive-compulsive disorder (OCD)   An anxiety disorder that causes a person to have disturbing repetitive thoughts (obsessions) and to perform rituals or routines (compulsions) to get rid of the obsessions. The disorder is diagnosed only when the repetitive behaviors consume many hours each day and interfere with daily life.

Oligospermia   A condition in which few sperm are produced in the semen. Oligospermia is often the cause of male infertility.

Opportunistic infections   Infections that seldom cause disease in people with normal immune function but "take the opportunity" to cause disease in people with a present illness or a lowered immune system, such as caused by HIV/AIDS.

Opposed estrogen   Estrogen replacement therapy that is taken with the opposing effects of progestin.

Oral contraceptives   Birth control pills that cause a woman's own reproductive hormone cycle to be suppressed by the synthetic estrogen and progestin. Without the natural signals, either the ovary egg follicle cannot mature and ovulation does not occur or implantation of a fertilized egg becomes impossible.

Oral sex   Stimulation of the genital or anal areas with the mouth or tongue. Unprotected oral sex can transmit sexually transmitted infections.

Organic brain syndrome (OBS)   A general term referring to physical disorders that cause a decrease in mental function, usually not including psychiatric disorders. OBS is a common "diagnosis" of the elderly. It is not an inevitable part of aging, however. OBS is not a separate disease entity but is a general term used to categorize physical conditions that can cause mental changes.

Orgasm   A series of muscular contractions of the pelvic floor muscles occurring at the peak of sexual arousal.

Orgasmic dysfunction   An inability to experience the orgasmic component of the sexual response cycle.

Orgasmic phase   Term used by Masters and Johnson to describe the third phase of the sexual response cycle in which the rhythmic muscular contractions of the pelvic floor occur.

Osteoarthritis   A disease in which the surface layer of cartilage erodes, causing bones under the cartilage to rub together. This friction results in joint pain, swelling, and loss of movement of the joints. Also called degenerative joint disease.

Osteopathic school   A school that focuses on natural medicine, which aims to restore function to the organism by treating the causes of pain and imbalance.

Osteopenia   Decreased calcification or density of bone. This descriptive term is applicable to all skeletal systems in which such a condition is noted.

Osteoporosis   An age-related debilitating disorder characterized by a general decrease in bone mass and structural deterioration of bone tissue.

Ova   Female reproductive cells that are released in single units from the ovary. Also called eggs.

Ovaries   Reproductive organs that produce ova, estrogen, and progesterone.

Overnutrition   A form of malnutrition caused by overeating, insufficient exercise, and excessive intake of vitamins and minerals. Overnutrition can lead to overweight and obesity.

Overweight   Having a body mass index (BMI) of 25 to 29.9.

Ovulation   The release of a mature ovum from the graafian follicles of the ovary.

Ovum   The female reproductive cell; an egg.

P

Panic disorder   An anxiety disorder characterized by periods of intense fear known as panic attacks that are accompanied by physical symptoms (pounding heart, sweating, dizziness, chest pain, and so on) and emotional distress.

Pap smear   A gynecological procedure in which a sample of cervical cells is examined for the presence of precancerous or cancerous cells.

Partial mastectomy   Surgery to treat breast cancer that involves the removal of some breast tissue and some of the surrounding lymph nodes. Also called segmental mastectomy.

Patent ductus arteriosus   A congenital condition common in premature babies in which the passageway between the pulmonary artery and aorta does not close.

Pelvic floor   The muscles that provide the basis of support for a woman's uterus, bladder, and rectum.

Pelvic inflammatory disease (PID)   A general term describing an infection of the internal female reproductive tract that can lead to infertility, chronic pain, or ectopic pregnancy. PID is usually caused by a sexually transmitted infection such as chlamydia or gonorrhea that spreads into the upper reproductive tract.

Perimenopause   Refers to the years immediately preceding and following the last menstrual period.

Perineal   Referring to the area of smooth skin between the vaginal opening and the anus, known as the perineum.

Perineum   The area of smooth skin between the vaginal opening and the anus.

Peripheral artery disease   A disease of the extremities (hands and arms but mainly in the legs and feet) in which the blood supply is diminished, and sufficient oxygen and nutrients do not reach these areas properly. Because waste is not removed from these areas effectively, the affected person may experience symptoms that range from cramping and numbness to gangrene (tissue death), which may require amputation of the extremity.

Personality disorders   Mental disorders that are characterized by distorted and inflexible thoughts and behaviors that make it impossible for a person to live a productive life or establish fulfilling relationships.

Phenylketonuria (PKU)   A genetic disorder in which a crucial liver enzyme is absent. It may result in severe mental retardation if left untreated.

Phobia   An anxiety disorder characterized by a powerful and irrational fear of a particular object or situation.

Phytochemicals   Plant chemicals found in fruits and vegetables that protect the body from cancer by blocking the carcinogenic activities of certain substances in the human body.

Phytoestrogen   Chemicals found in plants that may act like the estrogen produced naturally in the body.

Placebo   A substance that is inactive but given in the same dose and form as a real medication.

Placenta An organ that develops after implantation where the embryo attaches via the umbilical cord for nourishment and waste removal.

Placenta previa A complication of pregnancy in which the birth canal becomes obstructed by the placenta.

Plaque Fatty deposits on the lining of arteries.

Platelets Disk-shaped structures in the blood needed for blood coagulation. Also called thrombocytes.

Pneumocystis carinii pneumonia (PCP) A lung infection that affects those with damaged immune systems; the most common AIDS-related opportunistic infection in the United States.

Pneumonectomy Removal of the lung.

Polycystic ovarian syndrome A condition that is associated with the overproduction of male hormones, failure to ovulate, formation of cysts on the surface of the ovaries, inability to become pregnant, and abnormal hair growth on the body. Polycystic ovary syndrome occurs most often in women who are obese, and it generally can be reversed with weight loss. Also called polycystic ovarian disease (PCOD).

Polyps Small benign growths that develop in the endocervical canal or colorectal region.

Polyunsaturated fats A type of fat that is liquid at room temperature and when refrigerated. Such fats help lower both LDL and HDL cholesterol.

Postmenopause Life after the final menstrual period.

Postpartum psychosis The most severe of the psychiatric disorders that can develop in women after delivery. Symptoms of postpartum psychosis include depression, anxiety, irritation, tiredness, and sleep disturbances as well as behavior that tends to change throughout the day from clear consciousness to total loss of reality.

Post-traumatic stress disorder (PTSD) An anxiety disorder that usually begins within three months after a traumatic event. Its symptoms include flashback episodes, nightmares, and emotional numbness.

Preeclampsia A complication of pregnancy characterized by high blood pressure, swelling caused by fluid retention, and high levels of protein in the urine. Also called toxemia.

Premature labor Labor that begins before the completed ninth month of fetal gestation.

Premenopause The entirety of a woman's reproductive life—from first menstruation to menopause.

Premenstrual dysphoric disorder (PMDD) A condition associated with severe emotional and physical problems that are linked closely to the menstrual cycle; a more severe form of premenstrual syndrome (PMS).

Premenstrual syndrome (PMS) A group of cyclic symptoms that occur in some women about a week before menstruation, including breast tenderness, abdominal bloating, fatigue, fluctuating emotions, and depression.

Premium In terms of health insurance, a regular periodic payment.

Prevalence The total number of people with a given condition at a point in time.

Primary prevention Prevention of disease by reducing exposure to a risk factor that may lead to the disease. Primary preventive measures include healthy nutrition, regular physical activity, cessation of smoking, and safe sexual practices.

Private health insurance Health insurance provided by third-party payers to individuals or employer groups either through indemnity or managed care systems.

Prodrome Period of infectiousness before the first signs of infection are present.

Progestational phase Second half of the endometrial cycle. Also known as the secretory phase.

Progesterone The hormone produced by the corpus luteum of the ovary that causes the uterine lining to thicken.

Progestin A natural or synthetic progestational substance that mimics some or all of the actions of progesterone. It is used in conjunction with estrogen in hormone replacement therapy.

Prolapsed cord A complication of pregnancy in which the umbilical cord comes through the pelvis before the baby. It can result in a disrupted flow of oxygen to the baby due to a compressed cord.

Proliferation phase The phase in the menstrual cycle in which the ovarian follicles mature.

Proportionality A term relating to one of the themes of the USDA's new MyPyramid, which replaces the food guide pyramid. Proportionality is displayed on the pyramid by the different widths of the food group bands. The widths suggest how much food a person should choose from each group. The widths are just a general guide, not exact proportions. For example, larger widths represent greater proportions of foods such as fruits, vegetables, and whole grains; smaller widths represent smaller proportions of foods that are high in saturated or trans fats or have added sugars, cholesterol, or salt.

Prostaglandins A family of hormones present in many body tissues. The release of prostaglandins as uterine cells are shed is believed to be the cause of menstrual cramping.

Protein A substance that is basically a compound of amino acids; one of the essential nutrients.

Protein-energy malnutrition (PEM) A deficiency syndrome caused by the inadequate intake of protein and/or energy intake. PEM, the most destructive form of malnutrition, mainly affects infants and young children.

Psychedelic   A drug that produces a heightened sense of reality with visual hallucinations and, sometimes, psychotic-like behaviors.

Psychological dependence   An emotional or mental attachment to the use of a drug. Also called habituation.

Psychosis   A severe mental disorder characterized by a loss of contact with reality and severe personality changes.

Puberty   The stage of life between childhood and adulthood during which the reproductive organs mature and secondary sexual characteristics begin to develop. For girls, it is the time of the onset of menstruation, the development of breasts and body hair, and usually some level of growth spurt.

Public health insurance   Health insurance provided by government sources including Medicare, Medicaid, the Department of Defense (DOD), Veterans Administration (VA), and the Bureau of Indian Affairs.

Pulmonary arteries   Vessels that receive blood from the right ventricle to carry to the lungs for oxygenation.

Pulmonary stenosis   A condition in which the valve between the ventricle and pulmonary artery is defective and does not open properly.

Pulmonary veins   Vessels that return oxygenated blood from the lungs to the left atrium.

Purging   The use of vomiting, laxatives, or diuretics after a bingeing episode. Purging is characteristic of the eating disorder, bulimia nervosa.

Pus   A substance composed of dead bacteria, dead white blood cells, and fluid that is most commonly the result of an infection process.

R

Radiation therapy   Treatment with high-energy radiation from X rays or other sources.

Radical mastectomy   Removal of the entire breast, underlying chest muscles, and underarm lymph nodes following a diagnosis of breast cancer.

Rape   Any unwanted sexual act, including forced vaginal or anal intercourse, oral sex, or penetration with an object.

Recommended Dietary Allowances (RDAs)   Daily nutrient allowances recommended for healthy adults by the National Research Council.

Recreational drugs   Drugs taken purely for fun.

Red blood cells   One of the formed elements in circulating blood. It contains hemoglobin and transports oxygen. Also called erythrocytes.

Reproductive health   The function, well-being, and control a person has over his or her reproductive system, including that person's ability to decide if, when, and how to engage in sexual contact and/or have children.

Reproductive tract infections (RTIs)   Infections caused by a variety of organisms that affect the upper reproductive tract, the lower reproductive tract, or both. Most infections are transmitted by sexual intimacy and, therefore, are referred to as sexually transmitted infections (STIs).

Retrovirus   A virus that has the ability to take over certain cells and interrupt their normal genetic function.

Rheumatic heart disease   A heart condition resulting from a bacterial infection (*Streptococcus*) that has been inadequately treated. The infection can develop into rheumatic fever and damage the heart valves.

Rheumatoid arthritis   Chronic inflammatory disease of the joints that results from an autoimmune response.

Rh incompatibility   A condition that occurs when an Rh-negative mother and an Rh-positive father conceive a baby who inherits the father's Rh-positive blood type. This situation may present problems during pregnancy, labor, and delivery if the fetus's Rh-positive blood cells enter the mother's bloodstream.

Right atrium   One of the two upper chambers of the heart. It collects deoxygenated blood from the body.

Right ventricle   One of the two lower chambers of the heart. It pumps blood from the heart to the lungs to collect oxygen.

Rubella   An infectious disease often causing birth defects in pregnant women. Also called German measles.

S

Sarcoma   A cancer that originates in the connective tissue, such as cartilage, tendons, and bone.

Saturated fats   Fats that come primarily from animal sources.

Schizophrenia   A type of psychosis representing a complex group of diseases with symptoms that may appear gradually or suddenly and include hallucinations or delusions, disordered thinking, and an impaired ability to manage emotions and interact with others. Schizophrenia is the most chronic and disabling of the severe mental disorders.

Scleroderma   An autoimmune disease that is characterized by a thickening of the skin and internal organs, and by blood vessel disturbances.

Seasonal affective disorder (SAD)   A form of depression caused by seasonal shifts in daylight hours that affect a person's sleep–wake cycle.

Secondary prevention   Early detection and prompt treatment of disease. Examples of secondary preventive measures include screening tools such as mammography and Pap smears, which may detect disease before it spreads and thereby prevent further complications from the disease.

Secondary sex characteristics   The physical characteristics other than genitals that indicate sexual maturity, such as breasts and body hair.

Secretory phase   The phase of the menstrual cycle in which the corpus luteum develops and secretes progesterone.

Sedative   A drug that depresses the central nervous system, resulting in sleep.

Segmental mastectomy   Surgery to treat breast cancer that involves the removal of some breast tissue and some of the surrounding lymph nodes. Also called partial mastectomy.

Segmentectomy   Surgery to remove a section of a lobe of a lung.

Selective estrogen receptor modulators (SERMs)   Compounds that bind with estrogen receptors and exhibit estrogen action in some tissues and anti-estrogen action in other tissues. Many menopausal women use SERMs as an alternative to estrogen replacement, and infertile women use them for ovulation induction.

Self-mutilation   Any self-directed repetitive behavior that causes physical injury. Self-mutilation acts are not usually suicide attempts but rather behaviors meant to express or release emotional turmoil. Examples include skin cutting with razors or knives (the most common pattern); burning or biting oneself; picking one's skin or hair; and extreme injuries such as auto-enucleation (self-removal of the eye), castration, or amputation.

Septum   A dividing wall, such as that between the right and left sides of the heart.

Serotonin   A neurotransmitter (brain chemical) known to affect appetite.

Sex   An individual's biological status as male or female.

Sexual assault   Conduct of a sexual or indecent nature toward another person that is accompanied by actual or threatened physical force or that induces fear, shame, or mental suffering. The term is frequently used as an all-encompassing term for any type of unwanted sexual advance.

Sexual dysfunction   The inability of an individual to function adequately in terms of sexual arousal, orgasm, or in coital situations.

Sexual health   A state of physical, emotional, and social well-being in relation to an individual's sexuality.

Sexual harassment   Behavior that may include unwanted sexual attention or advances and/or the use of threats or bribery to obtain sexual favors. The offensive conduct often interferes with a person's ability to perform regular duties at work and creates an intimidating or hostile working environment.

Sexual health   A state of physical, emotional, mental, and social well-being related to sexuality.

Sexual orientation   One's erotic, romantic, and affectional attraction to people of the same sex, to the opposite sex, or to both sexes.

Sexually transmitted infections (STIs)   Infections of the reproductive tract that are transmitted by sexual intimacy. STIs include chlamydia, gonorrhea, syphilis, herpes, genital warts, hepatitis, and human immunodeficiency virus (HIV) infections.

Sickle cell anemia   A debilitating genetic disorder of the blood characterized by sickle-shaped red blood cells, primarily affecting African Americans.

Sigmoidoscopy   A procedure that uses a thin lighted tube to examine the rectum and lower colon.

Sign   Evidence of a disease or injury that an outside observer can notice, such as swollen glands, dilated pupils, or bruising.

Simple carbohydrate   A sugar. It provides the body with glucose and a quick spurt of energy.

Simple mastectomy   Complete removal of the breast but not the lymph nodes under the arm or chest muscles following a diagnosis of breast cancer.

Sitz bath   A tub in which one bathes in a sitting position with hips and buttocks under water and legs out.

Sjögren's syndrome   A chronic autoimmune disorder characterized by dry eyes and dry mouth and caused by decreased tear and salivary gland functioning.

Sodomy   A legal term used to define sexual activities, often including oral and anal sex, deemed undesirable or immoral. Sodomy laws once existed in many states, but these laws currently are rarely, if ever, enforced.

Spermicide   A chemical that breaks down the cell walls of sperm. It often is used in conjunction with barrier contraception methods.

Sphygmomanometer   A cuff device connected to a hose and measuring device to ascertain blood pressure.

Spina bifida   A neural tube defect in which the spine does not close during fetal development and exposed nerves are thereby damaged, possibly causing paralysis and life-threatening infections.

Spontaneous abortion   Unintentional ending of pregnancy before a fetus is viable; miscarriage.

Sputum   A secretion that is produced in the lungs and the bronchi (tubes that carry the air to the lung). This mucus-like secretion may become infected, become bloodstained, or contain abnormal cells that may lead to a diagnosis. Sputum is what comes up with deep coughing.

Squamous cell carcinoma   A nonmelanoma skin cancer that begins in the squamous cells of the outer layer of skin (epidermis). It usually first appears on areas of the skin exposed to the sun, such as the face, ear, neck, lip, and back of the hands, but it also can develop where skin has been injured, such as within scars, burns, or skin ulcers.

Staging   The process of learning whether cancer has spread from its original site to another part of the body.

Stalking   Behaviors directed toward a specific person that involve repeated visual or physical proximity; nonconsensual commu-

nication; verbal, written, or implied threats; or a combination of these behaviors that would cause fear in a reasonable person.

Statins   A class of cholesterol-lowering drugs.

Stent   An implantable steel screen that is placed at the site of arterial narrowing to keep an artery open.

Sterilization   The permanent, often surgical, end to fertility by interrupting the mechanisms of normal reproductive action.

Sternum   The breastbone.

Stillbirth   Death occurring before or during birth of a fetus of sufficient size and age to be otherwise expected to survive.

Stimulants   Drugs that affect the central nervous system and increase the heart rate, blood pressure, strength of heart contractions, blood glucose level, and overall muscle tension.

Stress   The response—be it physical, mental, or emotional—that a person displays when subjected to any type of stressor. Stressors can range from daily hassles to life-altering events, and they are experienced and perceived by people in very different ways.

Stress urinary incontinence   The involuntary release or leaking of small amounts of urine; usually associated with sudden exertion.

Stroke (cerebrovascular accident)   A condition in which blood vessel damage occurs in the brain.

Substance abuse   The overuse, misuse, and/or addiction to any chemical substance such as alcohol, tobacco, or drugs, including over-the-counter medications, prescription medications, and illicit drugs.

Sudden infant death syndrome (SIDS)   The diagnosis given for the sudden death of an infant younger than one year of age that remains unexplained after a complete investigation, which includes an autopsy, examination of the death scene, and review of the symptoms or illnesses the infant had prior to dying and any other pertinent medical history. Because most cases of SIDS occur when a baby is sleeping in a crib, SIDS also is called crib death.

Suffragist   An advocate of the right to vote and the ability to exercise that right.

Superior vena cava   The venous trunk draining blood from the head, neck, upper limbs, and thorax to the heart.

Surrogacy   A procedure for treating infertility in which a woman is artificially inseminated with the sperm of an infertile woman's partner. She then carries the pregnancy to term for the infertile couple.

Synovium   The cells lining the inside of the joint capsule that surround and protect the joint. The synovium is responsible for creating synovial fluid, which provides protective lubrication to the joint.

Symptom   Something a person feels in response to a disease or injury. Examples of symptoms include headache, a sore throat, or sharp pains.

Syphilis   A sexually transmitted bacterial infection that causes small, painless sores in the genital area, a rash, flu-like symptoms, and, after many years, systemic damage.

Systolic   First reading of blood pressure that represents the amount of pressure the blood exerts against the wall of the artery when the heart contracts.

T

Tamoxifen   An antiestrogen drug that is used as a treatment for breast cancer; may also inhibit breast tumor growth.

Target heart rate   A rate of 60% to 90% of the maximum heart rate at which the maximum benefit is derived from exercise.

Tay-Sachs disease   A genetic disorder characterized by the inability to process fat, ultimately resulting in death. It occurs almost exclusively among Jews of Eastern European ancestry.

T-cell   A cell that governs the immune system and assists the B-lymphocyte in producing antibodies; T-cells are reduced in a person with AIDS.

Tendonitis   Inflammation caused by friction from overuse of tendons (connective tissues that attach muscle to bone).

Teratogenic   The characteristic of producing a permanent abnormality in structure or function, causing growth retardation, or causing death when an embryo or fetus is exposed to a certain substance, organism, or physical agent.

Tertiary prevention   Prevention measures that take place once a disease has advanced. They may involve alleviating pain, providing comfort, halting progression of an illness, and limiting disability that may result from disease.

Testosterone   A male sex hormone that plays a role in the development of functionally mature sperm and is responsible for the development and maintenance of male secondary sexual characteristics such as the deepening of the voice and the growth of facial hair. Also secreted in small amounts by women.

Tetrahydrocannabinol (THC)   The primary psychoactive ingredient in marijuana and hashish.

Third-party payer system   A payment system whereby an insurer (or third party) pays for services rendered to an individual by a provider of care.

Thrombocytes   Disk-shaped structures in the blood needed for blood coagulation. Also called platelets.

Thrombus   A blood clot that blocks an artery.

Thrush   A yeast infection that infects the mouth.

Thyroid disease   Disease of the thyroid gland, often occurring from excess production of thyroid hormones (hyperthyroidism) or decreased production of thyroid hormones (hypothyroidism).

Thyroiditis   An inflammation of the thyroid gland. Chronic thyroiditis frequently results in lowered thyroid function (hypothyroidism).

Title IX The portion of the Education Amendments of 1972 that prohibits gender discrimination in educational institutions that receive any federal funds. If educational institutions are found to violate Title IX, their federal funding can be withdrawn.

Tolerance The body's ability to withstand the effects of a drug. Continued use of a drug may result in increased tolerance and decreased responsiveness.

Total hysterectomy and bilateral salpingo-oophorectomy Surgical removal of the uterus performed in conjunction with the removal of both ovaries and the fallopian tubes.

Toxemia A complication of pregnancy characterized by high blood pressure, swelling caused by fluid retention, and high levels of protein in the urine. Also called preeclampsia.

Toxic shock syndrome (TSS) A rare but serious infection caused by strains of the bacteria *Staphylococcus aureus* (*S. aureus*). For reasons not fully understood, these bacteria release toxins (poisons) into the bloodstream after deep wounds, surgery, or tampon use (especially high-absorbency tampon use).

Toxoplasmosis A disease that is caused by the parasite *Toxoplasma gondii*, which is associated with contaminated cat litter or soil containing cat feces. Infection by this parasite can cause problems with the fetus during pregnancy. It also can affect a person with a compromised immune system and is considered an opportunistic infection of HIV/AIDS.

Trafficking In regard to women, the use of force and deception to transfer women into situations of extreme exploitation; the recruitment, transportation, transfer, harboring, or receipt of persons by the threat or use of force or the abuse of power for the purpose of exploitation.

Trans fats Fats that are formed when vegetable oils are processed into margarine or shortening. Trans fats are found in snack foods such as potato chips, commercial baked goods with "partially hydrogenated vegetable oil" or "vegetable shortening," many types of fast food (e.g., french fries and onion rings), stick margarine, and some dairy products. These fats are solid or semi-solid at room temperature and raise levels of LDL cholesterol.

Transdermal therapy Treatment applied to the skin; the medicine or substance is absorbed through the skin and enters the bloodstream.

Transgender Anyone whose behaviors, thoughts, or traits differ from those traditionally ascribed to the person's sex.

Transient ischemic attack (TIA) An event in which an artery closes momentarily in a spasm and may result in a brief memory lapse or garbled speech.

Transitioning The process in which transsexuals work to change their appearance and societal identity so as to match their gender identity.

Transvaginal ultrasound A method of imaging the genital tract in women. The ultrasound machine sends out high-frequency sound waves, which bounce off body structures and thereby create a picture. With the transvaginal technique, the ultrasound transducer (a hand-held probe) is inserted directly into the vagina.

Trichomoniasis A vaginal infection caused by *Trichomonas vaginalis*, a single cell protozoan parasite with a whip-like tail that it uses to propel itself through vaginal and urethral mucus.

Tricuspid valve A heart valve that has three points or cusps and is situated between the right atrium and the right ventricle.

Triglycerides Fatty substances found in the body's fatty tissues. High levels of triglycerides are associated with an elevated risk of heart disease.

Tumor An abnormal mass of tissue that results from excessive cell division. It may be either benign or malignant.

U

Ultrasound A procedure that uses high-frequency sound waves to project an image of structures inside the body, such as an organ or a fetus during pregnancy.

Underinsured For the purposes of this book, a person who technically has health insurance but whose coverage is not enough to cover his or her regular medical expenses or whose coverage would not allow a person to afford adequate care in the event of a serious disease or illness.

Undernutrition Poor health resulting from the depletion of nutrients due to inadequate nutrient intake over time.

Underweight An individual who is below the acceptable average weight for his or her height or body type.

Universal health insurance A system by which the government provides health insurance to all citizens, thereby controlling health insurance at the federal level.

Unopposed estrogen Estrogen replacement therapy that is taken without the opposing effects of progestin.

Unsaturated fats Fats that come from plants and include most vegetable oils.

Urethra The tube through which urine passes from the bladder to outside the body. In men, semen also passes through the urethra.

Urethritis Inflammation of the urethra, often caused by infection in the bladder or kidneys.

Urinary incontinence The inability to control the flow of urine from the bladder.

Uterus A hollow, muscular organ located in the pelvic cavity of females in which the fertilized egg becomes implanted and develops; also called the womb.

V

Vacuum curettage The most widely used abortion technique in the United States. In this procedure, the cervix is first dilated. A vacuum curette—an instrument consisting of a tube with a scoop attached for scraping away tissue—is then inserted through the cervix into the uterus. The other end of the tube is attached to a suction-producing apparatus, which aspirates the contents of the uterus into a collection vessel.

Vagina A moist canal in females extending from the labia minora to the uterus.

Vaginal atrophy A condition often associated with menopause that refers to the thinning of the vaginal lining.

Vaginismus A relatively rare form of sexual difficulty in which a woman experiences involuntary spasmodic contractions of the muscles of the outer third of the vagina.

Varicocele A mesh of varicose veins in and around the testicle, which is associated with infertility and may have to be treated with surgery.

Vasectomy A male sterilization method whereby one or two small incisions are made just through the skin of the scrotum. The vas deferens is lifted through the incision, and the two ends are tied or cauterized to seal them.

Vasocongestion The engorgement of blood vessels in particular body parts in response to sexual arousal.

Vasoconstrictor A compound that results in narrowing of blood vessels.

Veins Blood vessels that carry blood from the capillaries toward the heart.

Ventricle The right or left lower blood-pumping chamber of the heart.

Ventricular fibrillation A disturbance in heart rhythm.

Venules Small veins.

Very-low-density lipoprotein (VLDL) A type of lipoprotein made up mostly of triglycerides. As with LDL, high levels of VLDL increase the risk of atherosclerosis.

Vestibular bulbs Part of the vast network of bulbs and vessels that engorge with blood during sexual arousal. Vestibular bulbs cause the vagina to increase in length and the vulvar area to become swollen.

Vestibule The area of the vulva inside of the labia minora.

Vestibulitis A recurring inflammation and burning sensation around the vaginal opening.

Villi Short vascular projections attaching the fetus to the uterine wall.

Viruses Small pathogens incapable of independent metabolism; can only reproduce inside living cells.

Vitamin An organic substance needed by the body in a very small amount. The various vitamins have many different functions in metabolism and nutrition.

Vulva The external genital organs of the female, including the labia majora, labia minora, clitoris, and vestibule of the vagina.

Vulvitis Inflammation of the vulva.

W

Water-soluble vitamins Vitamins used up or excreted in urine and sweat; must be replaced daily.

Western blot test Laboratory test used to detect antibodies; Western blots are performed after two positive ELISA tests to test for HIV.

White blood cells Elements in circulating blood that protect the body against pathogenic microorganisms. Also called leukocytes.

Y

Yeast infection A vaginal infection caused most commonly by the fungal organism, *Candida albicans*. Symptoms of yeast infections include abnormal vaginal discharge; vaginal and labial itching and burning; redness and inflammation of the vulvar skin; pain with intercourse; and painful urination.

Yo-yo dieting The practice of losing weight and then regaining it, only to lose it and regain it again. This practice makes it more difficult to succeed in future attempts to lose weight because thyroid hormone levels may drop very low in subsequent dieting, thereby significantly slowing basal metabolism.

Z

Zygote intrafallopian transfer (ZIFT) A method of assisted reproductive technology in which a fertilized egg is placed in the fallopian tube, allowing the zygote to continue its cell division and become implanted in the uterus naturally.

Zygote A fertilized egg.

INDEX

C

Cade, Yvette, 416
Calcium, 142, 236, 237, 238
Calendar method, 97
Cancer
  breast, 286–290
  cervical, 187, 291–293
  colorectal, 297–298
  costs of, 285–286
  decisions regarding, making, 299–300
  defined, 282–283
  globally, 286
  lung, 296–297
  ovarian, 295–296
  racial differences, 285
  screening guidelines, 300–301
  skin, 298–299
  smoking and, 371
  statistics, 283–285
  uterine tumors, 294–295
  types of, 283
Cannabis, 387
Capillaries, 266
Carbohydrates, 228–230
Carcinogenesis, 283
Carcinogenic, 373
Carcinogens, 283
Carcinoma, 282
Carcinoma in situ, 291
Cardiovascular disease (CVD)
  acute coronary syndrome, 269
  angina pectoris, 270
  cerebrovascular accident (stroke), 270–273
  congenital heart disease, 269–270
  congestive heart failure, 269
  coronary heart disease, 268–269
  costs of, 265
  defined, 264
  gender differences, 280–281
  globally, 265–266
  heart, 266–273
  metabolic syndrome, 270
  peripheral artery disease, 270
  racial differences in, 265, 281–282
  rheumatic heart disease, 270
  risk factors, 273–280
  smoking and, 266, 274, 370–371
  statistics, 264–265
Cardiovascular endurance, 240–241
Cardiovascular system, 266, 267
Carpal tunnel syndrome, 429, 430

Centers for Disease Control and Prevention
  biomedical research, 8, 9
  role of, 35
Centers for Medicare & Medicaid Services (CMS), 36
Cephalopelvic disproportion, 156
Cerebrovascular accident/disease (stroke), 270–273
Cervical cancer
  risk factors, 2911
  screening and diagnosis, 187, 291–292
  stages, 291
  treatment, 292–293
Cervical caps, 92, 104–105, 125
Cervical changes, benign, 290–291
Cervical dysplasia, 291
Cervical mucus method, 97, 98
Cervicitis, 292
Cervix, 74
Cesarean delivery, 156–157
Chan, Margaret, 56
Chantix, 375
Chemicals/toxins, in the workplace, 430
Chemotherapy, 290
Child abuse
  causes of, 407–408
  defined, 406
  global, 402
  statistics, 406–408
Child Abuse Prevention and Treatment Act, 406
Childbirth
  cesarean, 156–157
  decisions regarding, making, 167–168
  episiotomies, 151, 155
  historical views on, 132–133
  issues, checklist of, 153
  labor and delivery, 152, 154–155
  pain relief in, 155–156
  premature labor, 148
  prepared (natural), 133
  preparing for, 152
  relaxation classes, 152
  stages of labor, 154–155
Child care, 427
Childhood, sexuality and, 81
Child pornography, 401
Chlamydia, 180, 201
Cholesterol, 232
  cardiovascular disease and, 275–277
  what do the numbers mean, 277
Chorionic villus sampling (CVS), 146, 147
Chromosomes, 135
Chronic bronchitis, 372

Chapter 8
Opener © Photodisc; **page 209** © Photodisc; **page 215** © Ryan McVay/Photodisc/Getty Images; **page 217 (top)** © Photodisc

Part Opener 3 © Photodisc

Chapter 9
Opener © Photodisc; **page 227** © Denis Pepin/ShutterStock, Inc.; **page 230** © Cre8tive Images/ShutterStock, Inc.; **page 231** © Digital Stock; **page 238** © Dennis MacDonald/age fotostock; **page 240** © Larry St. Pierre/ShutterStock, Inc.; **page 242 (top)** © image100/age fotostock; **page 242 (bottom)** © Philip Date/ShutterStock, Inc.; **page 244** © Photodisc; **page 246 (top)** © Photodisc; **page 246 (bottom)** © Patrick Tuohy/ShutterStock, Inc.; **page 247** © Photodisc; **page 252** © Photodisc; **page 255** © Yui Monk/PA Photos/Landov

Chapter 10
Opener © Photodisc; **page 267** © Franc Podgorsek/ShutterStock, Inc.; **page 272 (top)** © Photodisc; **page 274** © Rob Marmion/ShutterStock, Inc.; **page 280** © Photos.com; **page 283** © Photodisc; **page 286** Courtesy of David Emanuel; **page 288** © Photodisc; **page 292 (left)** © Sadie Dayton, sadiephotography.com; **page 292 (right)** © Maurice Reed Photography; **page 298** Courtesy of National Cancer Institute

Chapter 11
Opener © Photodisc; **page 312 (left and right)** © Fred Hossler/Visuals Unlimited; **page 314** © Photodisc; **page 315** Courtesy of the National Fluid Milk Processor Promotion Board; **page 316** © Catalin Petolea/Dreamstime.com; **page 319** Courtesy of Jim Gathany/CDC; **page 323** © NMSB/Custom Medical Stock Photo; **page 325** © Chet Childs/Custom Medical Stock Photo; **page 326** © Photodisc

Chapter 12
Opener © Photodisc; **page 335** © Jeff Greenberg/age fotostock; **page 336** © PhotoCreate/ShutterStock, Inc.; **page 337** © David R. Frazier Photolibrary, Inc./Alamy Images; **page 339** © absolut/ShutterStock, Inc.; **page 341** © Francisco Caravana/ShutterStock, Inc.; **page 346 (top)** Courtesy of Andrea Booher/FEMA; **page 346 (bottom)** Courtesy of Gunnery Sgt. Katesha Washington/U.S. Marines; **page 352** © AbleStock; **page 354** © Bill Aron/PhotoEdit, Inc.

Part Opener 4 © Courtnee Mulroy/ShutterStock, Inc.

Chapter 13
Opener © Courtnee Mulroy/ShutterStock, Inc.; **page 362** © Filipe Raimundo/ShutterStock, Inc.; **page 364** Courtesy of Orange County Police Department, Florida; **page 367** © Simone van den Berg/ShutterStock, Inc.; **page 369** © Michael Newman/PhotoEdit, Inc.; **page 372** © Pixtal/SuperStock; **page 377** © Ingram Publishing/Index Stock Imagery, Inc.; **page 383** © Photos.com

Chapter 14
Opener © Courtnee Mulroy/ShutterStock, Inc.; **page 401** © Anton Albert/ShutterStock, Inc.; **page 404 (left)** Courtesy of The National Center for Victims of Crime; **page 404 (right)** Courtesy of the Family Violence Prevention Fund (www.endabuse.org); **page 406** © Photodisc; **page 410** © Christine Gonsalves/ShutterStock, Inc.; **page 415** Courtesy of The National Center for Victims of Crime

Chapter 15
Opener © Courtnee Mulroy/ShutterStock, Inc.; **page 420 (top)** © Dhannte/ShutterStock, Inc.; **page 420 (bottom)** © Photodisc; **page 423 (top)** Courtesy of the Pacific Northwest National Laboratory; **page 423 (bottom)** © Masterfile; **page 424** © Photodisc; **page 427** © Ryan McVay/Photodisc/Getty Images; **page 429** © Keith Brofsky/Photodisc/Getty Images; **page 432** © Photodisc; **page 434** © Semen Lixodeev/ShutterStock, Inc.